Complementary Sports Medicine

Philip Maffetone, DC

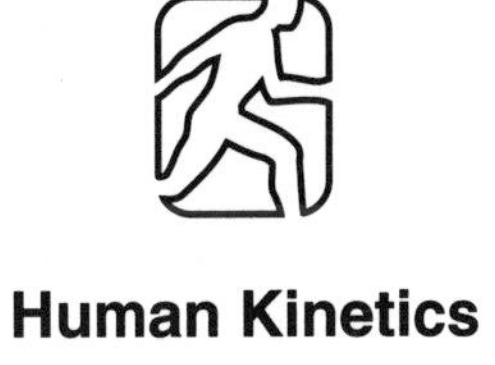

Human Kinetics

Library of Congress Cataloging-in-Publication Data

Maffetone, Philip.
Complementary sports medicine / Philip Maffetone.
p. cm.
Includes bibliographical references and index.
ISBN 0-88011-869-5
1. Sports medicine. 2. Alternative medicine. 3. Athletes--Wounds and injuries--Alternative treatment. I. Title.
[DNLM: 1. Sports Medicine. 2. Alternative Medicine. 3. Athletic Injuries--therapy. QT 261 M187c 1999]
RC1210.M24 1999
617.1'027--dc21
DNLM/DLC 98-52399
for Library of Congress CIP

ISBN: 0-88011-869-5

Acquisitions Editor: Loarn Robertson
Developmental Editor: Kristine Enderle
Assistant Editor: Amy Flaig
Copyeditor: Joyce Sexton
Proofreader: Erin Cler
Indexer: Pilar Wyman
Graphic Designer: Robert Reuther
Graphic Artist: Stuart Cartwright
Cover Designer: Keith Blomberg
Photographer (interior): Photos on p. 11 © Rich Cruse/RC Photo, p. 80 © AeroSport, Inc., pp. 328 and 329 © Hyperbaric Technologies Incorporated. All other photos by Tom Roberts.
Mac Illustrator: Sharon Smith
Medical Illustrator: Kristin Mount
Line Illustrator: Roberto Sabas
Printer: Edwards

Printed in the United States of America

10 9 8 7 6 5 4 3 2 1

Human Kinetics
Web site: http://www.humankinetics.com/

United States: Human Kinetics, P.O. Box 5076, Champaign, IL 61825-5076
1-800-747-4457
e-mail: humank@hkusa.com

Canada: Human Kinetics, 475 Devonshire Road Unit 100, Windsor, ON N8Y 2L5
1-800-465-7301 (in Canada only)
e-mail: humank@hkcanada.com

Europe: Human Kinetics, P.O. Box IW14, Leeds LS16 6TR, United Kingdom
+44 (0)113-278 1708
e-mail: humank@hkeurope.com

Australia: Human Kinetics, 57A Price Avenue, Lower Mitcham, South Australia 5062
(08) 82771555
e-mail: humank@hkaustralia.com

New Zealand: Human Kinetics, P.O. Box 105-231, Auckland Central
09-523-3462
e-mail: humank@hknewz.com

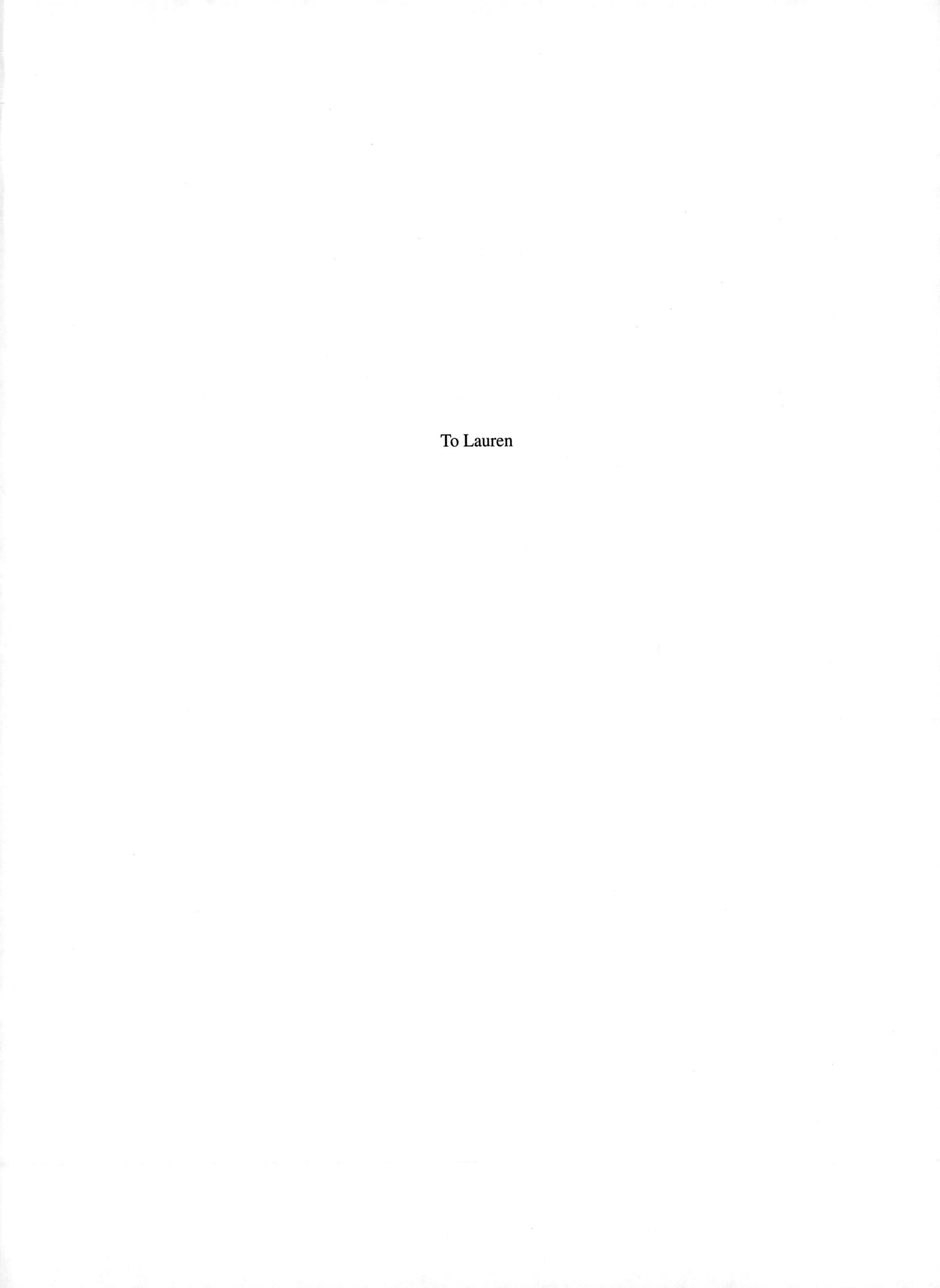

To Lauren

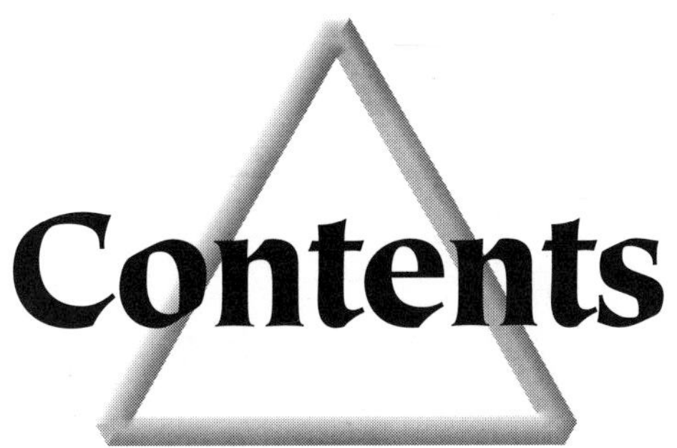

Contents

Preface vii

Acknowledgments ix

1 Philosophy of Complementary Sports Medicine 1

2 Definitions for Complementary Sports Medicine 9

3 Complementary Medicine Specialties 15

4 Metabolism and Energy Production 25

5 Neuromuscular Systems 33

6 Hormonal Systems 41

7 Patient History and Dialogue 53

8 Functional Testing and Interpretation 69

9 Assessing Posture, Gait and the Neuromuscular System 85

10 Muscle Testing Procedures 105

11 Applied Kinesiology Assessment 191

12 Assessments of Aerobic and Anaerobic Function 207

13 Heart Rate Monitor Assessments 213

14 Treatment of Muscle and Neurological Dysfunction 225

15 Treatment of Cranial and Pelvic Dysfunction 237

16 Treatment of Vertebral and Extravertebral Dysfunction 249

17 Pain and Pain Control 261

18 Diet Therapy 273

19 Nutritional Supplement Therapy 293

20 Ergogenic and Therapeutic Nourishment 311

21 Practitioner's Role in Training and Competition 319

22 Training and Competition Schedules 331

23 The Overtraining Syndrome 337

24 Training and Competitive Footwear 345

25 Carbohydrate Intolerance in Athletes 351

26 Weight and Fat Control 363

27 The Athlete's Triad of Dysfunction .369

28 Physical, Chemical, and Mental/Emotional Injuries: A Retrospect 375

References **388**
Index **417**
About the Author **429**

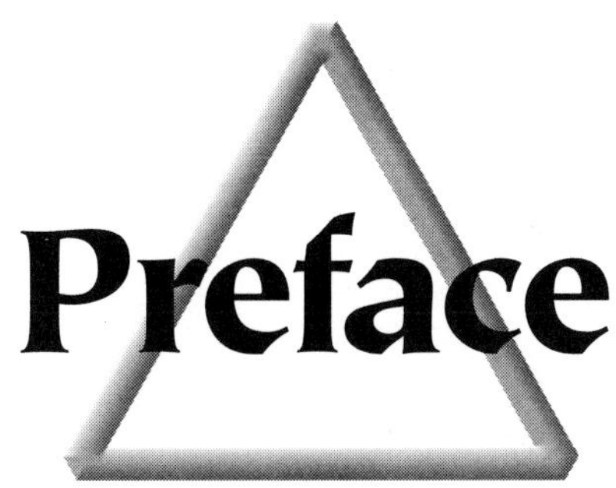

Preface

This text reflects my twenty years as a complementary sports medicine practitioner. My patients have included a range of chronically injured people, from those who were unable to work out at all to world-class champions. *Complementary Sports Medicine* offers a strategy for combining many nontraditional therapies into a complete individualized approach. These therapies include various hands-on techniques that address the acupuncture system, the neuromuscular and skeletal systems, diet and nutrition, training, and lifestyle issues—all with a focus of bringing forth healthier and more fit athletes who will remain free of injury and reach their performance potentials.

Complementary sports medicine may be hundreds of years old; its modern formats have evolved from a combination of alternative medicine, exercise physiology and biochemistry, and clinical experience. The word *complementary,* as used in the title and throughout the text, implies that the information can be used *with* more traditional approaches to sports medicine, rather than in place of them.

The ability to determine which therapy will work best for a given patient, as opposed to reliance on a predetermined cookbook approach, is a unique feature of complementary sports medicine. This therapy can be applied in an office setting, on the field, or on the road if one is traveling with a team or an individual athlete. In addition, this approach places significant emphasis on the interactive practitioner-patient relationship in which the practitioner is seen not only as a problem-solver but also as a teacher.

This text is designed for professionals and students in the sport and health fields. Those in complementary sports medicine now have a comprehensive text that provides referenced materials for clinical use and teaching purposes. Those in medicine, athletic training, alternative medicine, and other fields may want to add certain techniques to their existing practice. Coaches may find particular chapters useful; this book should help them make better decisions about referring athletes to the appropriate professional. Students will find in this text an introduction to a field they may not have been exposed to during their traditional courses.

I would like to encourage the reader to become a "patient." You and your staff and/or family may want to apply appropriate recommendations from the text to experience the process and be better able to relate these issues to other "patients." This text uses the words *patient* and *athlete* interchangeably, as all individuals are potential patients, and all people are athletes.

Acknowledgments

An endeavor such as this has involved many people and experiences that have influenced me throughout my professional life. I owe thanks to Dr. George Goodheart, who not only helped restore my health and fitness many years ago, but also taught me about complementary medicine. To Dr. Walter Schmitt, also my mentor, who reviewed the entire manuscript and helped me maintain a balance between art and science. And to all my patients, both the successes and failures, who helped me understand the real meaning of clinical outcome. In an indirect way, they are part of a process that will help other practitioners and patients.

In addition, special thanks go to Dr. David Seaman, who was most helpful in our in-depth discussions about the scientific literature; and Dr. Jerold Morantz who provided his clinic for photo sessions and his expert assistance in assuring accurate portrayal of the techniques. And to his associate, Dr. Eric Schwartzberg, and to Maria M. Hernandez for their modeling. A special thanks also goes to all those who perform in the splendid game of research—without them our clinical ideas and observations would not have a scientific component.

And finally, thanks to the people at Human Kinetics who took a chance on publishing a major work such as this—the first of its kind. The dissemination of educational information is the foundation of improving people's health and fitness.

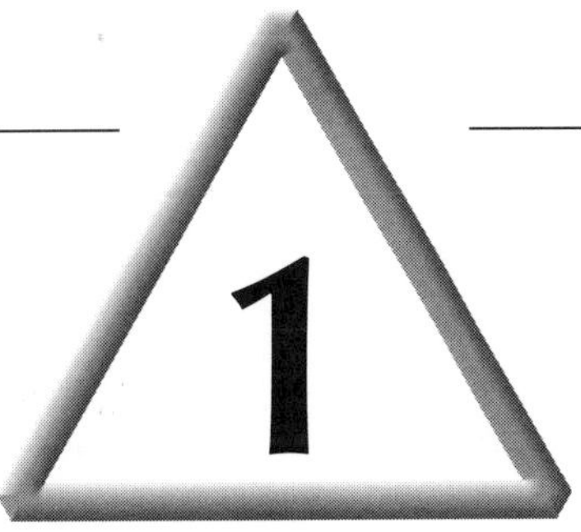

Philosophy of Complementary Sports Medicine

Like all other fields, complementary sports medicine is associated with a specific philosophy. This philosophy includes the ethics, theoretical concepts, and conviction of the individuals who make up the profession—a profession whose roots go back thousands of years. Early Hindu writings describe a balance between the body and mind that reveals the universe and living nature (or organisms and body systems) to be interacting wholes as opposed to a mere sum of elementary parts (Snook 1984). The book of Kung Fu expressed this as unity of the body and mind. In ancient Greece, analogously, sport was an integral part of a person's upbringing and not a separate activity in one's life (Leadbetter and Leadbetter 1986). This philosophy is maintained today in complementary sports medicine.

These ancient cultures produced the philosophical foundation of complementary sports medicine. Their approach to athletic care made use of many therapeutic tools and rendered particular care ranging from rest to activity, from diet to herbs. When needed, surgery was performed, usually by specialists. Only with the advent of modern medicine within the past century has there been a division of sports therapy into two distinct and competitive arenas. Today, one area of sports therapy is more Western and allopathic, and the other is often referred to as "alternative." Complementary sports medicine brings together the best of both.

COMPLEMENTARY SPORTS MEDICINE TODAY

A number of important modalities are associated with complementary sports medicine, although these are not necessarily limited exclusively to this field. Complementary sports medicine uses a hands-on approach, through specific therapies, assessment processes, and work with many other aspects of the patient's lifestyle and exercise training. This makes for an approach more like that of the general practitioner than that of the specialist. The complementary sports medicine professional treats not only high-level professional athletes, but also the average local sport enthusiast—both the weekend warrior and the beginner. Complementary practitioners develop a one-on-one relationship with the patient rather than using a team or group approach. They spend more time in assessing, treating, and educating each patient. Sometimes a specialist is needed. In this case, the complementary practitioner works simultaneously with the specialist. Thus in contrast to alternative medicine, complementary sports medicine is linked with, rather than segregated from, traditional modern medicine.

Perhaps more importantly, the assessment, treatment, and work with lifestyle factors in complementary sports medicine focus at least as much on the functional aspect of patients as on their specific injury or condition of ill health. In addition, the approach is function oriented rather than symptom directed. Complementary practitioners will often adopt information from clinical research and investigation to explore new areas of treatment when working with a patient.

The practitioner in this field not only approaches the patient differently than the traditional sports medicine and alternative medicine professional, but also sees himself or herself as an instructor or guide for the patient—part of the process of improving health and fitness. For example, the assessment and treatment processes are interactive; the patient is educated about the body and is required to share some of the responsibility. Practitioners play an active role in patient care and instruct patients to take an active role in their recovery and treatment. Ideally, complementary practitioners are also athletes on some level. Therefore practitioners can better relate to the patient and benefit from the experiences of their own knee pain, Achilles tendon problems, fatigue, and other ailments. This helps them to better understand patients and appreciate the healing process and the joy of getting better.

Today one can choose from so many specialties, with so much diversity within each profession, that many patients are unknowingly choosing their own therapies. If a tennis player develops a chronic shoulder pain, at some point he or she makes a decision to walk into a professional's office. That professional will most often render his or her specialty for the shoulder problem. If the office is that of an acupuncturist, the patient gets acupuncture. If the professional is a chiropractor, the patient will get spinal manipulation; if a medical doctor, usually drugs are given. The best care, however, may be a combination of therapies. With a more balanced approach and greater awareness and cooperation between professions and professionals, patients can receive superior care. More importantly, the complementary sports medicine practitioner may be able to provide a variety of different but appropriate therapies required by the patient.

Today, many professionals are incorporating techniques from other fields into their approach. Some orthopedics are using nutrition, chiropractors are providing dietary guidelines, and many doctors are considering how mental/emotional stress impacts their particular type of therapy.

THE HOLISTIC VIEW

Although the word "holistic" has been overused, abused, and misunderstood for the past few decades, it remains an appropriate word to use when one is referring to the field of complementary sports medicine. The true holistic approach of complementary sports medicine is one in which all aspects of the patient are considered. The information value of signs and symptoms is important; no sign or symptom is insignificant. Lifestyle, diet, and mental/emotional state are considered as well as competition and training schedules. In addition, the practitioner uses a holistic approach when helping and treating a patient, and considers the science of such therapy. In contrast, science and mainstream medicine usually focus on fragments of the whole by looking at signs of a disease and treating particular symptoms. As Willis W. Harman (1991) writes in his "A Re-Examination of the Metaphysical Foundations of Modern Science,"

> There is increasingly widespread agreement that science must somehow develop the ability to look at things more holistically. In a more holistic view, where everything, including physical and mental/emotional, is connected to everything, a change in any part affects the whole. In a holistic science there is no cause and effect—only a whole system evolving. Only when a part of the whole can be sufficiently isolated from the rest that reductionistic causes appear to describe adequately why things behave as they do, do the ordinary concepts of scientific causation apply. In general, causes are limited "explanations" that depend upon context. (pp. iii-iv)

A complementary practitioner working with a runner who has chronic low back pain considers many factors beyond the low back. Whether this pain is due to a muscle imbalance, ligament sprain or strain, or joint dysfunction, the back pain itself may be an end result of a variety of imbalances that could have developed over a long period of time. It is not unusual for an asymptomatic foot problem to not only contribute to, but also cause, a low back problem. In some patients, muscle imbalance in the temporomandibular joint (TMJ) may be a primary factor. In others, several causative factors may exist—all far from the site of back pain. By assessing the patient in a holistic way, through a complete inventory of the whole body and not just the low back, the practitioner can find and correct these obscure but often primary problems.

THE HOLISTIC PARADIGM AS AN EQUILATERAL TRIANGLE

Another way of looking at the holistic approach is to view it as an equilateral triangle as described by Walther (1988). Each equal side represents one important aspect of the patient's health: structural, chemical, or mental/emotional health. Figure 1.1 represents this paradigm.

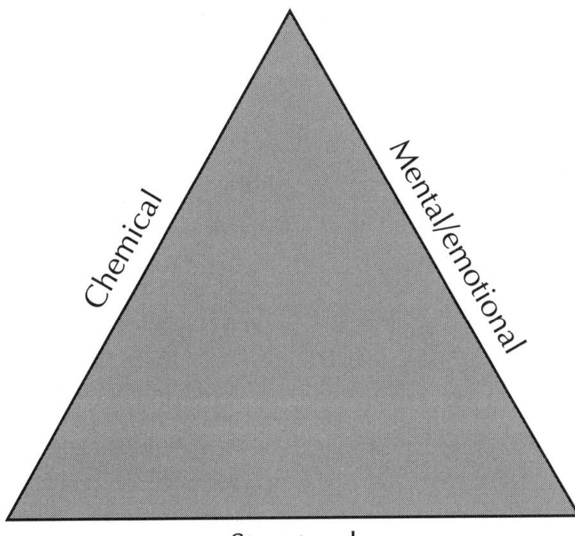

Figure 1.1 In complementary sports medicine, structural, chemical, and mental/emotional aspects of patient care are balanced as in an equilateral triangle.

The equilateral triangle concept is a simple representation and does not convey the complex interrelationships that exist throughout the body. For example, within the structure of the muscles are intricate chemical reactions that allow the muscle to function. Our thoughts are also chemical reactions. And without the structural aspect of intestinal absorption, the function of the villi, our nutritional status would be severely compromised. However, the triangle concept provides a starting point for discussion.

Structural Health

One side of the triangle portrays the person's structural health. This includes the skeleton, muscles, ligaments, and tendons. The functions of all our structural parts are very much dependent upon each other. For example, the tibialis posterior muscle plays a major role in the bony stability of the foot. And the physical equilibrium of the bony pelvis, itself dependent upon good muscle balance, has an indirect but significant impact on neck motion. Our whole body is a kinematic chain that acts as one complex functional unit. Although we study the body in separate and distinct parts, we cannot treat it successfully that way in the clinic.

The structural aspect of the body is often tended to by specific types of practitioners or specialists. Chiropractors, osteopaths, physical therapists, and massage therapists are among those professionals who focus much or all of their care on the structural aspects of their patients. Surgeons are also clearly structurally oriented.

With complementary sports medicine and its holistic approach, caring only for the structural aspect of a patient may be less than adequate even if the problem appears to be purely structural. A recurrent painful spinal imbalance, for example, is often associated with inflammation. If one treats only the inflammation with a local therapy such as aspirin or another anti-inflammatory medicine, the problem may not completely resolve. The patient's back may feel better, but the root of the problem has not been discovered. Perhaps the patient is wearing poorly fitted shoes or has a TMJ imbalance. In some situations, the complementary sports medicine practitioner can work with a medical practitioner in his or her expertise. For example, after surgery on a torn meniscus, the patient may greatly benefit from specific nutrition to help the healing process. The complementary practitioner looks at a person's entire structure.

Chemical Balance

The chemical side of the triangle incorporates all the biochemical aspects of the individual. Specific foods, nutrients, or drugs will have certain effects within the body. Consider the wide-ranging effects of caffeine or other drugs, or the effect of diet on energy production. As with structural health, one facet of body chemistry can influence many others. For example, eating a large, highly refined carbohydrate meal before exercise may have an adverse effect on the use of fats for energy and endurance. Also, emphasizing either protein or carbohydrate may favor the specific production of neurotransmitters in the brain like norepinephrine and serotonin, and this may influence concentration—a vital aspect of many sports.

Many professionals attempt to manipulate the body's biochemical systems. They do this with drugs, diet, nutritional supplements, and other approaches including homeopathic remedies, herbs, and other substances. Traditionally, nutritionists, naturopaths, homeopaths, and practitioners of Chinese medicine are the more conservative practitioners in this field, with many medical doctors and osteopaths frequently employing drugs.

As with strict adherence to structural health therapy, caring only for the chemical aspects of the body may not be most desirable even when the problem appears to be only chemical. People's chemistry can affect their structure, as is easily seen in the relationship between hormonal and nutritional status of the bones and the onset of osteoporosis. Conversely, people's structure can affect their biochemistry. For example, for an athlete who has difficulty chewing because of TMJ or tooth problems, eating certain healthy foods or properly digesting them may be difficult, affecting the nutritional status.

Mental/Emotional Wellness

The mental/emotional side of the triangle incorporates the behavioral aspects of the patient. The mental state may be referred to as cognition—sensation, perception, learning, concept formation, and decision making. It is important for the practitioner to understand these aspects of the patient, since they can affect overall health and fitness. The emotional state, the affective aspect of the patient, may include pain, moods of anxiety or depression, and loss of enthusiasm or motivation.

Traditionally, mental/emotional wellness is addressed by psychologists, psychiatrists, and counselors. Certainly all professionals are trained to be aware of the mental and emotional aspects of patients. For many patients, mental/emotional stress comes from trying to schedule training in relation to work and family obligations, from competitive anxiety, or from a pattern of frequent injuries. Complementary practitioners work with patients to balance their workout and competition schedules with structural health and chemical aspects as well as with their day-to-day life and family obligations. Complementary practitioners play a key role in helping to reeducate patients of all ages. In part, this is necessary because our society has promoted sport to an unhealthy level. Many young people think that playing hurt is good because of what they see and hear on television and radio; they think being all bandaged up in a game is a sign of superiority. And pushing oneself beyond the limit is something to strive for, people are told. Ad campaigns consisting of images that are not real are thrown at us and our children daily. This has helped to create attitudes and perceptions that contribute to the increase in sport injuries. Complementary sports medicine helps balance the message.

Case History

Jane was very frustrated by the many professionals she had seen over a period of about two years. This young woman, who played tennis three times a week and biked four times weekly, had sought care for her thoracic spine pain from an orthopedist whom her husband had once seen for his knee problem. The doctor ruled out structural causes and found no reason for the intermittent debilitating pain. Jane next saw a chiropractor. Although she gained relief, it never lasted more than a few days, so she saw an internist who did blood and urine tests and an upper gastrointestinal series. The doctor could not find a problem but prescribed antacids, which gave only minor relief. Jane then went to a nutritionist who did a bone-density test, which was normal. She saw the tennis pro to rule out mechanical problems; and then, on the advice of her family doctor, went to a psychologist. I saw Jane several weeks later. By now the pain was more diverse, with seemingly no pattern. Stress seemed to be the only common denominator, and I tested her adrenal hormones—cortisol, which was abnormally high, and dehydroepiandrosterone sulfate [DHEA(S)], which was abnormally low. It was clear that excess adrenal stress was a problem, although it was difficult to say whether it was the cause or the effect. Through the combined use of several approaches, including acupressure, nutrition, and dietary changes along with modification of her workout intensity, Jane was asymptomatic within two weeks, and in six months her adrenal hormone levels were normal. My impression was that she required the right combination of structural, chemical, and mental/emotional therapies suited to her unique, multifactorial problem.

EVERYONE IS AN ATHLETE

Another important aspect of this holistic approach is the fact that we are all athletes. We tend to categorize the patient population into athletes and nonathletes. But "couch potatoes" are in actuality just out-of-shape, inactive athletes who are literally a step away from being more athletic. Because of the potential health benefits, such a patient is perhaps the most important one to help. Many patients are reluctant to start exercising because they perceive this activity as a situation of "no pain, no gain." They see runners along the road who appear to be struggling, aerobic dance classes that look too advanced, and weight rooms that are full of sculptured bodies. If these patients understood that gradually working up to a 30-min easy walk, four or five times a week, would dramatically improve their health, many would happily comply. In addition, many patients are intimidated (and embarrassed) to work out where others with seemingly "ideal" bodies are also working out. Education becomes an important tool for these patients.

Likewise, we should not separate an athletic injury from all the rest. The patient who complains about shoulder pain from spring cleaning may have developed an imbalance not unlike that of the baseball pitcher who overworks the shoulder in spring training. We should not treat a "sports injury" but rather the person attached to it, regardless of the activity or situation that created the imbalance or dysfunction. Worse yet is the fact that too often a name is assigned to an injury so that a predetermined therapy can be given. Athletes are not the only ones who can benefit from complementary medicine. The fact is, every rotator problem in the shoulder is unique, every fascitis is different, and no two Achilles tendinitis problems are exactly the same. It follows that each patient is different and individual.

Early sports medicine doctors viewed their patients as athletes; they trained patients in addition to treating them. In Greece, athletes developed their skills under the direct supervision of sports physician trainers or gymnasts, who were involved in all aspects of the athlete's program (Leadbetter and Leadbetter 1986). This practice has been lost in recent times, as training has been given to specialists, including coaches, athletic trainers, and others who may not be aware of the functional status of the patient. Too often, communication between the therapy specialist and training specialist regarding an athlete's function or dysfunction, as well as his or her specific needs, is not efficient or is altogether absent.

In complementary sports medicine, variations in training specifically tailored to each athlete are an important part of the therapeutic process. Although in many cases the practitioner may not be with the athlete during the actual training, there is a clear understanding about each workout, and the goals are precise regardless of the level of sports training. More importantly, techniques such as biofeedback are used during training so that both caregiver and patient are more objectively informed about the training quality.

Whether it is walking for the beginner or training for an Ironman competition, the patient's program can be made more therapeutic with a variety of assessment workouts that give both practitioner and patient a clearer understanding of the program's efficiency and direction. We should not have to wait for a symptom to occur, for performance to falter, or for another end-result indicator to appear to find out that a patient's program does not match that person's specific needs. There are a variety of indicators, discussed throughout this text, that can be used to help round out the practitioner's holistic approach.

ART AND SCIENCE

The complementary sports medicine approach derives from both an art and a science perspective. The art is in the experience, expertise, and outcome, while the science includes basic physiology and its many models of energy production, neuromuscular actions, and biomechanical activity. An individual human being, however, may not always fit perfectly into a particular model. Work with an athlete cannot be accomplished effectively by either art or science alone; rather, a blending of the two helps make the outcome more successful. A practitioner who exemplifies this approach is like Michelangelo, whose knowledge about human anatomy is paralleled by his ability to portray the body in his paintings; the practitioner's artwork is a demonstration of his or her intellect. It is hoped that all clinicians practice both the art and science of their field through awareness of the uniqueness and beauty of the human body.

The art of complementary sports medicine includes the practitioner's ability to observe, experiment, and implement to find the optimal therapeutic outcome. This may be through diet, nutrition, exercise, or other therapy, but more often it is the proper combinations that best match the patient's needs. Art is in the ability to recognize when the body needs help—beyond what the patient tells us. Complementary sports medicine is an art also in the sense that some of the tools used in clinical practice have not been subjected to scientific scrutiny. Many assessment and treatment tools have not been researched; others have not been investigated thoroughly enough to establish why they might produce their results. Thus a tool may not have scientific acceptance. Instead of relying on science alone, then, the practitioner needs to be able to judge a tool by its usefulness for improving a specific clinical picture. In abstract terms, art is the body's dance, with full orchestra.

This dance can be analyzed with numbers; this is the science. The science lies in the objective ability to measure the human body's activity to determine its needs—and most importantly to develop theories about the mechanisms behind the activity. Science is the knowledge we gain by studying textbooks and journals—and it begins as art. An observation is made, but it may be years or centuries before the observation is scientifically substantiated. Knowledge about dietary fiber is a good example. Some 150 years ago, Dr. John Kellogg and Sylvester Graham, separately and through observation, proclaimed that fiber could reduce the risk of intestinal problems, cancer, and heart disease (McGee 1984). By 1974, science began to accept these observations when British surgeons, writing in the Journal of the American Medical Association, reported that fiber could reduce the risk of atherosclerosis and intestinal disease, including cancer (Burkitt et al. 1974). Today, it is a well-accepted fact that fiber is a crucial part of our diet.

Of increasing concern is the fact that today, many art forms are being abandoned for high technology. One example is acoustic assessment of fractures. According to Siffert and Kaufman (1996) at New York's Mount Sinai Medical Center, "The technique has become a relatively 'lost art' as more sophisticated X-ray and other imaging techniques have been developed" (p. 614). The authors encourage the use of this art, along with new technology, stating, "Auscultatory percussion is a useful tool in clinical fracture management, and particularly where roentgenographic facilities are inadequate or not available" (p. 614).

Combining art and science in the clinical realm makes for a more efficient and holistic approach, shifting the emphasis to the outcome as opposed to understanding and accepting the mechanism of a particular therapy. Today, more than ever, our approach to sports medicine is highly fragmented, with specialties and subspecialties that sometimes involve more competition among the professionals than among the athletes. It is important to be familiar with each specialty; these will be discussed in chapter 3.

FUNCTION AND DYSFUNCTION

In clinical practice, some patients present with clear problems of injury such as a fracture or a meniscus tear. However, many others do not have distinct injuries or diseases, but typically have complaints related to vague and less well-defined symptoms. The same pattern may exist for chemical and mental or emotional "injuries." These are referred to as functional problems, or a state of dysfunction, and are by far the most common problems seen in a complementary sports medicine practice. For example, a person may complain of low back pain but show no positive neurological or X-ray findings. Another person may experience fatigue but show normal values in blood tests. Yet another patient has acute diminishing athletic performance but by all standard medical assessments continues to be in optimal health. In addition, some patients possess various signs not related to an injury or disease state. Orthostatic or postural hypotension is common in athletes with heavy workout schedules; resting heart rate is elevated in others, and very low body temperatures are recorded in still others. In many cases, these signs and symptoms are manifestations of the preinjury state. To a complementary sports medicine practitioner, this body language indicates that if a person goes unchecked, he or she may develop more traditional, more obvious injuries, or even disease (see figure 1.2).

In the early functional stages of an injury, often no particular names are given to these imbalances—we simply say there is a functional problem, or a dysfunction. We could use the phrase "functional injury" or, in the case of an illness, "functional illness." In this situation it is better to describe the signs and symptoms, or preferably the clinical findings or neurophysiological dysfunction, than to apply a name to the condition. For example, we would say, "The patient's right latissimus dorsi is inhibited with a concurrent overfacilitation of the right pectoralis major muscle, producing shoulder joint

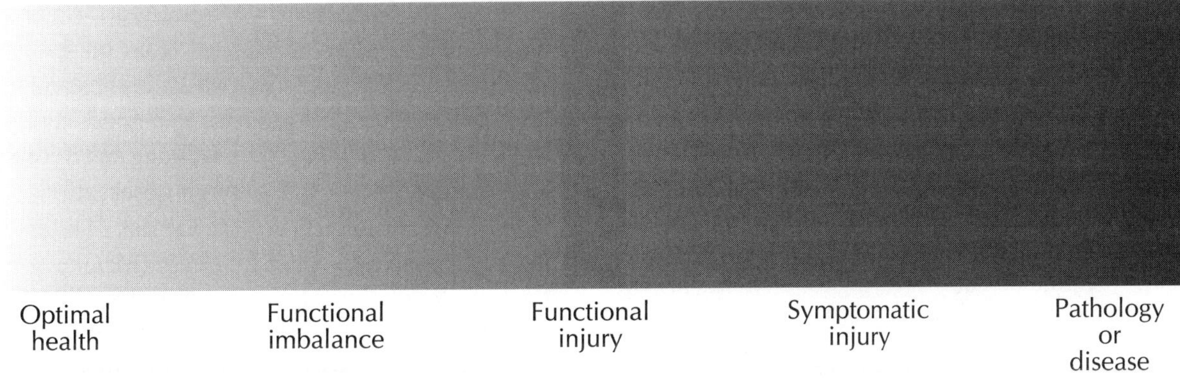

Figure 1.2 The "black and white" model of functional injury and traditional injury definitions

dysfunction." This athlete complains of an inability to throw the ball, rendering her unable to play effectively. Patients with functional problems do not necessarily fit into classical injury models; typically microtrauma exists without the classic cell atrophy, inflammation, or degenerative changes. In most cases, early injury is without pain.

It is also important to emphasize that an injury is not always synonymous with pain, trauma, or obvious debilitation. It is possible for an injury to be an asymptomatic dysfunction, one accompanied by more subtle and abnormal changes in joint motion, power output, or eye-hand coordination.

The first scientific observation of functional problems may have been made by Hans Selye (1976). In the 1920s, while still a student, Selye observed these general patterns of signs and symptoms and termed this a syndrome of "just being sick." He eventually showed that there were clear physiological responses to a variety of stressors, all mediated through the adrenal glands, taking place before a clear illness began. Today, we can measure adrenal hormones and discover in some cases that they are not within normal limits in athletes who do not have pathology but do show various signs and symptoms—indications of dysfunction (see figure 1.2).

A functional injury is a dysfunction in the body's structural, chemical, or mental/emotional process. It is somewhere between the state of optimal health or excellent function and some frank injury or disease. In some cases, the symptoms are very minor or vague and are ones traditionally discounted by many doctors. More importantly, subtle states of dysfunction may not produce any signs or symptoms in the patient. In this case, it is up to the practitioner, through a complete assessment, to find and correct these relatively minor but important imbalances. All of these problems can not only affect sport performance but also interfere with the quality of life.

THE NEED FOR BALANCED CARE

It would be wrong to think that only conservative therapy should be used in caring for all patients in a complementary sports medicine practice. Likewise, many problems seen in athletes do not require surgery or drugs. The fact is that there will be times when the use of more radical care is necessary and times when a conservative approach will be successful. In instances in which a specialist is needed, especially if the need is for surgery or if one's license does not permit writing a prescription, the referral process not only is a necessary part of complete therapy but also contributes to harmony among all branches of health care. Presently, health care providers are as fractionated as ever, even within the same profession. Competition seems to sometimes supersede the need to share information and refer to someone who can help in the assessment process or apply a more useful therapy.

Referrals to specialists should also be accompanied by an understanding, on the part of all involved, that possibly during or after the work of the specialist, more conservative services may be very valuable. For example, a patient who requires knee surgery may benefit from specific dietary or nutritional factors, such as omega-3 oil that can increase natural anti-inflammation production, helping in the recovery process. Immediately afterward, improving muscle function through acupressure or muscle therapy can help with postural balance and speed recovery, sometimes dramatically.

CONCLUSION

The concept of balance in all that is done in assessment, therapy, and especially lifestyle work is the highlight of complementary sports medicine. Whether the philosophy comes from Chinese medicine (the balance of yin and yang) or considers simple mechanical balance of muscle groups or nutritional balance, the final goal is the same: the optimal balance of the whole person. Natural balance in sports medicine was also recognized by the early Greeks (Leadbetter and Leadbetter 1986), who wrote of too much or too little of any component, referred to as disharmony. Around 1910, chiropractic borrowed the philosophy of "too much or too little nerve energy." Modern physiology uses the word homeostasis. Whatever the philosophy, the idea of balance is now universally accepted.

2

Definitions for Complementary Sports Medicine

As complementary sports medicine is a holistic discipline, much of the phraseology used in this field brings together otherwise disparate terminology. As such, many terms are defined in pairs: clinical and academic, health and fitness, aerobic and anaerobic, function and dysfunction. Like the Chinese yin and yang, many paired terms relate to the need for balance within the body and mind, and not just to the concept that they are opposites or mirror images. In addition, the words within each pair of terms complement each other. While definitions of some of the terms used in complementary sports medicine are similar or identical to the modern traditional definitions, other terms are interpreted differently. These definitions reflect a philosophical divergence and are part of the whole complementary paradigm. With such a strong emphasis on lifestyle and education of the patient, definitions become useful, easy to understand, and practical for the patient and practitioner alike.

CLINICAL AND ACADEMIC

Complementary sports medicine makes an important distinction between the words *clinical* and *academic*. *Clinical* pertains to the observation and treatment of patients, and *academic* relates to the theoretical and basic sciences. With few exceptions, definitions used in this text are based on clinical observation with an understanding of and respect for the fact that there is also an academic component. For example, in most clinical situations there is an academic element, and for a practitioner to better understand academic information, he or she must be able to relate to it clinically.

HEALTH AND FITNESS

As is the case with many terms, health and fitness are so casually and globally defined, both professionally and publicly, that many people are not clear on their precise definitions. As a result, the two terms are often combined into one and their meanings are interchanged.

Optimal health is an ideal state one can strive for but will not necessarily be able to obtain. It is more conditional and relative than the mere absence of disease or a subjective state of just feeling good. Optimal health is the perfect balance and function of all the systems of the body working in harmony, including the nervous, skeletal, muscular, hormonal, intestinal, and all other systems.

Fitness, which is more definitive, relates to a person's athleticism. It implies the ability to perform work effectively. A runner who completes a marathon in under 3 hr is more fit than the one who finishes in 3.5 hr. Fitness does not necessarily imply competition; the walker who exercises five days per week is more fit than the sedentary individual.

The most common misconception about health and fitness is that the two always exist simultaneously. Many believe that athletes possess more health because of their fitness training. Unfortunately this is sometimes, but not always, the case. Proper sports training can and should provide great health and fitness benefits, but many people do not reap these benefits because of some disharmony in the process, such as preexisting physical imbalances, overtraining, or failure to meet nutritional demands. Millions of people who begin to exercise in hopes of getting healthy find out they become more fit, but their health has suffered as a consequence. Injury, ill health, and other signs and symptoms that result from exercise imbalance are indications that overall health has suffered. Moreover, during this health-reducing process, fitness can even improve. The athlete who develops to a world-class level, only to find that he or she experiences fatigue and has allergies and chronic knee pain, is the classic patient seen in a complementary sports medicine practice. These individuals are fit but unhealthy. Ultimately, an unhealthy athlete will lose fitness, although this may take a long time. Often a young athlete who sacrifices health for fitness may not show signs or symptoms for years. Consider college and professional football, basketball, and hockey players for example. But for many people with average fitness potential who take up tennis, running, or cycling, the same process can occur.

Among athletes, coaches, and other professionals focused on improving performance, (which emphasizes fitness), health is sometimes neglected. A primary concern for the complementary sports medicine professional is the balance of health and fitness. This is accomplished by looking at the whole person and improving areas that are not functioning optimally. Not only will doing so lead to enhanced performance, but this athletic improvement will continue for a longer time period than one might expect.

It is important, then, that all the work done in training also be health promoting. An important long-term goal in training, in addition to improved performance, is to increase the quality of a person's life—not just for the moment but throughout the person's life span. This is accomplished by correcting and preventing an imbalance between health and fitness.

PREVENTION

Various professions define prevention differently. In many cases, modern medicine sees prevention as the process of screening for disease. Annual physicals, mammograms, and blood tests check for diseases in their earliest stages. For a middle-aged overweight patient who wants to begin an exercise program, a physical examination is recommended—an important first step in the process. This evaluation screens for heart disease, diabetes, anemia, and other disease states. But while the screening process may uncover a cardiac problem, for example, it may not find functional problems, many of which may be the precursor to a more serious future injury.

Sometimes prevention is defined as avoidance of disease. Philosophically, this is the other extreme of the medical definition. But heart disease, cancer, and other degenerative processes may actually be a "normal" part of the aging process.

Avoiding disease completely may not be a reality. But outliving disease is a reality. Many people maintain very good function through their 80s and 90s and die from nonspecific causes despite having evidence of heart disease, cancer, or other conditions. Complementary sports medicine prefers a definition of prevention that incorporates the functional aspect of the patient and refers to the postponement or slowing of the onset of dysfunction and disease. Postponing dysfunction and disease occurs when we maintain a higher quality of life throughout our lifetime.

Epidemiologists refer to this concept as "squaring the survival curve," an idea advanced by Fries and Crapo (1981). According to this concept, relatively high levels of structural, chemical, and mental/emotional function are maintained throughout life and are diminished only at the very end of the life span; in some cases the diminution may not even be obvious (see figure 2.1). When applied to an athlete, function relates not only to health but also to fitness. Healthy and fit athletes maintain a high level of competitiveness for a much longer-than-average period, without injury (see figure 2.2).

Through prevention, we can also improve the quality of our lives. More importantly, each person—doctor and patient—must take responsibility for his or her own health and fitness. For the professional, educating the patient in this regard is an important part of the complementary sports medicine approach.

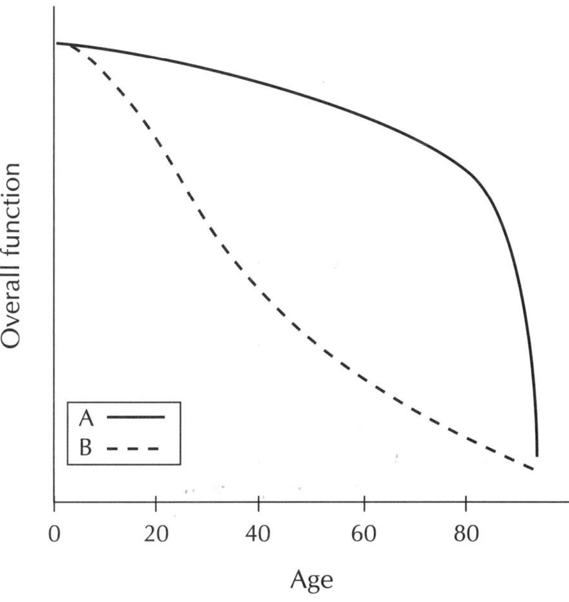

Figure 2.1 "Squaring the survival curve" refers to maintaining a high level of structural, chemical, and mental/emotional function throughout life. A) A person maintaining a higher level of function throughout life. B) A person with loss of function earlier in life.

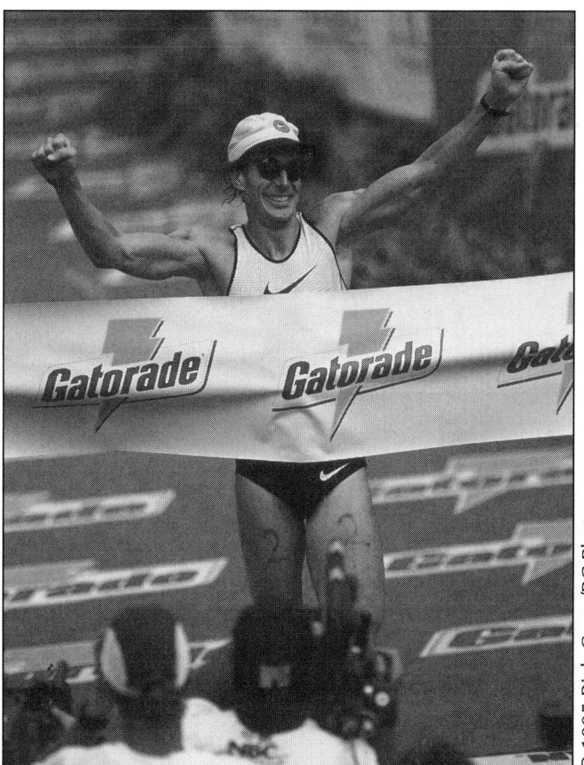

© 1995 Rich Cruse/RC Photo

Figure 2.2 Mark Allen winning the 1995 Ironman World Championships at age 37. Allen is a six-time winner of the Ironman Triathlon Championship.

Consider the definition of the word *doctor*, which means teacher. By teaching their patients how to be both healthy and fit, practitioners serve a vital role that goes beyond correcting someone's knee problem or even improving human performance.

TRAINING

Training defined more holistically refers to both health and fitness, with patients ultimately understanding balance and having an appreciation of bodily function. When defining training, complementary sports medicine looks at the whole process rather than just the actual workout time. An equally important aspect of training is the rest phase. The complete definition of training includes the workout plus the rest necessary for proper recovery, as seen in the equation Training = Work + Rest.

The work is the actual workout—the specific training routine that builds muscles and improves their efficiency, increases oxygen uptake, improves cardiac function, and so on. This part of training is sometimes referred to as the overload, and with effective training comes a progressive increase in overload. For example, muscles must be worked slightly harder than normally in order to rebuild and improve their function. In many people we see undertraining or training deficiency—the lack of activity. The human body is made for activity, and without activity we can suffer imbalances and ill health.

The balance of training can also be seen physiologically as an equilibrium between anabolic and catabolic metabolism. Training can be seen as a continuum of building up and tearing down. This balance is controlled by many factors, including genetics, type of training, and hormonal activity.

When one looks at the patient holistically, working out is not always limited to an athletic training overload. For many people housework, yard work, or office work is an activity that may evoke a physical overload or other stress in the form of a chemical or mental/emotional overload. This activity works the muscles, stimulates the metabolism and nervous system, and may even increase blood lactate. Although such work may not necessarily help in a given athlete's specific training, it must still be considered part of the training program because it is work.

Rest is the other part of balanced, holistic training. During the rest phase, the body recovers from training overload and prepares for the next session. During rest, there should be no real training, even in the form of other lifestyle activities that induce overload. Included in this phase is the need for sufficient sleep. For patients who are unable to successfully rest and recover from their workout, the alternative is to reduce their workout time and/or intensity to maintain a balanced training equation. This is one of the most important mechanisms used to help the patient secure a balance of health and fitness.

OVERTRAINING

An imbalanced training equation is the simple definition of overtraining. The most common cause of excessive or imbalanced training is overloading of the body to the point of trauma or abuse, or beyond the point where an effective recovery can take place before the next workout. This may result from too much work, too frequent workouts, too little rest, or a combination of these. Unfortunately, many believe the only way to reach their potential is to train more—an attitude of, or obsession with, "no pain, no gain." And clinically, we know that this attitude can lead to structural, chemical, or mental/emotional injuries. The concept of "no pain, no gain" has been scientifically refuted. For example, Costill et al. (1991) showed that for a group of swimmers who trained twice as long as a second swim group, there were no additional improvements in the group performing the longer training. It is the author's opinion that overtraining, including the mildest form of overtraining, is found in 60-75% of the athlete population. Overtraining is not only a common precursor to injury but also the most common cause of diminished performance. Both these problems occur only after overtraining has gone on for a period of time—sometimes a long period.

Overtraining must be distinguished from overreaching. While overtraining produces imbalance, overreaching refers to a short-term period of increased training volume, increased intensity, or both. If the period of overreaching causes a physical, chemical, or mental/emotional imbalance in the individual, as it frequently does, it has turned into functional overtraining. As discussed in later chapters, a number of diagnostic markers are available to determine when and if overreaching has turned into overtraining.

AEROBIC AND ANAEROBIC

Two key words used throughout this text are *aerobic* and *anaerobic*. The systems designated by these terms form the basis for a person's being both healthy and fit. *Aerobic* and *anaerobic* are frequently defined according to their oxygen relationships—aerobic referring to oxygen utilization and anaerobic to the absence of oxygen. Traditionally, athletes have sometimes been placed into one of two groups and thought of as aerobic or anaerobic athletes. The fact is that both systems work in any individual, both at rest and during activity.

However, in complementary sports medicine, a clinical definition of each term is employed—one that is more useful and that allows easier measurement in an office setting. In this case, the aerobic and anaerobic systems are defined based on the origin of their chief source of energy for adenosine triphosphate production. Fatty acids are the potentially predominant source of aerobic energy, while glucose is the primary anaerobic energy source. Aerobic refers to the increased utilization of fatty acids, and anaerobic to the increased utilization of glucose by the body.

Even in people who utilize a high percentage of fat for energy, there is still a significant contribution from glucose, especially to maintain beta oxidation. This contribution from glucose may be relatively small if activity is minimal, and large during times of higher-intensity workouts. (In some sprint and power sports, glucose [and creatine phosphate] are the exclusive fuels.) As workout intensity increases, so does the demand for more glucose as the dominant fuel, with less reliance on fatty acids. In this instance our definitions are still useful. As exercise intensity increases, the individual becomes more anaerobic and less aerobic; low-intensity workouts are generally more aerobic.

What makes these definitions relate more closely to an athlete's functional state is the fact that many lifestyle factors can significantly influence our ability to utilize fatty acids for energy. Some of these include the macronutrient makeup of the diet, training intensities, and stress.

Complementary sports medicine's definitions of aerobic and anaerobic are useful to both clinician and patient. For the average athlete, the definition of anaerobic as "without oxygen" is not precise in relation to performance. During any activity, including rest, the body cannot survive without oxygen for more than a couple of minutes. In the case of microorganisms, however, the definition "without oxygen" would be most appropriate.

ENDURANCE

If we define endurance as the time during which a given exercise intensity can be sustained, it still does not reflect the important aspect of endurance: fuel utilization. Clinically, endurance is also an expression of aerobic function, including the quality and quantity of that aerobic function, in an individual. Most importantly, with improved aerobic function and endurance comes the ability to utilize more fatty acids for energy. For the athlete, endurance is the ability to perform more work (e.g., to sustain a more rapid pace) while remaining at the same level or at relatively low levels of intensity (i.e., heart rate). This is accompanied by a reduced respiratory quotient (increasing the percentage fat utilization for energy) and a diminished dependence on carbohydrate utilization.

Traditional definitions of endurance vary greatly. McArdle et al. (1991) define endurance as "the time limit of a person's ability to maintain either a specific isometric force or a specific power level involving combinations of concentric or eccentric muscular contractions" (p. 756). Wilmore and Costill (1994) describe it as the ability to resist fatigue; includes muscular endurance and cardiorespiratory endurance. Endurance is traditionally evaluated using aerobic power as measured by $\dot{V}O_2max$. However, not only is this impractical for the average clinician and athlete, but endurance can vary greatly among individuals with an equal $\dot{V}O_2max$ (Coyle et al. 1988).

AEROBIC SPEED

Through proper aerobic training comes more endurance, which has just been defined as the ability to perform more work with the same or less effort. In the case of a runner, for example, this increased work capacity takes the form of more aerobic speed. Using the heart rate as a measure of effort, suppose a runner can go 5000 m in 18 min. After four months of improving endurance, he or she can run that same distance in 17 min. The concept of aerobic speed is also applicable to other sports. During the course of a game, the basketball player maintains the ability to run up and down the court faster with less effort (i.e., utilizing less energy) and fatigue. The distance cyclist, swimmer, or cross-country skier can go faster with the same or less energy and for longer periods. This gain in aerobic speed is accomplished by increasing the utilization of fatty acids for energy as shown in a decreased respiratory quotient. This form of speed is distinguished from anaerobic speed, which is called sprinting—here a short burst of energy is provided through glycolysis (and creatine phosphate) and is limited to 2 to 4 min.

The following list shows actual changes in an endurance runner over a four-month period. These 1-mile measurements were taken after a warm-up while the athlete maintained a heart rate of 145 beats per minute.

April	8:21
May	8:11
June	7:57
July	7:44

CONCLUSION

Alternative definitions effectively combine the philosophical, assessment, and therapeutic aspects of complementary sports medicine. Though the deviation from academic definitions is not dramatic, the clinical emphasis allows for a more practical, patient-centered practice.

3

Complementary Medicine Specialties

Within the health care community are many specialties collectively referred to as alternative therapies, alternative medicine, or, more properly, complementary medicine. While many practitioners within these professions attend to the needs of athletes, no definitive statistics are available regarding the popularity of the practice among the many sports. Eisenberg et al. (1993) demonstrates that Americans made more visits to providers of alternative medicine (425 million visits a year) than to all U.S. primary care physicians (388 million annual visits). In Europe (Christie 1991; Himmel et al. 1993), Canada (Verhoef and Sutherland 1995), Israel (Bernstein and Shuval 1997), and many other areas of the world, these therapies are referred to as complementary medicine.

Many complementary and alternative therapies encompass practices outside the medical mainstream. However, certain specialties, such as physical medicine and rehabilitation, have long included many of the therapies now being categorized as "alternative" (Kronenberg et al. 1994). In addition, even the nomenclature used in relation to diagnosis is quite varied and nonstandardized. Cashman (1988) showed that medical, osteopathic, and chiropractic nomenclatures describing very similar anatomical distortions of the spine contained 10 separate terms that were currently being employed. These variations in terminology only create more barriers between professions and the patients who seek improved care.

CATEGORIES OF COMPLEMENTARY SPECIALTIES

Three general categories of complementary medicine specialties comprise practitioners or subgroups that provide sports medicine care. The first category consists of practitioners who predominantly provide hands-on care: chiropractic, traditional osteopathy, massage therapy, and other manual therapies. The second category includes those professionals who deal with lifestyle factors; they offer dietary or nutritional advice, or dispense other types of non-drug supplements (i.e., homeopathics, herbs, and other remedies). This group includes specialists in the fields of nutrition, diet, homeopathy, and sport psychology. The third category includes professionals who incorporate most if not all of the methods mentioned into one approach—utilizing both hands-on techniques and lifestyle improvement, including nutritional, herbal, or other types of non-drug supplementation. The three predominant groups within this category are Chinese medicine, applied kinesiology, and naturopathy. While many people are not familiar with these professions, most are familiar with some of their individual elements. For example, Chinese medicine was the first to utilize acupuncture, herbology, manipulation, nutrition and diet, music and color therapy, and many other individual techniques. Applied kinesiology employs acupressure, diet, nutrition, manipulation, and similar hands-on techniques. Naturopathy involves a similar approach to patient care.

To sum up, the three major categories of complementary therapies are these:

- Practitioners who predominantly or exclusively use hands-on techniques, such as chiropractors, traditional osteopaths, and massage therapists
- Professionals who predominantly or exclusively use lifestyle-oriented treatments, such as nutritionists, dietitians, nurses, homeopaths, and sport psychologists
- Professionals who combine hands-on and lifestyle-improvement techniques, such as applied kinesiologists, naturopaths, and Chinese medicine practitioners

This list is not meant to be all-inclusive. Hundreds of professionals and paraprofessional groups have evolved from the field of complementary medicine and are seeking autonomy, many dealing with the care of athletes. Some of these other approaches are Ayurvedic medicine (the original Hindu medical system based on body balance); biofeedback (the use of visual or auditory information about body function); herbology (the use of botanicals to treat the body); meditation (including many types such as transcendental meditation and other techniques for personal relaxation and spiritual exploration); orthomolecular medicine (the use of high-dose vitamins, minerals, trace elements, amino acids, enzymes, hormones); sensory deprivation (the use of flotation tanks); and many types of yoga (for physical and spiritual discipline). There are also groups of professionals from mainstream medicine who are claiming their independence in the complementary field, including nurses (Geddes and Henry 1997). Moreover, many medical practitioners are utilizing nutrition and diet, acupuncture, or other complementary therapies in their existing practices, sometimes as an adjunct to their current approach or as a replacement for their previous specialty.

At times, professionals in one field implement therapies more often used in another. For example, although most chiropractors perform spinal manipulation, some also utilize diet and nutrition, acupuncture, or other modalities. Also, many professionals incorporate sports training into their therapeutic regime, while many more review a patient's training as part of an evaluation of the whole person.

METHODS OF ASSESSMENT

On a basic level, methods of assessment help define the various practitioners and health care professionals. Many such disciplines use a symptom-based assessment approach, in which a specific treatment or remedy is given for a particular symptom. For example, calcium is often used by nutritionists when the athlete has tight muscles. A similar version of a symptom-based approach is providing a particular remedy for a specific condition—the sum of certain symptoms gives rise to a named condition. For example, iron supplements are given to a patient with hypochromic-microcytic anemia. Symptom-based assessments are most effective when all the patient's symptoms are correlated with other findings during an examination of the whole person.

Instead of using symptom-based assessments, complementary sports medicine professionals apply physiologically-based diagnostic methods, usually in conjunction with a complete inventory of symptoms and other findings and lifestyle factors. For example, the athlete who complains of muscle tightness may have muscle imbalance as described by Walther (1988) and Janda (1996). Often there is a muscle inhibition opposing the overfacilitated muscle. In many cases, the muscle inhibition is more primary and asymptomatic, with the symptomatic muscle tightness as a secondary problem. One of the most frequently seen examples is tightness in the low back muscles; here abdominal muscle inhibition is common. In such a patient, giving calcium for tight muscles may or may not provide some symptomatic relief. In either case the primary cause has not been addressed. In the case of supplementing iron for patients with anemia, this treatment may not be completely effective if malabsorption or blood loss is the cause and this primary issue has not been addressed.

Recently, however, many holistic approaches have turned into symptom-based approaches. Acupuncture (part of Chinese medicine) is traditionally practiced by determining which meridians are out of balance, regardless of the patient's complaints. Today, acupuncture is often practiced by symptoms: points a, b, and c are treated for symptom X or condition Y. Other examples of symptom treatment include diet ("cholesterol-lowering diet," "weight-loss diet," "pregame meal," etc.) and nutrition (vitamin C for colds, creatine phosphate for energy, chromium for fat burning, etc.). It is unfortunate that so many professionals and individuals have turned to this "cookbook" style of health care when complete assessment and individualized care considering all of the body's symptoms can be much more effective.

EXAMPLES OF COMPLEMENTARY SPECIALTIES

What follows is a brief discussion of some of the major complementary medicine professions. There are many others that are usually some variation of the ones described here. Table 3.1 lists some complementary medicine approaches and the related assessment, treatment, and lifestyle-improvement methods they typically employ. It should be emphasized again that in many cases, a professional in a particular field may incorporate assessment methods, therapies, and lifestyle recommendations from another discipline.

Table 3.1 Complementary Sports Medicine Disciplines and the Related Primary Assessment, Therapy, and Lifestyle Methods Employed

Discipline	Primary assessment	Primary therapy	Primary lifestyle
Applied kinesiology	Muscle testing with all other standard methods	Many	All aspects
Naturopathy	All forms of standard methods	Many	All aspects
Chinese medicine	Pulse and facial diagnosis	Acupuncture, herbs, massage/manipulation, qigong	All aspects
Diet/Nutrition	History, diet assessment	Dietary recommendations, nutritional supplements	Diet
Sport psychology	History, consultation	Counseling, visualization, mental imaging	Mental/emotional stress
Chiropractic	Palpation, X-rays	Spinal manipulation	Posture
Traditional osteopathy	Palpation, posture, X-rays	Cranial-sacral therapy, spinal manipulation	Depends on practitioner
Massage therapy	History	Massage	Relaxation, posture
Homeopathy	History	Homeopathic remedies	Depends on practitioner

Chiropractic

While manipulation of the spine has been used for centuries, the chiropractic profession, which specializes in this technique, dates back to 1895. Chiropractors believe that spinal vertebra misalignments, called chiropractic subluxations, interfere with the normal activity of the nervous system to cause functional problems on a physical, chemical, or mental/emotional level. The term *subluxation* in chiropractic has more functional meaning than the standard definition, which refers to a partial or incomplete dislocation (*Dorland's Illustrated Medical Dictionary* 1994). Subluxation refers to a joint that is dysfunctional within its normal range of motion. This joint dysfunction may not necessarily cause pain, but will usually have some adverse effect on the person's physical, chemical, or mental/emotional state. In this text, these types of spinal and other joint problems are referred to as a joint complex dysfunction as discussed by Seaman (1997).

Some chiropractors also address imbalances associated with other joints including the temporomandibular joint and the joints of the feet, knees, wrists, and so on. Chiropractors have successfully treated patients with conditions ranging from back and neck pain to intestinal disorders and allergies. In the United States, chiropractors must receive a doctoral degree (DC) in a rigorous education nearly identical to that of medical school except that it does not include studies in surgery. Some chiropractors are also trained in other complementary disciplines, including diet and nutrition, applied kinesiology, and Chinese medicine.

In the 1950s and 1960s, Major Bertrand DeJarnette (1979), both a chiropractor and an osteopath, developed his "Sacro Occipital Technique", which included many manipulative therapies, especially non-force techniques for improving pelvic and cranial function. DeJarnette categorized pelvic distortions that are often primary structural faults causing other, secondary, mechanical problems. This technique is primarily used today by complementary medicine professionals.

Over the past several decades, chiropractic sports medicine and rehabilitation have been emerging fields within complementary medicine. Many professional, collegiate, and amateur teams and individual athletes utilize chiropractic care as a major part of their sports programs, with chiropractors becoming more accepted by mainstream practitioners.

Osteopathy

Traditional osteopathy is a manipulative-based therapy using a conservative non-drug approach. There is a stronger focus on the bones of the head and neck and the musculoskeletal system in general; but other therapies are used by some osteopaths, including acupuncture, diet and nutrition, and applied kinesiology. Osteopathy was developed in the 1890s by Andrew Taylor Still, but by the 1950s the majority of osteopaths were incorporated into mainstream medicine. Today, most osteopaths in the United States practice like medical doctors, having abandoned their traditional techniques. Their doctor of osteopathy degree (DO) is nearly identical to a medical degree. In many parts of the world, especially Europe, many osteopaths have maintained their traditional roles, often utilizing other complementary approaches.

Cranial osteopathy, developed in 1939 by William Sutherland, DO, is a subspecialty within osteopathic manipulative medicine. A cranial osteopath focuses particularly on the movements of the cranial bones and their relationships with the spine and sacrum. This is referred to as the cranial-sacral mechanism. This mechanism is described as a dynamic force within the living human body: the qi or energy of the central nervous system. Osteopaths describe precise movements of all 26 cranial bones, which constitute a significant part of the body's self-healing mechanism. This cranial bone motion is associated with the breathing mechanism as certain bones move in particular fashion with both inhalation and exhalation. The amount of movement is in the range of fractions of a millimeter. Concomitant with this movement is an oscillation of the cerebral spinal fluid, which is also in a rhythmic motion with the cranium and sacrum.

Cranial osteopaths do not view the adult skull as a fused mass. They describe the cranial bones as fitting together with various grooves and gearlike articulations with each other. The sutures are comprised of connective tissues, membranes, and blood vessels with elastic tissue that is identifiable microscopically. Holding this mechanism together is the dura mater, which is attached at the foramen magnum, the second and third cervical vertebrae, and the sacrum. Cranial osteopaths believe that any disruption in cranial movement may have an adverse effect on any part of the mechanism, interfering with the body's self-healing abilities. Problems within the cranial-sacral mechanism can occur as a result of trauma (beginning with birth), daily microtrauma, breathing irregularities (especially improper breathing), muscular strain, or other imbalances.

Assessment is done by palpation of the cranium, sacrum, and spine; by postural evaluation; and by other approaches depending on the practitioner. Correction of cranial-sacral problems is accomplished manually by applying gentle pressures at certain points on the cranium and sacrum, often in conjunction with inhalation or exhalation, or through manipulation of certain spinal vertebrae. The goal is to correct an imbalanced cranial-sacral mechanism.

In the 1930s, Frank Chapman, DO, theorized that specific reflex points on the body were related to certain organs and glands and that stimulating these reflexes might improve lymphatic drainage of the related organs or glands. These points are referred to as Chapman's reflexes. George Goodheart, DC, later developed Chapman's work and incorporated it into applied kinesiology with other traditional osteopathic techniques.

Massage Therapy (Therapeutic Massage)

The profession of massage therapy comprises trained, licensed practitioners who provide various types of massage techniques. Massage therapy is being prescribed increasingly by both mainstream and complementary practitioners to supplement their own therapies for all types of patients, including athletes. Massage focuses on increasing blood circulation and lymph flow, reducing muscle tension and spasm, improving range of motion, and helping to reduce pain. It involves soft tissue manipulation of the body and aids in stress reduction, which can aid in recovery from training and competition or from injury. Smith et al. (1994) found reductions in delayed-onset muscle soreness and in creatine kinase and cortisol levels following massage therapy. Field et al. (1996) found that massage therapy can reduce anxiety, and Ironson et al. (1996) showed a positive effect on the immune system. All these are key issues for athletes.

A variety of techniques are used in sports massage, including different types of Swedish massage. This sports massage includes the use of standard effleurage, petrissage, and vibration techniques; cross-fiber massage that involves friction techniques applied to create a stretching and broadening effect in large muscle groups; and trigger-point massage, which involves specific finger pressure into myofascial trigger points in muscle and connective tissue to reduce hypersensitivity and muscle spasms. Trigger points may cause restricted and painful movement of muscles, ligaments, and tendons, as well as referred pain, and were first described by Travell and Rinzler (1952). More recently, Lewit (1991) stated that trigger points are bands of muscular tissue that appear contracted while the rest of the muscle is quiescent. In addition to massage therapy, other methods described in this text can help relieve trigger points.

Massage therapists can perform regular maintenance care, treatments for specific athletic injuries, and massage before and after athletic events or training.

Nutrition and Diet

Nutritional and diet therapy is widely used by so many professionals that it is difficult to categorize. Many within the field do not consider it an alternative technique. For example, nurses and dieticians who work in an institution have been applying basic nutrition for decades as part of mainstream medicine. In addition, MDs and DOs who work in hospitals may use dietary or nutritional recommendations as appropriate for certain types of conditions. This work encompasses parenteral nutrition and addresses special needs of cardiac, diabetic, arthritic, and other patients. The differences between mainstream nutrition and diet therapy and the complementary approach are many; most importantly, practitioners of the latter consider the functional aspect of the patient and specific nutrients that may improve function, rather than waiting for a clear deficiency state before implementing treatment. Most importantly, the approach should be individualized: all patients are unique in their dietary and nutritional needs. When nutritional recommendations are applied, other aspects of the patient often need to be considered, such as stress, training, intestinal function, and so on.

Another clear division in the field of diet and nutrition is between so-called natural or unprocessed foods and processed foods. The same division applies in the arena of vitamin and mineral use; some products are real, natural food supplements, and others are isolated or synthetic versions of what nature provides. Within the field of diet and nutrition, significant scientific and clinical data have emerged regarding sport performance enhancements with the use of various nutritional remedies and dietary changes.

Homeopathy

The history of homeopathy begins with its founder, Samuel Hahnemann (1755-1843), a German physician. Hahnemann coined the word "homeopathy" (homoios in Greek means "similar"; pathos means "suffering") to refer to the pharmacological principle, the "law of similars," that is its basis. Homeopathy evolved in the United States through the work of Hans Gram, a Dutch homeopath, who emigrated to the United States in 1825. Today, homeopathy is widespread throughout the world, especially in Europe, Asia, the Far East, Central and South America, Australia, and Russia.

Homeopathy is based on the "law of similars" that was described by Hippocrates and has been utilized by people of many cultures, including the Chinese, Greeks, and Native American Indians. Hahnemann developed the "law of similars" into a systematic medical art and science. Immunizations, allergy treatment, and other medical approaches are based on this "law of similars."

The homeopath uses extremely low-dose substances to treat a person's problems. In effect, the practitioner seeks to find a substance that, if given in overdose, would produce symptoms similar to those a sick person is experiencing. The most controversial aspect of homeopathy is the dosages.

Homeopathic doses are produced by a series of dilutions that result in an exceedingly low-dose substance. This process is called "potentization" and refers to a specific procedure of serial dilution in which 1 part of a medicinal substance is diluted with 99 parts distilled water or ethyl alcohol; 1 part of this latter solution is then diluted further with 99 parts distilled water or ethyl alcohol. This process of dilution may be continued to different numbers of dilutions, most commonly 3, 6, 9, 12, 30, 200, 1000, 10,000, 50,000, or 100,000. When a homeopathic medicine is labeled "C," this means that the medicine was diluted 1:99. A medicine labeled "X" or "D" was diluted 1:9. When a medicine is described as a "30X," this means it was diluted 1:9 and that the dilution was repeated 30 times. If a medicine is labeled "LM," it was diluted approximately 1:50,000. Homeopaths have observed that the more a medicine has been potentized, that is, diluted in this fashion, the longer it generally acts and the fewer the doses needed to be effective.

More startling is the fact that while homeopaths and scientists agree that solutions diluted beyond 24X or 12C may not have any molecules of the original solution, they assert that "something" remains: the essence of the substance, its resonance, its energy. Homeopaths generally assess patients using history of symptoms.

Naturopathic Medicine

Naturopathy is the holistic practice of natural therapeutics, or natural medicine, which works with a variety of hands-on and lifestyle factors including diet, nutrition, herbal medicine, homeopathy, acupuncture, physical medicine, exercise, and others. In addition to treating a variety of imbalances, the naturopath focuses on functional problems to prevent future illness and injury. These practitioners assess patients through physical examinations, blood and urine tests, nutritional and dietary evaluations, and other methods.

Naturopathy began in the United States in the early 1900s, when many natural therapies that had previously existed were joined together. By the mid-1900s, naturopathy rapidly declined as allopathic medicine was flourishing. Today, the naturopathic physician must obtain an ND degree from a four-year graduate-level naturopathic college. In the United States, only eight states license naturopaths: Alaska, Arizona, Connecticut, Hawaii, Montana, New Hampshire, Oregon, and Washington. Naturopathy is growing again as the complementary movement has expanded.

Chinese Medicine

This approach is one of the oldest known systems of assessment and therapy, and was perhaps the first true "holistic" method because it addressed every aspect of the patient's life, including wellness treatments to maintain good health. Chinese medicine includes four main aspects: acupuncture; massage and manipulation; herbal medicines; and exercise disciplines called qigong, the most popular form being tai chi.

A key focus in Chinese medicine is assessment, which relies heavily on observation and on palpation of the radial pulses. In addition to pulse diagnosis, important tools include observation of the face (facial diagnosis), the texture and look of the skin, and the odor of the breath. Pulse diagnosis is the foundation of Chinese medicine assessment. In this approach, the radial pulse is palpated with three fingers, with the practitioner feeling a separate pulse in each. Each pulse also has a superficial and deep quality (each considered a separate pulse), providing 6 pulses on each wrist. These 12 pulses relate to the 12 "meridians" that according to Chinese theory are the channels in which energy (called qi) flows through the body. (Chinese medicine is often called meridian therapy.) On each meridian, there are many different points that can be stimulated by manual pressure (acupressure), needles (acupuncture), heat (through the burning of the moxa herb, referred to as moxibustion), and electricity (electroacupuncture). These are called meridian therapy points, or acupuncture points (the term used in this text). The Chinese also incorporate herbal therapy, music and color therapy, and even psychotherapy to help balance qi.

The basic theory in Chinese medicine is that an imbalance of qi—which consists of yin and yang energy—is the cause of dysfunction and ultimately disease. The balancing of yin and yang energy is therefore the goal of the practitioner, who may use any or all of the therapeutic tools to accomplish this depending on which is most applicable to the patient's needs based on assessment. This balance does not stop with the individual but continues into society as a whole. The individual, as well as the surrounding society, is a delicate balance of yin and yang. Yin represents water, quiet, substance, and night; yang represents fire, noise, function, and day. The two are polar opposites, and therefore one of them must be present to allow the other to exist; for instance, how can you experience joy if you do not understand sorrow? More interesting is the fact that many ancient Chinese visited their practitioners when they were well, paying the practitioner a retainer to keep them healthy. If they became ill, they stopped paying until wellness returned.

Applied Kinesiology

Like Chinese medicine and some other approaches already described, applied kinesiology (AK) combines many existing therapies into one system. Applied kinesiology is unique due to its use of manual muscle testing as part of an assessment process that focuses on the functional aspect of the patient's structure, chemistry, and mental/emotional state. These assessment methods help the practitioner find the therapies that best match the patient's specific needs. This process is done each and every time practitioner and patient come together. Between visits to the practitioner—referred to as sessions in this text—the patient makes appropriate lifestyle changes as recommended by the practitioner according to previous assessments.

Through evaluation of the function of certain muscles pre- and posttreatment, therapeutic efficacy can be evaluated. Applied kinesiologists theorize that physical, chemical, and mental/emotional imbalances are associated with secondary muscle dysfunction—specifically a muscle inhibition (usually followed by overfacilitation of an opposing muscle). Applying the proper therapy results in improvement in the inhibited muscle. Leisman et al. (1995) showed that AK muscle testing procedures can be objectively evaluated through quantification of the neurologic electrical characteristics of muscles, and that the course of AK treatments can be objectively plotted over time. Another theory within AK is that specific muscles are associated with specific areas of the body: there are organ-muscle, gland-muscle, meridian-muscle, spine-muscle, and reflex-muscle relationships. (The relationships between specific spinal nerves and specific muscles are better known.)

There is not a specific academic degree for AK—rather, AK is practiced by those already possessing a license to practice in another field. Applied kinesiology is utilized worldwide mostly by chiropractors, medical doctors, and osteopaths, along with a variety of other practitioners. Courses and certifications are given by the International College of Applied Kinesiology, which has chapters throughout the world. Individuals either practice as applied kinesiologists or use AK as an adjunct to their particular specialty. For example, chiropractors, medical doctors, or osteopaths may predominantly practice their specialty but utilize AK assessment and treatment methods as an adjunct. This blending is very feasible because AK is an open system based on sound physiological principles, and many therapeutic approaches can be incorporated according to the doctor's expertise and interests.

Applied kinesiology was developed by George Goodheart, DC, beginning in 1964. Goodheart noticed that significant postural improvements could be made immediately following manipulation of an inhibited muscle, specifically through stimulation of the muscle's neurological components: Golgi tendon organs or spindle cells. Gradually, a variety of existing modalities including acupressure, osteopathic techniques, nutrition, and many others were combined as treatment options, with use of manual muscle testing as one of the diagnostic aids. Goodheart added a muscular relationship to Chapman's reflexes, theorizing that organ or glandular dysfunction was followed by specific muscle inhibition and observed that manually stimulating specific Chapman's reflexes improved the related muscle function (and body posture). Today, it can also be confirmed clinically that adrenal dysfunction, for example, such as excess cortisol production or diminished dehydroepiandrosterone sulfate [DHEA(S)], is associated with muscular inhibition of the sartorius or tibialis posterior muscle(s).

Acupuncture meridians were also correlated with muscles; each meridian was found to have one or more corresponding muscles that reacted to the state of the meridian. For example, if a meridian was low in qi, the related muscle was usually inhibited, and the corresponding meridian with too much qi was associated with an overfacilitated muscle.

In addition to Chapman's reflexes, acupuncture points, and muscle neurological reflexes, AK incorporates manipulation of the cranium, spine, and extravertebral joints as described by the chiropractic and osteopathic professions. In addition, many other techniques have been borrowed, refined, and incorporated into AK, including those directed at the nervous system, temporomandibular joint, and diaphragm muscle, as well as a system of nutritional assessment. The tool used most often to help the practitioner match the optimal therapy with the patient's needs is manual muscle testing, which is always done in conjunction with other methods of diagnosis, including blood and urine tests, blood pressure measurement, and standard orthopedic, neurologic, and physical examinations.

Sport Psychology/Sport Awareness

In 1956 Roger Bannister wrote, "Though physiology may indicate respiratory and circulatory limits to muscular effort, psychological and other factors beyond the ken of physiology set the razor's edge of defeat or victory and determine how close an athlete approaches the absolute limits of performance" (Newsholme 1996, p. 246). Sport psychology is not necessarily considered an alternative medicine, but clearly it can be used in conjunction with both complementary and mainstream medicine. A variety of psychological-type therapies are often considered alternative, including hypnosis, use of mental/emotional imagery, biofeedback, and meditation. Hampf (1993) states that in "chronic pain cases, alternative [psychological] therapies merit consideration, even though they may generally be rejected by Western medicine as unscientific" (p. 15). But according to Crossman (1997), "Medical professionals realize the importance of incorporating psychological strategies into rehabilitation from athletic injury, but often feel they lack the knowledge to do so" (p. 333).

Communication between caregiver and patient, an important component of "bedside manner," is the first step to improved awareness by the patient of his or her body and mind. As Laemmel (1996) writes, "The very earliest myths relating to the art of healing give great weight to the vital importance of human dialogue" (p. 863). Too many practitioners are unwilling to talk with their patients—a primary complaint of patients.

Under the rubric of sport psychology and awareness can also be placed many mental/emotional aspects of sports medicine, including one rarely considered a sport psychology issue—education. Through lack of basic understandings about body function, athletes can bring on themselves significant stress. Likewise, when they obtain incorrect or improper information, for example when influenced by advertising or social trends, athletes can become more stressed. Obsession on the part of an athlete with dieting, bingeing and purging, or overtraining is an obvious example. Forming balanced goals and having a purpose for working out and competition are also key priorities for athletes. In many cases, athletes are unaware of their purpose in sports. For some, this may eventually lead to significant mental/emotional stress.

As described earlier and as will be elaborated in more detail in a later chapter, stress plays a major role in sport and is a significant contributory factor in physical, chemical, and mental/emotional injuries.

All practitioners can play a vital role in helping with sport awareness when working with athletes. Helping athletes to understand their body's normal and abnormal function, including nutritional needs and exercise physiology, can help them overcome social pressures, media and advertising distortion, and other problems they may encounter.

CONCLUSION

Millions of athletes, from professionals to local enthusiasts, seek care from complementary practitioners each year. Most of these practitioners come from existing alternative or complementary medicine circles, although more mainstream medical doctors are now entering the arena. With the dramatic rise in interest on the part of both patients and professionals in the United States, complementary therapies are now being taught in nearly 30% of medical schools and family practice residency programs, with another 12% of such institutions planning or considering offerings in some complementary therapies (Carlston et al. 1997).

Whether one uses Chinese medicine, AK, or some combination of therapies, the important concern is outcome: Has the whole patient improved? This question can and should be asked and answered by both the practitioner and patient. If the question is to be answered properly, outcomes must also include reassessments. If an injury causes pain and dysfunction, an effective therapy results not only in the elimination of pain but also in the restoration and improvement in function as evidenced by the same method of assessment originally used to diagnose the problem. This adds an important measure of objectivity to clinical practice. Later chapters in this book present a number of assessment methods useful for evaluating function and dysfunction, and outline ways in which these methods can be employed to continually monitor the athlete.

4 Metabolism and Energy Production

This chapter is an overview of the mechanisms by which the body derives energy, an important aspect of athletic function. The efficient conversion of macronutrients to energy—from the processes of beta oxidation, glycolysis, and protein degradation through the Krebs cycle (also called the citric acid or tricarboxylic acid cycle) and electron transport chain—is one of the key components in improving athletic efficiency. Improving the function of this system can be a powerful therapy to increase physical, chemical, and mental/emotional balance and athletic performance.

The body has two general "energy systems" that it uses to convert fatty acids and carbohydrates into energy. These are the aerobic and anaerobic systems, which encompass both structural and chemical aspects of an individual. The systems generate energy from fatty acids and glucose to produce movement.

ENERGY FROM MACRONUTRIENTS

The ability to generate energy from food not only propels an athlete to the finish line, but is the force used by the body for all activities, from postural muscle tone during resting to breathing and daily chores. If this energy-producing mechanism is somehow disturbed because of nutritional, dietary, or other factors including stress, energy production can be impaired. The result will be an imbalance and dysfunction in the individual. This may produce almost any pattern of signs and symptoms ranging from fatigue to depression, from poor performance to a physical injury or a variety of compounding problems—any of which will become the patient's complaints.

Our body's three important macronutrients are fats, carbohydrates, and proteins; these are the sources of all energy used for daily activity, exercise, and recovery. In their natural state, these macronutrients also contain the vital micronutrients and phytochemicals necessary if energy production and other bodily processes are to proceed efficiently. The first step in optimizing this energy-producing process is choosing the foods that contain the needed nutrients. The next two steps are of critical importance and are often neglected in our society as a whole and by practitioners: aiding the efficient mechanism of digestion and the absorption of food into the nutrients used by the body.

A variety of factors may adversely affect digestion, the most common ones being stress and exercise. Any dysfunction in the process of digestion may significantly affect the absorption of nutrients from food. For example, a patient who is under excess stress may not digest a protein meal efficiently because of reduced stomach hydrochloric acid, resulting in less absorption of amino acids.

Once the body ingests food as fats, carbohydrates, and proteins, these substances undergo a variety of biochemical transformations. Carbohydrates are broken down to glucose and undergo glycolysis. Fat is broken down to fatty acids and glycerol, with the fat portion going through the process of beta oxidation, and glycerol to glycolysis. Proteins are degraded into their base components of amino acids. All macronutrient by-products enter into the Krebs cycle. This process results in the release of hydrogen's electrons in the electron transport chain with the final production of adenosine triphosphate (ATP).

Certain vitamins and minerals are necessary in order for the Krebs cycle to function. These include riboflavin, niacin, thiamin, and pantothenic acid and the minerals magnesium, manganese, and iron (Mayes 1993).

ENERGY PRODUCTION

All students learn about these energy-producing cycles and reactions. However, frequently many of the cofactors—in the form of micronutrients—are less familiar. In complementary sports medicine, understanding the ways in which these micronutrients play their crucial role can help in the improvement of the patient's function. Figure 4.1 shows each aspect of this scheme in more detail.

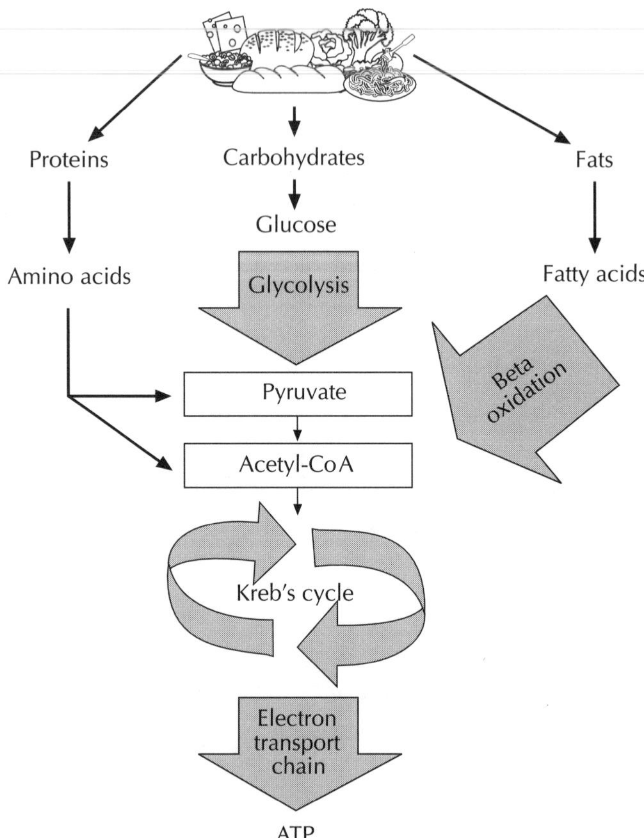

Figure 4.1 General scheme of the Krebs cycle with macronutrient associations

Fats

Triglycerides obtained from fat are a major source of energy. Lipoprotein lipase mediates the breakdown of circulating triglycerides into fatty acids that can be used by skeletal muscles for energy (Borensztajn 1979). The fatty acid molecules are carried by the blood, where they are called free fatty acids, to the muscle cell. Fatty acids enter the cell by diffusion. If the concentration of fatty acids is higher in the blood than inside the cell, more fatty acid will enter the cell and be available for energy. Factors that increase or decrease levels of fatty acids in the blood can have a significant impact on the availability of fat for energy production. For example, a proper warm-up can increase free fatty acids. Excess insulin, which may be produced from excess carbohydrate consumption or in people who are insulin resistant, may diminish blood fatty acids.

Two other factors are significantly related to the utilization of fat for energy. First, the process of beta oxidation occurs in the mitochondria, making the aerobic muscle fibers the chief site of energy production from fat. Second, these triglycerides are carried to the muscles in the blood, so improved circulation favors more fat transport with the potential of more fat utilization for energy. Any factor that adversely affects the muscle fiber or its mitochondria or the blood flow to the muscle can have a negative impact on the utilization of fat for energy. Such effects may relate to contractibility of the muscle (which requires calcium), uptake of the fatty acid into the mitochondria (which requires carnitine), and circulation as impacted by a variety of nutrients (such as iron and hydration). Glucose utilization is also important for maintaining the use of fat for energy. The number of aerobic muscle fibers (compared to anaerobic), as well as efficient circulation, is important for effective glucose uptake and metabolic efficiency of insulin action (Utriainen et al. 1996).

Finally, the fatty acid molecule undergoes transformation to acetylcoenzyme A (acetyl-CoA), completing beta oxidation. This process can also be influenced by coenzymes. Both flavin adenine dinucleotide ($FAOH_2$) and nicotinamide adenine dinucleotide (NAD+) are coenzymes needed in order for beta oxidation to proceed; $FAOH_2$ is formed from the vitamin riboflavin, and NAD+ is formed from the vitamin niacin. Levels of these nutrients in the diet that are below what the individual requires can affect the process of beta oxidation.

Carbohydrates

Vital to the process of aerobic function and fatty acid utilization is the continued catabolism of glucose. The breakdown of fats can continue only if sufficient oxaloacetic acid is produced in the Krebs cycle to combine with acetyl-CoA formed during beta oxidation.

The process of generating energy via glucose is referred to as glycolysis. It involves a variety of steps, ultimately leading to the production of acetyl-CoA and oxidation in the Krebs cycle. Although glucose is the predominant sugar, this is also the primary pathway for both fructose and galactose from the diet. These sugars are ultimately converted to glucose.

Glucose begins the process of glycolysis by phosphorylation to glucose 6-phosphate via the enzyme hexokinase (and in the liver and pancreas as glucokinase). A variety of nutritional factors are important in order for this process to proceed. The reaction involves not only a phosphate donor, but also magnesium, as Mayes (1993) emphasizes. Low levels of dietary magnesium, or poor absorption, may have a negative impact on this mechanism. In addition, NAD+ plays a vital role, requiring niacin; fluoride has an inhibitory effect on enolase, a necessary enzyme in the middle of the glycolytic pathway.

The production of lactic acid is a characteristic feature of glycolysis. Lactic acid is formed from pyruvic acid. This step requires lactate dehydrogenase. Lactate dehydrogenase requires niacin for its function. Pyruvic acid is also converted to acetyl-CoA, and this requires pyruvate dehydrogenase, a thiamin (vitamin B1)-dependent enzyme. If thiamin is not available, more pyruvic acid will convert to lactic acid.

Lactic acid is continually produced by the muscles. When workout levels are low to moderate, the production is equal to the rate of its removal; only when intensity levels rise will lactic acid accumulate. Quantitatively, the production of lactic acid can vary greatly from person to person, depending on stress levels, nutritional state, and workout intensity.

Excess lactic acid from the muscle is diffused into the circulation where it is buffered to form sodium lactate. Sodium lactate reacts with oxygen and NAD+ and is oxidized in the liver. Lactic acid is an important pathway for energy production through its reconversion to pyruvic acid and ultimately glucose. Through this mechanism (called the Cori cycle), lactic acid helps maintain effective blood sugar and muscle glycogen levels.

Another important aspect of glycolysis is that it is regulated by the enzyme phosphorylase. This enzyme can be influenced significantly by the hormone epinephrine, which is produced from increased sympathetic nervous system activity and is elevated during any stress.

Proteins

Protein is a required component of the diet, but its role in supplying energy is limited, though still important. Up to about 10-15% of an athlete's energy needs may be supplied from protein during very long workouts or very intense training. Protein (through a series of intermediate reactions) may be converted to glucose in the process of gluconeogenesis. The gluconeogenic pathway converts pyruvate into glucose. The precursors of glucose are lactate, glucogenic amino acids, and glycerol. As previously discussed, lactate is formed by active muscles when the rate of glycolysis exceeds the metabolic rate of the Krebs cycle and electron transport chain. Amino acids are derived from proteins in the diet. The hydrolysis of triglycerides generates glycerol. Certain amino acids undergo a chemical transformation (transamination) and are used as intermediates in the Krebs cycle. For example, after losing two amine groups, glutamine forms alpha-ketoglutaric acid, aspartate forms oxaloacetic acid, and alanine forms pyruvic acid.

Any disruption in the process of protein utilization can have a negative effect on the metabolism's ability to produce energy. For example, if dietary protein is too low or is not effectively digested, amino acid absorption may be inadequate. In addition, specific nutritional substances are required for many reactions. In the deamination of glutamate to alpha-ketoglutarate, for example, niacin is required for NAD+. These are examples of dietary or nutritional factors that may be related to a patient's fatigue during the day and not necessarily directly related to working out. During athletic competition, fatigue may develop because of the accumulation of by-products. Lactic acid, for example, may lower the pH of the muscle, limiting energy for muscle contraction.

ENERGY SYSTEMS

Traditionally, some texts list the production of energy from three systems. McArdle et al. (1991), for example, discuss the immediate-energy or ATP-creatine phosphate system, the short-term energy or lactic acid system, and the long-term energy or aerobic system. In this text, the immediate-energy and short-term energy systems are referred to as the anaerobic system, and the long-term energy system is called the aerobic system.

The Aerobic System

In their evolution as hunter-gatherers, humans became highly dependent upon the aerobic system. For the hunter-gatherer of thousands of years ago, being physically active for extended periods of time required a significant amount of energy from the aerobic muscle fibers; the modern marathon runner has the same requirement. These aerobic muscle fibers, a predominant feature of the aerobic system, are also referred to as type I fibers. In addition to their ability to utilize large amounts of fatty acids for energy, they can utilize carbohydrates and amino acids for energy. These fibers are highly vascularized, surrounded by a much larger number of capillaries than anaerobic fibers are.

The fatty acids used by the aerobic muscle fibers come from both endogenous (intramuscular lipid reserves) and exogenous (adipose tissue) sources. Gollnick (1985) and Karlsson et al. (1974) showed that the capability to utilize more fats for energy was dependent upon the type of training, with lower-intensity training increasing fatty acid utilization. The ability of endurance training to accomplish this task is attributable to the increased enzymes necessary for lipid oxidation (Hurley et al. 1986), specifically by the high concentrations of mitochondria containing oxidative enzymes such as succinate dehydrogenase.

Stored fat represents a tremendous reserve of potential energy, even for a lean athlete: up to 100,000 kcal of energy. For an 18-carbon fatty acid molecule, 147 molecules of ATP are generated through the combined efforts of beta oxidation, the Krebs cycle, and the electron transport chain. Because of its greater quantity of hydrogen molecules, fat contains more potential energy than the other two macronutrients combined; each gram of dietary fat has potentially 9 calories of energy, with carbohydrate and protein providing 4 each. This contrast is put into clinical perspective by Newsholme (1977), who presents that the energy reserves from fat in a healthy athlete can power a run for 119 hr, with reserves from glucose allowing the energy for only a 1.6-hr run.

During rest, fat may contribute significant amounts of energy, up to 60-80% of the amount needed. This may also be true during light and moderate workouts, and even during longer training periods and competitions, especially in athletes with good function. From an athletic performance standpoint, Lambert et al. (1994) and Muoio et al. (1994)

demonstrated improvements in performance after consumption of a diet higher in fat, which makes more fat available for energy. And Vukovich et al. (1993) showed that an increase in dietary fat spared stored glycogen during exercise, an important function for endurance and competition.

Much of this action of fat is highly dependent upon the health of the individual, the pre-workout meal, and the person's fitness level. Hughes et al. (1994) showed that in certain individuals with impaired glucose tolerance, the beneficial effects of exercise on lipid indexes are not observed. Foster et al. (1979) showed that feeding of glucose 30-45 min before endurance exercise increases the rate of glucose utilization but impairs mobilization of free fatty acids and reduces the exercise time to exhaustion. An athlete's level of fitness is an important factor when one considers whether a higher amount of fat can be used for energy. Improvements in aerobic function including that of the aerobic muscle fibers, avoidance of training stress, and proper nutrition are necessary for utilization of more fats for energy.

The extensive number and volume of the mitochondria are a dominant feature of the aerobic muscle fiber. Many other factors that allow this process to continue are important in order for the aerobic muscle fiber's mitochondria to generate energy from fats. These factors include dietary and nutritional considerations, stress factors, and training. But none of these processes can function effectively if sufficient oxygen is not delivered to the cells.

The Anaerobic System

When short-term speed and power are required, the anaerobic system is well suited to the task. While anaerobic muscle fibers are much larger than their aerobic counterparts, their actions are very short-lived.

The anaerobic muscle fibers are also referred to as type II fibers and are further divided into three separate groups based on their metabolic properties. The type IIa fiber contains anaerobic qualities but has a high capacity for aerobic function. This fiber's aerobic qualities, combined with the great potential of type I fibers, allow tremendous possibilities for the utilization of fats for energy in most people. The only possible exception is the sprinter who is genetically endowed with a high number of type IIb fibers and does not train his or her aerobic system.

The type IIb fiber contains the true anaerobic trait, generating energy only from glycolysis. While these fibers are found in all people, they are more numerous and better developed in sprint and power athletes. They have the ability to supply energy for short periods of time, but anaerobic fibers are not endowed well with capillaries. These fibers not only have less blood supply, but "may have no associated capillaries at all" (Mountcastle 1974, p. 620). Bonde-Petersen and Robertson (1981) demonstrated in the cat that relative ischemia exists in anaerobic fibers, but not in aerobic ones, during both isometric and isotonic muscle contractions. Colliander et al. (1988) states that "The higher the fast twitch fiber composition, the lower the attendant capillary density and content of aerobic enzymes, and thus the greater is the force loss and the less the recovery" (p. 84). Although these fibers do not depend on oxygen, the need for other nutrients still exists. Since all the different types of fibers are mixed within a given muscle in humans, it appears that the anaerobic fibers (especially type IIb) are dependent on the aerobic fibers' blood supply (see table 4.1). The type IIc muscle fiber is not discussed much in the literature.

Table 4.1 Three Commonly Recognized Muscle Fibers in Humans

	Type I	Type IIa	Type IIb
Other names	Aerobic	Mixed (aerobic and anaerobic)	Anaerobic
Potential energy source	Fatty acids	Fatty acids	Glucose

The amount of energy available for aerobic and anaerobic metabolism varies considerably. The availability of energy from carbohydrates is very limited. Only 36 molecules of ATP are generated through the combined work of glycolysis, the Krebs cycle, and the electron transport chain. Recall that a molecule of fat produces about four times this amount of ATP—or more, depending on the specific fatty acid.

In addition to the short-term energy potential of the anaerobic system, an immediate-energy system exists that is not dependent on glycolysis. This simpler mechanism utilizes phosphocreatine, sometimes called creatine phosphate. In this anaerobic mechanism, the enzyme creatine kinase quickly converts phosphocreatine to ATP. Like glycolysis, this process does not require oxygen. The production of ATP through this action is very limited to only a few seconds of activity.

TRAINING EFFECTS ON ENERGY SYSTEMS

Training plays a major role in enhancing both the structural and chemical aspects of an individual's muscle fibers. For example, endurance training will improve aerobic muscle fiber function, including increasing the number of mitochondria and the enzymes that convert more fat to energy. The type IIa fiber will also benefit from endurance training. However, this training will not develop the anaerobic type IIb fibers.

All muscles contain all the types of fibers; the proportions found in any one person are not determined by genetics alone. While genes may play a role, our environment (e.g., training) may be even more important. Simoneau et al. (1985) showed that after 15 weeks of training, the proportions of fiber types changed. Specifically, endurance training significantly increased the proportion of type I fibers and decreased the proportion of type IIb fibers. Abernathy et al. (1990) discussed a variety of transitions between aerobic and anaerobic fibers based on the type of training; sprint training decreased type I fibers, and endurance training may convert type IIb to IIa fibers and increase type I fibers.

In addition, inactivity can affect muscle fiber population. Haggmark et al. (1986) showed that in one athlete immobilized for surgery, decreases occurred in type I fiber content, from 81% to 58% after six weeks. Training restored the type I fiber content to 85%. It is also possible that those individuals who are not physically active also have reduced type I fiber content in their muscles, rendering them aerobically deficient.

One goal of training is to improve long-term endurance and overall function. Unfortunately, short-term training of almost any type will result in improvements in a number of important factors, including $\dot{V}O_2$max, oxygen consumption, muscle strength, and muscle glycogen content, but not neccessarily improve long-term endurance. Fox (1979) showed an approximately 10% increase in $\dot{V}O_2$max during three types of training schedules—two, four, and five days per week. All participants increased $\dot{V}O_2$max to approximately the same extent during the training period. On average, all participants achieved a peak level of $\dot{V}O_2$max after about seven weeks.

Clinically, we know that many individuals who show short-term benefits will not continue their programs. Beginning exercisers will often give up a program because of discomfort or lack of enjoyment. More serious athletes will sometimes become overtrained or injured and be forced to stop or greatly modify their workouts. Obtaining benefits from exercise is only the first step and by no means indicative that a particular program is effective. An individual's needs will be constantly changing, and these needs must be continually assessed and modified, when necessary, before signs or symptoms of imbalance occur. In this way the person will be less likely to give up and will continue to obtain benefits, without dysfunction, for years and decades rather than weeks or months. This type of care is an important component of complementary sports medicine.

Dysfunction of the aerobic system may result from a variety of factors. Nutritional issues are important, as already mentioned. In addition to niacin, riboflavin, thiamine, and magnesium, carnitine serves as a carrier for the entrance of fatty acids into the mitochondria. Dietary factors, such as too little fat or protein or too many carbohydrates, may influence available fatty acids. These dietary and nutritional factors are discussed in chapters 18 and 19. Hormonal factors are also important for aerobic function; insulin is important, for example, because higher levels may promote carbohydrate use and lower levels may result in a greater amount of fat utilization. In addition, adrenal hormones, especially epinephrine and norepinephrine, play a significant role in aerobic function. Cortisol and other adrenal hormones are important also and play a key role during stress. These are all factors that can greatly influence the function of the aerobic system; they are discussed in more detail in the appropriate chapters.

CONCLUSION

A working knowledge of the body's metabolism, as well as an understanding of how energy is produced, is important, since manipulating these areas may prove to be a valuable therapy. Key areas include the energy potential of fats and carbohydrates, their use by aerobic and anaerobic muscle fibers, and the role of certain nutrients in making energy available. The ability to apply these aspects of physiology enables the practitioner to avoid "cookbook" therapies and to treat each patient as an individual, meeting the specific needs of each. Understanding how fats and carbohydrates are used by the aerobic and anaerobic systems will better prepare the practitioner to utilize specific complementary assessment methods, therapies, and training techniques.

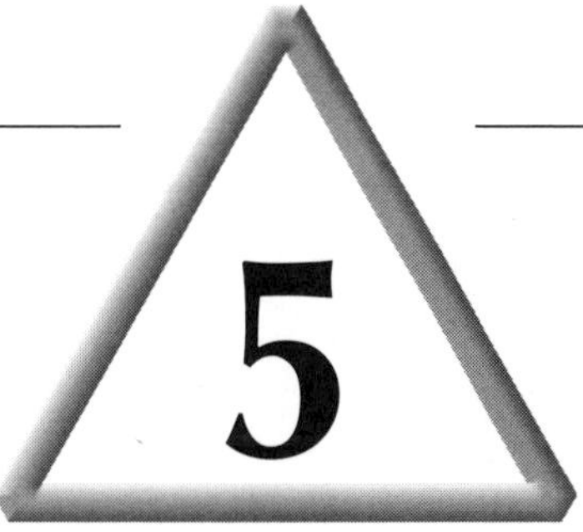

Neuromuscular Systems

The nervous system is a major player in all athletic functions. In complementary sports medicine, use of the neuromuscular system is a vital aspect of both the assessment and the therapeutic processes. The behavior of this system is sometimes referred to as "body language." Interpretation of the body's posture and gait, as well as the use of manual muscle testing, is an important part of the assessment process. Dietary and nutritional changes to influence the chemical components of the neuromuscular system, as well as certain types of exercise training, are among the therapeutic options. The neurological model presented here also helps explain how muscles are influenced by a variety of lifestyle factors, such as stress, diet, and nutrition.

FACILITATION AND INHIBITION

Complementary sports medicine uses the words *facilitation* and *inhibition* to describe the contraction and lack of contraction of skeletal muscles, respectively. It is understood that even though the central state of the alpha motoneuron is a reflection of multiple facilitatory and inhibitory effects, the final outcome is either facilitation or inhibition. Excitation occurs when facilitation reaches the threshold for depolarization, where the "all-or-none" phenomenon takes place and a muscle contracts. (The terms *conditionally facilitated* or *conditionally inhibited* might be more neurologically correct, but in this text the words *facilitated* and *inhibited* are used.)

Facilitation occurs at the neuromuscular junction, with an action potential traveling the length of the muscle fiber resulting in facilitation and contraction. Inhibition of the motoneuron occurs postsynaptically (and presynaptically on some neurons) and results in the decreased likelihood of contraction of the muscle.

NEUROMUSCULAR JUNCTION

The connection between the motoneuron and the skeletal muscle fiber is a highly specialized region referred to as the neuromuscular junction (sometimes called the motor end plate). Each muscle fiber usually contains its own neuromuscular junction, which functions to transmit a nerve impulse from the axon of the nerve to the muscle. This area also changes the electrical impulse of the neuron to a chemical impulse in the muscle fiber. This is accomplished by the neurotransmitter acetylcholine, which causes excitation (followed by muscle contraction) in the muscle.

Acetylcholine is manufactured in the cytosol of the nerve terminal by the reaction of acetylcoenzyme A and the nutrient choline.The release of acetylcholine is triggered by the uptake of calcium. Acetylcholine is quickly broken down by the enzyme cholinesterase. Sodium also plays a key role by diffusing inside the neuron to create an electrical potential.

The amino acids gamma aminobutyric acid (GABA) and glycine play a major role in neuromuscular inhibition by increasing the permeability of the neuron to potassium and chloride. Inhibition is important in controlling the smoothness of actions in some sports and helps protect the muscle from overcontraction.

NEUROLOGICAL MECHANISMS WITHIN THE MUSCLE

Specific sensory areas within the muscle and tendon are responsible for facilitation and inhibition of the whole muscle. These are the muscle spindle cells and Golgi tendon organs, and they are described by Guyton (1986). These receptors have an important protective action, providing the central nervous system with information about the muscles, joints, and limbs.

Muscle Spindle Cells

Sensory information about changes in the length of the muscle fibers is provided by muscle spindles, and their reactions are facilitatory (see figure 5.1). Through their action, a muscle that is stretched will react with more contraction to increase power and function and is protected from damage.The muscle spindles are important in regulating posture and gait.

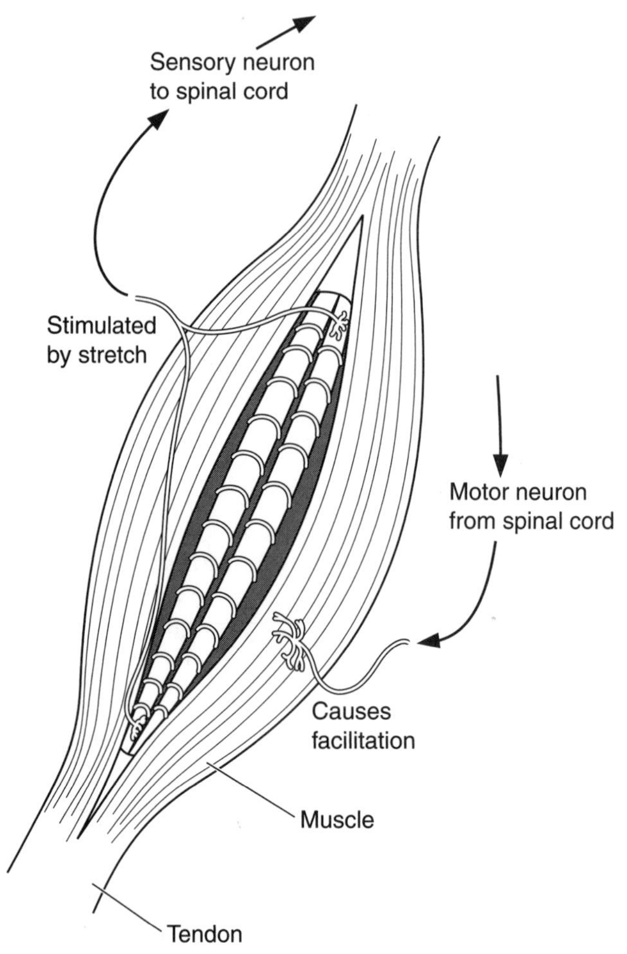

Figure 5.1 The muscle spindle cell mechanism

Golgi Tendon Organs

The tension and stretch of the muscle are detected by Golgi tendon organs, which are found within the tendon. When stimulated, these produce inhibition of the muscle (see figure 5.2). These sensory receptors react when a muscle is shortened, and in passive stretching, protecting the muscle and ligament from potential injury during overload.

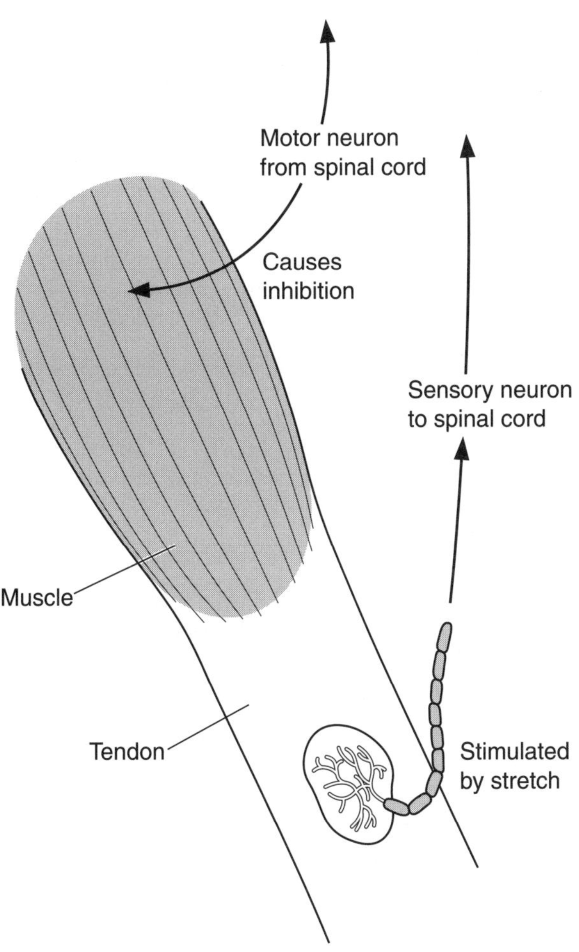

Figure 5.2 The Golgi tendon organ mechanism

MUSCULAR IMBALANCES

Muscular imbalance refers to a deviation from the expected normal facilitated or inhibited muscle and is described by Janda (1986), Jull and Janda (1987), and Sahrmann (1987). This imbalance often begins as a muscle inhibition, due to some physical, chemical, or mental/emotional stress, and it may cause secondary muscle overfacilitation followed by dysfunction in the related joint(s). In some cases, muscle inhibition is secondary to joint dysfunction. This was described as early as 1965 by DeAndrade et al., and it has been more recently characterized by others (Fisher et al. 1997; Spencer et al. 1984). Physical causes of muscle inhibition are attributable to an imbalance between the external demand and the functional capacity of the muscle as described by Liebenson (1996). For example, overtraining in running, cycling, or weight lifting may result in localized microtrauma that leads to a protective response and an abnormal muscle inhibition. Macrotrauma is more easily observed and usually more acute. This is common in contact sports like football, hockey, and boxing.

We can use lifting a weight with the biceps brachii muscle as an example of the common neuromuscular mechanisms of facilitation and inhibition. In this action, the biceps muscle is normally facilitated. At the same time this action takes place, however, the triceps brachii, the antagonist, becomes inhibited, allowing facilitation of the biceps and the lifting of the weight (see figure 5.3). In most actions in the body, this balance of normal facilitation and inhibition exists. When there is a neuromuscular imbalance, there is an abnormal facilitation or inhibition—typically both. The result is muscle imbalance that can adversely affect posture, gait, and joint function; athletic performance is compromised. For example, if a patient's pectoralis major clavicular (PMC) muscle is abnormally inhibited, the antagonist—the latissimus dorsi—is often overfacilitated. In this case, movement of the shoulder joint is compromised and over time this can

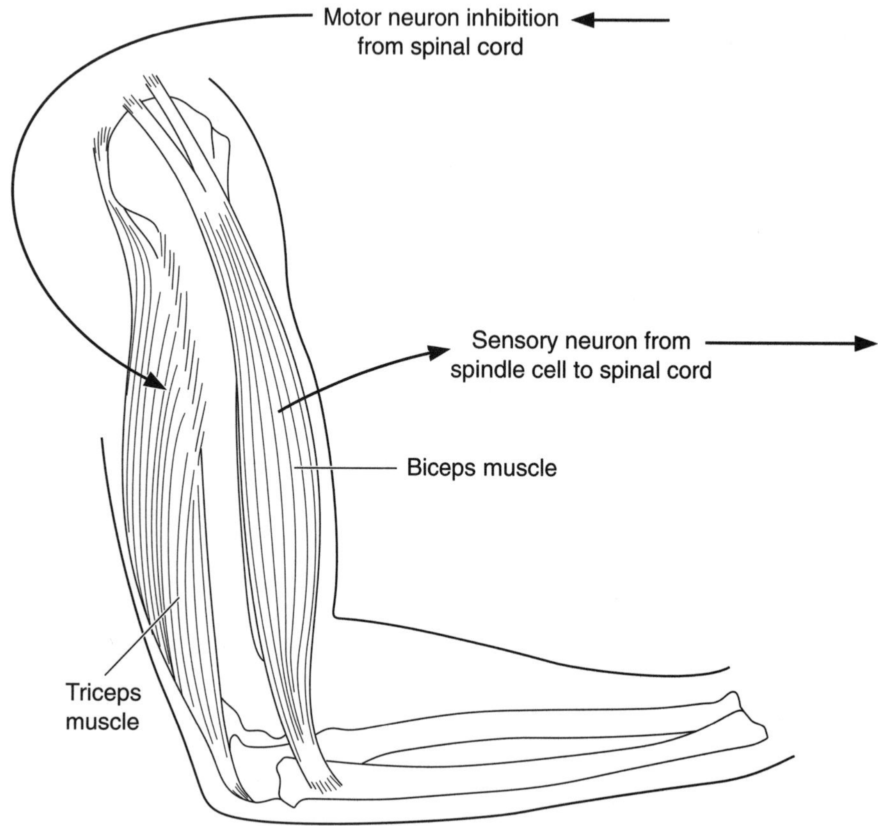

Figure 5.3 Example of normal muscle facilitation and inhibition using the biceps and triceps.

produce dysfunction, including inflammation or possibly other damage. In later stages of the problem, patients will usually complain of joint pain, but in the early stages they will typically feel the overfacilitated muscle as a "tightness" but not the inhibited muscle.

As for the chemical aspect of neuromuscular function, nutritional and dietary factors play an important role. Poor intake or absorption of calcium or choline, for example, may contribute to dysfunction of facilitation. Poor protein digestion may result in less-than-optimal amounts of certain amino acids, which may interfere with the chemistry of inhibition. Even lifestyle stress may affect muscle function through the adrenal cortex hormones that control sodium and potassium metabolism.

NEUROMUSCULAR RELATIONSHIPS WITH GAIT AND POSTURE

One of the most important tools used in evaluating a patient is observation of both static posture and gait. Understanding the normal or expected state of the neuromuscular system will help one discover the abnormal, imbalanced condition. What follows is a discussion of gait and posture in the normal and in the dysfunctional state. In this text, dysfunctional muscles include those normal (nonpathological) muscles that are not receiving the proper signals, usually because of a nonpathological neurologic dysfunction. This problem may originate in the nervous system, within the muscle, or in other systems, such as the hormonal, gastrointestinal, or immune systems. In addition, as discussed in other chapters, the acupuncture system, cranial-sacral mechanism, and other nontraditional sources may also influence neuromuscular function. Pathological muscular dysfunction is beyond the scope of this text and is not discussed here.

Normal Gait

If we observe an athlete in a walking or running posture (see figure 5.4), we will see a continual pattern of facilitation and inhibition. If a patient is placed in a gait position in which the right upper limb and left lower limb are flexed and the other two limbs are extended, we can assume the following neuromuscular state: the right upper limb flexor muscles are facilitated along with the left lower limb flexors, while in the same limbs the respective antagonists are inhibited. Likewise, the left upper limb flexors and the right lower limb flexors are inhibited while those extensors are facilitated. Table 5.1 lists specific muscles that match this example.

More importantly, we can clinically evaluate the relative function of the flexors and extensors on the field or in the office by manually muscle testing the athlete in a gait position. Manual muscle testing, as described by Kendall et al. (1993) and Walther (1988), is a clinical tool used to determine the function of the specific muscle. Taking the example just given, the right PMC muscle can be manually tested while the athlete is positioned in the gait. Figure 5.5a–b shows how the practitioner performs this test using two methods, with the patient standing and lying. If the muscle is functioning normally, it will be facilitated.

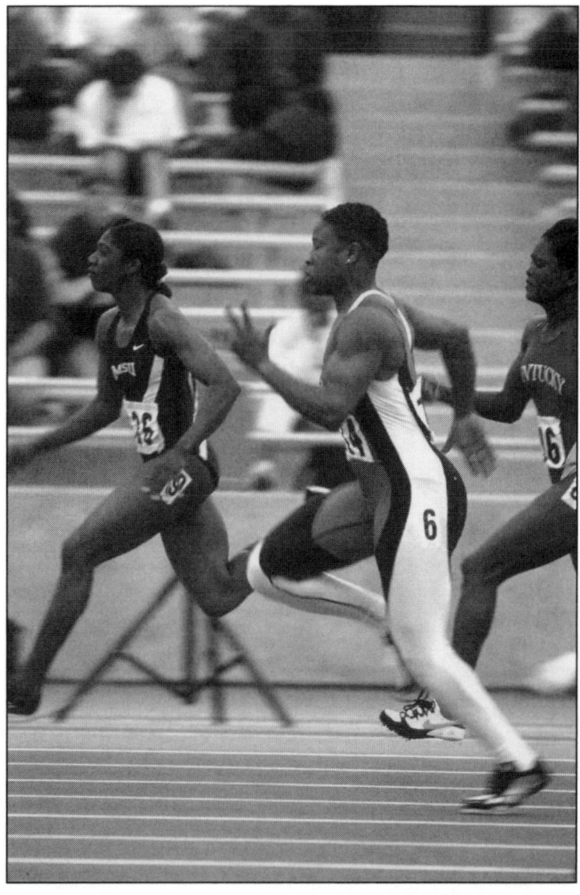

Figure 5.4 This runner shows flexor activity in the right hip and left shoulder muscles, and extensor activity in the left hip and right shoulder.

Table 5.1 Some Muscles That Are Normally Facilitated and Inhibited During Gait

	Facilitated	Inhibited
Right upper limb	Pectoralis major clavicular	Latissimus dorsi
Left lower limb	Psoas major/Quadriceps	Hamstrings
Left upper limb	Latissimus dorsi	Pectoralis major clavicular
Right lower limb	Hamstrings	Psoas major/Quadriceps

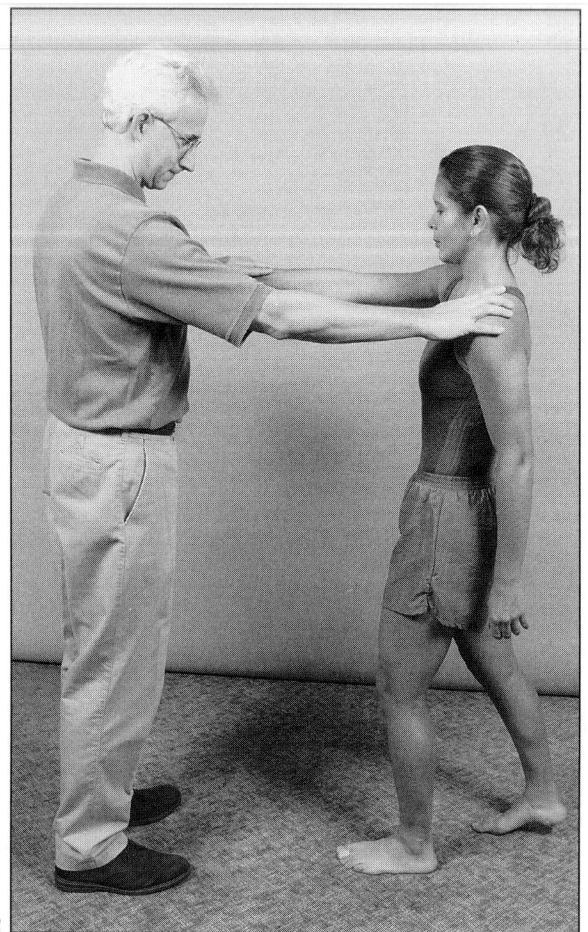

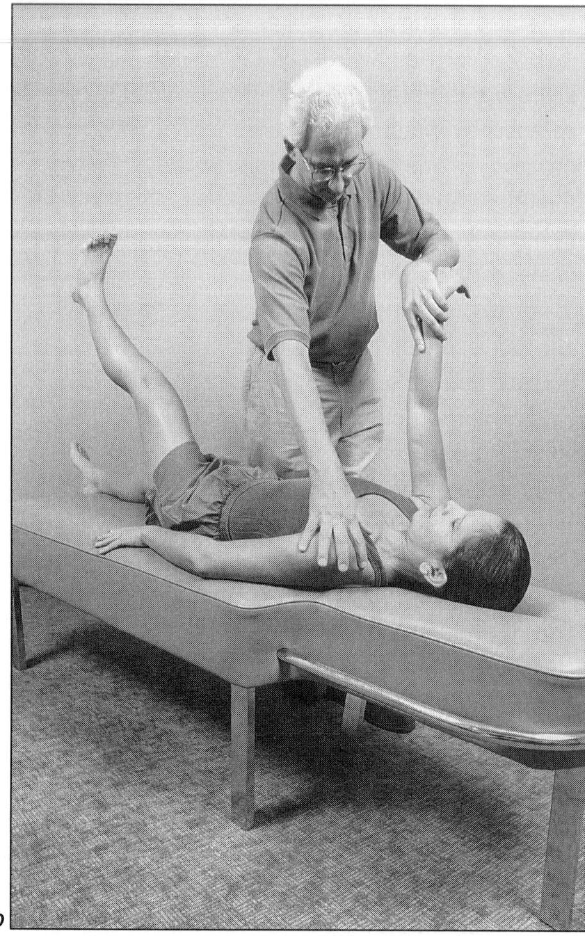

Figure 5.5a–b The practitioner is testing the patient's right PMC (*a*) standing and (*b*) lying while in a gait position.

Abnormal Gait

Close observation of an athlete's gait will often reveal muscular imbalances. These may be the result of muscles that are facilitated or inhibited at the wrong time. For example, in figure 5.5a–b, the right PMC should be facilitated; this allows the arm to flex during the normal gait. If this facilitation does not occur, the flexion of the arm may not be compensated for by other flexors. The result is observed in the gait as a decreased forward action of the right arm during flexion as compared to the left (if the left shoulder muscles are normal). When this problem occurs, manual muscle testing will reveal an inhibited right PMC when the person is being tested in a gait position.

In other cases of abnormal gait, a muscle that is normally inhibited may be facilitated. As in the preceding example, this can be diagnosed using both observation and manual muscle testing. For example, when the right PMC is facilitated in the flexed limb, the right latissimus dorsi is normally inhibited. While in the gait position, the person's latissimus dorsi can be manually tested to determine whether it is normally inhibited or abnormally facilitated.

Many times, testing a patient's posture in a neutral position—with the person either lying on an office examination table (or on the ground on the playing field) or standing—can reveal muscle facilitation or inhibition that is normal or abnormal.

Normal Posture

Like the gait, a person's posture is generally reflected in their neuromuscular function. Observing the static posture may disclose imbalances that can then be verified with manual muscle testing. For example, the practitioner can observe for shoulder balance by placing one finger on each acromion process. If one shoulder is noticeably higher than the other, a muscular imbalance may be the cause. Some instances of a previous bone fracture, surgery, or osseous anomaly may also result in a postural distortion. But the majority of postural deviations are the result of muscles being abnormally inhibited and abnormally overfacilitated. Normal posture occurs when neuromuscular function is balanced and all muscle tests in the standing position are normal, that is, when none show inhibition.

Abnormal Posture

If neuromuscular function is compromised, certain muscles will be abnormally inhibited and others abnormally overfacilitated during testing with the patient in the standing or lying position. Sometimes muscle testing in certain postural positions will show a pattern similar to that of a specific gait. For example, if a patient has an inhibition of the right latissimus dorsi, the left hamstrings, the left PMC, and the right psoas, it is as if the person's neuromuscular system is in the gait position depicted in figure 5.5a–b—even though the actual physical position is obviously not that way. This is the typical state of dysfunction that precedes an injury and often continues after injury, helping maintain its chronicity.

Once specific muscle imbalance is determined, correction of the neuromuscular system is accomplished with specific therapeutic neurologic input. This may include manual stimulation of an acupuncture point, Golgi tendon organs or muscle spindles, or other therapies described in later chapters. Whatever the case, in most instances if an effective therapy is applied, the neuromuscular system will immediately change and function will return to normal. In the case of a PMC that is abnormally inhibited, applying the proper therapy should result in an immediate change so that when the muscle is tested after the therapy, it will be normally facilitated. Only occasionally is there a need for prolonged rehabilitation in a patient who has been physically active. In the case of a patient beginning an exercise program, walking can serve both as exercise and as an effective therapeutic tool.

STRENGTH, POWER, AND FUNCTION

In all the relationships with muscle evaluations that we have considered, function is what is being evaluated, rather than strength or power. Muscular strength is the maximum force generated by the muscle. In a more clinical definition, strength is the maximum weight a person can lift at one time. The definition of power includes a time component. Power is the combination of strength and speed of the movement.

Function relates to the normal movement of the muscle and appropriate balance of facilitation and inhibition, regardless of strength and power. A muscle that functions well may have a high or low level of power or strength. Even a very powerful weight lifter has muscle inhibition, and the weakest, most out-of-shape elderly patient has muscle facilitation.

If a patient has neuromuscular dysfunction, treatment is directed at finding the cause. This may relate to local problems with Golgi tendon organs or muscle spindle cells or to other problems described in later chapters. However, treatment of this dysfunction is usually not effective if the therapy is lifting weights or performing other activities that increase power and strength: the result will be a patient who has more strength but still possesses neuromuscular dysfunction.

AUTONOMIC BALANCE

Throughout this text, reference is made to the autonomic nervous system and to the balance of sympathetic and parasympathetic function. For the practitioner, especially noteworthy are the relationships of the autonomic nervous system to training and overtraining, adrenal function, the insulin mechanism, and others. Certain structural, chemical, and mental/emotional signs and symptoms may be attributed to autonomic imbalances. For example, increased sympathetic activity may be associated with specific types of overtraining, whereas other overtraining patterns correspond to a parasympathetic-dominant state (Lehmann et al. 1997). These are reflected in an increased resting and training heart rate with excess sympathetic stress or in a diminished resting heart rate with a parasympathetic dominance. Blood sugar-handling stress may induce various signs and symptoms due to increased sympathetic activity (Tepperman and Tepperman 1987). Hydrochloric acid dysfunction and secondary malabsorption may result in either diminished production, or in some cases an excess due to autonomic imbalance (McColl 1997). Malabsorption can lead to nutritional imbalances.

The endings of the parasympathetic nerves secrete acetylcholine (requiring choline), and most sympathetic nerve endings secrete norepinephrine (requiring tyrosine) (Guyton 1986). In general, sympathetic activity increases adrenal (medullary) function and catecholamine output, prolonging sympathetic stimulation, and increases the metabolic rate of all cells. It also increases muscle strength, an important sign of overtraining, and raises blood sugar. The parasympathetic system increases gastrointestinal function, which is required for digestion and absorption of nutrients.

Both aspects of the autonomic system are functioning at all times; this state is referred to as sympathetic or parasympathetic tone. The nervous system maintains a certain level of tone that is also influenced by various structural, chemical, and mental/emotional stresses. These may be either beneficial or harmful. For example, the onset of exercise, and especially the mental/emotional stress of competition, result in an increase in sympathetic tone. This allows for a variety of important actions including shunting blood to the working muscles, raising blood glucose, and increasing muscle strength—all necessary for training or competing. Excess or unnecessary (unused) sympathetic tone, however, can be harmful, as already noted. This excess sympathetic stimulation was referred to by Selye (1976) as the alarm reaction, especially in relation to its effect on the adrenal glands, discussed in the next chapter.

CONCLUSION

By understanding normal neuromuscular mechanisms and being able to physically evaluate them, the practitioner can specifically determine areas of dysfunction and can further individualize the therapeutic component. More importantly, the neuromuscular system should be used interactively (by practitioner and patient) as a key element in assessment and treatment of the functional aspects of the patient. This interaction helps the practitioner to assess the actions of the neuromuscular system and to measure the immediate outcome of a particular therapy. This ability to manipulate the neuromuscular system, change the patient's function, and measure the outcome is an important part of complementary sports medicine.

6

Hormonal Systems

Physical, biochemical, and mental/emotional stresses have significant influence on athletic function. Hormonal systems react to all stress, including exercise activity, and provoke the body's adaptation response. By understanding the normal function of the adrenal glands and other hormonal systems, the practitioner can best evaluate, then deter or correct much of the hormonal dysfunction seen in patients while in its earliest stage. This discussion of hormonal function will not include pathology.

This chapter will also present a discussion of prostaglandins (though technically not hormones, these act like local hormones) and related compounds such as leukotrienes and thromboxanes, collectively known as eicosanoids. The ability of the practitioner to manipulate these chemicals in the patient, through diet and nutritional intervention, can have a great impact on the balance of inflammatory and anti-inflammatory activity and other problems common in athletes. In addition, the importance of immune function in sport will be considered, along with the subject of oxygen free radicals and their related antioxidants.

ADRENAL GLAND HORMONES

Adaptation to training and competition is a fundamental requirement to the success of any training program and to the success of all sport performance. The optimal function of the adrenal hormones is vital for training and competitive achievement and for prevention of physical, chemical, and mental/emotional injuries. Any dysfunction in the hormonal system may affect the function of lipase and the whole spectrum of utilization of fat for energy. Cortisol and dehydroepiandrosterone sulfate (DHEA[S]) are important adrenal cortex hormones—ones not only modified by training and competitive stress but also easily measured in the clinical setting. While the adrenal cortex produces over 50 steroid hormones, those that are important for our discussion belong to three classes: glucocorticoids, mineralocorticoids, and androgens. The adrenal medulla also produces an important group of hormones called catecholamines.

Glucocorticoids

Collectively, glucocorticoids increase hepatic glycogen, promote lipolysis in the extremities, and promote protein metabolism. Cortisol is the dominant glucocorticoid, responsible for gluconeogenesis. It is elevated with increases in structural, chemical, and mental/emotional stress, which excites the hypothalamus to produce adrenocorticotropic hormone. This anabolic effect may reverse to a catabolic effect if cortisol levels are physiologically high, as seen in patients with excess stress (Bernton et al. 1995) including overtraining (Hoogeveen and Zonderland 1996). In addition, the high cortisol in these patients can promote lipogenesis in the face and trunk. In some patients over the age of 35-40, an accumulation of fat in the face and especially the abdomen is not uncommon, and may indicate high cortisol levels. Of great importance is the fact that increased production of cortisol reduces the output of other adrenal cortical hormones, including DHEA(S) and aldosterone (Parker et al. 1985).

Mineralocorticoids

The mineralocorticoids, predominantly aldosterone, are important for the retention of sodium and the excretion of potassium in the kidney. This is vital since neuromuscular activity would not take place without regulation of these minerals. Indirectly, aldosterone also assists in the balance of potassium and pH, since the kidneys exchange potassium or a hydrogen ion for each sodium ion reabsorbed. In addition, aldosterone increases blood volume, and cardiac output.

Androgens

The most common androgen is DHEA(S), which is a precursor to other androgens—mainly those in extraadrenal tissues, namely estrogen and especially testosterone. These adrenal steroid hormones are synthesized from cholesterol that is obtained almost exclusively from plasma.

Testosterone is an androgen important for a number of physiological activities, including control of muscle growth (hypertrophy), growth and maturation of the skeleton, and increased protein synthesis. It is especially important for recovery through its anabolic action. Testosterone may increase or decrease in athletes during training, depending on the individual and a variety of factors including genetics, nutritional state, and training.

Catecholamines

The catecholamines, predominantly epinephrine and norepinephrine, are two other important adrenal hormones and are among those synthesized in the gland's medulla region. The medulla is actually part of the sympathetic nervous system, since preganglionic fibers from the splanchnic nerve end here. With appropriate neurological stimulation from the hypothalamus and brainstem, epinephrine and norepinephrine are produced. For these and other reasons, when looking at a patient clinically, we must view the hormonal and nervous systems as one "neuroendocrine" system.

Along with those of the adrenal cortex, the hormones of the medulla are a vital part of the adaptation process observed in exercise, eliciting the so called "fight-or-flight" mechanism. This is especially true in the serious athlete who undergoes intense physical, chemical, and mental/emotional stress in the context of competition. These neurological and hormonal responses in such athletes are not unlike those of the overworked and overstressed executive who may also exercise and become a patient.

The catecholamines are synthesized from the amino acid tyrosine in a series of steps; the release of epinephrine and norepinephrine is calcium-dependent. Evaluations of overtrained athletes have shown that many patients have an increased need for calcium in the diet or in the form of nutritional supplementation. More important is the increased need to utilize calcium once it is consumed. This includes its efficient digestion and absorption (which are diminished by stress) and removal by excess dietary glucose (typically through sports drinks), since glucose interferes with the tubular reabsorption of calcium in the kidney (Lemann et al. 1969).

The catecholamines produce a variety of actions, including increased glycogenolysis in liver and muscle, increased metabolic rate, increased respiration and heart rate, release of free fatty acids (activating triglyceride lipase), and shunting of blood at the onset of exercise from the organs and glands to the working muscles. About 80% of the catecholamines are in the form of epinephrine. Levels of this hormone increase with higher levels of exercise—generally around 70%-75% of $\dot{V}O_2$max—and in longer bouts of exercise, as described by Wilmore and Costill (1994). This may have significant implications for training heart rate levels. In healthy athletes, training results in lower resting epinephrine levels (Bove 1984). This lowering of hormone is followed by a lowered resting heart rate and blood pressure as frequently seen with exercise programs. But in some athletes who train at high levels of intensity, the resting levels of epinephrine may become elevated (Kirwan et al. 1988) and can serve as a marker for overtraining. These athletes usually show an elevation of the resting heart rate.

TRAINING EFFECTS ON ADRENAL HORMONES

During exercise, there is a normal rise in cortisol levels, especially during the first 60 min (Wilmore and Costill 1994). The degree of elevation is related to the individual's conditioning, with untrained subjects showing higher cortisol responses (McArdle et al. 1991). Stallknecht et al. (1990) showed that more intense exercise produced not only more cortisol but also produced adrenal gland enlargement due to hypertrophy and hyperplasia. In patients who have trained too intensively and may be overtrained, measurement of cortisol may help assess the overtraining.

Barron et al. (1985) showed that the impaired hormonal response in overtrained athletes indicated hypothalamic dysfunction. The whole mechanism of adrenal stress is initiated in the brain; the hypothalamus (and sympathetic nervous system) is activated during exercise, stimulating the pituitary, which in turn stimulates the adrenal glands. This system is referred to as the hypothalamic-pituitary-adrenal axis.

Exercise-induced high cortisol levels have also been associated with amenorrhea (Ding et al. 1988). In addition, De Cree et al. (1995) reported that in women who exercise, this problem may result in decreased bone density. High cortisol levels can also affect males, with a potential impact on their reproductive status. Roberts et al. (1993) showed that overtraining significantly increased cortisol and lowered testosterone levels in men; findings included a 47% reduction in sperm counts.

Under high levels of chronic stress, including intense exercise, DHEA(S) levels are often reduced. For that reason, DHEA(S) has become very popular with athletes in recent years, with this product now available over the counter. Orentreich et al. (1984) showed that DHEA(S) diminishes with age; the highest levels occur between ages 20 and 30, and then there is a 10% decline each decade. With reduced DHEA(S), lower levels of testosterone and estrogen are observed. Belanger et al. (1994) showed that in men, DHEA(S) contributed to about half the circulating testosterone; in women, DHEA(S) may contribute to 100% of the estrogen.

Reduced DHEA(S) is an indication of potential overtraining, chronic stress, or both. In addition, insulin levels above normal can suppress DHEA(S) production and increase its clearance by the liver. Administration of DHEA(S) also lowers insulin levels and significantly increases testosterone. Buster et al. (1992) demonstrated a nearly 300% increase in testosterone in women after oral DHEA(S) supplementation. These and other reasons are given by athletes for self-prescribing DHEA(S). The author's clinical experience agrees with the position of Nestler (1994) and of Bland (1997), who states, "Given these observations, a better method for controlling DHEA(S) would not rely upon giving supplementary doses but on the ability of the body to regulate its own DHEA(S) levels through proper regulation of serum insulin levels and glucose management" (p. 33). In this case, this means assessing athletes and helping them correct their dietary, nutritional, training, and lifestyle imbalances.

Hakkinen et al. (1988) showed that certain types of training affect hypothalamic and pituitary function, with resulting increases in testosterone. However, Keizer et al. (1989) reported that testosterone was diminished during certain periods of training in male runners. Hoogeveen and Zonderland (1996) use diminished testosterone, along with elevated cortisol, as indicators of overtraining. Testosterone is also diminished during tetracycline therapy (Pulkkinen and Maenpaa 1983).

Adrenal hormone dysfunction is also related to seasonal affective disorder (SAD) as described by Rosenthal et al. (1984) and its prevalence in athletes as outlined by Rosen et al. (1996). In the latter study, symptoms occurring mostly in the fall and winter months associated with SAD included impaired social functioning, depression, poor sleep patterns, lowered energy and libido, decreased physical capacity, and increased cravings for carbohydrates. Of the 65 college hockey players evaluated, almost half were classified as having some form of SAD: 51% were asymptomatic, 11% met the obvious criteria for SAD, and 39% were classified as having a functional problem referred to as "subsyndromal seasonal affective disorder." Kasper et al. (1988) and Rosenthal et al. (1984) describe the use of light therapy to successfully treat SAD.

PANCREATIC HORMONES

Two pancreatic hormones, insulin and glucagon, are important in athletes. The onset of exercise normally increases glucagon and diminishes the production of insulin. This action by the pancreas promotes hepatic glycogenolysis, maintains glucose homeostasis, and increases the utilization of fatty acids for energy (Wasserman et al. 1995). Insulin is predominantly a regulator of glucose metabolism, allowing transport of glucose across the cell membrane. Insulin is also responsible for the filling of glycogen stores and for allowing amino acids to enter muscle cells, and it increases the activity of potassium and calcium at the cellular level. Separately, glucagon stimulates gluconeogenesis during exercise, enhances the oxidation of fat in the liver, increases the hepatic amino acid metabolism, and may play a role in nitrogen excretion. According to Wasserman et al. (1995), "Because of the important roles that glucagon and insulin play, any physiological or pathological condition that affects their secretion or efficacy will impact on the metabolic response to exercise" (p. 22).

Pancreatic Hormones and Diet

One key factor affecting pancreatic hormone function is the diet. Granner (1993) describes insulin's action on a glucose meal as follows: approximately 50% of the glucose is carried into the cells and converted to energy via glycolysis, up to 10% is converted to glycogen when these stores require replenishment, and approximately 40% or more of the glucose is converted to fat for storage. More importantly, insulin's effect on glucose metabolism can vary dramatically from person to person (Reaven 1995). Coulston et al. (1993) showed that a high-carbohydrate diet increases insulin production even in relatively healthy men and women.

A number of other factors may affect insulin production. Certain hormones including cortisol, epinephrine, growth hormone, estrogens, and progesterone in high physiological amounts can increase insulin production, possibly resulting in hyperinsulinemia. Increases in these insulin-stimulating hormones may come from overtraining, stress, or use of birth control pills. In turn, excess insulin is associated with significant hormonal imbalance, including lowered DHEA(S) production (Nestler and Jakubowicz 1996; Nestler and Strauss 1991). Excess insulin and high-carbohydrate diets have been implicated in a number of disease states (Reaven 1997), including heart disease, breast cancer, polycystic ovary disease, non-insulin-dependent diabetes, obesity, hypertension, in addition to high blood cholesterol and triglycerides. This group of conditions originally was termed Syndrome X by Reaven (1988).

Hyperinsulinemia

Hyperinsulinemia can impair the normal glucose mechanism and is associated with insulin resistance—a dysfunction of the normal biologic response to insulin (Reaven 1995). Insulin resistance occurs when the mechanism that recognizes insulin is no longer operative, reducing the number of functional receptors for insulin and reducing the amount of glucose entering the cell. This problem can occur at an early age and potentially increase through life, resulting in disease. The author (Maffetone 1997) has termed the full spectrum of this condition beginning in its earliest functional stage as carbohydrate intolerance, which will be discussed in detail in chapter 25.

Carbohydrate Intolerance

Carbohydrate intolerance (CI) can result in a continuing vicious cycle of increased insulin production and insulin resistance, and often increases with age (Broughton and Taylor 1991). Di Pietro and Suraci (1990) showed that a family history of diabetes mellitus can be a risk factor for insulin resistance even in the presence of normal glucose metabolism. According to Groop et al. (1997), first-degree relatives of patients with non-insulin-dependent diabetes mellitus (NIDDM) have a 40% risk of developing NIDDM, with the risk being higher if the disease was inherited from the mother rather than the father.

Carbohydrate intolerance is relatively common in the population; exact numbers vary depending on definitions, opinions of its incidence, and when the condition can first be assessed. Potentially, up to three-quarters of the population, including athletes, have CI. Moreover, many patients who require an effective exercise program already have more advanced stages of CI. In competitive athletes, CI can have a significant impact on sport performance (Maffetone 1997). In some of these patients, normal glucose tolerance tests are obtained in the presence of excess insulin, indicating insulin resistance (Zimmet et al. 1992). In other cases, normal insulin levels exist in the presence of slightly impaired glucose tolerance (Swinburn et al. 1995). Bassett et al. (1990) demonstrated the existence of a category of patients who are "otherwise normal" but have carbohydrate dysfunction as indicated, sometimes transiently, by a distinct pre-beta band on lipoprotein electrophoresis (these are very low density lipoproteins). These authors considered this a transitional state between normal and abnormal. The existence of a pre-beta lipoprotein may also be considered diagnostic of type IV hyperlipoproteinemia (Berkow 1992), another named condition within the full spectrum of CI.

Patients with CI are at great risk for developing diseases in later years (Hughes et al. 1994). For example, patients with CI have an estimated 10-fold greater risk for developing NIDDM. Some of these patients who become diabetic have had clearly measurable CI and hyperinsulinemia for up to 20 years before the onset of diabetes (Zimmet et al. 1992). It is difficult to estimate the number of dysfunctional but disease-free years there have been previous to the onset of the early overt manifestations.

It is clear that exercise in general can slow the age-related insulin resistance common in the population. But Seals et al. (1984) showed this to be the case only for some individuals. Hughes et al. (1994) demonstrated that carbohydrate-intolerant subjects do not obtain some of the beneficial effects of exercise training. Craig et al. (1989) reported that exercise training improved glucose tolerance in younger and older athletes, but the response of older athletes was well below that of the younger group and the changes did not affect the age-related differences in glucose tolerance.

One important aspect of sport is the possibility of inactivity as a result of competitive off-seasons, injury, or other factors, especially in amateurs who work full-time. Rogers et al. (1990) showed that some masters athletes had a deterioration in glucose tolerance after only 10 days of inactivity. In clinical practice, it is not unusual to have patients who are former competitive athletes to now be out of shape, overweight, and sometimes obese. Improvement in lifestyle factors, including properly matched training, can usually begin to improve the patient's overall condition almost immediately.

FATTY ACIDS, EICOSANOIDS, AND INFLAMMATION

Physiological damage to tissues results in the process of inflammation. This damage is produced during all exercise, especially exercise of high intensity and during competition. Acute intense exercise induces immune and inflammatory responses comparable to those in infections and trauma (Konig et al. 1997). The process of inflammation, however, has three beneficial features in that it is the start of a complex recovery or healing process; it prevents the spread of damaged tissue to other areas, which potentially can cause secondary problems; and it disposes of local cellular debris. Following damage, a number of chemicals are released, including prostaglandins, thromboxanes, and leukotrienes. Edema follows the flow of fluid into interstitial spaces, white blood cells increase, and ultimately fibroblasts continue the process of recovery with collagen synthesis. In the normal situation, this balanced mechanism results in healing. However, a number of factors may cause an imbalanced response to tissue damage, resulting in poor recovery or continued inflammation. Some of the important chemicals produced by the body in response to injury—prostaglandins, thromboxanes, and leukotrienes—are produced from certain dietary fatty acids and are referred to as eicosanoids (Mayes 1993).

In addition to their role as an energy source, as a structural component of many cell walls, and as an integral part of the mitochondrial membrane, dietary fatty acids are important in the inflammatory process. Most importantly for the inflammation response, some of these fatty acids undergo enzymatic changes—desaturation (adding a double bond between carbon atoms) and elongation (adding a pair of carbon atoms to make the fatty acid longer)—that result in the production of various pro- and anti-inflammatory chemicals.

In addition to certain adrenal hormones that have anti-inflammatory effects, eicosanoids play a major role in recovery from exercise and in correction of micro- and macrotrauma. Because of the extensiveness of the fatty acid cascades and the fact that eicosanoid terminology is not standardized, this topic is simplified here. Readers who wish to pursue the topic further are urged to consult the references in this text, as well as others on the subject.

In clinical practice, it is relatively easy to manipulate the patient's fatty acid balance to create specific effects, especially to increase levels of those chemicals that produce powerful anti-inflammatory eicosanoids and to reduce levels of those that are pro-inflammatory. This also helps increase the pain threshold. These inflammatory and anti-inflammatory substances are produced by the body from specific dietary fatty acids. According to Mayes (1993), "By varying the proportions of the different polyunsaturated fatty acids in the diet, it is possible to influence the type of eicosanoids synthesized, indicating that it might be possible to influence the course of disease by dietary means" (p. 232). Konig et al. (1997) demonstrated positive therapeutic effects through changing dietary fatty acid composition in those with chronic inflammatory conditions. Gray and Martinovic (1994) saw significant improvement with the use of essential fatty acids in patients who had chronic fatigue syndrome. The relationship of certain fatty acids to CI has been demonstrated by Simopoulos (1994) and is discussed in chapter 25. Clinically, practitioners in complementary sports medicine have found these techniques very useful in all types of inflammatory conditions, in certain ailments and injuries that produce pain, and in CI and insulin resistance (including diabetes mellitus).

It is clear that a certain balance of fatty acids produces specific inflammatory and anti-inflammatory activity through the action of eicosanoid synthesis and metabolism (Innis 1996). Most importantly, reduced essential fatty acid intakes increase the pro-inflammatory eicosanoids (Blond and Bezard 1991) as will be discussed later. This condition can occur in athletes consuming a low-fat diet. Two of these fatty acids are considered essential since the human body cannot synthesize them—linoleic acid and alpha-linolenic acid. A third, arachidonic acid, can be synthesized from a by-product of linoleic acid metabolism, dihomo-gamma-linolenic acid, and it is also found in the diet. Dietary eicosapentaenoic acid can also play a role in eicosanoid production.

For the clinician, a general understanding that these three fatty acids are found in three distinct groups of dietary fats, and that they are converted to three separate groups of eicosanoids, will make applying these potentially complex biochemical cascades to a patient's condition much easier. In this text, the three groups of dietary fats are referred to as Groups A, B, and C, and the chemicals they produce as the Series 1, 2, and 3 eicosanoids. Each eicosanoid series contains prostaglandins, thromboxanes, and leukotrienes. More specifically, the Group A end products produce the Series 1 eicosanoids, the Group B end products produce the Series 2 eicosanoids, and the Group C end products produce the Series 3 eicosanoids. Series 1 and 3 eicosanoids are anti-inflammatory, and Series 2 are inflammatory (see figure 6.1).

Group A Fats

Group A includes most of the omega-6 fats (those with a double bond located six carbons from the methyl end of the chain) and includes the essential fatty acid, linoleic acid (LA). These fats are found in most vegetable oils, especially corn, peanut, and safflower oil, with smaller amounts in the vegetables themselves. Other sources of LA include production from the bacteria *Escherichia coli* found as part of the normal flora of the large intestine and large adipose tissue stores that may have accumulated due

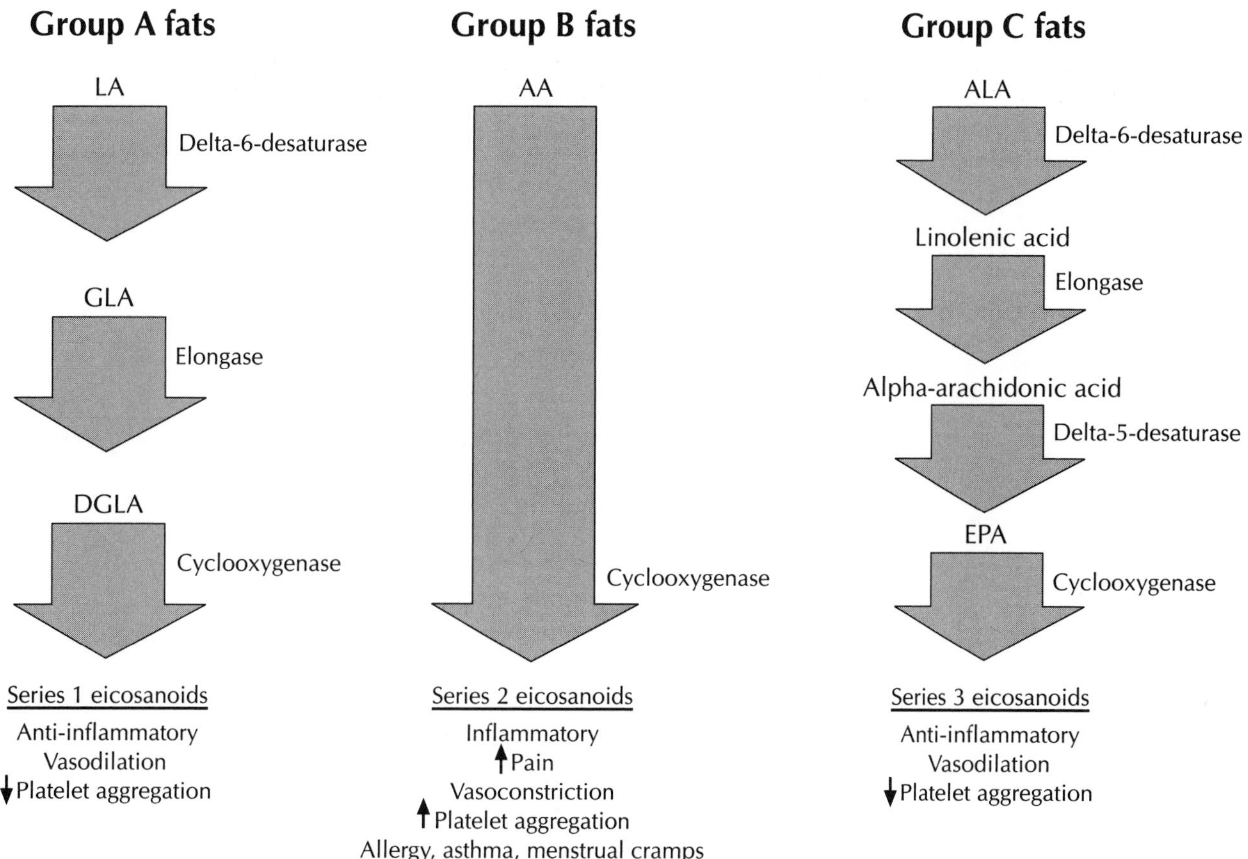

Figure 6.1 Conversion of dietary fats to eicosanoids, and the required enzymes.

to excess dietary intake (Mantzioris et al. 1995). Group A fats are desaturated and elongated to form the Series 1 eicosanoids. The process begins with the conversion of LA to gamma-linolenic acid (GLA) by the action of the delta-6-desaturase enzyme. The GLA is then converted to dihomo-gamma-linolenic acid (DGLA), which requires elongase, before being converted to the Series 1 eicosanoids. This last step requires the cyclooxygenase enzyme.

Group B Fats

Group B fats are synthesized to the Series 2 eicosanoids, which provoke inflammatory, allergic, and hypersensitivity (including asthma and menstrual cramps) responses. Group B fats contain arachidonic acid (AA), also an omega-6 fat, and are found in meats, dairy foods, and shellfish. Unlike what occurs with the Group A and C fats, there is only one main step from AA to the Series 2 eicosanoids, cyclooxygenase enzyme. A unique feature of this cascade is that AA can also be produced from DGLA, with the enzyme delta-5-desaturase required for this activity. Stimulation of this enzyme can cause increased conversion of DGLA to AA, resulting in more inflammatory Series 2 and fewer Series 1 eicosanoids (Medeiros et al. 1995). This enzyme activity is increased with insulin and thyroxin (Bezard et al. 1994). Estrogen decreases both delta-5- and delta-6-desaturase enzymes, and increases in delta-5-desaturase are seen in aging (Medeiros et al. 1995).

The Series 2 eicosanoids encompass two separate pathways. One results in the production of leukotrienes (requiring the lipooxygenase enzyme) and the other results in the Series 2–related pros-

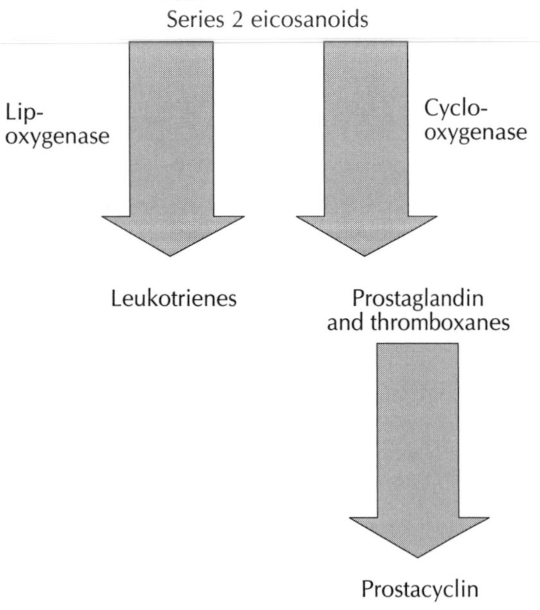

Figure 6.2 Series 2 eicosanoids are further broken down.

taglandins and thromboxanes, which may produce prostacyclin (requiring the cylooxygenase enzyme) (Koester 1993). Figure 6.2 shows these relationships.

Leukotrienes activate leukocytes and stimulate their movement to areas of inflammation and injury. Thromboxanes stimulate platelet aggregation, and the Series 2–related prostaglandins mediate inflammation and sensitize pain receptors. Prostacyclin is an inhibitor of platelet aggregation and a vasodilator, countering the inflammatory and pain-producing effects of the other Series 2 eicosanoids. It may also promote the repair of cartilage (Dajani et al. 1991)—another reason athletes may not want to severely restrict or avoid foods containing AA. Prostacyclin is inhibited by aspirin (through Series 2 eicosanoid inhibition), as discussed later.

Group C Fats

The Group C fats take a path similar to that of the A fats, but contain the essential fatty acid alpha-linolenic acid. These are sometimes referred to as omega-3 fats because each has a double bond located three carbons from the methyl end of the chain. Alpha-linolenic acid is converted to linolenic acid through the action of the delta-6-desaturase enzyme, to alpha-arachidonic acid by elongase, and to eicosapentaenoic acid (EPA) by delta-5-desaturase. Conversion of EPA to Series 3 eicosanoids is stimulated by the cyclooxygenase enzyme. Like the Series 1 eicosanoids, the Series 3 end products have significant anti-inflammatory action. In addition, this process is preferred over the Group A conversions (Umeda-Sawada et al. 1995).

IMBALANCE IN DIETARY FATS

It is important to note that all three series of the eicosanoids produced by dietary fatty acids have beneficial effects in the body. Only when there is an imbalance is there the great possibility of biochemical dysfunction. For example, Funk (1993) showed that the Series 2 eicosanoids in the brain are important for the normal response of the nervous system to pain. Locally, however, an excess production of the same Series 2 eicosanoids increases inflammation and the pain associated with it. Other actions of the Series 2 eicosanoids include vasoconstriction of the blood vessels and the promotion of platelet aggregation. Series 2 eicosanoids are also important for absorption of zinc from the small intestines (Song et al. 1998), and possibly other nutrients as well. Desimone et al. (1993), however, showed that these chemicals could produce systemic bone loss, another example of the effect of excess Series 2 eicosanoids. Some fats are also vital in improving mineral metabolism. For example, increased levels of essential fatty acids increase both calcium absorption and bone calcium (Claassen et al. 1995). Krieger (1997) demonstrated, however, that calcium transport is inhibited by the Series 2 eicosanoids. Series 1 and 3 eicosanoids balance the Series 2 eicosanoids; Series 1 and 3 have anti-inflammatory effects, vasodilate blood vessels, and prevent platelet aggregation.

A variety of physical, chemical, and mental/emotional factors may influence the production of eicosanoids. Eicosanoid production is influenced by training itself, especially with regards to intensity. Dietary manipulation also can affects eicosanoid balance, as can certain hormones. In addition, mental/emotional stress in athletes also affects the production of eicosanoids. Physical activity by itself has a substantial influence on the production of the Series 2 chemicals, resulting in inflammation. Almekinders et al. (1993) showed that human tendon fibroblasts produced a significant amount of Series 2 eicosanoids following repetitive motion. This effect increases with higher levels of intensity. Patients who walk, run, lift weights, or perform any other repetitive-motion action produce these pro-inflammatory hormones as part of the normal process of recovery, which also depends on the anti-inflammatory Series 1 and 3 eicosanoids.

A number of biochemical factors influence eicosanoid production. As already noted, dietary manipulation can do so. Bezard et al. (1994) and Bouziane et al. (1994) reported that low-protein diets increase essential fatty acid requirements; the latter demonstrated that protein-deficient diets increase the Series 2 eicosanoids. According to Rudin (1982), low dietary fiber increases the demand for essential fatty acids.

In addition, the use of specific nutritional supplements can influence eicosanoid production as discussed in chapter 19; that is, GLA, alpha-linolenic acid, and EPA can significantly increase their respective levels of eicosanoids (Johnson et al. 1997). Certain vitamins, including niacin (Mayes 1993), vitamin E (Despret et al. 1992), vitamin C (Gardiner and Duncan 1988), and vitamin B6 (Maranesi et al. 1993), can increase Series 1 and 3 eicosanoids. Magnesium (Mahfouz and Kummerow 1989) and zinc (Eder and Kirchgessner 1996) also influence the conversion of fatty acids to eicosanoids. Most of these factors influence eicosanoid balance through their effects on the desaturase and elongase enzymes. The activity level of desaturation and elongation may be different in different organs and glands (Lopez et al. 1993).

Other foods and hormones can inhibit delta-6-desaturase. Among these are EPA, AA, excess alcohol, glucose and fructose (Bezard et al. 1994), testosterone (Marra and de Alaniz 1989), thyroxin (Ves-Losada and Peluffo 1993), and epinephrine (Bezard et al. 1994). An increased intake of Group A fats can also inhibit this enzyme (Storlien et al. 1997), as can obesity (Blond et al. 1989). An excess amount of dietary salt in hypertensive animals has also been shown to inhibit delta-6-desaturase (Poisson et al. 1993). In addition, steroids and lithium may inhibit the desaturase enzymes, as can fasting (Bezard et al. 1994).

Aging also reduces some of the desaturase enzymes (Bordoni et al. 1988). The effect of age, however, is more significant in the delta-6-desaturase activity of Group C fats (Ulmann et al. 1991); delta-5-desaturase increases with age. As a result, AA may increase with age (Maniongui et al. 1993). The delta-6 enzyme activity of Group A fats is also more sensitive to seasonal factors, with diminished activity in the spring and fall. In addition, dietary fats may adversely affect the desaturase activity of Group C fats more than that of Group A. Other factors such as aging, seasons, and other diet issues can also affect eicosanoids.

The delta-5-desaturase enzyme is a key factor in eicosanoid balance. As noted earlier, the conversion of Group A fats to Group B fats (i.e., DGLA to AA) requires the delta-5-desaturase enzyme. This enzyme may be activated by insulin (Medeiros et al. 1995). Increased insulin production may occur in those with CI, as previously discussed. Even in healthy individuals, increased insulin can also be produced from consumption of a high-carbohydrate diet (Coulston et al. 1993). Sesamin, a component of sesame seed oil, inhibits the action of delta-5-desaturase (Chavali et al. 1997). This response, however, is most active in the conversion of DGLA to AA and, for unknown reasons, does not seem to affect the production of EPA (Umeda-Sawada et al. 1995). In addition, EPA inhibits the delta-5-desaturase enzyme.

Other dietary factors also influence the essential fatty acid cascades, the most important being trans fats, which are contained in large amounts in hydrogenated and partially hydrogenated oils such as margarine (Mayes 1993). These fats are manufactured by the chemical conversion of Group A fats but do not possess the functions of an essential fatty acid. Moreover, they can exacerbate essential fatty acid deficiency. Most importantly, trans fats can inhibit delta-6-desaturase and elongase enzymes and may stimulate delta-5-desaturase, causing eicosanoid imbalance (Simopoulos 1997). This can inhibit the production of anti-inflammatory Series 1 and 3 eicosanoids and potentially result in a relative increase in inflammatory Series 2 eicosanoids.

Mental/emotional stress can also have a negative effect on eicosanoid balance by inhibiting the delta-6-desaturase enzyme. This may be due to the sympathetic nervous system reaction and the accompanying production of catecholamines (Mills et al. 1994).

Among substances that inhibit the conversion of fatty acids to eicosanoids, the most commonly used are aspirin (acetylsalicylic acid) and other nonsteroidal anti-inflammatory drugs (NSAIDs). This is accomplished by inhibition of the cyclooxygenase enzyme, and it results in inhibition of not only the pro-inflammatory eicosanoids but also the anti-inflammatory ones. (Some inflammation, however, continues through the lipooxygenase pathway, which is not inhibited by NSAIDs.) The analgesic and antipyretic effects of aspirin are the most easily obtained; anti-inflammatory effects occur only with higher doses of NSAIDs (Amadio et al. 1993). A variety of side effects are attributed to the use of NSAIDs including delayed soft tissue, cartilage, and bone healing; as well as muscle dysfunction and others as described in chapter 17.

Clinically, athletes who symptomatically improve after using aspirin or another NSAID, or those with chronic inflammation as measured by C-reactive protein or erythrocyte sedimentation rate, may require balancing of essential fatty acids through the diet or through supplementation to accomplish similar or identical outcomes without the dangers of the side effects of the drugs.

TRAINING EFFECTS ON IMMUNITY

Cortisol and other glucocorticoids have a specific inhibitory effect on the immune system (Granner 1993). In general, this effect is anti-inflammatory through inhibition of the release of Series 2–related prostaglandins and leukotrienes. Physiologically high levels of cortisol may be related to overtraining and the suppression of the immune system. Accompanying the rise in cortisol in training is a diminished testosterone level (often due to a decrease in DHEA[S] as discussed earlier). Hoogeveen and Zonderland (1996) showed that a lowered testosterone/cortisol ratio may be related to overtraining. Testosterone and cortisol are competitive agonists at the receptor level of muscle cells, and their measurement can be used as an indication of the anabolic/catabolic balance (Urhausen et al. 1997).

In their experiments, Shepard and Shek (1996) showed that the onset of exercise is associated with the release of pro-inflammatory eicosanoids and is accompanied by immune dysfunction in some athletes. A high-intensity workout, for example, can suppress the immune system, but a light to moderate workout may stimulate it (Konig et al. 1997). Immune dysfunction is generally less pronounced in very young individuals. According to Pedersen et al. (1996), the immunosuppressive effect of high-intensity workouts includes "suppressed concentration of lymphocytes, suppressed natural killer and lymphokine activated killer cytotoxicity and secretory IgA in mucosa" (p. 236). Neutrophil activity can also be adversely affected, increasing with high-intensity exercise. Both of these types of white blood cells are easily measured in the clinical setting, and abnormal levels are not uncommon in athletes. These problems are often associated with upper respiratory tract and other infections seen in athletes. Upper respiratory illness can change an athlete's gait and increase the risk of injury (Weidner et al. 1997). In addition, immune suppression is amplified one to two weeks after competitive events.

During light to moderate training, the immune system can be enhanced (Pedersen et al. 1996). Athletes who train for up to 1 hr and at intensities of 60%-70% $\dot{V}O_2max$ often have improved immunity and fewer infections throughout the year. Immune dysfunction and associated infection including colds, flu, or other immunosuppressive signs or symptoms—even the most mild problems—may be an indication of chronic overtraining.

It is important to note that the immunosuppressive action of intense training does not mean that athletes should never train intensely. Rather the implication is that after a bout of intense training, proper recovery is necessary so that the immune system returns to normal before the next intense session. On the other hand, if the same athletic end result can be achieved without such intense training, then more training should be of the less intense type.

A number of nutritional factors are associated with immune function. Cordova and Alvarez-Mon (1995) discussed the fact that zinc levels in athletes can be very low. Not only can low zinc diminish endurance, zinc is also important for the production of anti-inflammatory Series 1 and 3 eicosanoids. Decreases in glutamine following intense training may also contribute to immune suppression since glutamine is essential for the normal function of immune cells (Newsholme 1994). Even a long endurance event such as a marathon run results in significant glutamine loss in plasma.

In addition to intense training, other factors are associated with immune suppression, including mental/emotional stress, nutritional imbalances, and quick weight-loss programs (Nieman 1997a, 1997b). The importance of considering the whole person is again emphasized.

OXIDATIVE STRESS

An important aspect related to immune function is the potential of increased oxidative stress—the cellular condition of elevated reactive oxygen radicals that cause significant damage. These are molecules converted from the O_2 form to a chemically unstable superoxide or the singlet oxygen state. Packer (1997) described a number of sources of this chemical stress, including mitochondrial superoxide production, ischemia-reperfusion mechanisms, and autooxidation of catecholamines. Oxidative stress increases with high-intensity or long-duration training and competition. Evidence of exercise-induced oxidative stress comes from measurements of free radicals, oxidized lipids, and DNA and the measurement of glutathione.

The continual production and action of oxygen radicals are balanced by our antioxidant defenses. This defense system acts against oxygen radical attack; it includes enzymes that scavenge harmful oxygen radicals and their by-products, as well as antioxidants. Two important enzymes in this system are superoxide dismutase and catalase. Both are contained in higher levels in the type I muscle fibers because of the increased mitochondria in this fiber type (Jenkins et al. 1984). Glutathione peroxidase is another important enzyme in the antioxidant system. Not only does light to moderate training not seem to create the same oxidant stress as high-intensity workouts, but Sen (1995) showed that submaximal training may even augment these antioxidant defenses. On the other hand, Tiidus et al. (1996) showed that not all who engage in light to moderate exercise of short duration derive these benefits. This may be attributable to a variety of lifestyle factors, including diet, nutrition, and stress.

The level of intensity is important in relation to oxygen radical formation and other immune dysfunction. Dillard et al. (1978) were the first to show that training at 75% $\dot{V}O_2max$ and higher significantly raised oxygen radical production as measured by expired pentane. Mills et al. (1996) showed in horses that oxidative stress induced by moderate training in a very hot and humid environment was at least equal to that induced by high-intensity exercise. The author (Maffetone 1996) developed a training heart rate formula to help determine optimal training intensities (using the heart rate) that are health promoting and theoretically do not raise oxygen radical production significantly.

Injury, poor performance, and even disease may arise from increased exposure to oxygen radicals or from impaired defense mechanisms. Lawler et al. (1997) discuss the relationships of oxygen radicals to skeletal muscle fatigue, especially in the diaphragm muscle. In addition, athletes with existing dysfunction may produce more oxygen radicals than normal. Laaksonen et al. (1996) found that young, moderately active and otherwise healthy diabetic men had increased resting and postexercise oxidative stress.

Many studies, such as that of Dekkers et al. (1996), show that various nutrients in supplement form (commonly called antioxidants) are protective against skeletal muscle damage and inflammation following training, including specifically vitamin C, vitamin E, and selenium. Ghiselli et al. (1997) reported that the Mediterranean diet, with its high intake of antioxidants, fiber, and raw foods, protects against oxygen radicals. Yu (1996) also showed that diet restriction without loss of nutrients can increase life span through improved control of oxidative stress.

In addition to exercise, other factors may also increase one's susceptibility to oxygen free radicals, including air pollution, excess alcohol, non-ionizing radiation (ultraviolet and microwaves), and psychological stress (Moller et al. 1996).

CONCLUSION

An understanding of the athlete's hormonal system is the first step in recognizing dysfunction and being able to manipulate and improve function. Adrenal hormone imbalance is essential not just for good health but also for optimal performance. Control of insulin can help to increase the amount of fatty acids and reduce reliance on glycogen during training and competition, improving endurance. The balance of fats and eicosanoids can affect inflammation and influence the immune system. Careful assessment of the patient's free radial status is important in helping to prevent injury and improve overall performance.

7

Patient History and Dialogue

Sir William Osler said, "Never treat a stranger" (Terezhalmy and Schiff 1986). This quote applies well to complementary sports medicine as one very important component is the relationship between practitioner and patient. Gathering information about an athlete's physical, chemical, and mental/emotional state will be at its most comprehensive during the history-taking process if this is done correctly. Too often, this procedure is abbreviated—or worse, the seemingly rambling testimony of the patient is ignored by the practitioner. Many pieces of evidence emerge as one listens to the patient, and knowing when to stop the process is an important aspect of the professional's art. To truly view the whole person, the practitioner may need to spend a significant amount of time in this initial appraisal of the patient. The only exception is during times of acute trauma when emergency care is the priority. Even then, certain information may be of great value if it is available.

TAKING A HISTORY

Perhaps the most important aspect of care is taking a complete and effective history. Skilled history taking, more than examinations or test results, is the key to a proper diagnosis (Fowler 1997). In a prospective study of 100 patients, Winkler (1979) showed that only 5% of the subjects that did evaluations other than the history established a diagnosis not made by history taking.

Because of our emphasis on advanced technology, practitioners are potentially given such extensive diagnostic information that the one-on-one history is losing significance in our health care system (Laemmel 1996). Not only are the art and science of taking a successful history important in an initial patient visit, but maintaining dialogue on all subsequent visits is also vital. As patients progress, many changes take place (all positive ones, it is hoped); this means that on subsequent visits their structural, chemical, and mental/emotional state will be slightly or significantly different from before. Assessment, treatment, and lifestyle relationships must keep pace.

Laemmel's (1996) comments are representative of an optimal approach to the care of patients in a complementary sports medicine practice: "In order to achieve a true dialogue, it is necessary that [the practitioner] abandon the role-playing so common to physician-patient relationships and that he meet his patient on a person-to-person basis. In this process he will reveal his self-perception, his relationship to fellow human beings and, not least, his idea of what it means to be a healer" (p. 863).

Like many practitioners, many patients have become "specialists" with regard to the types of problems they complain of. For example, it is not uncommon for athletes to complain about their knee pain while not considering gastrointestinal stress, insomnia, or other seemingly unrelated problems they also have. Some patients may not want to discuss their other problems. In complementary sports medicine, the whole patient is assessed, including the workout history, athletic goals, stress, and other issues. It is important for the patient to understand this concept from the beginning of the relationship.

There are two important aspects of taking a history. The first aspect is the relationship developed in the one-to-one encounter between practitioner and patient. It is not possible to provide a minimum time frame for this. However, at least a 30- to 60-min history and sometimes longer, may be necessary in order for practitioner and patient to understand each other. An important part of this dialogue is that it allows the practitioner to obtain more information than has been noted on the patient's forms.

The second aspect is the use of forms. Much of the information obtained in the dialogue may also be revealed on the written forms. This repetition can be helpful rather than a waste of time. The duplication helps confirm or verify the complaint or condition. In addition, some patients are likely to write more information on a form than they will give during dialogue—although in other cases, the converse is true.

The additional time spent (usually much more than in mainstream medicine) and the more extensive use of forms (usually in much more depth than in mainstream medicine) are part of the difference and uniqueness of complementary sports medicine history taking. However, the most important difference is in the questions asked through the forms and the interpretation of the answers—specifically the relationship of these questions and answers to functional problems rather than disease. Most of the forms contain questions that refer to functional signs and symptoms.

HISTORY FORMS

This chapter provides examples of history forms, such as the symptom survey, merely to illustrate a complementary medicine approach to assessing the physical, chemical, and mental/emotional aspects of each patient. Many different types of history forms may work well. Some practitioners find that they work best from a form tailored to their specific needs. Symptom surveys have proven both reliable and valid for workplace ergonomics programs (Baron et al. 1996), as a discomfort and pain index (Franzblau et al. 1997), and as a questionnaire for musculoskeletal disorders (Laubli et al. 1991).

These and other forms allow patients to state their main problems and to recall problems they may not think are important or do not think of as abnormal. For example, joint pain or insomnia may be more common in people over the age of 40 or 50 than when they were younger, and some think of these as a normal part of the aging process. In addition, the practitioner needs to know everything about the patient—not just about the pain, but also about drugs or nutrients taken, family history, stress levels, and the like. In addition to duplication with the dialogue, a particular form may contain questions similar to those on other forms. This redundancy can also serve a purpose in ensuring that patients are consistent in their complaints and helping to place stress on the importance of particular questions.

It is often best to give forms to patients before their initial appointment, with instructions to complete in full. In most cases this can be accomplished by sending the forms to the patient after the initial contact to schedule an appointment. This allows the patient to spend adequate time answering the questions. The examples provided in this chapter consist of four different forms totaling about nine pages. As the accuracy of information is vital, allowing patients enough time in their own environments to complete forms properly can be important. In some types of practices, having the patient send back the forms ahead of the scheduled appointment also has its advantages, allowing the practitioner adequate time to read them. In either situation, it is important for the practitioner to see the forms before having the dialogue.

At the end of this chapter, there are four forms that might serve as a beginning of the assessment process. Within the chapter are a description of each form and an interpretation of some content areas. These forms allow patients to write about their main complaints along with other problems they may have. In addition, as already mentioned, responding to forms prompts patients to think about other areas that they may not have considered talking about or areas they did not think were related to their problems. For example, a patient with low back pain may not have thought to consider a potential temporomandibular joint problem, which may turn out to be related to the back problem. Or people who are always fatigued may not think it is abnormal to get sleepy after meals. On the basis of the patient's responses, or lack of responses, the practitioner can ask more specific questions during the initial visit that will allow a fuller understanding of the patient's system, how it reacts to stress and training, and possibly how the person would respond to certain therapies.

GENERAL INVENTORY

Form 7.1 is an illustration of a general form used in private practice. It inventories most of the systems from muscles and joints, to eyes, ears, nose, and throat, to the gastrointestinal system, and so on. Patients can mark any area that pertains to them. On the second page are specific questions about the main complaint, secondary complaints, operations, medications, nutritional supplements, and other pertinent topics.

This type of form serves as part of the general screening process, especially to help rule out more serious conditions that may not be appropriate for complementary sports medicine practitioners to deal with. These include disease processes. The general inventory form makes patients think about all the areas of the body, prompting them to note a variety of symptoms.

SYMPTOM SURVEY

In previous chapters, we considered the usefulness of looking at all symptoms that the body creates rather than one symptom in one area. A four-page form (see form 7.2) is an example of an inventory of a number of common symptoms that in many cases may reflect body dysfunction more than disease. The form presents items divided into groups based on certain very general physiological indicators, and it may be useful to help one ascertain certain patterns of problems and their origins. These groups of symptoms may be caused, in part, by specific nutritional, dietary, or other imbalances that need to be addressed. Note that a particular imbalance can produce symptoms that may be clustered in more than one group. For example, those with increased sympathetic tone (Group One) may also have blood sugar-handling stress (Group Three). The following listing corresponds to the groups on the Symptom Survey:

- Group One symptoms are sometimes associated with excess sympathetic and/or diminished parasympathetic tone.
- Group Two symptoms may be associated with excess parasympathetic and/or diminished sympathetic tone.
- Group Three contains symptoms common in some patients with blood sugar-handling problems.
- Group Four symptoms are related to some cardiovascular complaints.
- Group Five contains some symptoms common to liver and gallbladder dysfunction.
- Group Six symptoms are associated with other gastrointestinal dysfunction.
- Group Seven symptoms may be associated with complaints from three hormonal systems: Subgroups A and B relate to hyper- and hypothyroid function, respectively; Subgroups C and D to hyper- and hypopituitary function, respectively; and Subgroups E and F to hyper- and hypoadrenal function, respectively.
- Group Eight A (Female Only) contains some symptoms that relate to general hormonal and menstrual problems.
- Group Eight B (Male Only) contains some symptoms related to general hormonal and prostate problems.
- Group Nine contains some symptoms of carbohydrate intolerance.
- Group Ten symptoms are associated with poor essential fatty acid metabolism.
- Group Eleven and Twelve symptoms are related to neurological dysfunction and potential nutritional needs for two distinct parts of the vitamin B complex.

Note that this form also includes a section in which patients list their five most important complaints. The responses here should correspond to the major and secondary complaints on the first form described (form 7.1). Some patients are unable to decide on these major complaints. They may change their mind each time they are asked about their biggest problem, sometimes producing a new list of complaints. This inability to decide may be associated with psychological or emotional stress.

The symptom survey type of form is also useful to review as treatment progresses, with the practitioner asking the patient about certain signs or symptoms that had been marked. Such a review can help to ensure that the patient's more subtle problems are improving. In addition, the patient can fill out a new form after two to four months of therapy to provide more objective feedback regarding the effectiveness of care.

NUTRITION QUESTIONNAIRE

Form 7.3 contains more than 40 questions about nutrition, diet, and other possible habits of the patient. As with the preceding two forms, there is some duplication between this form and others. This document is useful for the practitioner in helping patients with their eating or nutritional habits. For example, question 3 concerns the amount of water consumed each day, and several other questions relate to caffeine and alcohol consumption—substances that may increase dehydration and offset water intake. This form may also be helpful for assessing certain metabolic problems. For example, question 26 is "Do you often feel hungry, no matter how much you eat?" This should prompt the practitioner to consider possible blood sugar or insulin problems, check the other forms for similar indications, ask the patient more specific questions, and begin to consider other tests to help rule in or out potential problems. As with the other forms, the questions here help both the practitioner and patient recall certain areas of diet and nutrition that may be relevant to the overall assessment process.

DIETARY ANALYSIS

Three basic types of dietary data collection tools are used by health care professionals and researchers. These include direct weighing of foods, which may be the most accurate but is expensive and time consuming and requires a high level of participation; the diet recall, which relies on the patient's memory; and the diet diary, which may distort usual food intake. Each method has inherent strengths and weaknesses, but they all still have good clinical value for both practitioner and patient. De Castro (1994) concludes that "the diet diary technique is the method of choice for investigations of the ingestive behaviors of free-living humans" (p. 179). Bingham et al. (1995) found that although weighed records were the most accurate method of dietary assessment, the only other method that could approach this level of accuracy was an estimated seven-day diary.

The seven-day diary form (see form 7.4) allows patients to write down everything they eat and drink over a period of up to seven days. Keeping the diary can benefit patients in that this is often the first time they have recorded what and how much (or little) they consume. Recording can help raise their awareness level regarding the quality and quantity of their diet. For many patients, just this simple action is often followed by improved eating habits. The practitioner can gain further understanding about the patient's physiology by seeing what foods are consumed. More importantly, computer analysis of the patient's diet can help determine the macro- and micronutrient status and any potenial imbalances. In many cases in which practitioners provide their patients with dietary recommendations, compliance is higher when patients see the outcome of their dietary analysis. Figures 7.1 and 7.2 illustrate information gained through the use of a simple computer program to analyze an athlete's diet, giving an average one-day profile.

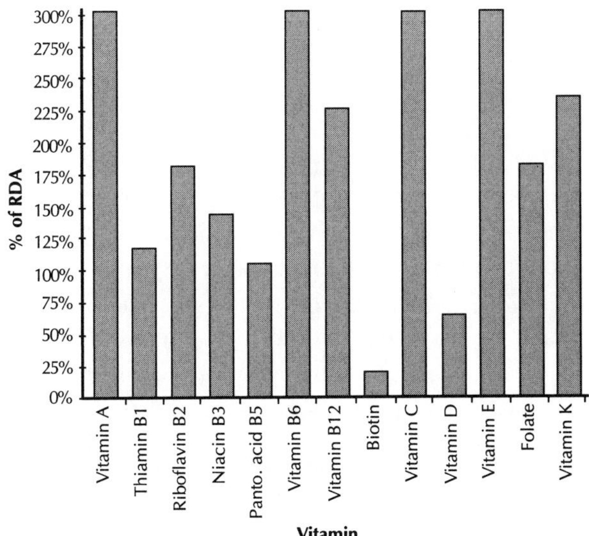

Figure 7.1 Dietary analysis allows a practitioner to gather data on vitamins in an individual's diet.
Reprinted by permission of NutrAnalysis, Inc.

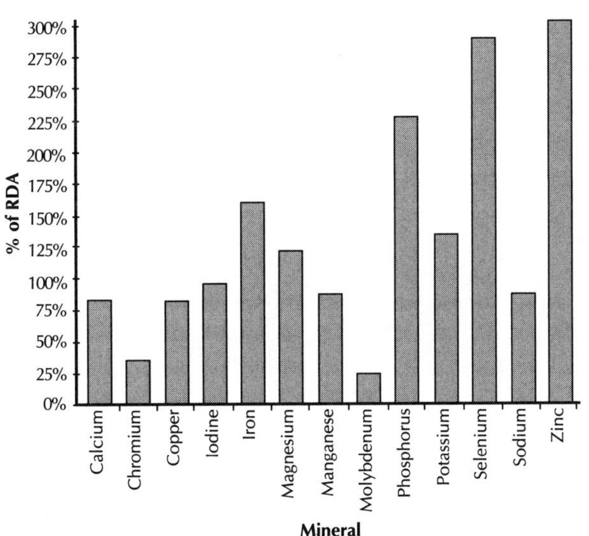

Figure 7.2 Dietary analysis also allows a practitioner to gather data on minerals in an individual's diet.
Reprinted by permission of NutrAnalysis, Inc.

TRAINING DIARY AND HISTORY

Many athletes maintain an exercise or training diary. This may consist of notes on the calendar or a more formal daily journal. For patients who keep any type of diary, it is important that they bring it for their initial visit. Those who do not maintain a diary should be encouraged to do so, as it can be a valuable part of the assessment process at all stages.

Making a copy of the patient's training diary for office records is also an important part of the history. If a patient does not maintain a complete diary, the practitioner should include an interview regarding the patient's program and should have the patient write out his or her current and/or past routine. Information should include at least the types of workouts (running, walking, biking, etc.), the total time of each workout, how the person felt during and after, and some measure of intensity (such as heart rate or perceived exertion). Other measures can include the distance covered, pace or speed, or other secondary variables. A list of competitions is also important, including all successes and failures, the patient's subjective feelings, and other such information.

An important item in a diary should be some goal orientation. This can relate to competition (i.e., completing a 10,000-m run in under 40 min), personal fitness (being able to swim 25 laps), health (losing 15 pounds), or some combination of such aspects of the patient's life. This goal setting is something the practitioner should carefully evaluate and discuss with the patient, especially with regard to how realistic a goal is and how well it matches the patient's structural, chemical, and mental/emotional state. If a patient has no defined goals, the practitioner should consider helping the person create some realistic goals that can be written in both the patient's diary and the office records.

In addition to the patient's exercise routine (or lack thereof), an important issue is equipment and location. This includes any mechanical apparatus used (bikes, treadmills, free weights, etc.) and the type of terrain if applicable (concrete streets, dirt roads, wooden gym floor, etc.). In addition, the patient should bring all training and competitive footwear to the first session for the practitioner to inspect. This issue is discussed in chapter 24.

CONCLUSION

After taking a comprehensive history, the practitioner must choose between two options: either accept or reject the patient. When patients are not accepted, they should be told why and should be given names of professionals whose work might fit better with their type of problem. In some cases, the patient's problem may be outside the scope of the practitioner's license or expertise. Occasionally, the practitioner may not feel comfortable with the mental/emotional relationship that developed, or did not develop, during the initial session.

Taking an effective history may be the most important aspect of patient care. History taking requires the allocation of adequate time for the initial dialogue and the completion of forms that prompt the patient to provide more information. In addition, the practitioner can use the completed forms as a guide through a more effective dialogue, asking the patient to expand on some of the important information presented. Each practitioner must decide which format to use to derive information from an initial visit, including the forms to be used, questions to be asked, and details to be gathered. Keeping accurate notes is an important aspect legally and ethically and also for good follow-up and future reference. Patients who are evaluated in a complete and efficient way will also generally have more respect for the practitioner, refer more patients, and more likely comply with any recommendations.

Form 7.1 General Survey

Name ____________________ Home phone ____________ Work phone ____________

Address ____

Date of birth ____________ Age _____ M _____ F _____ Marital status ____________ No. of children _____

Occupation ____________________ Referred by ____________________

Please check the appropriate space for any of the following symptoms that you now have or have had previously. This is a confidential health questionnaire.

O = Occasional F = Frequent C = Constant

O	F	C	**General**
☐	☐	☐	Allergy
☐	☐	☐	Chills
☐	☐	☐	Convulsions
☐	☐	☐	Dizziness
☐	☐	☐	Fainting
☐	☐	☐	Fatigue
☐	☐	☐	Fever
☐	☐	☐	Headaches
☐	☐	☐	Insomnia
☐	☐	☐	Excess weight loss
☐	☐	☐	Excess weight gain
☐	☐	☐	Nervousness
☐	☐	☐	Depression
☐	☐	☐	Sweats
☐	☐	☐	Tremors

O	F	C	**Muscle and Joint**
☐	☐	☐	Arthritis
☐	☐	☐	Foot trouble
☐	☐	☐	Hernia
☐	☐	☐	Low back pain
☐	☐	☐	Neck pain
☐	☐	☐	Poor posture
☐	☐	☐	Sciatica
			Pain/Numbness in:
☐	☐	☐	Shoulders
☐	☐	☐	Arms
☐	☐	☐	Elbows
☐	☐	☐	Wrist/Hand
☐	☐	☐	Hips
☐	☐	☐	Legs
☐	☐	☐	Knees
☐	☐	☐	Feet

O	F	C	**Gastrointestinal**
☐	☐	☐	Belching or gas
☐	☐	☐	Colitis
☐	☐	☐	Constipation
☐	☐	☐	Diarrhea
☐	☐	☐	Indigestion
☐	☐	☐	Distension
☐	☐	☐	Excess hunger
☐	☐	☐	Gallbladder problems
☐	☐	☐	Hemorrhoids
☐	☐	☐	Liver problems
☐	☐	☐	Nausea
☐	☐	☐	Stomach pain
☐	☐	☐	Poor appetite
☐	☐	☐	Vomiting

O	F	C	**EENT**
☐	☐	☐	Asthma
☐	☐	☐	Colds/Flu
☐	☐	☐	Crossed eyes
☐	☐	☐	Deafness
☐	☐	☐	Dental decay
☐	☐	☐	Ear problems
☐	☐	☐	Enlarged glands
☐	☐	☐	Eye pain
☐	☐	☐	Near-sightedness
☐	☐	☐	Far-sightedness
☐	☐	☐	Gum problems
☐	☐	☐	Hay fever
☐	☐	☐	Hoarseness
☐	☐	☐	Nasal obstruction
☐	☐	☐	Nosebleeds
☐	☐	☐	Sinus problems
☐	☐	☐	Sore throats

O	F	C	**Cardiorespiratory**
			Blood pressure:
☐	☐	☐	High
☐	☐	☐	Low
☐	☐	☐	High cholesterol
☐	☐	☐	Chest pain
☐	☐	☐	Poor circulation
☐	☐	☐	Rapid pulse
☐	☐	☐	Slow pulse
☐	☐	☐	Ankle swelling
☐	☐	☐	Chronic cough
☐	☐	☐	Difficulty breathing
☐	☐	☐	Wheezing
			Spitting up:
☐	☐	☐	Blood
☐	☐	☐	Phlegm

O	F	C	**Skin**
☐	☐	☐	Boils
☐	☐	☐	Bruise easily
☐	☐	☐	Dryness
☐	☐	☐	Hives or rash
☐	☐	☐	Itching
☐	☐	☐	Varicose veins

O	F	C	**Genitourinary**
☐	☐	☐	Bed-wetting
☐	☐	☐	Blood in urine
☐	☐	☐	Frequent urination
☐	☐	☐	Painful urination
☐	☐	☐	Pus in urine
☐	☐	☐	Kidney stones
☐	☐	☐	Prostate problems

For women only:

Date of last period (day 1): ____________

Birth control: ____________

O	F	C	
☐	☐	☐	Menstrual problems
☐	☐	☐	Hot flashes
☐	☐	☐	Irregular cycle
☐	☐	☐	Menopausal symptoms

(continued)

Form 7.1 *(continued)*

What is your major complaint? ______

How long have you had this condition? ______

Have you had this or similar conditions in the past? ______

Is this problem getting worse? ______ Constant? ______ Worse in morning? ______ Evening? ______

Is this interfering with work? ______ Sleep? ______ Exercise? ______ Other? ______

What do you believe is wrong with you? ______

List other problems you have now ______

______

List past operations and dates ______

______

Have you ever been hospitalized other than for surgery? ______

Have you ever had any mental or emotional disorder? ______

Have you had any other injury in the past two years? ______

Are you taking medication? ______ Describe ______

Are you taking nutritional supplements? ______ Describe ______

______

Are you allergic to any foods, drugs, etc? ______

Do you have any dental problems? ______ Dr.: ______

Do you wear arch supports? ______ Heel lifts? ______ Special shoes? ______ What is your shoe size? ______

Date of your last physical exam? ______ Dr.: ______ Blood test? ______

Habits (describe with amounts):

Alcohol ______ Coffee ______

Cigarettes ______ Drugs not listed above ______

Describe your present exercise habits (or attach additional page): ______

______

Please list the main health problems in your family:

Name: Relation: Problem:

______

______

______

In case of emergency, please list the name and number of a friend or relative NOT living with you:

______

Your signature: ______ Date: ______

Form 7.2 Symptom Survey *(Restricted to professional use)*

Patient ______________________ Doctor ______________________ Date ______________

Instructions: Number the boxes that apply to you. Use (1) for MILD symptoms (occurring once or twice a year), (2) for MODERATE symptoms (occurring several times a year), and (3) for SEVERE symptoms (you are aware of the symptom almost constantly).

GROUP ONE

1 ☐ Acid foods upset
2 ☐ Get chilled often
3 ☐ "Lump" in throat
4 ☐ Dry mouth/eyes/nose
5 ☐ Pulse speeds after meal
6 ☐ Keyed up—fail to calm
7 ☐ Cuts heal slowly
8 ☐ Gag easily
9 ☐ Unable to relax; startle easily
10 ☐ Extremities cold, clammy
11 ☐ Strong light irritates
12 ☐ Urine amount reduced
13 ☐ Heart pounds after retiring
14 ☐ "Nervous" stomach
15 ☐ Appetite reduced
16 ☐ Cold sweats often
17 ☐ Fever easily raised
18 ☐ Neuralgia-like pains
19 ☐ Staring, blink little
20 ☐ Sour stomach frequently

GROUP TWO

21 ☐ Joint stiffness after arising
22 ☐ Muscle/leg/toe cramps at night
23 ☐ "Butterfly" stomach, cramps
24 ☐ Eyes or nose watery
25 ☐ Eyes blink often
26 ☐ Eyelids swollen, puffy
27 ☐ Indigestion soon after meals
28 ☐ Always seem hungry; feel "lightheaded" often
29 ☐ Digestion rapid
30 ☐ Vomiting frequent
31 ☐ Hoarseness frequent
32 ☐ Breathing irregular
33 ☐ Pulse slow; feels "irregular"
34 ☐ Gagging reflex slow
35 ☐ Difficulty swallowing
36 ☐ Constipation, diarrhea alternating
37 ☐ "Slow starter"
38 ☐ Get "chilled" frequently
39 ☐ Perspire easily
40 ☐ Circulation poor, sensitive in cold
41 ☐ Subject to colds, asthma, bronchitis

GROUP THREE

42 ☐ Eat when nervous
43 ☐ Excessive appetite
44 ☐ Hungry between meals
45 ☐ Irritable before meals
46 ☐ Get "shaky" if hungry
47 ☐ Fatigue, eating relieves
48 ☐ "Lightheaded" if meals delayed
49 ☐ Heart palpitates if meals missed or delayed
50 ☐ Afternoon headaches
51 ☐ Have bad reaction to overeating sweets
52 ☐ Awaken after few hours sleep—hard to get back to sleep
53 ☐ Crave candy or coffee in afternoon
54 ☐ Moods of depression—"blues" or melancholy
55 ☐ Abnormal craving for sweets or snacks

GROUP FOUR

56 ☐ Hands and feet go to sleep easily, numbness
57 ☐ Sigh frequently, "air hunger"
58 ☐ Aware of "breathing heavily"
59 ☐ High-altitude discomfort
60 ☐ Open windows in closed room
61 ☐ Susceptible to colds and fevers
62 ☐ Afternoon "yawner"
63 ☐ Get "drowsy" often
64 ☐ Swollen ankles, worse at night
65 ☐ Muscle cramps, worse during exercise; get "charley horses"
66 ☐ Shortness of breath on exertion
67 ☐ Dull pain in chest or radiating into left arm, worse on exertion
68 ☐ Bruise easily, "black and blue" spots
69 ☐ Tendency to anemia
70 ☐ "Nosebleeds" frequently
71 ☐ Noises in head, or "ringing in ears"
72 ☐ Tension under the breastbone, or feeling of "tightness," worse on exertion

(continued)

GROUP FIVE

73 ☐ Dizziness
74 ☐ Dry skin
75 ☐ Burning feet
76 ☐ Blurred vision
77 ☐ Itching skin and feet
78 ☐ Excessive falling hair
79 ☐ Frequent skin rashes
80 ☐ Bitter, metallic taste in mouth in mornings
81 ☐ Bowel movements painful or difficult
82 ☐ Worrier, feel insecure
83 ☐ Feeling queasy; headache over eyes
84 ☐ Greasy foods upset
85 ☐ Stools light-colored
86 ☐ Skin peels on foot soles
87 ☐ Pain between shoulder blades
88 ☐ Use laxatives
89 ☐ Stools alternate from soft to watery
90 ☐ History of gallbladder attacks or gallstones
91 ☐ Sneezing attacks
92 ☐ Dreaming, nightmare-type bad dreams
93 ☐ Bad breath (halitosis)
94 ☐ Milk products cause distress
95 ☐ Sensitive to hot weather
96 ☐ Burning or itching anus
97 ☐ Crave sweets

GROUP SIX

98 ☐ Loss of taste for meat
99 ☐ Lower bowel gas several hours after eating
100 ☐ Burning stomach sensations, eating relieves
101 ☐ Coated tongue
102 ☐ Pass large amounts of foul-smelling gas
103 ☐ Indigestion 1/2-1 hour after eating; may be up to 3-4 hours
104 ☐ Mucous colitis or "irritable bowel"
105 ☐ Gas shortly after eating
106 ☐ Stomach "bloating" after eating

GROUP SEVEN

(A)

107 ☐ Insomnia
108 ☐ Nervousness
109 ☐ Can't gain weight
110 ☐ Intolerance to heat
111 ☐ Highly emotional
112 ☐ Flush easily
113 ☐ Night sweats
114 ☐ Thin, moist skin
115 ☐ Inward trembling
116 ☐ Heart palpitates
117 ☐ Increased appetite without weight gain
118 ☐ Pulse fast at rest
119 ☐ Eyelids and face twitch
120 ☐ Irritable and restless
121 ☐ Can't work under pressure

(B)

122 ☐ Increase in weight
123 ☐ Decrease in appetite
124 ☐ Fatigue easily
125 ☐ Ringing in ears
126 ☐ Sleepy during day
127 ☐ Sensitive to cold
128 ☐ Dry or scaly skin
129 ☐ Constipation
130 ☐ Mental sluggishness
131 ☐ Hair coarse, falls out
132 ☐ Headaches upon arising, wear off during day
133 ☐ Slow pulse, below 65
134 ☐ Frequency of urination
135 ☐ Impaired hearing
136 ☐ Reduced initiative

(C)

137 ☐ Failing memory
138 ☐ Low blood pressure
139 ☐ Increased sex drive
140 ☐ Headaches, "splitting or rending" type
141 ☐ Decreased sugar tolerance

(D)

142 ☐ Abnormal thirst
143 ☐ Bloating of abdomen
144 ☐ Weight gain around hips or waist
145 ☐ Sex drive reduced or lacking
146 ☐ Tendency to ulcers, colitis
147 ☐ Increased sugar tolerance
148 ☐ Women: menstrual disorders
149 ☐ Young girls: lack of menstrual function

(E)

150 ☐ Dizziness
151 ☐ Headaches
152 ☐ Hot flashes
153 ☐ Increased blood pressure
154 ☐ Hair growth on face or body (female)
155 ☐ Sugar in urine (not diabetes)
156 ☐ Masculine tendencies (female)

GROUP SEVEN *(continued)*

(F)

157 ☐ Weakness, dizziness
158 ☐ Chronic fatigue
159 ☐ Low blood pressure
160 ☐ Nails weak, ridged
161 ☐ Tendency to hives
162 ☐ Arthritic tendencies
163 ☐ Perspiration increase
164 ☐ Bowel disorders
165 ☐ Poor circulation
166 ☐ Swollen ankles
167 ☐ Crave salt
168 ☐ Brown spots or bronzing on skin
169 ☐ Allergies—tendency to asthma
170 ☐ Weakness after colds, influenza
171 ☐ Exhaustion—muscular and nervous
172 ☐ Respiratory disorders

GROUP EIGHT A: Female Only

173 ☐ Easily fatigued
174 ☐ Premenstrual stress
175 ☐ Painful menses
176 ☐ Depressed feelings before menstruation
177 ☐ Menstruation excessive
178 ☐ Painful breasts
179 ☐ Menstruate too frequently
180 ☐ Vaginal discharge
181 ☐ Hysterectomy/ovaries removed
182 ☐ Hot flashes
183 ☐ Menses scanty or missed
184 ☐ Acne, worse at menses
185 ☐ Depression long-standing

GROUP EIGHT B: Male Only

186 ☐ Prostate trouble
187 ☐ Urination difficult or dribbling
188 ☐ Night urination frequent
189 ☐ Depression
190 ☐ Pain on inside of legs or heels
191 ☐ Feeling of incomplete bowel evacuation
192 ☐ Lack of energy
193 ☐ Migrating aches and pains
194 ☐ Tire too easily
195 ☐ Avoid activity
196 ☐ Leg nervousness at night
197 ☐ Diminished sex drive

GROUP NINE

198 ☐ Sleepy after meals
199 ☐ Bloated after meals
200 ☐ Poor concentration after meals
201 ☐ Diabetes in family
202 ☐ High blood pressure, cholesterol, or triglycerides
203 ☐ Always hungry
204 ☐ Fingers swollen or tight after exercise
205 ☐ Heart disease, stroke, breast cancer in family

GROUP TEN

206 ☐ Aspirin improves symptoms
207 ☐ Menstrual cramps
208 ☐ Chronic inflammation
209 ☐ Dry itchy skin or scalp
210 ☐ React badly to sweets or excess carbohydrates
211 ☐ Eat restaurant or fast food often
212 ☐ Spring allergies

GROUP ELEVEN

213 ☐ Low blood pressure
214 ☐ Poor circulation
215 ☐ Slow metabolism
216 ☐ Intolerant to noise
217 ☐ Slow or irregular heartbeat
218 ☐ Headaches with feeling of tight band around head
219 ☐ Carbohydrate intolerance

GROUP TWELVE

220 ☐ Tense, irritable, and high-strung
221 ☐ High blood pressure
222 ☐ Poor fat metabolism
223 ☐ Restless, jumpy, and shaky legs
224 ☐ Overreact to caffeine
225 ☐ Tendency to spasm
226 ☐ Rapid heartbeat

(continued)

Form 7.2 Symptom Survey *(continued)*

Important: Please list below the five main complaints you have in order of their importance.

1. ____

2. ____

3. ____

4. ____

5. ____

(Please do not write below this line.)

Doctor's notes:

Form 7.3 Nutrition Questionnaire

Name ______________________ Case No. ________ Age ________ Sex ________

1. Are you taking medication? . . . . Yes ________ No ________
   If yes, list the kind and dosage and whether it is taken on a regular basis. ______________________
   ____
   ____
   ____
   Do you feel the medication is helping you? ______________________
2. Are you taking nutritional supplements? . . . . Yes ________ No ________
   If yes, list the kind and dosage and whether they are taken on a regular basis. ______________________
   ____
   ____
   ____
   Do you feel the nutritional supplements are helping you? For example, do you notice a specific improvement in the way you feel? ______________________
3. Approximately how many regular-size drinking glasses of water do you drink per day? ________
   Is the water usually regular tap water, or special water such as distilled or well water? ______________________
   ____
4. If you are a smoker, what do you smoke (cigarettes, pipe, etc.) and how many daily? ______________________
   ____
5. How often do you consume alcohol?
   Never ________ Once in a while ________ Often ________ Daily ________
6. How many cups of regular coffee (caffeinated) do you drink daily? ________
7. How many cups of decaffeinated coffee do you drink per day? ________
8. How many cups of tea or glasses of iced tea do you drink per day? ________
9. Approximately what percentage of your food is of the "convenience" variety? (Examples: Hamburger Helpers, TV dinners, frozen pot pies, etc.) ______________________
10. When you eat out, do you prefer the "quick food" approach, such as McDonald's, Burger King, etc? ________________
    ____
11. Do you use extra salt on your food at the table? . . . . Yes ________ No ________
12. Do you eat a lot of condiments such as catsup and other spicy foods? . . . . Yes ________ No ________
13. Do you like sour foods such as lemon (unsweetened), dill pickles, and other pickled foods? Yes ________ No ________
14. Do you avoid or cut fat from your meat? . . . . Yes ________ No ________
15. Do you use butter or margarine? . . . . Yes ________ No ________
16. Do you like oil-type dressings on your salad? . . . . Yes ________ No ________
17. Do you enjoy eating cheese? . . . . Yes ________ No ________
18. Do you drink milk? . . . . Yes ________ No ________
    How much per day? ___________ Is it pasteurized? . . . . Yes ________ No ________
19. Do you like foods that have a high sugar content, such as pastries, donuts, etc.? . . . . Yes ________ No ________
20. When you eat a donut, do you prefer to have it plain, with frosting, or filled? ______________________
21. Do you eat sugar-coated cereal? . . . . Yes ________ No ________
    When you eat cereal, how many teaspoons of sugar do you use on an average-size serving? ________
22. How many teaspoons of sugar do you use in coffee or tea? ________
23. How many soft drinks do you consume daily? ________

(continued)

Form 7.3 *(continued)*

24. Do you try, as often as possible, to drink sugar-free soft drinks and use artificial sweeteners with coffee and food? . . . . Yes ________ No ________
25. What kind of fruit do you prefer to eat? . . . . Fresh ________ Canned ________ Sugar-free ________
26. Do you often feel hungry, no matter how much you eat? . . . . Yes ________ No ________
27. When you eat bread, is it white or whole wheat? ________
28. Do you usually eat breakfast? . . . . Yes ________ No ________
29. Do you usually feel better after eating? . . . . Yes ________ No ________
30. Do you usually feel worse after eating? . . . . Yes ________ No ________
31. Do you snack a lot between the three major meals? . . . . Yes ________ No ________
32. When you have a snack, what type of food do you prefer? For example, sweet roll, cookies, cheese, crackers, fruit, vegetables. ________
33. Do you frequently skip meals? . . . . Yes ________ No ________
34. Do you have to watch what you eat to avoid gaining weight? . . . . Yes ________ No ________
    Do you have to watch what you eat to avoid losing weight? . . . . Yes ________ No ________
35. Do you have more than one meal per day that lacks a vegetable other than corn, potatoes, peas, or green beans? . . . . Yes ________ No ________
36. Are there days when you do not eat any raw vegetables? . . . . Yes ________ No ________
37. Do any foods seem to irritate you in some way? . . . . Yes ________ No ________
    If yes, name the foods and describe the problem. ________
38. What foods do you especially like? ________
39. What foods do you dislike? ________
40. Do you feel that your diet is excessive in some respect? . . . . Yes ________ No ________
    If yes, describe. ________
41. Do you feel your diet is deficient in some respect? . . . . Yes ________ No ________
    If yes, describe. ________

Notes ________

Form 7.4 Dietary Analysis

So that your diet can be accurately evaluated, write down everything you eat for one week. It is important to put down *everything,* including snacks, candy, coffee, and the amount of water you drink. Include the approximate amounts of the food, such as 2 tbsp. peas; 1 large hamburger patty; small glass orange juice. If the information is not typical of your normal diet—for example, if you are not feeling well and your appetite is poor—include this information either in the block for that day or attach an additional page.

1st day—	2nd day—	3rd day—	4th day—	5th day—	6th day—	7th day—
Date ________	Date ________	Date ________	Date ________	Date ________	Date ________	Date ________
Breakfast	Breakfast	Breakfast	Breakfast	Breakfast	Breakfast	Breakfast
Snack	Snack	Snack	Snack	Snack	Snack	Snack
Lunch	Lunch	Lunch	Lunch	Lunch	Lunch	Lunch
Snack	Snack	Snack	Snack	Snack	Snack	Snack
Supper	Supper	Supper	Supper	Supper	Supper	Supper
Snack	Snack	Snack	Snack	Snack	Snack	Snack

Reprinted, by permission, from D. Walther, 1988, *Nutrition questionnaire* (Pueblo, CO: Systems DC).

8

Functional Testing and Interpretation

Certain tests not commonly applied (or no longer used) in mainstream medicine may give general clues about the patient's functional state. These evaluations have been used in complementary medicine for many years and can be performed by a trained assistant, paraprofessional, or practitioner, depending on local laws that may govern their scope and usage. When taken individually, none of these tests should be construed as having significant meaning. Rather, they are meant to complement other findings made by the practitioner or signs and symptoms of the patient.

These tests are reproducible and therefore can be used throughout a treatment period with confidence for the purpose of comparison and to measure treatment efficacy. Although the main reason for utilizing these tests is to obtain more information about the functional status of the patient, in some cases, such as measuring exercise blood pressure in normotensive individuals, the observation of dysfunction may also predict potential future disease (Mundal et al. 1994). Some tests described here are routine office assessments; these are suggested for use during every new patient examination and some follow-up evaluations. Others are more specialized and are useful in certain kinds of cases as described further on.

ROUTINE OFFICE ASSESSMENTS

It is recommended that routine office assessments be part of each initial examination, as they may provide clues to the patient's functional state and are relatively accurate and reproducible. They can also provide a relatively objective marker for patient progress. Tests showing results that are not within normal limits can be repeated on each visit until the patient shows a normal test for three or more visits. In some cases, repeating all the tests periodically may be helpful.

Postural Blood Pressure

In addition to blood pressure measurements to rule out hyper- and hypotension, evaluation of potential orthostatic hypotension and its functional orthostatic hypotension is important for patients in a complementary sports medicine practice. The standard position for measuring blood pressure is with the patient seated with feet flat on the floor; the left arm is used. After this, the assessment method to rule out postural hypotension involves measuring blood pressure in the lying position first and then immediately measuring it in the standing position. A decrease or lack of increase especially in the systolic blood pressure on standing should be considered abnormal. Pressure measurements can vary, depending on the patient's structural, chemical, and mental/emotional state, and it is recommended that postural pressures be evaluated on each visit on all patients. Results should be carefully recorded for future comparisons. Berkow (1992) defines orthostatic hypotension as a fall in blood pressure of about 20/10 mmHg on assuming an upright posture. This is not a disease but rather a dysfunction of the mechanisms involved in regulating blood pressure. Functional aspects of this condition are much more common and can be seen with a fall of less than 20/10 mmHg. Normally, the postural change (increased gravity stress) results in an increase in systolic blood pressure of approximately 8 mmHg (Walther 1988). Failure of this rise is sometimes referred to as orthostatic hypotension, postural hypotension, or Ragland's sign.

The mechanisms involved in the normal changes of blood pressure include pooling of blood in the vessels of the abdomen and pelvis, which lowers the heart rate. The body compensates with increased baroreceptor activity in the aortic arch and carotid bodies, which speeds up the heart rate and raises blood pressure. This compensation is due to a sympathetic-mediated vasomotor response and an increase in catecholamines, predominantly norepinephrine.

Other hormonal activity—including that of aldosterone from the adrenal cortex—is followed by a slight sodium and water retention. According to Berkow (1992), "When hormonal responses are faulty, these homeostatic mechanisms may be inadequate for restoring the lowered blood pressure" (p. 434). If blood pressure is not compensated upon standing, the lack of orthostatic tolerance may cause the patient to experience light-headedness; but other symptoms may include visual changes, head and neck discomfort, palpitations, anxiety, and in some cases syncope (Jacob et al. 1997). De Lorenzo et al. (1997) discuss the association of orthostatic hypotension with chronic fatigue syndrome; highly trained athletes have this problem more often than average fit individuals (Convertino 1993).

Patients with orthostatic hypotension may have a number of problems. Ruling out people with serious conditions (such as hypovolemia and central nervous system disorders) and drug side effects (from diuretics, antihypertensives, and monoamine oxidase inhibitors), as well as others reacting adversely to nonsteroidal anti-inflammatory drugs (NSAIDs) (which may cause renal sodium retention and inhibition of vasodilation by prostaglandins), the relatively healthy patient may often have a functional adrenal problem as described by Walther (1988). Orthostatic hypotension is common in patients with chronic autonomic failure and is especially aggravated with the ingestion of large meals (Puvi-Rajasingham and Mathias 1996). Yang and Chang (1990) showed that disease-free patients with orthostatic hypotension had normal epinephrine levels in the recumbent posture but that this adrenal hormone failed to rise upon standing. Polinsky et al. (1980) studied 16 patients with orthostatic hypotension; 12 had deficient plasma catecholamine responses to hypoglycemia, and of these, 7 had almost no plasma epinephrine response.

Frequently, patients with orthostatic hypotension will manifest other signs or symptoms relating to functional adrenal problems. These include symptoms in Group Three (blood sugar dysfunction) and Group Seven F (adrenal dysfunction) on the Symptom Survey shown in the previous chapter, especially an increased craving for salt. Researchers suggest salt as the first line of treatment in some patients with orthostatic intolerance.

McCarthy et al. (1997) showed that despite increases in blood volume (which is expected to improve orthostatic tolerance), resistance training did not improve orthostatic tolerance. Levine (1993) discussed the frequent association between orthostatic hypotension and long-term endurance-trained athletes. Raven and Pawelczyk (1993) showed that those endurance athletes with higher $\dot{V}O_2max$ levels (above 65 ml × kg^{-1} × min^{-1}) were more likely to have an intolerance to orthostatic hypotension. These findings support results of authors who observed that more than half of new patients had some degree of orthostatic hypotension.

Exercise Blood Pressure

Another important blood pressure assessment can be made during exercise. Exercise blood pressure normally increases with the type of exercise and correlates with intensity. In most test situations, an increased systolic pressure may be as high as 180-190 mmHg, with diastolic changes increasing by less than 10 mmHg. Exaggerated blood pressure responses in normotensive patients may be considered a predictor of future hypertension (Nazar et al. 1997). These blood pressure increases during exercise are in the range of >200 mmHg for systolic pressure at a workload of 150 W. These patients also show slightly higher cortisol and catecholamine levels and relatively higher heart rates, possibly indicating an early stage of overtraining. Mundal et al. (1994) showed that rises in systolic pressure of 48.5 mmHg during bicycle ergometer exercise at a workload of only 100 W was a significant predictor of cardiovascular mortality. Occasionally, a diminished blood pressure increase takes place during exercise. This poor exercise response may be due to a diminished cardiac reserve (McArdle et al. 1991).

Oral pH

The use of pH paper in the office setting permits a simple test that can be performed on each athlete. Allow at least 10-15 min after the patient has had anything to eat or drink and have the patient moisten a small (at least 1 cm) strip of pH paper with saliva for about 5 sec. Compare the color change with the color-coded indicators on the pH dispenser. Record the pH in the patient's file and recheck regularly.

The oral pH is regulated by the pH of the saliva and to a lesser degree by food remnants. According to Mayes (1993), the pH of the saliva is usually about 6.8 but may vary on either side of neutral; on the other hand, lingual gland fluid pH may be as high as 7.5. Hendrix (1974) states that salivary amylase is active up to a pH of 11.0. The salivary pH as it relates to and reflects body function has been used in complementary medicine since Hawkins (1947), a dentist, first described it. His claims have been clinically validated through many years of use. Hawkins theorized that in the adult, salivary pH should be approximately 7.6, and in children slightly higher, 7.8. At these levels, very little tooth decay or periodontal disease occurred. If the pH was above or below this level, Hawkins proposed that certain dietary changes would help return the pH to its normal levels. If the pH is above 7.6, patients should add more carbohydrate foods—potatoes, fruits, cereals, breads, and grains. If the pH is below 7.6, more protein foods (meats, fish, cheese), fats, and oils are recommended.

Improvements in pH may take up to several weeks depending on what changes are required to correct the imbalances causing the abnormal pH. It may be associated with diet, exercise training, stress factors, and nutritional needs. It is possible, however, sometimes to quickly change oral pH after one session, especially when treatment results in improved autonomic nervous system balance.

The state of the autonomic nervous system has a significant effect on salivary quality and quantity. Anderson et al. (1984) showed that parasympathetic stimulation produced large amounts of saliva low in protein, whereas sympathetic stimulation evoked lesser amounts of saliva high in protein. Asztely et al. (1996) demonstrated that circulating catecholamines from adrenal, extraadrenal, and extragland-ular sources reduced parotid acinar granules in rats. Chorot et al. (1992) found an inverse relationship between heart rate and salivary pH, possibly demonstrating a reduced pH in those with increased sympathetic activity. This low pH may be an important finding in the early, functional stages of overtraining.

These dietary recommendations also seem to correlate very well with the metabolic state of the individual. Unpublished data by the author comparing salivary pH with respiratory quotient showed that people with a higher respiratory quotient generally had a lower salivary pH, indicating that those who utilized more carbohydrates and less fats for energy (as indicated by a higher respiratory quotient) had a lower salivary pH.

Temperature

Body temperature is another easy measurement that can be made initially; it is a good general screening measurement. Taking the oral (under the tongue) temperature will show a normal temperature of 37 °C (98.6 °F), an above-normal reading, or a below-normal reading. Rectal temperatures are typically 0.6 °C (1 °F) higher than oral readings. Normal daily variations of perhaps a few tenths may exist, with morning readings being the lowest and late-afternoon temperatures the highest. Nighttime temperatures may also drop slightly, and stimulate sleep onset (Murphy and Campbell 1997).

In addition to measurement of the patient's temperature in the office, axillary temperatures can be recorded by some patients at home for several days up to one month. In some patients, below-normal temperatures may occur only at certain times of the week or month. Form 8.1 is a form commonly used by patients to record basal axillary temperatures at home. In this instance, the patient takes his or her temperature in the morning upon awakening, before getting out of bed. Once the person gets up to move around, body temperature may rise slightly. Patients are instructed to keep the thermometer under the armpit for a full 10 min and to record the result on the chart. The basal axillary temperature range is 36.5 to 36.7 °C (97.8 to 98.2 °F) (Barnes and Barnes 1972).

Raised Temperature

Temperatures above normal may indicate infection, inflammation, or other serious problems (although in the very young and elderly, and in some alcoholics, infections or inflammation may lower body temperature). A higher-than-normal temperature in an athlete may indicate a need for rest. Above-normal temperature is a strong indication to cease all training until the problem is found or the temperature returns to normal. The only exception would be immediately after training or competition. For example, distance runners can have very high rectal temperatures of 41 °C (over 105 °F) after races of 5000 m, or after about 12 to 15 min of maximum effort (McArdle et al. 1991). Increases in core temperature most likely reflect the normal compensation for intense activity. Saltin and Hermansen (1966) found that increases in body temperature paralleled oxygen (O_2) uptake and exercise intensity. Exercise at 50% $\dot{V}O_2$max can raise temperatures to about 37.3 °C (99 °F), and intensities of 75% $\dot{V}O_2$max can elevate temperatures to about 38.5 °C (101 °F). Patients who are working in a very physical job, people under emotional stress, and active children may also show slightly elevated temperatures (Guyton 1986). All these factors should be considered when temperature is assessed.

Lowered Temperature

Below-normal temperatures may indicate thyroid dysfunction or a subclinical hypothyroidism even when thyroid blood indexes are normal (Northover et al. 1983; Vana et al. 1990). Sehnert and Croft (1996) also showed that the temperature is a sensitive screening test, along with laboratory analysis, for the hypothyroidism seen following trauma, which they termed "posttraumatic hypothyroidism." These observations of the relationship between body temperature and thyroid dysfunction were initially made by Barnes (1942), who eventually associated this problem to cardiac dysfunction (Barnes and Barnes 1972). The relationship between subclinical thyroid dysfunction and cardiac performance has also been described by Foldes et al. (1987). Saito et al. (1983) showed a close relationship between hypothyroidism and hypertension.

Below-normal temperatures may be associated with symptoms noted by the patient on the Symptom Survey, Group Seven B. In addition to low temperature as a potential sign of a subclinical hypothyroid state, there are other symptoms that may be related to this imbalance. They include mental and physical fatigue, weight gain, depression, cold hands and feet, and crying spells. Those who feel good only after exercise stimulation may also have a subclinical hypothyroid condition. Skin problems are very common (skin that is dry and chapped with frequent cracking around the heels and on the hands), as is hair loss, especially thinning of the lateral one-third of the eyebrow.

Nonsteroidal anti-inflammatory drugs, including aspirin, inhibit prostaglandin production, which can affect thermoregulation (Murphy et al. 1996) with the result of decreasing body temperature.

Form 8.1 Basal Temperature

Case No. ____________ Name ______________________________________ Dates started/ended______________________

Directions

1. Shake down your thermometer and put it close to your bed.
2. Before getting up in the morning, put the thermometer in your armpit touching the skin.
3. Keep it there for 10 minutes; minimize movement. Read your temperature and record it.
4. Indicate the first and last days of your menstrual cycle (if applicable).
5. If a day is skipped for any reason during the month of charting, note it on the chart.

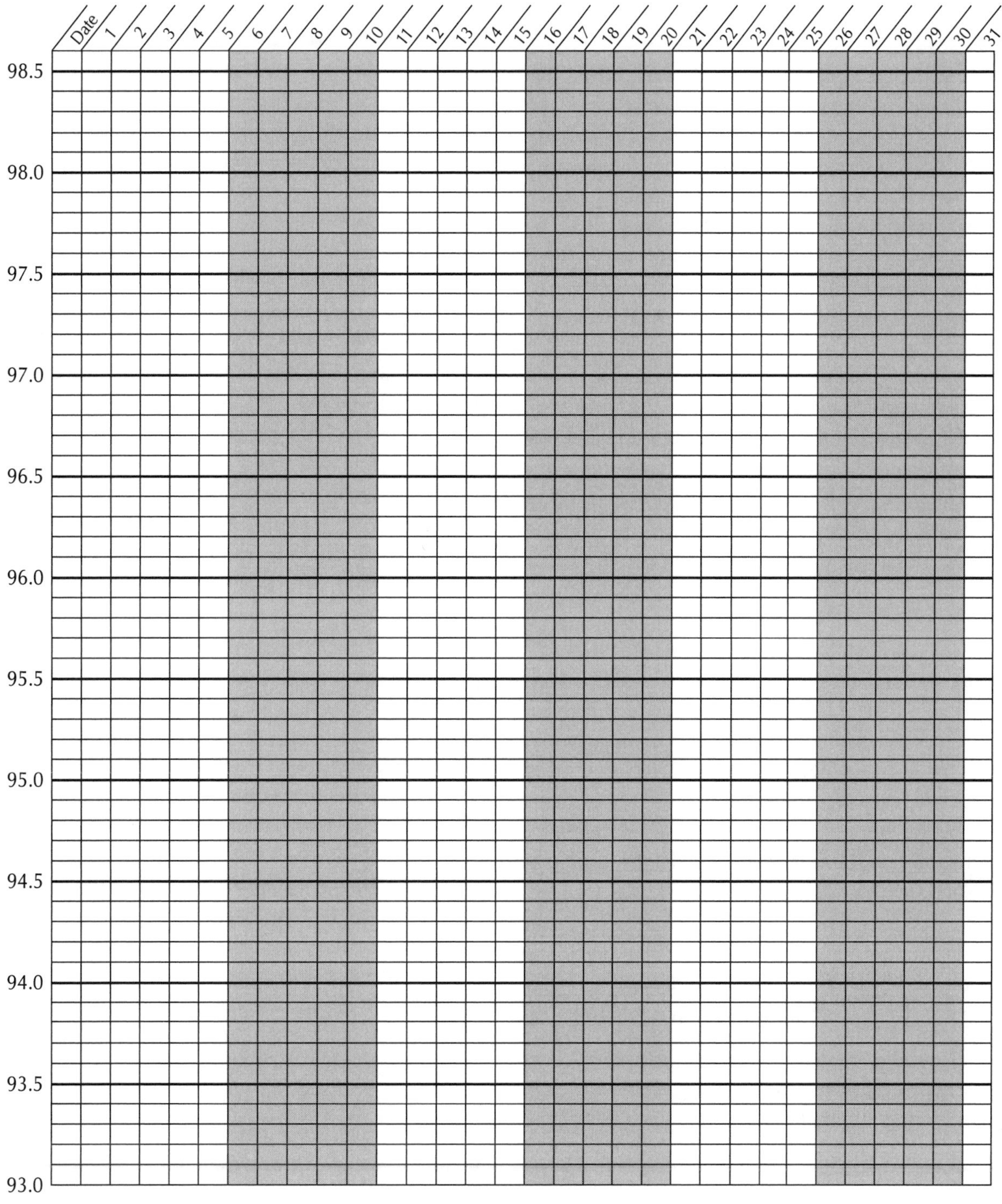

Reprinted by permission of AeroSport, Inc.

Training Effects

Inactive patients with thyroid dysfunction often have high respiratory quotient values and could benefit greatly from exercise, which raises body temperature. O'Malley et al. (1980) reported that raising body temperature had a positive influence on thyroid-stimulating hormones in hypothyroid patients. More importantly, thyroid hormones have a positive effect on mitochondrial function; Muller and Seitz (1984) showed that T3 (triiodothyronine) directly stimulated mitochondrial respiration and the synthesis of adenosine triphosphate (ATP).

Vital Capacity

The total volume of air that can be forcibly exhaled in one breath is called the forced vital capacity. This can be measured in the office or field setting with a small handheld spirometer. The vital capacity is differentiated from total lung capacity, which is the vital capacity plus the residual lung volume (the volume of air that remains in the lungs after forced exhalation); assessing total lung capacity requires more elaborate equipment. Also commonly measured is the forced expiratory volume in 1 sec (FEV1), which also requires more specialized equipment.

When measuring vital capacity in patients, it is best to do the testing in one posture, as different positions produce different results. The recommendation is the standing position whenever possible. Sitting postures produce lower vital capacity measurements. Patients should take as deep a breath as they can and exhale into the spirometer as hard, as fast, and as completely as possible. Perform three completed tests, recording all results. If the patient is unable to complete three tests, none of the measurements should be taken as valid. Spirometry measures the vital capacity in cubic centimeters (cc), which can then be converted to a percentage by considering the patient's height. The absolute vital capacity can be useful for monitoring each patient's progress. Tables for this conversion accompany spirometers.

Indication of Functional Capacity

Spirometry is used in complementary sports medicine as a general indicator of the functional capacity in patients, especially with regard to the strength of their respiratory muscles and pulmonary compliance (distensibility of the chest and lungs). Benfante et al. (1985) showed that vital capacity was directly associated with overall health. When the patient's pretreatment vital capacity is low, increased vital capacity after therapy is a general measure of success. Increases of 20% or more have frequently been observed by the author and other practitioners who measure vital capacity during the course of therapy. This increase can often be seen after one session of successful therapy. In addition, the author (Maffetone 1996) has found that brief exposures to a mild hyperbaric chamber (without added O_2) can increase vital capacity significantly.

Unfit patients with lowered vital capacity should be encouraged to start or increase exercise training. While training may not significantly change vital capacity, endurance training in older athletes appears to slow the decline with aging (Hagberg et al. 1988). More importantly, slowly warming up with low-intensity activity before training results in a significant increase in vital capacity during the training session (Kesavachandran and Shashidhar 1997), making training more efficient.

Generally, vital capacity significantly increases from late childhood through adolescence, independent of growth (Burrows et al. 1983). From late adolescence into the early to mid-30s, little change takes place, but by the mid-30s the vital capacity begins to diminish with age. Sparrow et al. (1993) showed that physiologic concentrations of cortisol may speed the deterioration of ventilatory function that occurs with aging. Hitsuda (1994) demonstrated a positive relationship between thyroid hormones (specifically T3) and vital capacity.

Exercise-Induced Asthma

Vital capacity may be useful in the assessment of exercise-induced bronchospasm or constriction, commonly called exercise-induced asthma. This condition is defined as a bronchial spasm or constriction, causing diminished airflow, with symptoms of wheezing, chest tightness, coughing, and difficulty breathing, that is triggered by exercise (Weiler 1996). Assessment of this condition can be made with an exercise challenge by measuring vital capacity before and after easy activity. As already noted, easy exercise should result in an increased vital capacity. In patients with exercise-induced asthma, the vital capacity does not increase after a warm-up of easy exercise, and the result is often a diminished vital capacity (Vacek 1997). In some cases, a hard effort may be necessary to allow observation of these abnormal changes (Schoene et al. 1997).

Other Dysfunctions

In addition to its relationship to health and fitness, vital capacity is associated with other factors and may indeed reflect dysfunction previous to the onset of more significant disease. Burchfiel et al. (1997) show that in men, vital capacity and other pulmonary function tests are negatively related to subscapular skinfold thickness, electrocardiogram abnormality, heart rate, white blood cell count, and eosinophil count, but positively related to height, grip strength, physical activity, and mean corpuscular hemoglobin concentration. A number of other health-related factors are also associated with vital capacity:

- An increased blood leukocyte count and diminished vital capacity are associated with increased total mortality (Weiss et al. 1995). Sparrow et al. (1984) also showed that the leukocyte count was inversely related to vital capacity.
- Vital capacity is inversely related to weight gain. Chen et al. (1993) showed that each kilogram of weight gain was associated with a loss of 26 ml in vital capacity.
- Nutritional factors are related to vital capacity. Van Antwerpen et al. (1995) showed a direct relationship between beta carotene levels and vital capacity in smokers. And Sparrow et al. (1982) found that copper was positively related to vital capacity.
- Lange et al. (1990) suggest that there is an accelerated decline in vital capacity at the onset of diabetes mellitus.
- Lower vital capacity is associated with the subsequent onset of hypertension (Sparrow et al. 1988).
- Chyou et al. (1996) reported that pulmonary function during middle age was a significant predictor of cognitive function later in life.
- There are a number of immune system associations with lowered vital capacity: increased levels of serum immunoglobulin (IgE) (Shadick et al. 1996), increased skin-test reactivity to common allergens (Gottlieb et al. 1996), and increased histamine response in the lungs (Rijcken et al. 1988).

In clinical practice, a portable, handheld spirometer to measure forced vital capacity is an accurate assessment tool (Rebuck et al. 1996). Measurements from these units should not be compared with measurements made with larger, more conventional devices. However, the accuracy of the smaller devices is echoed by Malmberg et al. (1993), who state, "The repeatability of the measurements with the pocket spirometer is close to that reported previously for flow-volume spirometry" (p. 89).

Breath-Holding Time

The breath-holding time, or breath-holding endurance, is a general test that measures respiratory reflexes and respiratory muscle function. It also reflects vital capacity (Feiner et al. 1995), is a valid measure of endurance of physical discomfort (Hajek 1989), is a simple test of respiratory chemosensitivity (Stanley et al. 1975), and can be used to measure the magnitude of dyspnea (Perez-Padilla et al. 1989). Evaluation of breath-holding time can be done early in the examination period—using the same postural position each time for consistency, since reevaluation will be necessary in some cases. The normal result used in complementary sports medicine for breath-holding time on inhalation is 50 sec. According to McArdle et al. (1991), breath-hold after normal exhalation is about 40 sec. Gay et al. (1994) showed that people who had pulmonary disease, those with congestive heart failure, and those who smoked had breath-holding times nearly half that of others without disease (25 sec vs. 45 sec); this study did not show any differences between breath-holding and age or sex. Taskar et al. (1995) demonstrated that breath-holding was lower in patients with sleep apnea compared to normal subjects, and Stanley et al. (1975) reported lower times in patients with chronic airway obstruction.

Breath-holding results are relatively consistent when obtained from visit to visit, but Barlett (1977) showed that the time can be increased with successive trials during a single session. Also, the Valsalva maneuver can increase breath-holding times. Alpher et al. (1986) reported that both a psychomotor task (hand dynamometer) and a mental performance task (mental arithmetic) during breath-holding increased the time. Madanmohan et al. (1992) found that 12 weeks of yoga significantly increased breath-holding time. Exercise training may improve breath-holding time, but only if the basic physical, chemical, or mental/emotional problems causing a low time have been corrected.

Waist-to-Hip Ratio

Tape measurement of the body can provide more information for the complementary sports medicine practitioner than scale weight alone. While a patient's weight has some significance, it is mostly a measure of water content, not percentage body fat or fat distribution. The waist-to-hip ratio is a measure of body fat distribution, and may reflect all-cause mortality including that from cardiovascular and noncardiovascular diseases (Duncan et al. 1995). Specifically, an abnormal ratio is often associated with carbohydrate intolerance.

Two separate tape measurements are required to obtain the waist-to-hip ratio: the first is a measure of the circumference of the patient's waist at the umbilicus (a), and the second is a measure of the hip circumference (b) (Nestler 1994). The ratio of a to b is noted (a divided by b). In men, a ratio greater than 0.9 and in women a ratio of 0.8 indicates android body type (sometimes referred to as android obesity—but many of these patients are relatively lean). The android body type is larger on top and is sometimes characterized as "apple shaped" in contrast to the gynecoid, or as a "pear-shaped" body type, which has a lower waist-to-hip ratio. In addition to inactive patients, many active, trained athletes have elevated waist-to-hip ratios.

Common Laboratory Tests

Traditional blood and urine tests are an integral part of a proper patient assessment in a complementary sports medicine practice. These include at least a complete blood count *and differential,* erythrocyte sedimentation rate, and a complete serum analysis. In addition, some patients may require further testing as an aid in the assessment process. C-reactive protein (a measure of inflammation), fasting insulin, glucose, and triglycerides (to consider carbohydrate metabolism disorders), and other values may provide additional vital information. Any abnormal or borderline result should be retested after a period of therapy.

As Bunch (1980) states, "Physicians are conditioned to interpret blood test results outside 'normal' limits as being signs of disease. In endurance-trained athletes, such 'abnormal' test results may instead be indications of physical activity" (p. 113). Bunch presents data illustrating that anemia, liver disease, myocardial ischemia, or renal disease might be diagnosed erroneously unless the physician is aware of the exercise habits of the patient. The most common example of this type of potentially misleading information is the levels of creatine kinase and creatine kinase MB band, which are released both after prolonged exercise and after an acute myocardial infarction. Staubli et al. (1985) showed that the levels of these two enzymes were similar in runners after a marathon and patients following an acute myocardial infarction.

Unfortunately, some patients have not been properly screened with laboratory evaluations. And some have previously been incompletely evaluated. In an evaluation of iron status, for example, in addition to the more common tests such as hemoglobin, hematocrit, and serum iron, a more comprehensive evaluation would include measuring ferritin, total iron-binding capacity and its percentage saturation, and transferrin.

While some athletes are truly anemic, practitioners should be cautious about presuming this condition in athletes on the basis of symptoms alone, especially in women, without having the benefits of laboratory results. Labeling athletes with traditional terms, such as "sports anemia," is contraindicated in many male and female athletes who more often have normal complete blood counts (Douglas 1989). Even some positive laboratory results may be an improper diagnosis because of when blood is drawn. Recent prolonged exercise may produce a "dilutional anemia" by increasing serum ferritin levels, masking a true iron deficiency; these changes may require up to six days to return to normal (Dickson et al. 1982). Scheduling and interpreting the patient's blood test should be done with care.

It should also be noted that blood tests for vitamins and minerals are commonly employed. However, these merely reflect a particular nutrient's level in the blood and not necessarily the level in the tissues. It is possible to have low tissue nutrient levels with normal blood tests (Miyajima et al. 1989) or deficient dietary intakes that are not reflected in a blood test (Lukaski and Penland 1996), which can adversely affect performance. The suggestion is that blood tests for nutrients may be useful as a screening process and *not* as an absolute indication of nutrient status.

Another common presumption made by some athletes and practitioners is that exercise automatically provides protection against conditions such as heart disease. As a result, sometimes certain tests are not performed. Blood tests in trained athletes to rule out potential disease are just as important as in people who are beginning an exercise program. Hubinger et al. (1995) failed to show, in athletes who averaged approximately 60 km (37 miles) per week, any improvements in lipoprotein(a). High concentrations of lipoprotein(a) are associated with increased risk of cardiovascular disease.

Body mass index, gender, and sport type are factors that may have varying degrees of relationship to blood test results. For example, Telford and Cunningham (1991) showed that hemoglobin concentration, hematocrit, and red cell count were higher in athletes with higher body mass index and that these measures varied between sports. Women generally had lower red blood indexes and higher white blood cell counts.

SPECIALIZED TESTS

In some situations, as the practitioner deems necessary, additional testing may be performed based on the patient's history and evaluations. This supplemental testing includes certain blood tests, the cold pressor test, salivary hormone evaluation, and respiratory quotient. These tests are used when additional information is needed regarding the patient's function.

Special Blood Tests

In certain groups of athletes, a higher incidence of some relatively uncommon problems is sometimes evident. In these cases, special blood or urine tests may be necessary. For example, lead levels may be a concern for patients who exercise in areas of high atmospheric lead. Orlando et al. (1994) found significantly higher blood lead levels in runners from various geographical locations in comparison to nonrunners. The levels in these runners significantly correlated with intensity and frequency of the workouts. Blood tests for lead may be important in such cases. Another example is kidney stones. Irving et al. (1986) found that marathon runners had a significantly higher incidence of renal stone formation than the general population. Urine tests for calcium may provide valuable information in these types of patients.

Other specialized blood tests may be used in patients suspected of having food sensitivities or allergies. Some patients absorb whole proteins resulting in the production of IgG, IgA, and IgE antibodies, which can be measured in the serum (Kolopp-Sarda et al. 1997). Common allergens include proteins from cow's milk, soy, and egg white. However, rather than routinely performing these tests, the practitioner may use them to verify the results of a good assessment process. In addition, proper treatment may eliminate most secondary food allergies, the type that is most common. Consequently these tests may be most useful in later sessions to assess any additional needs or in cases in which patients are not responding to the therapy.

Cold Pressor Test

The cold pressor test helps determine whether the patient has sympathetic dysfunction; it is performed if one suspects a significant autonomic imbalance. One of the patient's hands (up to the wrist joint) is immersed in ice water of about 8 °C (46 °F) for 2 min (Mishra and Mahajan 1996), and blood pressure is then measured. This produces a sympathetic/adrenergic reaction resulting in vasoconstriction, tachycardia, and transient hypertension and serves as a general test for vasomotor function and sympathetic responsiveness (van den Berg and Smit 1997). Shimizu et al. (1992) demonstrated a significant increase in both epinephrine and norepinephrine following the cold pressor test in normal subjects.

While the cardiovascular responses to the cold pressor test are reproducible (Rashed et al. 1997), there may be considerable individual differences (Fasano et al. 1996)—some resulting from fitness levels, diet (i.e., caffeine intake), stress, and other lifestyle factors at the time of the test. In general, some patients show higher levels of sympathetic drive and increased response to the adrenergic stimulation of the cold pressor test (Herkenhoff et al. 1994). Typically, patients who are more fit have higher muscle sympathetic nerve activity both at rest and during the cold pressor test (Ng et al. 1994), but their cardiovascular responses may be significantly attenuated (Brandon et al. 1991).

Individuals who *do not* exhibit an increase in blood pressure during or immediately after the cold pressor test may exhibit reduced sympathetic nervous system function (Sakai et al. 1996). As this test does not indicate what may be causing the dysfunction, the problem must be discovered by other assessment methods. In diabetes, the initial blood pressure response is significantly lessened (Luft et al. 1996). According to Sanderson et al. (1997), "In Syndrome X patients there is coronary endothelial dysfunction which is apparent in response to physiological stimuli induced by the cold pressor test" (p. 414). Instead of the normal dilation of the coronary arteries, these patients showed vasoconstriction with a significant decrease in blood flow.

Given the variety of factors associated with the cold pressor test, no normal ranges are established. However, Seals (1990) showed in healthy subjects that systolic blood pressure increased an average of 24 mmHg and heart rate increased an average of six beats with a 90-sec test using one hand. (In this same study, muscle sympathetic nerve activity increased by 187%.) Changes above or below these general numbers may indicate dysfunction in the sympathetic nervous system, hormonal system, or both.

Salivary Hormone Tests

It is possible to successfully and accurately measure certain hormone activity through saliva. Peters et al. (1982) showed that in the case of cortisol, salivary assay may provide results of greater diagnostic significance than plasma concentrations. Salivary profiles for specific hormones may be extremely useful in a complementary sports medicine practice; these include cortisol, DHEA(S), estrogens, progesterone, and testosterone—all measurable through salivary means. Salivary collection, as opposed to drawing blood, is also useful since it samples patients in their own environments rather than in a doctor's office, laboratory, or hospital, where they are often feeling added stress—which may affect the outcome of the test. In some cases, it may be most advantageous to measure these hormones four times over a 24-hr period. This is almost a priority for hormones such as cortisol, since cortisol level varies through the day and a patient may be normal in the morning but have a very high cortisol level at noon, at 4 P.M., or in the evening. In other cases, when regular hormone evaluation is necessary, such as during brief but high-stress training periods prior to a competitive season, the convenience of salivary testing is clear. In difficult cases, hormones such as estrogen can be measured for longer periods, for example during part or all of a menstrual cycle.

Impaired hormonal function may be a diagnostic marker for overtraining (Barron et al. 1985), a common problem in sport. Various hormone tests, including measures of cortisol, DHEA(S), and the testosterone/cortisol ratio, can be used as an indication of the anabolic/catabolic balance of the athlete (Urhausen et al. 1997). O'Connor et al. (1989) found that depression and cortisol levels were significantly higher during overtraining, and Ding et al. (1988) reported that high cortisol was also associated with exercise-related amenorrhea. This is in agreement with results of De Cree et al. (1995), who showed that high-intensity activities are associated with low estrogen. According to Keizer et al. (1989), DHEA(S) seems to be an even more useful marker during training than cortisol. Even patients with painful injuries, such as temporomandibular joint dysfunction, can show significantly higher cortisol levels due to pain (Jones et al. 1997).

Salivary samples are collected with a kit containing vials for each collection time. Each vial contains compact cotton. Patients place the cotton in the mouth, moisten it thoroughly, and place it back in the vial. When all samples have been taken, the kit is returned to the laboratory for evaluation. Avoidance of certain foods and drinks during the test period is specified by the laboratory in written instructions. Throughout this text we will consider functional imbalances associated with abnormal hormone levels, especially cortisol and dehydroepiandrosterone sulfate (DHEA[S]).

Respiratory Quotient

As noted earlier, the vast majority of our energy comes from the metabolism of carbohydrates and fats. About 40% of the breakdown of glucose and fatty acids is converted to adenosine triphosphate, with the remaining 60% being dissipated as heat. The conversion of glucose and fatty acids to energy depends on O_2 availability, with the reaction producing carbon dioxide (CO_2) and water; both of these gases are exchanged in the lungs. This pulmonary transaction normally equals the amount exchanged by the body's tissues (Wilmore and Costill 1994). Direct calorimetry measures this heat loss as a way to obtain information about energy production. This is expensive and not practical for the clinician, who can use indirect calorimetry to obtain similar information. Indirect calorimetry is a useful means of acquiring data on the amount of energy production from both glucose and fatty acids.

By measuring gas exchange in the lungs, that is, the CO_2 exhaled in relation to the O_2 consumed, it is possible to determine the amount of glucose and fatty acid used for energy during rest or activity. This ratio of CO_2 to O_2 is referred to as the respiratory quotient (RQ) or respiratory exchange ratio. During the complete oxidation of a molecule of glucose, six molecules of CO_2 are produced and six molecules of O_2 are consumed. The RQ, then, for glucose is determined: $6\ CO_2/6\ O_2 = 1.0$.

More O_2 is required to oxidize fat, with different fatty acids yielding slightly different results. Palmitic acid, for example, produces 16 CO_2 molecules for every 23 molecules of O_2: $16\ CO_2/23\ O_2 = 0.69$. The RQ for fat is usually considered to be 0.7. It is highly unlikely that a person would be utilizing 100% carbohydrate or 100% fat for energy (an RQ of 1.0 or 0.7); rather it will be a combination of the two that is used. Therefore, the RQ for a given individual is usually between 1.0 and 0.7. In chapter 2 we noted the importance of utilizing lower RQs for both endurance sports and overall health.

Table 8.1 Percentage of Kilocalories Derived From Carbohydrates and Fats

RQ	% Carbohydrates	% Fat
0.7	0	100
0.72	5	95
0.74	12	88
0.76	19	81
0.78	26	74
0.80	33	67
0.82	40	60
0.84	47	53
0.86	54	46
0.88	61	39
0.90	67.5	32.5
0.92	74	26
0.94	81	19
0.96	87	13
0.98	94	6
1.0	100	0

Adapted, by permission, from W. McArdle, F. Katch and V. Katch, 1991, *Exercise physiology,* 4th ed. (Baltimore: Williams & Wilkins), 153.

By means of the chart shown in table 8.1, the RQ can also be converted to a percentage of glucose and fatty acids used as energy, making it a more helpful tool for educating patients. For example, in a person obtaining about half of his or her energy from carbohydrates and half from fats, the RQ would be 0.85; 40% carbohydrates and 60% fats is an RQ of 0.82. This method of determining the percentage of kilocalories from carbohydrates and fats does not consider protein sources of energy (which are generally very small). Table 8.1 gives some of the nonprotein RQ equivalents as a percentage (McArdle et al. 1991).

Using Respiratory Quotient

The practitioner may have many reasons to use RQ as an assessment tool. It is an accurate method of determining substrate utilization; it ensures that the patient is building a high level of endurance; it monitors people attempting to lose body fat; and it may help assess imbalances in patients with recurrent structural, chemical, and mental/emotional injuries. It is also useful as a general screening tool and one that can be used for comparison with the Maximum Aerobic Function test described in chapter 13.

Testing with a gas analyzer at one time was an optional assessment due to reduced availability and expense. With the advent of portable, accurate equipment and lower costs, determining the RQ may be more practical and an evaluation to consider with many patients. Compact and user-friendly equipment enables practitioners to measure RQ with a gas analyzer in a clinical setting or sports environment (see figure 8.1). This technology allows the user to perform the test on a treadmill, on an ergometer, or on most exercise equipment (or at rest) and provides a printout of the results, which, in addition to RQ, may include heart rate, volume of oxygen ($\dot{V}O_2$), volume of carbon dioxide ($\dot{V}CO_2$), and other results depending on the specific type of equipment used. Table 8.2 is an example of a printout obtained with an AeroSport.

When evaluating patients with a gas analyzer, it is important to adhere to a strict protocol, especially in doing reevaluations. Time of day, previous meal, and training schedule relationships must be consistent. During the evaluation, warm-up, workload, heart rate, and other issues should be consistent. The type of footwear the patient is using should also be noted, as oversupported shoes affect O_2 uptake (Jorgensen 1990). Correlating the RQ with a specific heart rate helps adjust to these many variables. For example, measuring the monthly RQ at specific heart rates during treadmill running is an effective tool for a runner training for competition. As RQ decreases at the same heart rate, the pace should improve (i.e., speed should increase).

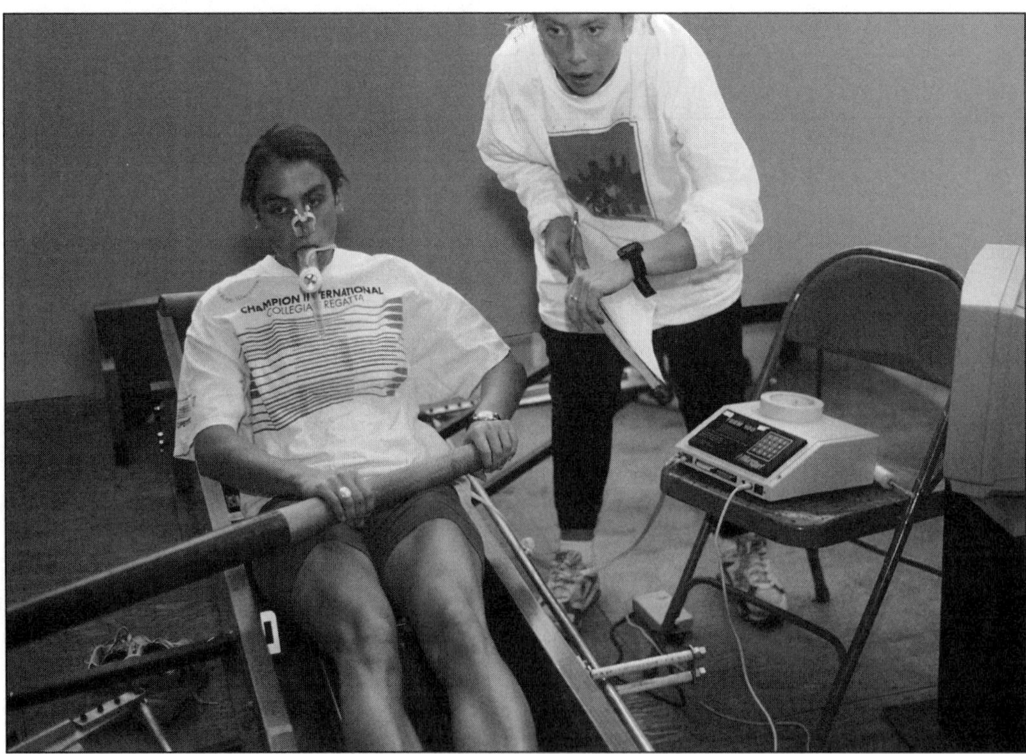

Figure 8.1 AeroSport gas analyzer
Reprinted by permission of AeroSport, Inc.

Table 8.2 AeroSport TEEM 100 Metabolic Analyzer

Patient ID# 1457	Weight kg 65.5 Height cm 175.3	Starting temp 20° Age 34 years	BP 734 mmHG Female
Predicted Values	BSA 1.892m^2 RMR 1450 kcal/24 hr	BMI 21.41 Max$\dot{V}O_2$ 1.85	BMR 33.53 MaxHR 186

Time	$\dot{V}O_2$	$\dot{V}CO_2$	VEs	RQ	VEb	CO_2%	O_2%	HR	TruO_2	O_2/kg	O_2/HR
1:20	1.03	.76	18.6	.74	23.4	4.14	15.67	120	5.56	15.7	8.6
1:40	.86	.65	15.7	.76	19.7	4.17	15.75	120	5.46	13.1	7.2
2:00	1.16	.89	20.6	.77	25.9	4.33	15.57	126	5.64	17.6	9.2
2:20	.98	.79	19.3	.81	24.2	4.11	16.04	126	5.10	14.9	7.8
2:40	.96	.79	18.7	.82	23.5	4.25	16.01	120	5.11	14.6	8.0
3:00	1.01	.84	19.8	.83	24.9	4.24	16.03	120	5.08	15.4	8.4
3:20	.94	.77	19.6	.82	24.6	3.96	16.32	132	4.79	14.3	7.1
3:40	1.13	.93	23.0	.82	28.9	4.09	16.18	132	4.93	17.2	8.6
4:00	1.13	.93	22.2	.82	27.9	4.23	16.03	135	5.09	17.2	8.4
4:20	1.15	.95	22.8	.83	28.6	4.20	16.08	138	5.03	17.5	8.3
4:40	1.38	1.15	27.7	.83	34.8	4.17	16.13	135	4.97	21.0	10.2
5:00	1.17	1.02	24.9	.87	31.3	4.14	16.34	144	4.72	17.8	8.1
5:20	1.25	1.11	26.5	.89	33.3	4.23	16.33	138	4.71	19.0	9.1
5:40	1.31	1.12	26.5	.85	33.3	4.28	16.13	144	4.95	19.9	9.1
6:00	1.36	1.20	28.6	.88	35.9	4.23	16.28	147	4.77	20.7	9.3
6:20	1.29	1.17	29.6	.91	37.2	3.98	16.66	153	4.35	19.6	8.4
6:40	1.68	1.52	36.9	.90	46.3	4.14	16.47	162	4.55	25.5	10.4
7:00	1.63	1.48	35.4	.91	44.5	4.22	16.42	159	4.59	24.8	10.3
7:20	1.84	1.72	41.0	.93	51.5	4.23	16.51	168	4.48	28.0	11.0
7:40	1.77	1.74	40.6	.98	51.0	4.33	16.58	168	4.36	26.9	10.5

Total calories = 95.31

Total grams fat = 2.27

Total grams CHO = 17.97

Peak $\dot{V}O_2$ = 2.66 and is 144% predicted

BP = barometric pressure; BSA = body surface area; BMI = body mass index; BMR = basal metabolic rate; RMR = resting metabolic rate; HR = heart rate; VEs = expired ventilatory volume per minute-BTPS (body temperature pressure standard); VEb = expired ventilatory volume per minute-STPD (standard temperature pressure dry); TruO_2 = true oxygen %; %CHO = % carbohydrate expended.

Table 8.3 The Relationship Between Heart Rate and Respiratory Quotient in a Highly Aerobically Fit Athlete

Heart rate	RQ
104	.74
114	.75
124	.79
127	.80
135	.82
137	.83
141	.84
153	.85
155	.87
169	.90

Table 8.3 shows actual relationships between an athlete's heart rate and RQ. Applying these ideas is very simple and is helpful especially for the practitioner who does not have a gas analyzer.

With the ease and convenience of these measurements come some limitations. As already mentioned, these determinations do not consider the protein contribution to energy. This can be determined by measuring nitrogen loss in urine and sweat, which is not possible for the average practitioner (and usually not necessary). Since the amount of energy derived from protein is very small, especially under the conditions of measuring RQ, this error becomes relatively insignificant.

Measurements of RQ should be made only during submaximal exercise or at rest. During high-intensity workouts, the CO_2 produced in the lungs may not reflect the amounts in the tissues, perhaps because of the deep breathing that accompanies a hard effort. In addition, if the workout intensity is high enough to produce excess blood lactate (so that production is greater than the breakdown), tissue pH is lowered and the body attempts to raise the pH by producing more CO_2. Despite these relatively minor problems, RQ is an excellent assessment tool in the clinical environment.

Certain dietary or nutritional imbalances may adversely affect RQ. In patients whose aerobic system functioning is low, the ability to utilize fatty acids is also low. This is reflected in a higher RQ. Athletes with higher RQs may have a higher rate of injury; patients who adhere to an effective program including training, diet and nutrition, and other lifestyle factors typically show lower RQs. Those needing to decrease body fat can be monitored to ensure that the appropriate metabolic changes are taking place, and overall good health may be reflected in a lower RQ.

Individuals who are more aerobically developed are generally healthier and more fit. As aerobic function improves, the patient's overall health improves. This correlation was shown by Leaf and Allen (1988), who demonstrated the relationship between RQ and lipid profiles. Maffetone (1997) also showed a relationship between RQ and the patient's subjective complaints. Table 8.4 provides some examples of this relationship.

Table 8.4 The Relationship Between Patients' Respiratory Quotients (as a Percentage of Substrate Utilization) at Rest and Their Subjective Complaints

Patient	RQ as percentage fat and sugar	Complaints
JC	88% sugar, 12% fat	Extreme fatigue, insomnia, 45 lb overweight
BK	74% sugar, 26% fat	Afternoon and evening fatigue, asthma, headaches
JO	62% sugar, 38% fat	4 P.M. fatigue, seasonal allergies, 10 lb overweight
PS	55% sugar, 45% fat	Chronic, mild knee pain; indigestion
MK	42% sugar, 58% fat	Occasional low back pain
BE	37% sugar, 63% fat	None

In addition to the assessment tools described in this chapter, practitioners may wish to include other common tests, such as range of motion, split weight measurements, Master 2–step tests, and others. Without a complete picture of the patient's physical, chemical, and mental/emotional state, therapy becomes less focused and less specific, more random and more expensive. It is also likely to be less successful, and progression or regression will be more difficult to evaluate.

Table 8.5 is a review of the tests described in this chapter.

CONCLUSION

Determining dysfunction begins with clues from the patient during the history-taking process, with additional information from a document like the Symptom Survey and various tests. For example, a patient who complains of fatigue as a primary problem may have checked many symptoms in Group Seven F (hypoadrenia). This makes the practitioner think of a possible adrenal dysfunction as associated with the patient's fatigue. This information is further verified by a functional orthostatic hypotension. With more indicators pointing to adrenal dysfunction, the

Table 8.5 Routine Office and Special Assessments

Name of test	Procedure	Expected or normal	Possible abnormal
Postural BP	Take BP lying, then immediately standing	Increased systolic pressure by 8 mmHg	Functional or orthostatic hypotension
Exercise BP	Compare BP at rest and during exercise	<200 mmHg systolic <10 mmHg diastolic	Possible cardiac problem; possible future hypertension
Cold pressor test	Hand in ice water for 2 min	Increased systolic pressure by 20-25 mmHg Increased heart rate by 6-8 bpm	If >, ↑ sympathetic tone; if <, ↓ sympathetic tone
Oral pH	Measure pH of saliva	7.6 (7.8 in children)	If low, ↑ protein and oils in diet; if high, ↑ carbohydrates
Temperature	Measure temperature	Oral: 37 °C (98.6 °F) Axillary: 36.5-36.7 °C (97.8-98.2 °F)	If low, thyroid dysfunction; if high, infection-inflammation
Vital capacity	Use spirometer with patient standing	Varies with height	General indicator of overall health
Spirometric reading	Measure vital capacity after warm-up	Should increase	If no change or decrease following exercise, consider exercise-induced asthma
Breath-holding time	Patient takes deep breath and holds	50 sec	General indicator of respiratory function
RQ	Use gas analyzer to measure CO_2/O_2	0.7-1.0	% carbohydrate and fat utilization
Salivary hormones	Moisten cotton with saliva and send to lab	Laboratory parameters	Overtraining

practitioner can be more confident that this is a significant functional problem.

After effective history taking, composed of a dialogue and history forms, a complete examination should help the practitioner confirm and isolate causes of imbalances that may be producing signs and symptoms. This begins with some routine assessments, followed by a decision whether other special tests are necessary. Other assessments follow, including posture, gait, and muscle testing as well as other heart rate tests as described in subsequent chapters.

9

Assessing Posture, Gait, and the Neuromuscular System

Among the important examination procedures for the complementary sports medicine practitioner is the evaluation of posture and gait, and of the neuromuscular system that controls them. An imbalance of these mechanisms, usually initiated by neuromuscular dysfunction, can lead to injury, ill health, or poor athletic performance. Locating faulty muscles that distort posture and gait, and being able to successfully and quickly improve their function, are important goals of the practitioner. This process begins with proper assessment of the neuromuscular system using posture, gait, and manual muscle testing as a guide. This interactive assessment of function is a major aspect of complementary sports medicine.

NEUROLOGICAL INFLUENCES ON POSTURE AND GAIT

One goal of observing posture is to obtain clues about individual muscles or groups of muscles that are not functioning normally. While postural distortions are sometimes attributable to other problems, such as past bone trauma, growth irregularities, and poor posture, a significant number of postural imbalances are due to muscle dysfunction as indicated by postural improvements after a successful treatment. Guskiewicz et al. (1997) reported that after incurring head trauma, athletes fail to use their visual system effectively (visual dysfunction), altering posture, and that the return of postural stability may provide clinicians with a tool for determining when an athlete may safely return to competition.

The examples used here of postural distortion due to specific muscle imbalance may not always appear so clear in clinical practice since it is common for more than one muscle inhibition to be related to postural distortion. Nonetheless, this guide can be useful in helping the practitioner obtain important information from a patient's posture. In addition, because posture is the sum of all neuromuscular function, analysis of posture both before and after treatment in each session can serve as a useful measure of therapeutic efficacy. The clinician should expect a noticeable or preferably a significant improvement in posture after any successful therapy, since all remedial treatment induces specific changes in the nervous system that can ultimately affect posture. If these changes are positive, an improvement in posture will usually be noted; if they are negligible, little or no change may occur; and if they are negative, they may worsen posture.

Human posture, whether static or moving, is a synthesis of neuromuscular function, including proprioceptive, vestibular, and visual inputs. Any disturbance in that function can adversely affect function elsewhere in the body. A variety of other normal actions, listed next, may also have an effect on posture and gait. These are all vital aspects to take into account when one is evaluating the whole person. Consider the following examples:

- Specific proprioception from the dorsum of the foot plays a significant role in posture and gait (Guyton 1986). Depending on where pressure is placed on the dorsum of the foot during gait, certain muscles will contract to control posture. This is called the magnet reaction and may be useful for assessing foot dysfunction.
- Modern athletic footwear impairs normal proprioception from the foot (Robbins et al. 1995).
- Age also affects proprioception. Petrella et al. (1997) found that proprioception diminishes with age but that regular exercise may attenuate this decline.
- The position of the head, as described later, is also important for posture, and it is related to the interpretation of vestibular signals and eye gaze. Shupert and Horak (1996) showed that the vestibular system plays an important role in both head and trunk stabilization. Head position may also influence thermoregulatory muscle tonus (Meigal et al. 1996), and hyperventilation disrupts mechanisms mediating vestibular compensation (Sakellari et al. 1997).
- Exercise affects postural control mechanisms. High-intensity exercise diminishes proprioceptive function (Lattanzio et al. 1997). Lepers et al. (1997) reported that athletes made less effective use of vestibular inputs after running than after cycling. Saxton et al. (1995) demonstrated significant impairment of neuromuscular function from adversely affected proprioception that was evident for 48 hr after weight lifting.
- Posture and gait dysfunction can occur with a variety of illnesses. Athletes with upper respiratory infection and fever may develop mechanical stress due to increased stride length and range of motion (Weidner et al. 1997). Diabetics may have altered posture and gait due to sensory deficits in the feet (Simmons et al. 1997); decreased cerebral blood flow in Alzheimer's patients may also cause gait dysfunction (Nakamura et al. 1997).
- Certain drugs affect postural balance. Li et al. (1996) found that tricyclic antidepressants impaired postural reflexes.

These and other factors further emphasize the need for a complete history of the patient.

STATIC POSTURE

One effective and simple way to observe static posture in a clinical setting is with the use of a plumb line for reference (see figure 9.1). This device is a cord suspended from a fixed point above (i.e., from the ceiling), with a weight attached to the end of the cord and hanging freely close to the floor. Evaluation must be done on a level floor with the patient barefoot, wearing minimal clothing, and in as relaxed a position as possible. The patient's breathing should be maintained, since breath-holding may influence muscle function as indicated by increased postural sway (Jeong 1991).

Posterior View

When one observes patients from the posterior, the patient should stand with their back to the plumb line with its weight midway between the heels. Observe for deviations from the normal, optimal posture: head tilt (compare mastoid processes), high or low shoulder level, scapula positions, high or low iliac crest, pelvic rotation, upper and lower extremity rotation, upper and lower extremity adduction and abduction, foot pronation, the line of the Achilles tendon, and any spinal deviations (scoliosis, hyper- or hypolordosis). Also note any significant muscle asymmetry or excess lateral sway.

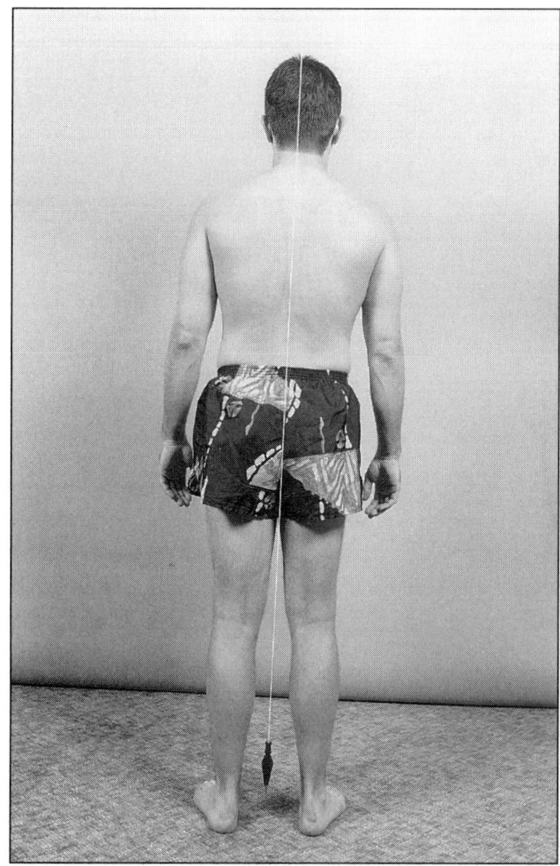

Figure 9.1 Observing a patient from the posterior using a plumb line

Lateral View

For observation of the lateral posture, on both left and right, the patient stands with the plumb line passing through a point just anterior to the lateral malleolus of the distal fibula (see figure 9.2). The plumb line should pass through the midcoronal plane, which hypothetically divides the body into anterior and posterior halves of equal weight. The plumb line should pass through the knee joint just anterior to its axis, just posterior to the hip joint, through the bodies of the lower lumbar vertebrae, and through the shoulder joint, the cervical vertebral bodies, and the external auditory meatus. Observe for and note any deviations from normal, including, among others, excess flexion or extension of the knee, shoulder, or elbow joints; abdominal protrusion; abnormality of breathing pattern; anterior-posterior sway; and excess spinal lordosis or kyphosis.

One should also observe from the anterior: the patient stands behind and faces the plumb line, with the plumb-line weight midway between the heels. The weight-bearing feet are more easily observed from this position; look at the toes, the arches (for excess pronation or supination), and any calluses. Observe femur rotation as indicated by the position of the patella; anterior or posterior tilt of the pelvis, shoulders, or head; or anterior or posterior position of the arms.

Examples of Postural Imbalance

Muscle inhibition is usually accompanied by a specific postural distortion, unless it is well compensated. A single muscle inhibition often creates a precise postural distortion, although looking at the effect of one muscle's inhibition on posture can be somewhat academic since there is usually more than one muscle inhibition at any one time and the body usually tries to compensate for any dysfunction. Both of these effects result in altered

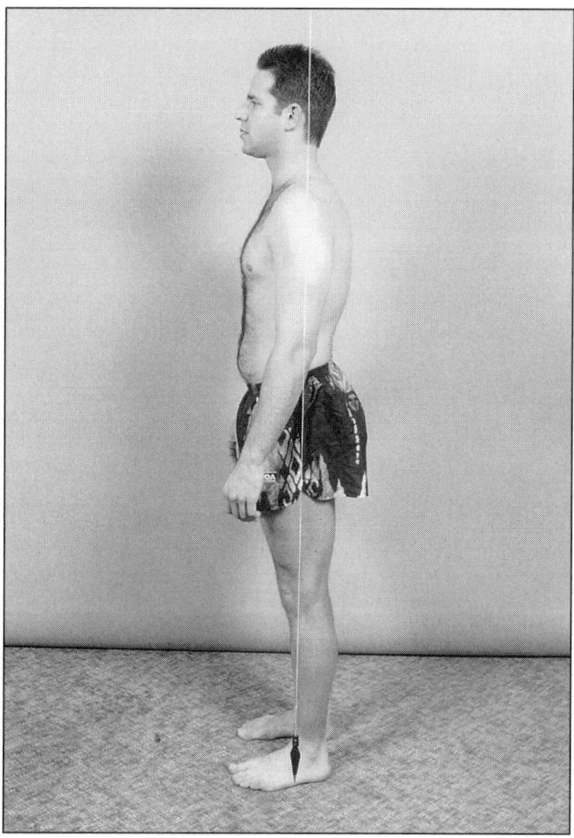

Figure 9.2 Observing the patient's lateral side using a plumb line

posture. Therefore, this discussion on postural imbalance is of general necessity, with potentially more than one postural distortion resulting from the same muscle imbalance. For example, psoas major muscle inhibition typically causes the pelvis to tilt. Specifically, the pelvis may rise on the side opposite the inhibition (i.e., the side of the overfacilitated psoas). However, in many cases, the reverse is true and the psoas inhibition is found on the side of the elevated pelvis. This may depend on which problem was primary and which secondary, how the foot reacts, what other muscles are compensating, and other factors.

When the practitioner observes a particular postural imbalance, the potential muscle inhibition associated with that imbalance can be manually tested to confirm or rule out the relationship. Normal posture is depicted in figure 9.3, and some of the more common distorted postures are represented in figures 9.4 through 9.23. All figures are shown from the patient's posterior to anterior or lateral as indicated. In these examples, one muscle is inhibited and the opposite one is overfacilitated or tight.

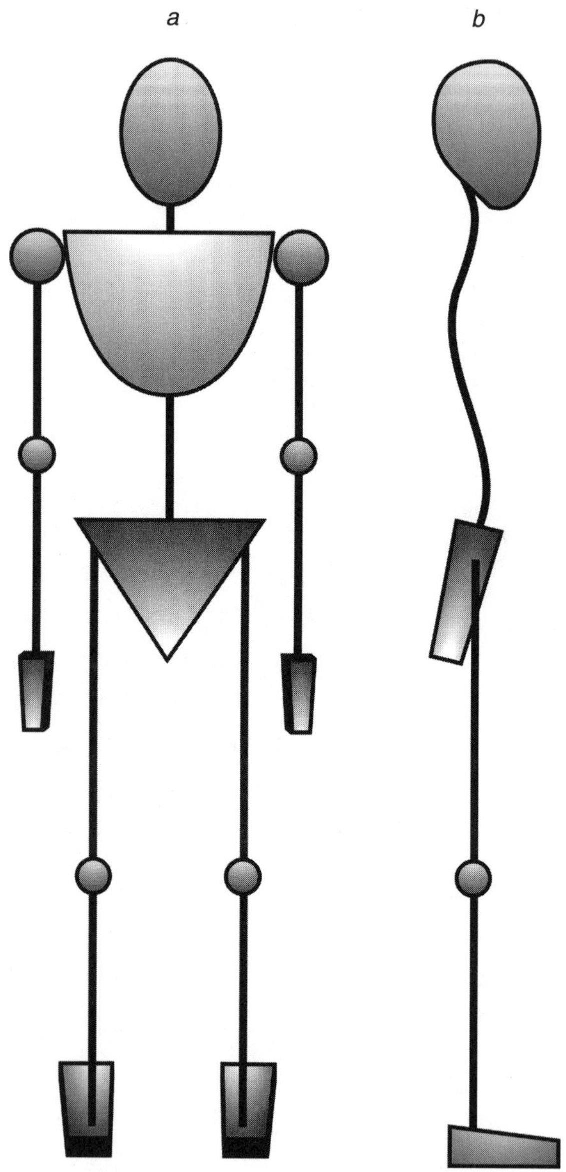

Figure 9.3a–b Normal posture depicted in (*a*) the posterior-to-anterior view and (*b*) the lateral view.

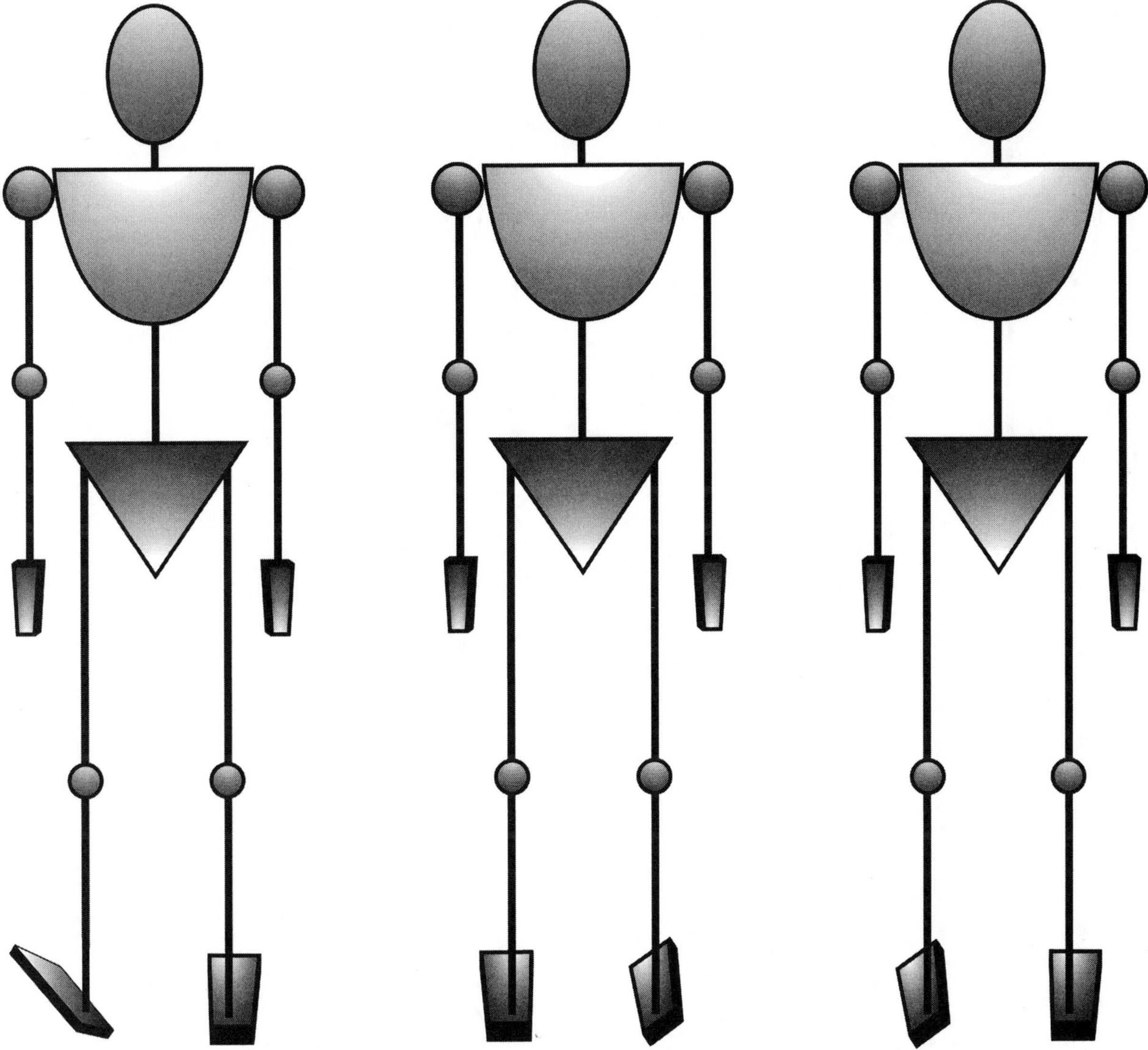

Figure 9.4 Inhibition of the left tibialis posterior may cause excess pronation and lateral foot rotation.

Figure 9.5 Right tibialis anterior inhibition may also result in excess pronation.

Figure 9.6 Left peroneus longus and brevis inhibition may allow excess supination.

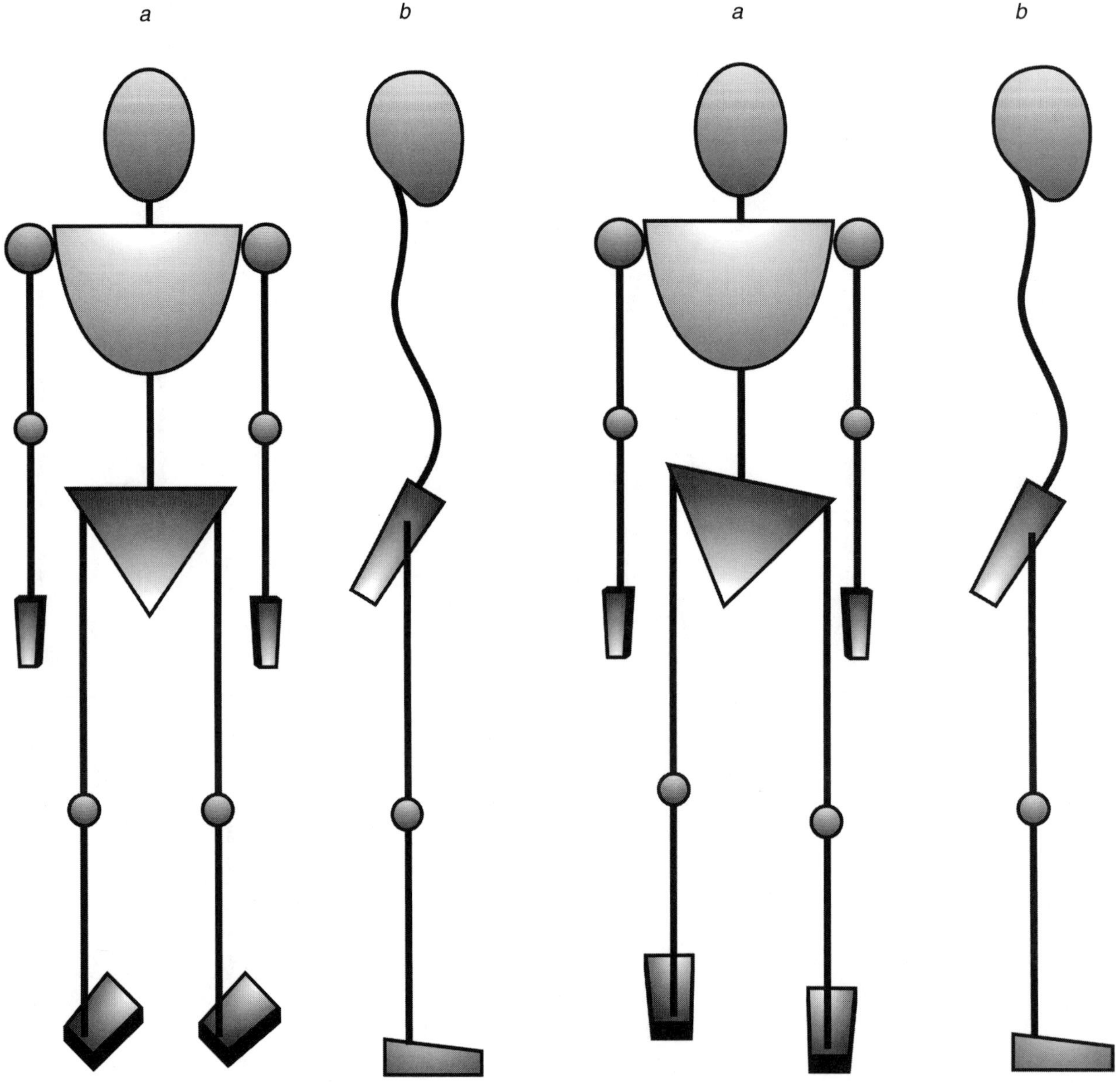

Figure 9.7a-b Inhibition of the hamstring; on left is biceps femoris allowing medial foot rotation. On right is semitendinosus and semimembranosus allowing lateral foot rotation. Pelvis tilts anterior on ipsilateral side with excess lumbar lordosis, especially if all hamstring muscles are inhibited. (*a*) Posterior-to-anterior view, (*b*) lateral view.

Figure 9.8a-b Left gluteus maximus inhibition may result in an elevation and anterior rotation of the pelvis on the ipsilateral side, with an increased lumbar lordosis. (*a*) Posterior-to-anterior view, (*b*) lateral view.

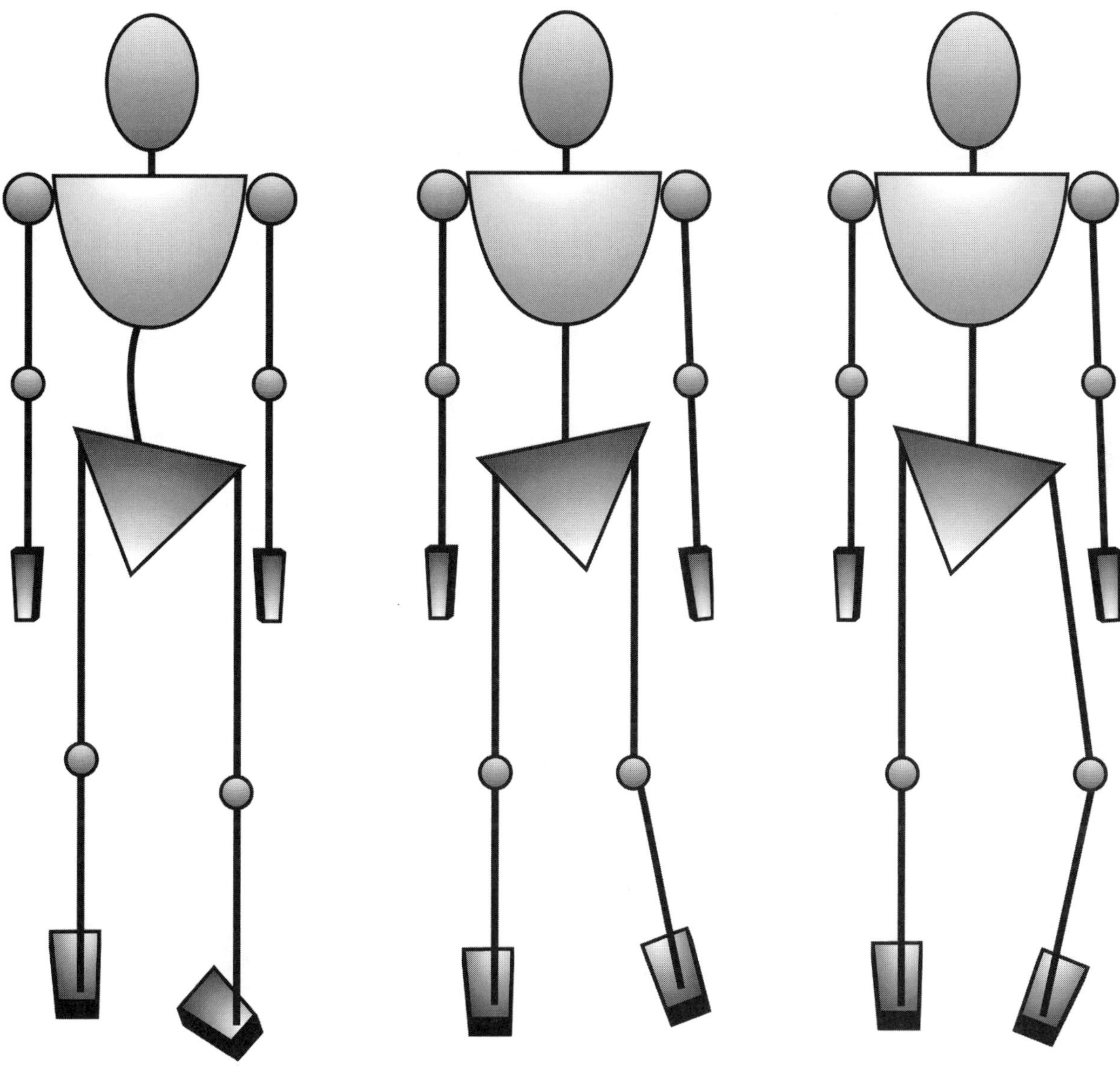

Figure 9.9 Psoas inhibition on the right may allow medial rotation of ipsilateral foot with excess pronation. Lumbar spine convex on contralateral side (tight psoas). Pelvis may be lower (sometimes higher) on ipsilateral side.

Figure 9.10 Right sartorius or gracilis inhibition may cause a posterior rotation of the pelvis seen as an elevation on the ipsilateral side and genu valgum.

Figure 9.11 Right adductor inhibition may cause elevation of pelvis on contralateral side and genu varum on ipsilateral side.

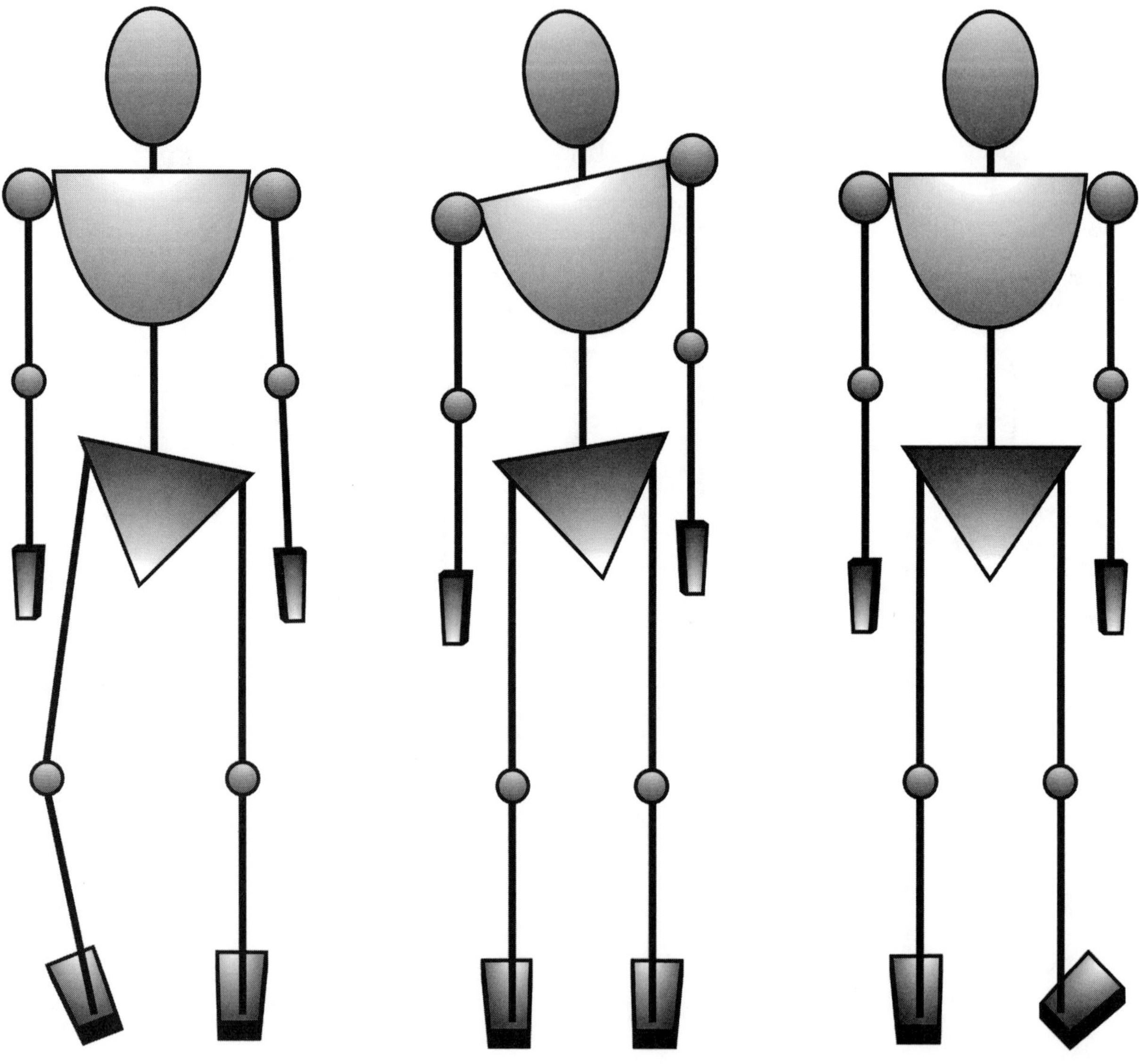

Figure 9.12 Left tensor fascia lata inhibition may cause elevation of pelvis on ipsilateral side and genu varum.

Figure 9.13 Inhibition of the right gluteus medius may result in elevated pelvis, shoulder, and head on right.

Figure 9.14 Left piriformis inhibition may cause the contralateral foot (tight piriformis side) to laterally rotate.

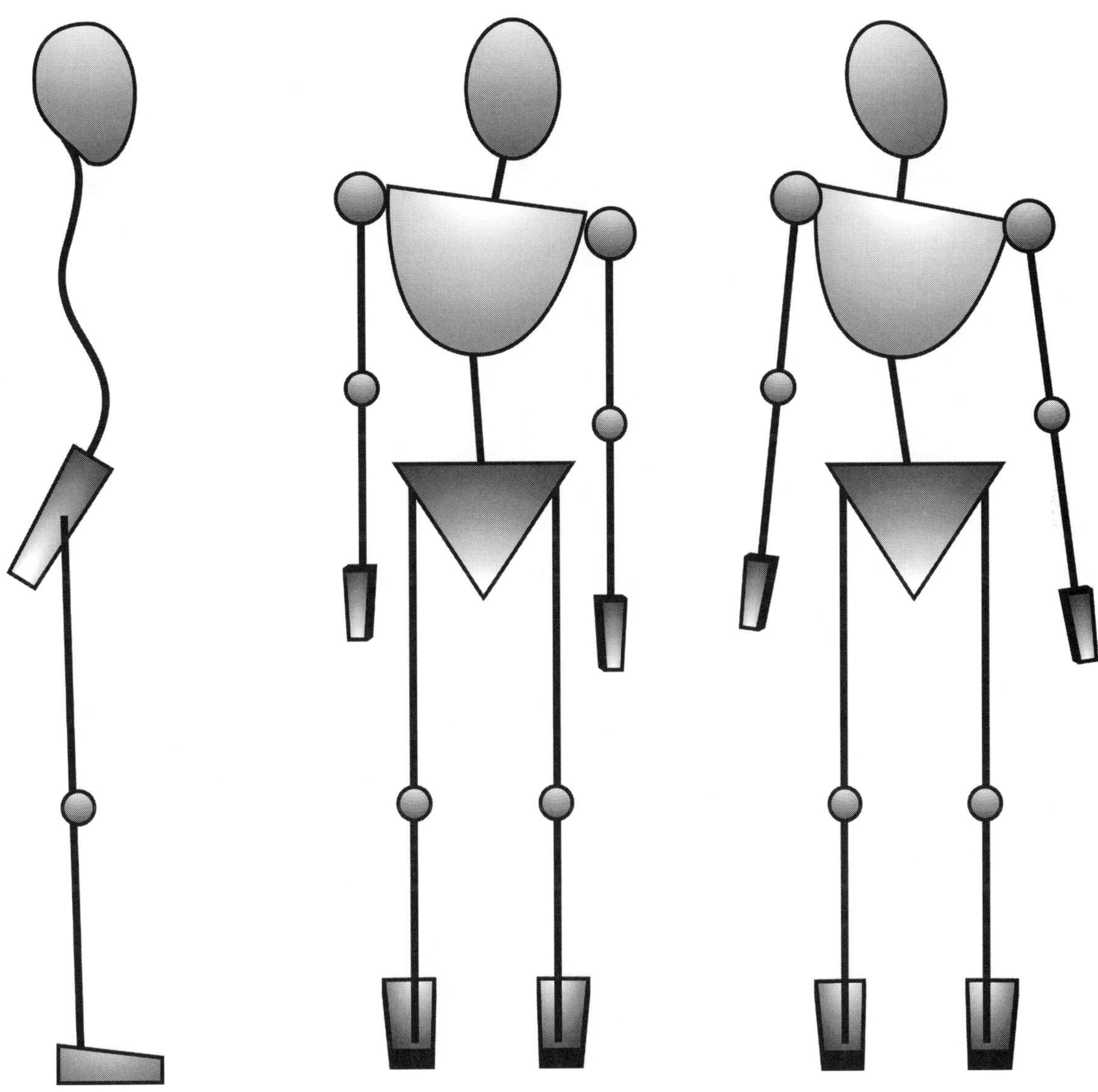

Figure 9.15 Abdominal muscle inhibition can produce increased lumbar lordosis and an anterior tilt in the pelvis.

Figure 9.16 Latissimus dorsi inhibition on the left may cause an elevation of the shoulder.

Figure 9.17 Inhibition of the right upper trapezius can elevate the head and depress the shoulder ipsilaterally.

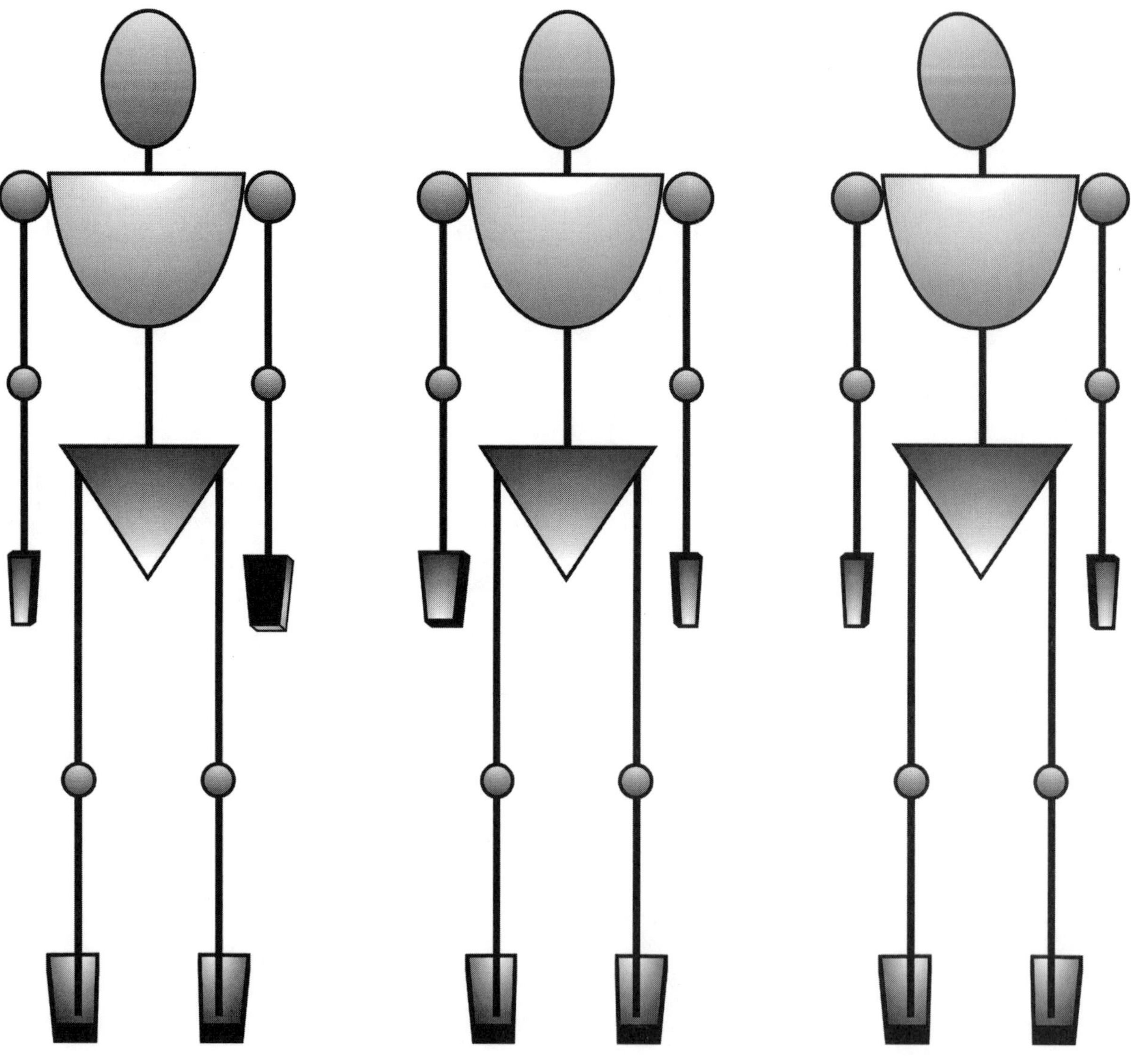

Figure 9.18 Inhibition of the right lateral rotators — teres minor, infraspinatus posterior deltoid, and supraspinatus — allows excess medial rotation of the shoulder, observed in the hand facing more posterior.

Figure 9.19 Inhibition of the left medial rotators — subscapularis, latissimus dorsi, pectoralis muscles — may allow excess lateral rotation of the shoulder, observed in the hand facing more anterior.

Figure 9.20 Unilateral neck flexor inhibition on the right can cause the head to tilt toward the contralateral side.

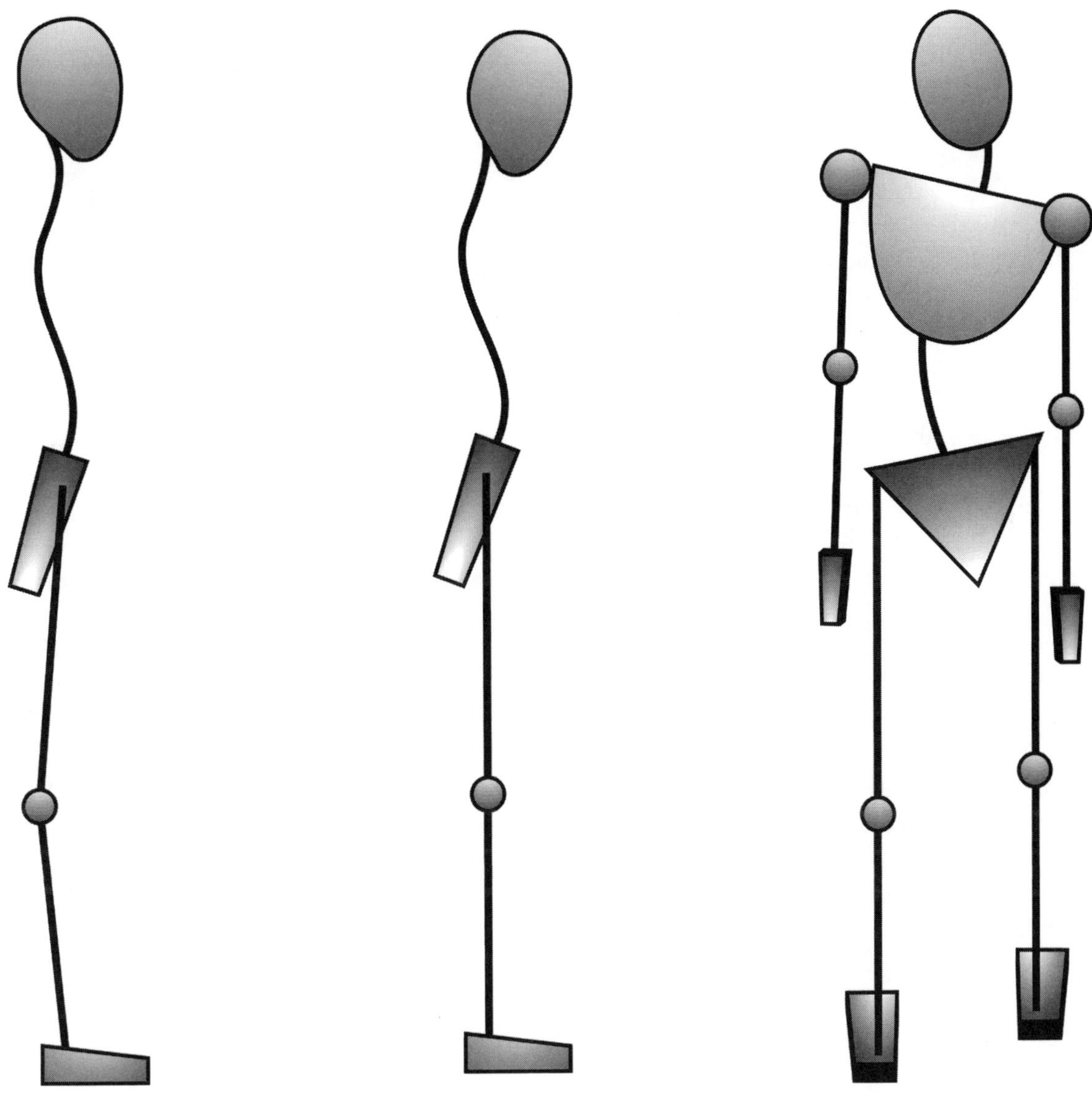

Figure 9.21 Inhibition of rectus femoris may cause posterior rotation of pelvis and hyperextension of the knee.

Figure 9.22 Bilateral inhibition of neck extensors allows excess flexion of head.

Figure 9.23 In a clinical situation, any one muscle inhibition, such as in the right sartorius in this example, can change body posture from head to feet. The specific postural deviation will vary depending on compensation.

Joint Complex Dysfunction

Altered posture is usually associated with joint dysfunction, which is often secondary to muscle inhibition. Joint complex dysfunction (JCD) refers to imbalances with structural, chemical, and mental/emotional components occurring in and around a joint that is not functioning properly. Joint complex dysfunction is not a dislocation or luxation, but a functional disruption of joint structures and related soft tissue, circulatory, and neurological aspects (Seaman 1997).

Among the common manifestations of JCD are pain and inflammation. Also with muscle imbalance comes secondary physical stress on the skeleton, especially the joints, ligaments, tendons, and other muscles. Subtle movements of the skeleton, including the bones of the skull, jaw joints, and spine, may become significantly distorted, resulting in a structural stress. This can adversely affect body movement, eye-hand coordination, and the ability to dissipate shock. These secondary factors may then allow other problems to develop. For example, the normal shock of running—which is usually well compensated—may cause injury in the athlete with previous muscle imbalance, followed by skeletal stress and poor shock-absorption capability. However, pain is not always associated with JCD, as an asymptomatic joint can produce dysfunction—that is, poor performance—and can also lead to other secondary imbalances. Joint complex dysfunction can result from trauma and/or neuromuscular imbalance or from inactivity or immobilization (Liebenson 1992).

For active athletes, the structural aspects of JCD can lead to chemical imbalances (i.e., inflammation), which can then trigger nociception and mechanical adaptations including additional muscle imbalances. Local and systemic autonomic reactions also accompany JCD, further complicating the syndrome (Seaman 1997). If and when the individual senses this dysfunction, disability, or discomfort, mental/emotional stress may follow; this could ultimately lead to further physical and chemical distress, maintaining a vicious cycle. One important goal of treatment is to break this cycle by restoring function, allowing the body to heal itself.

MANUAL MUSCLE TESTING

Frequently employed neurological tests evaluate for general muscle function, or pathology; for instance, one may ask patients to shrug their shoulders to determine whether cranial nerve XI is intact. Muscle testing in complementary sports medicine looks at functional relationships.

Muscle function can be assessed as normal or abnormal. The normal response to a muscle test is normal facilitation or normal inhibition. Abnormal test outcomes include abnormal facilitation, where the muscle is overfacilitated, or abnormal inhibition, where the muscle's inhibited state is not what is expected. In this way, muscle testing reflects a person's neurological state. The muscle testing procedures in this text come from the work of Kendall et al. (1993) and Walther (1988), and also from the experience of the author and others with extensive clinical backgrounds. As described earlier, many practitioners use the terms "weak" and "strong" when referring to inhibition and facilitation muscle testing outcomes, respectively. While not technically correct and perhaps confusing, the words "weak" and "strong" have also been used in relation to abnormal and normal outcomes, as well as to electromyography differences (Lawson and Calderon 1997; Perot et al. 1991; Leisman et al. 1995, 1989).

Performing a Test: Muscle Evaluation

A normal response to a muscle test is exemplified when the muscle can successfully function despite the stress placed on it in the form of an opposing force from the practitioner. Since the patient is positioned so that only one muscle or muscle group is being tested, the practitioner must judge by experience and take care to avoid applying too much force. The amount of force the practitioner utilizes will depend upon the ability of the patient's muscle to maintain resistance. Likewise, if a muscle is unable to maintain its normal function while maintaining the correct test position, it is testing abnormally.

Abnormal responses observed in muscle testing may possibly be the result of an inhibition of the central integrated state, or functional status, of the muscle's motoneuron pool despite conscious descending excitatory inputs. Leisman et al. (1995) found significant electromyography differences between normal and abnormal muscle tests and also identified differences in somatosensory evoked potentials between these two states (Leisman et al. 1989).

It is vital that the practitioner use proper and effective methods in testing muscles. This methodology comes both from a knowledge of anatomy and physiology and from experience. Through use of these methods, an effective assessment process evolves, and the likelihood of a more successful therapeutic outcome is increased.

Another important issue to consider during muscle testing evaluations is the position of the patient in relation to the type of muscle being tested. The vestibular mechanism—the tonic labyrinthine reflexes—helps maintain the position of the eyes and body as the head moves. In part, specific changes take place in the body relative to head movements. There are four positions of the head that can influence these changes: head face down, head face up, right-side head down, and left-side head down. If a person begins to fall forward, for example, with the head facing downward, there is an increased facilitation of all the limb flexors to help prevent falling. During an examination when the patient is in a similar face-down position, as in lying prone, the same mechanism functions: the flexor muscles of the limbs are normally more facilitated. Likewise, when the head is face up or when the patient is lying supine, the extensors of all the limbs are facilitated.

When the left side of the head is down (left ear down), the left limb extensors and right flexors are facilitated and the right extensors and left flexors are inhibited. The opposite reaction takes place when the right side of the head is down; the right extensors and left flexors are facilitated and the left extensors and right flexors are inhibited.

The effects of the labyrinthine mechanism apparently are not significant enough to cause normal inhibition using muscle testing; but the normal facilitation effect can overcome an existing inhibition, and this can be demonstrated using muscle testing. For example, if a standing patient has an abnormal inhibition of a muscle that has extensor function, such as the latissimus dorsi, placing the patient in a supine position should result in a normal facilitation of that muscle (negating the inhibition); placing the patient in a prone position should inhibit the latissimus dorsi.

Muscle testing serves as a screening assessment—one that reflects neuromuscular activity. If normal function does not exist, as in the case of some patients, this neuromuscular dysfunction can have a significant impact on future assessment and treatment effectiveness. Patients with these problems may also be predisposed to diminished performance and physical injury because the normal mechanisms that control posture and gait are disrupted.

An example of the vestibular reflexes in action is seen in sprinting athletes, who thrust their head forward in rhythm with the whole body in a sometimes subconscious attempt to continuously stimulate flexor activity in the limbs. But if there is existing muscle imbalance that distorts the head, normal vestibular activity may not take place, adversely affecting posture and gait. A common example of this phenomenon is abnormal inhibition of the right neck flexors with secondary overfacilitation of the left neck extensors causing postural distortion of the head (and often neck pain).

As the head position changes from the vertical, messages are sent from the vestibular apparatus to the brain, resulting in body-position adaptations. Sports necessitating precise balance—including those requiring increased eye-hand coordination or rapid changes in head and body position, and others such as diving, gymnastics, and tennis—require optimal function of this mechanism. In short, all sport activities depend on this mechanism, even during resting conditions.

As described previously, many physical, chemical, and mental/emotional states can affect muscle function, and it is important that the practitioner be aware of these.

The elicitation of pain during muscle testing may also be a factor in the assessment process. In most cases, painful muscle testing is still effective, unless the pain is severe.

Examples of Muscle Tests

The two muscles discussed here, the pectoralis major clavicular division and the latissimus dorsi (see figures 9.24 and 9.25), will serve as an introduction to muscle testing; the discussion is continued in the next chapter. In addition to their importance in all sport activities, these two muscles are useful for evaluating the function of the patient's gait. These muscles can be used to help develop the art of muscle testing in practitioners who are just learning these techniques.

Pectoralis Major Clavicular

The pectoralis muscle has two parts that are differentiated by specific movement, anatomy, and neurological innervation. This discussion focuses on the upper or clavicular portion of the muscle, referred to as the pectoralis major clavicular (PMC); we will consider the lower or sternal portion in the next chapter. Dysfunction of the PMC can create a variety of symptoms, especially in the shoulder joint and during movement of the humerus. Difficulty or pain when one attempts to touch the opposite shoulder may be a clue to PMC inhibition.

Action

The PMC is a flexor of the shoulder joint and an adductor and medial rotator of the humerus. It is an important part of the running and swimming gait, bench press, push-ups, and all throwing motions and is an important stabilizer in activities such as cycling. It also assists in elevation of the thorax on forced inspiration.

Origin

Medial one-third to one-half of the clavicle

Insertion

Lateral lip of the humerus

Nerve

C5-7

Testing

Patient is supine or standing with shoulder flexed to 90°. Elbow is fully extended with near-maximum but comfortable internal rotation. The practitioner uses the left hand to test the right PMC, with the right hand supporting the contralateral shoulder. Contact is made proximal to the wrist joint with testing pressure in the direction in line with the muscle fibers—abduction with very slight extension. The patient must avoid flexing the elbow (which recruits the biceps), flexing the contralateral shoulder, or rotating the trunk. Note: In addition to their individual tests, both PMCs can be tested at the same time. Position both limbs as described above. Testing pressure is the same.

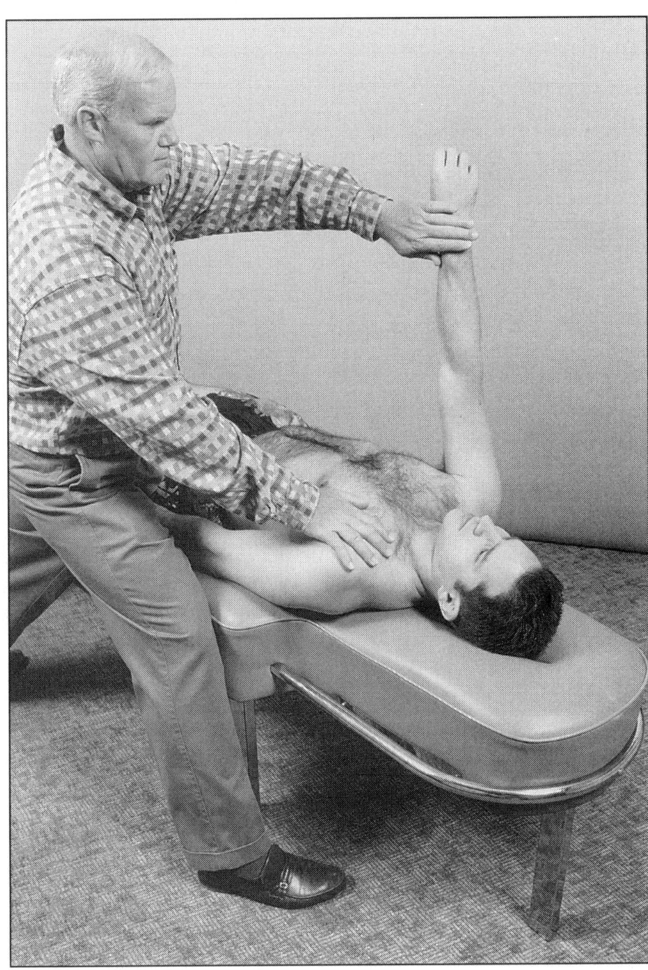

Figure 9.24 Practitioner testing the patient's right PMC

Latissimus Dorsi

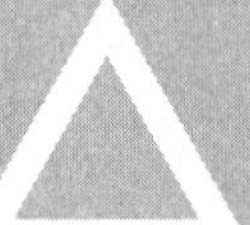

This muscle is important for proper arm movement during swimming, rowing, walking, and running, as well as for low back flexion and extension motion, and is a middle and low back stabilizer. It may be inhibited in patients who have pain or difficulty when placing their hand on their lumbar region and in people with low back pain.

Action

The latissimus dorsi is a medial rotator, adductor, and extensor of the shoulder; it depresses the shoulder joint. It also assists in anterior and lateral pelvic flexion and in hyperextension of the spine.

Origin

Spinous processes of T6-12, L1-5, and the upper sacral vertebrae; the thoracolumbar fascia of ribs 9-12 (and with connections to slips of origin of the external oblique abdominal muscle); the posterior third of the medial iliac crest; and occasionally on the inferior angle of the scapula.

Insertion

The muscle forms a tendon that passes (with the teres minor tendon) through the axillary region to attach on the intertubercular groove of the humerus.

Nerve

C6-8

Testing

Patient is prone or standing with the elbow locked in extension, the arm in medial rotation with slight extension and in full adduction. Contact is made proximal to the wrist joint, and pressure is applied in the direction of abduction and slight flexion.

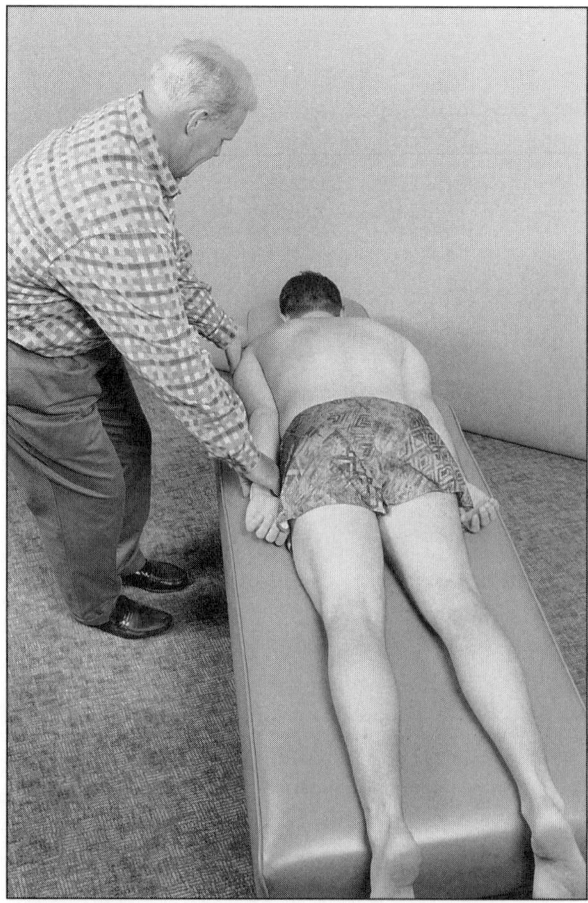

Figure 9.25 Practitioner testing the patient's left latissimus dorsi

The next chapter provides similar descriptions of tests for an extensive list of muscles, with the addition of some of the common therapeutic reflex points and acupuncture meridian associations.

Interpreting a Muscle Test

When testing muscles and gathering an inventory of normal and dysfunctional ones, recall that the body is a whole functional unit, with all areas reacting to and with all other areas. For example, abnormal muscle inhibition is often followed by abnormal overfacilitation (i.e., muscle "tightness") of another muscle (typically its antagonist). This simple pattern of muscle imbalance may sometimes be amplified many times to create a seemingly abstract tangled web of dysfunction. But this state is one that is organized by the body, and it is the job of the practitioner to make sense of it so that an assessment can be made and an appropriate therapy applied.

When patients have muscle inhibition, their body attempts to compensate by incorporating other muscle activity, which, among other things, slightly distorts their posture and gait. This may also happen during the evaluation of a patient. During testing of a muscle that proves to be abnormally inhibited, the patient may consciously or subconsciously attempt to compensate for that dysfunction by substituting or "recruiting" other muscles of similar action. Patients usually do this (consciously or subconsciously) by trying to change their posture to adequately incorporate other muscles into the action. It is the job of the practitioner to be aware of any attempt at recruiting during testing if an effective evaluation is the goal.

An important aspect of muscle testing is objectivity—at least inasmuch as can be achieved when one is working with human subjects. Predetermining that a muscle is abnormally inhibited or facilitated does not support objective analysis: this is the most common error people make when learning muscle testing. Properly applying the art and science of muscle testing can result in as much objectivity as any other aspect that the physical examination permits.

Muscle Testing Devices

Muscle testing can be performed with use of the practitioner's hands, an isokinetic machine, and other handheld devices. However, isokinetic machines and other equipment for more objective testing of muscles have not been shown to be suitable for clinical use (Kendall et al. 1993), for the reason that these types of equipment are expensive and difficult to use in the clinical environment. This equipment may be useful for research purposes, however. Using force measurements from both practitioner and patient, Perot et al. (1991) demonstrated a significant difference in "strong" versus "weak" muscle testing outcomes and showed that these changes were not attributable to decreased or increased testing force from the practitioner performing the tests. Using electromyographic studies, Leisman et al. (1995) showed distinctions between inhibited and facilitated muscles, as well as between muscle inhibition and muscle weakness due to fatigue.

Marino et al. (1982) and Wadsworth et al. (1987), however, showed significant reliability between handheld devices and manual muscle testing. Regarding the optimal approach for clinical use, Kendall et al. (1993) state, "Our hands are the most sensitive, fine tuned instruments available" (p. 7); and according to Walther (1988), " presently the best 'instrument' to perform manual muscle testing is a well-trained examiner, using his perception of time and force with knowledge of anatomy and physiology of muscle testing" (p. 277).

OTHER TYPES OF MANUAL MUSCLE TESTING

The time element is another important aspect of manual muscle testing. Nicholas et al. (1978) found that the duration of the tester's effort was a significant factor in ratings. Showing a similar relationship, Hsieh and Phillips (1990) found a difference between patient-initiated and practitioner-initiated methods of testing.

Schmitt (1996) described three different types of muscle tests: Type 1, practitioner initiated; Type 2, patient initiated; and Type 3, patient initiated to maximum contraction. All three types measure the response of the muscle during eccentric contraction. Each type differs in the level of preloading of the muscle prior to eccentric testing. It is possible to have an inhibition of a given muscle using one testing method but not another. Type 1 is a pure eccentric test, with the practitioner starting the test and the test continuing with the patient's contraction of the muscle. In the Type 2 test, the patient starts contracting initially (concentric contraction), pushing against the tester's hand. Before the patient applies maximum force, the practitioner applies pressure (eccentric test). Type 3 is similar to Type 2 except that the practitioner waits for maximum contraction (full isometric contraction) from the patient before applying force. Abnormal results from each type of test have certain assessment and therapeutic possibilities. For example, Type 1 problems may be associated with joint dysfunction, the need to stimulate acupuncture points, or the need to treat specific muscle points such as Golgi tendon organ or spindle cells. Type 2 problems may be associated with certain injuries, allergy and hypersensitivity reactions, and endocrine problems. Type 3 findings may be related to suprasegmental problems, including temporomandibular joint dysfunction, cranial-sacral imbalances, autonomic dysfunction, and nutritional problems.

MUSCLE TESTING AND GAIT

In addition to being evaluated through static testing, many muscles can be evaluated in specific gait positions. The two muscles described earlier can be tested in the normal walking/running gait position to determine whether normal neuromuscular activity is taking place during gait.

In the normal walking/running gait, when the right arm and left leg are flexed and the left arm and right leg are extended, specific facilitative and inhibitory actions are attributed to the PMC and latissimus dorsi. In this gait position, the practitioner expects to find that the right PMC has increased facilitation (to promote flexion) and that the right latissimus is inhibited (to allow flexion). The contralateral arm is in the opposite state: the left PMC is inhibited (to allow extension) while the left latissimus dorsi is more facilitated to promote extension. These normal neuromuscular conditions can be evaluated and confirmed with manual muscle testing as follows.

The practitioner must confirm that the PMC and latissimus dorsi are in a normal state in the standing (neutral) position before placing the patient in a gait position.The patient is placed in the appropriate gait position as previously described. In doing so, the practitioner makes sure that the right (forward) knee is slightly flexed and the right foot is bearing enough weight to simulate walking or running (see figures 9.26 and 9.27). Both PMC and both latissimus dorsi

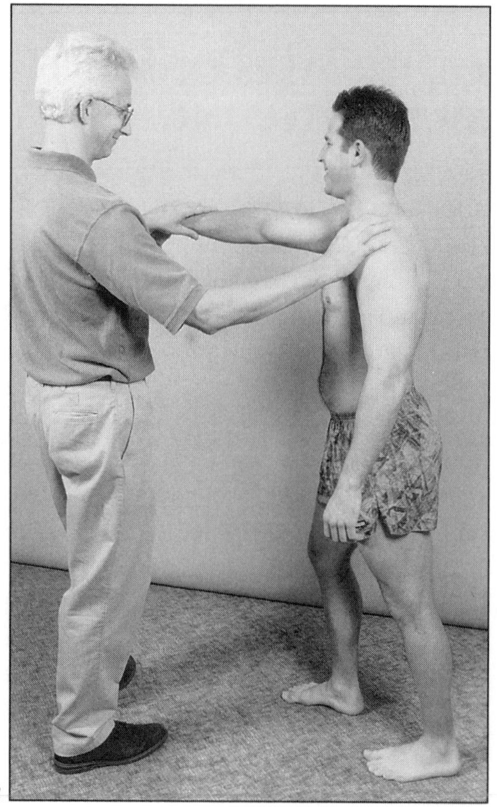

a

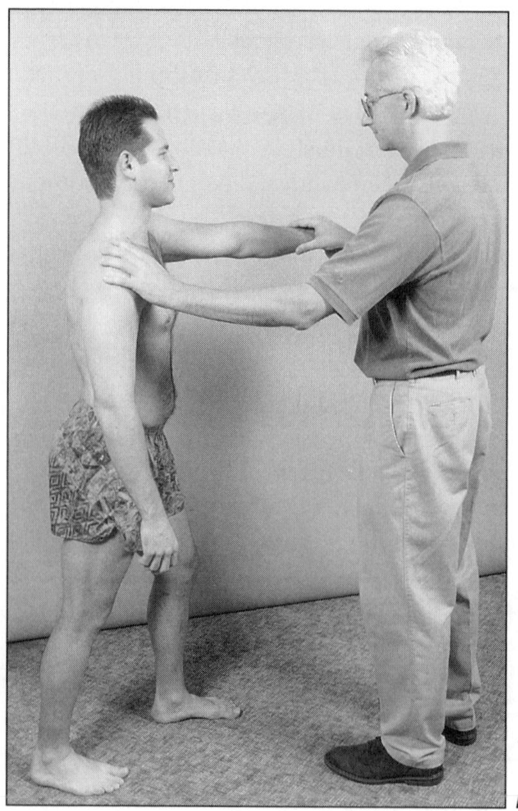

b

Figure 9.26a–b Practitioner performing (*a*) gait testing with right PMC and (*b*) gait testing with left PMC

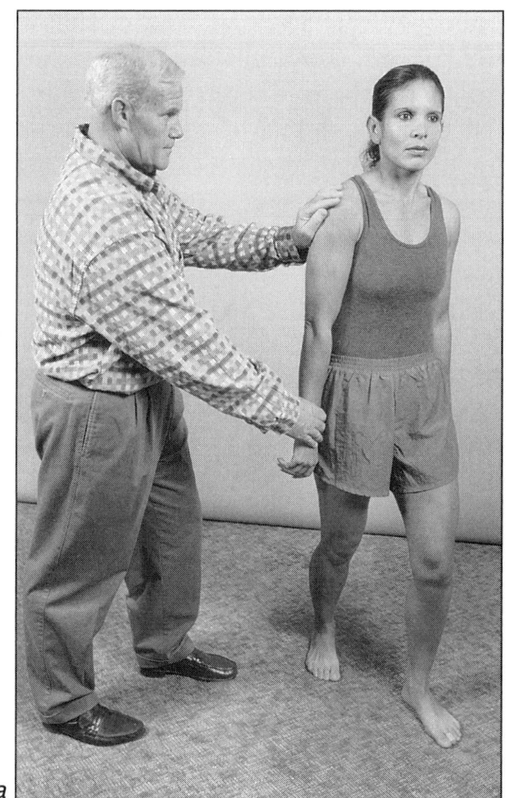
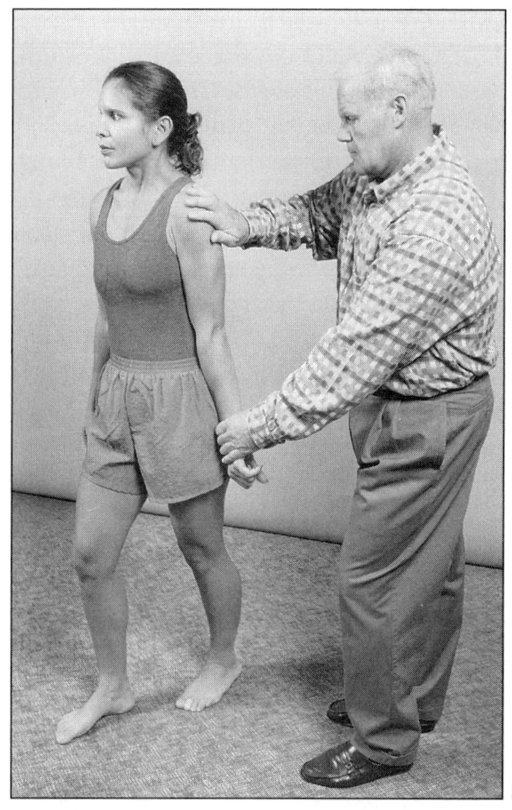

Figure 9.27a–b Practitioner performing (*a*) gait testing with right latissimus dorsi; (*b*) gait testing with left latissimus dorsi

muscles are tested and the results are noted. Any differences between the expected results and the actual results are noted. The practitioner during the testing process must maintain objectivity by making no assumptions regarding the expected outcomes.

If the expected outcomes are the same as the actual ones (a facilitated right PMC and left latissimus dorsi and an inhibited left PMC and right latissimus dorsi), neuromuscular function in these muscles during this gait is considered normal. In some patients, however, the expected and actual results are different. For example, if the right PMC is inhibited, this is an abnormal response; any test result not in accord with the expected results is abnormal. In most cases, these abnormal neuromuscular states are not pathological but functional disturbances.

Recall the evaluation of the patient in the standing (normal) position. Some patients may have abnormal function of one or more muscles. In this position, for example, if a patient has an abnormal inhibition of the left PMC and right latissimus dorsi, this constitutes a problem: the neuromuscular system is acting as if the body is already in a specific gait position. In other words, the muscles are acting as if the body is taking a step with the right leg as described earlier. This type of imbalance could have significant consequences on all movement and is an example of a neuromuscular imbalance causing a musculoskeletal stress.

In addition to the PMC and latissimus dorsi, many other muscles function in a precise neurological pattern with gait. For example, as the right arm flexes during gait, the head turns toward the right through facilitation of the left sternocleidomastoid muscle (with inhibition on the right side) in the neck. At the same time, the left upper trapezius and neck extensors are inhibited (with facilitation on the right). In some instances, these muscles (described in the next chapter) can also be tested with the patient in the appropriate gait position to evaluate proper neuromuscular function, although using the PMC and latissimus dorsi to screen for proper neuromuscular gait function is the most effective and easiest approach.

A faulty neuromuscular mechanism, as described earlier, can add physical stress to joints, ligaments, tendons, and bones. This can also create, aggravate, or maintain a physical injury. In addition, chemical stress in the form of inflammation, for example, can be maintained with the real possibility of producing a mental/emotional stress due to the consequences of the physical and chemical handicap placed on the individual, especially in athletes who compete. Failure of this neuromuscular mechanism to function properly could place excessive stress on the cranium, temporomandibular joint, and the visual and vestibular mechanisms controlling posture, which can continue the vicious cycle.

Practitioners just learning how to muscle test will find this gait testing very helpful for developing their skills. For any practitioner, using these simple tests during an initial exam can help differentiate normal neuromuscular function from abnormal. When abnormal neuromuscular function exists anywhere in the body, it has the potential to affect other areas as well. For most if not all types of patients, correcting this dysfunction becomes a primary concern—before any other therapy is considered. The method of correction may be as simple as stimulating certain therapeutic reflexes or acupuncture points, as described in the next chapter, or using other complementary sports medicine skills.

CONCLUSION

Manual muscle testing during the examination is of great importance in assessing neuromuscular function. Testing of muscles is done in specific positions, such as in the normal posture or in gait position. In addition, testing muscles in conditions that mimic the athlete's specific sport, or even at the athlete's site of competition, can be useful. However, proper muscle testing is a key to an effective examination. Poor or careless testing often results in misinformation or wrong choice of therapies. As with all other examination procedures, the most objective approach possible is the most effective.

10

Muscle Testing Procedures

Muscles often lose function and become inhibited because of structural problems like trauma or a chemical imbalance due to a hormonal influence. Other times, mental/emotional stress can lead to muscle dysfunction. The resulting muscle inhibition can cause such problems as disruption of normal posture and gait, loss of joint support, and diminished performance. Determining which muscles are dysfunctional is a vital part of the assessment process in many patients.

In many cases, muscle testing is also useful in helping to determine conditions of imbalance elsewhere in the body. For example in patients with mechanical imbalance in the pelvis, spine, or hips, and especially the ankles, weight bearing through these areas may cause a variety of normal muscles to become inhibited; but this does not occur when gravity stress is removed. As described in the next chapter, muscles are also useful as part of a challenge mechanism to help the practitioner assess for chemical and mental/emotional dysfunction throughout the body. Correction of muscle dysfunction can be accomplished with a variety of hands-on techniques, including application of certain pressure to the muscles—directly affecting specific joints in the spine, pelvis, and extravertebral joints—and cranial manipulation.

This chapter describes muscle testing for more than 40 muscles. Included in each description is information about the importance of the muscle's action in sport, its anatomical and neurological associations, and how to test it.

Before discussing the muscle test, we will look two different types of therapeutic reflexes (acupuncture points and Chapman's reflexes), each related to each muscle being considered. These reflexes are specific points on the skin, often found far from the related muscle, that when stimulated may improve the function of that muscle.

ACUPUNCTURE POINTS

These areas can be treated with finger pressure (sometimes referred to as acupressure) using moderate pressure (4-5 lb or less—the amount of pressure you would use to ring a doorbell) on the body point for about 15 sec. In some cases, rapid tapping with a fingertip for 20-30 sec is an alternative, especially with the use of these points for pain control. In traditional acupuncture, points are often treated with needles, but these techniques require special training and licensure, and discussion of them is beyond the scope of this text. In almost all cases, however, finger pressure (or tapping) is as effective.

Each muscle is associated with one of the muscle meridians located throughout the body; the meridian for each muscle is listed in the description of the testing for that muscle. The names of all the acupuncture meridians and the abbreviations used in this text are as follows:

Lung (LU)
Kidney (KI)
Large intestine (LI)
Circulation sex (CX)
Stomach (ST)
Triple heater (TH)
Spleen (SP)
Gallbladder (GB)
Heart (HT)
Liver (LV)
Small intestine (SI)
Conception vessel (CV)
Bladder (BL)
Governing vessel (GV)

The locations of some important acupuncture points described in this chapter are as follows (also see figure 17.2):

LU 9: Anterior wrist at the most lateral end of the wrist crease

LI 11: Lateral end of the elbow crease found during elbow flexion

ST 41: Mid-dorsum of foot at anterior ankle flexure, lateral to the tibialis anterior tendon

SP 2: Medial edge of big toe at base of the proximal phalanx

HT 9: Just proximal to the nail of the fifth finger on radial side

SI 3: Medial side of hand just proximal to head of the fifth metacarpal

BL 67: Just lateral to the fifth toenail

KI 7: Three finger-widths above and slightly posterior to the medial malleolus

CX 9: Just proximal to the nail of the third finger on radial side

TH 3: Posterior hand just proximal to the fourth metacarpal head on the ulnar side

GB 43: Lateral to the proximal end of the fourth proximal phalanx (gait reflex is GB 42)

LV 8: Medial knee just posterior to the medial meniscus (intertubercular space)

In traditional Chinese medicine, these particular points are referred to as tonification points. The reader should note that different texts on acupuncture may show slightly different locations for certain points because of variation in the interpretation of older writings and the experiences of various authors.

CHAPMAN'S REFLEXES

These areas are treated with moderate finger pressure or rubbing for about 15 sec, although occasionally these reflexes require much longer therapy. Again, the amount of pressure used is approximately 4 lb or less, the amount you would use to ring a doorbell. There are usually two Chapman's reflexes for each specific muscle, one anterior and one posterior, with both on the ipsilateral side for most muscles. These reflexes are usually a single point, but some are larger areas. These, along with any exceptions, are noted in the section for each muscle. Muscles that share the same anterior and posterior Chapman's reflexes (with organ or gland relationships given in parentheses) are as follows:

Sartorius; gracilis; tibialis posterior (adrenal)

General neck flexors, including sternocleidomastoid and extensors (stomach)

Gluteus medius and minimus; piriformis; peroneus longus and brevis (reproductive organs and glands)

Pectoralis major sternal (liver/gallbladder)

Latissimus dorsi; middle and lower trapezius; triceps (spleen/pancreas)

TREATMENT OF REFLEX POINTS WITH MUSCLE TESTING

Treatment of one or more reflex points may benefit a given muscle. In the case of the acupuncture points, some of the most frequently successful ones are listed under each muscle described. It is important to note that since each patient's set of imbalances is unique, it is best that the practitioner take time to find the most successful therapeutic point(s). Clinical methods of determining these are described in the next chapter. In addition, acupuncture point locations vary slightly from one patient to another. Palpation is an important tool when one is locating these points. They are more often located in a slight depression in soft tissue than on a bony prominence or tendon, and they are generally tender when palpated as compared to surrounding tissue.

For convenience, in the following sections the muscles are listed by their most common test body positions, although a muscle can usually be tested with the patient in more than one position. Sometimes people can be tested standing, as described earlier for the evaluation of gait. In other situations, patients may be tested in the sitting position or in a specific position that an athlete may assume during training or competition. There are times when it is valuable to assess a patient in these special positions; sometimes a muscle will dysfunction only during a specific postural stress. For example, a race car driver may have a normally functioning pectoralis major clavicular muscle in the standing and supine positions and will manifest inhibition only when tested in the driver's seat. A cyclist may have a normally functioning latissimus dorsi but show abnormal inhibition of this muscle when in a poor position on the bike.

Sternocleidomastoid Muscle

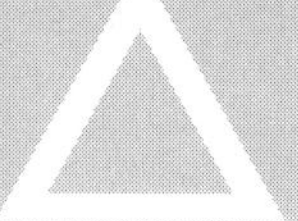

The sternocleidomastoid (SCM) muscle and other neck flexor muscles are often inhibited in whiplash-type injuries, and sometimes in rotational trauma; typical examples are seen in football, boxing, hard contact when the athlete is hit without warning, and skiing falls. All neck flexors may be less functional if the rectus abdominis muscle is weak or inhibited.

Action

Turns the head to the contralateral side, draws it to the ipsilateral shoulder, and flexes it, especially during bilateral contraction. The SCM is important for quick movements in sport and for balance and helps stabilize the head for efficient eye-hand coordination.

Origin

Sternal head of the muscle attaches to the manubrium; clavicular head attaches to the medial aspect of the clavicle.

Insertion

Temporal bone on the lateral side of the mastoid process; occiput on the lateral half of the superior nuchal line

Nerve

C2, 3, cranial nerve XI

Therapeutic Reflexes

Chapman's—Anterior: a point just below the middle of the clavicle where the pectoralis major clavicular attaches; posterior: over the laminae of C2

Acupuncture meridian—stomach

Common acupuncture points—ST 1, 41

Testing Position

Supine

Testing

Patient is supine with shoulders abducted to 90° and elbows flexed. Shoulders and thorax must remain on the table. An attempt to raise shoulders or contract abdominal muscles may indicate recruitment, especially if there is inhibition of the SCM. Practitioner uses fingertips placed on the forehead with pressure into extension.

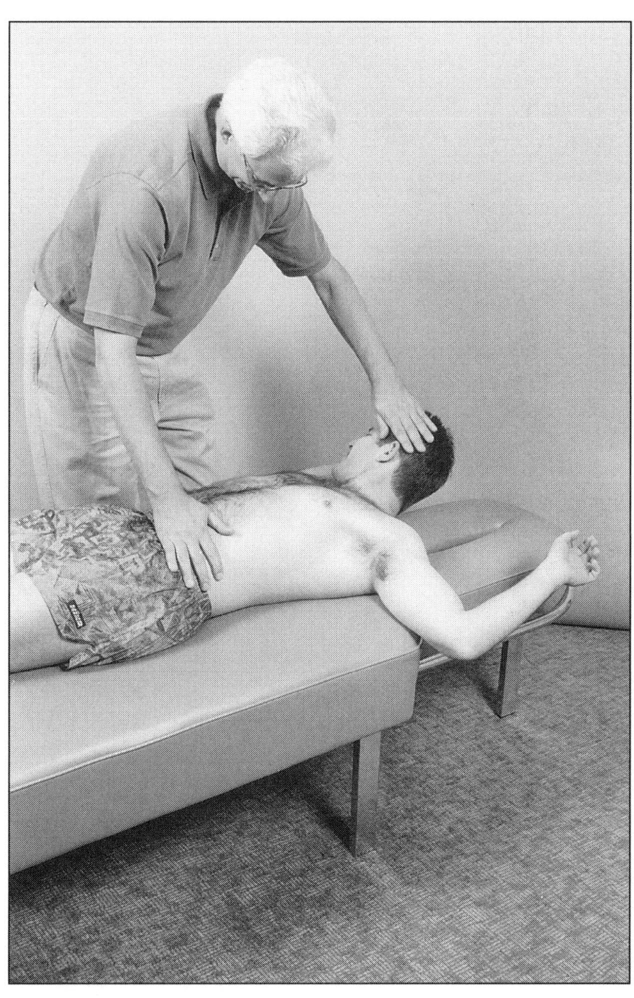

Medial Neck Flexors

(Includes Scalenus Anticus, Medius, and Posticus)

As with the SCM muscle, the scalenus anticus, medius, and posticus muscles are often inhibited in whiplash-type injuries and sometimes in rotational trauma. All neck flexors may be less functional if the rectus abdominis muscle is weak or inhibited.

Action

These muscles flex the head and provide slight head rotation. They stabilize the head during quick movements.

Origin

Transverse processes of C2-7

Insertion

Anterolateral portion of the first and second rib

Nerve

C3-8

Therapeutic Reflexes

All reflexes are the same as for SCM.

Testing Position

Supine

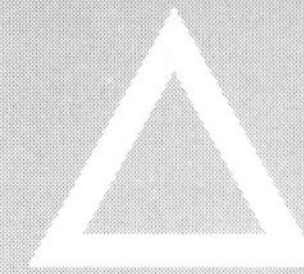

Testing

Same position as for SCM except that the head is only slightly rotated (10-15°) away from side to be tested.

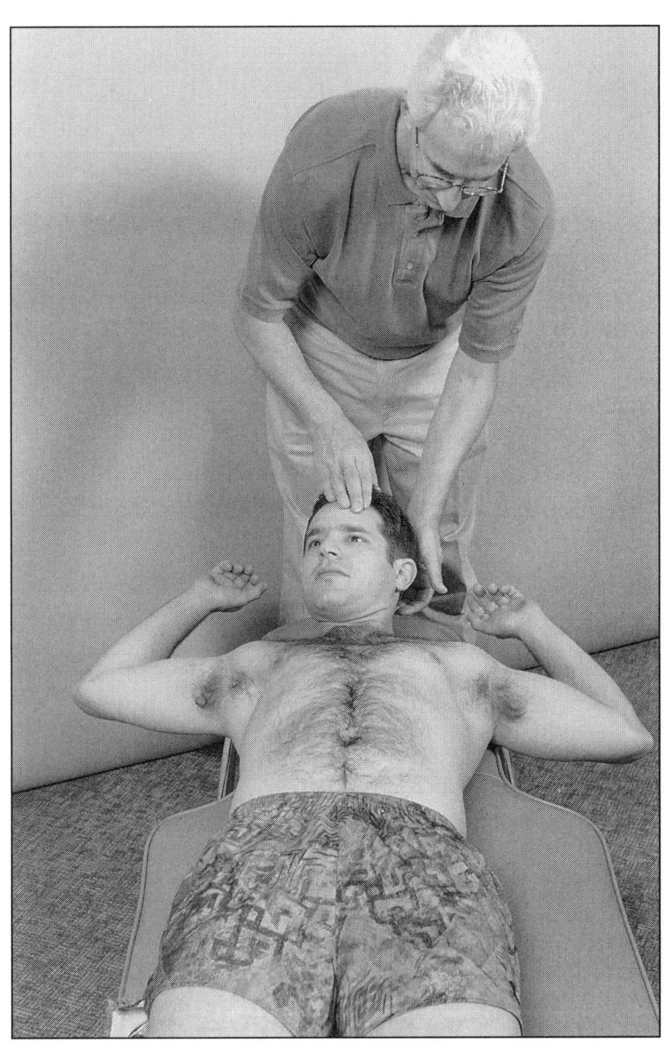

Pectoralis Major Clavicular Muscle

The pectoralis muscle has two parts that are differentiated by specific movement, anatomy, and neurological innervation. This discussion focuses on the upper or clavicular portion of the muscle. Dysfunction of the pectoralis major clavicular (PMC) can create a variety of symptoms, especially in the shoulder joint and during movement of the humerus. Difficulty or pain when one attempts to touch the opposite shoulder may be a clue to PMC inhibition.

Action

Flexes the shoulder joint and adducts and medially rotates the humerus. The PMC is an important part of running and swimming gait, bench press, push-ups, and all throwing motions, as well as an important stabilizer in activities such as cycling. It also assists in elevation of the thorax on forced inspiration.

Origin

Medial one-third to one-half of the clavicle

Insertion

Lateral lip of the bicipital groove of the humerus

Nerve

C5-7

Therapeutic Reflexes

Chapman's—Anterior: sixth (sometimes fifth) intercostal space from sternal junction to lateral chest wall (left side only); posterior: T6,7 laminae on left only. These reflexes are for both left and right PMC.

Acupuncture meridian—stomach

Common acupuncture points—ST 1, 41

Testing Position

Supine

Pectoralis Major Clavicular Muscle

Testing

Patient is supine or standing with shoulder flexed to 90°. Elbow is fully extended with near-maximum but comfortable internal rotation. The practitioner uses the left hand to test the right PMC, with the right hand supporting the contralateral shoulder. Contact is made proximal to the wrist joint with testing pressure in the direction in line with the muscle fibers—abduction with very slight extension. The patient must avoid flexing the elbow (which recruits the biceps), flexing the contralateral shoulder, or rotating the trunk. Note: In addition to their individual tests, both PMCs can be tested at the same time; both limbs are positioned as described above. Testing pressure is the same.

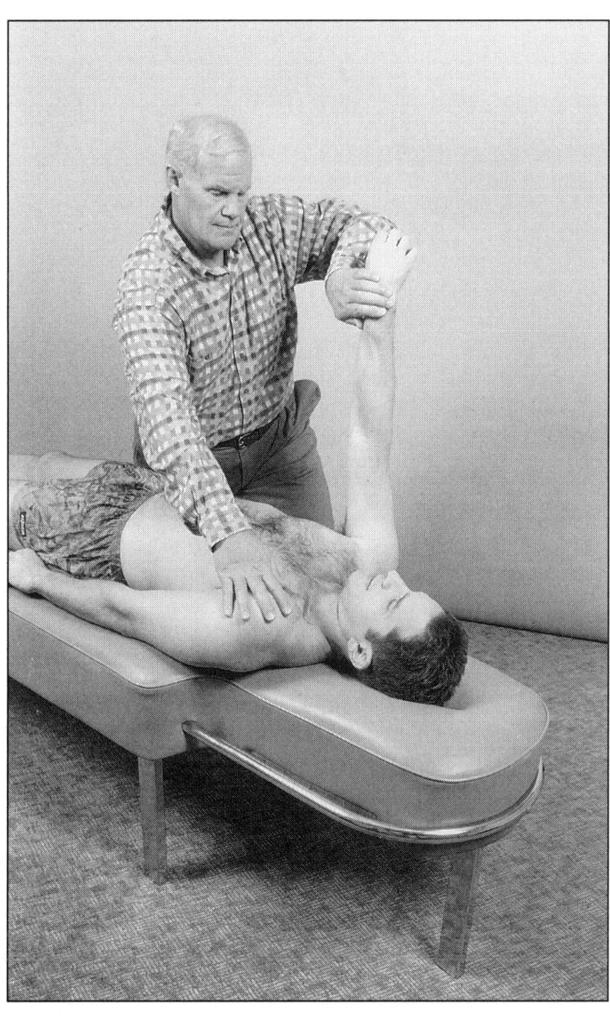

Pectoralis Major Sternal Muscle

This is the lower portion of the pectoralis major muscle. The clinical features are similar to those of the PMC, especially with regard to importance in the throwing motion, climbing, and swimming gait and for shoulder stability.

Action

Adducts and medially rotates the humerus, flexes the shoulder and extends it from a flexed position; assists in elevation of the thorax on forced inspiration

Origin

Anterior surface of the sternum and cartilages of ribs 1-6 (sometimes 7) and the aponeurosis of the external oblique

Insertion

Lateral lip of the bicipital groove of the humerus (same as PMC)

Nerve

C6-8, T1

Therapeutic Reflexes

Chapman's—Anterior: fifth (sometimes sixth) intercostal space from sternal junction to lateral chest wall (right side only); posterior: T5-7 laminae on right only; right-side reflexes are for both left and right pectoralis major sternal (PMS).

Acupuncture meridian—liver

Common acupuncture points—LV 3, 8

Testing Position

Supine

Testing

The patient's shoulder is flexed to 90°. Elbow is fully extended with near-maximum but comfortable internal rotation. The practitioner uses the left hand to test the right PMS, with the right hand supporting the contralateral pelvis. Contact is made proximal to the wrist joint with testing pressure in the direction in line with the muscle fibers—abduction obliquely away from the contralateral hip. The patient must avoid flexing the elbow (which recruits the biceps), flexing the contralateral shoulder, or rotating the trunk.

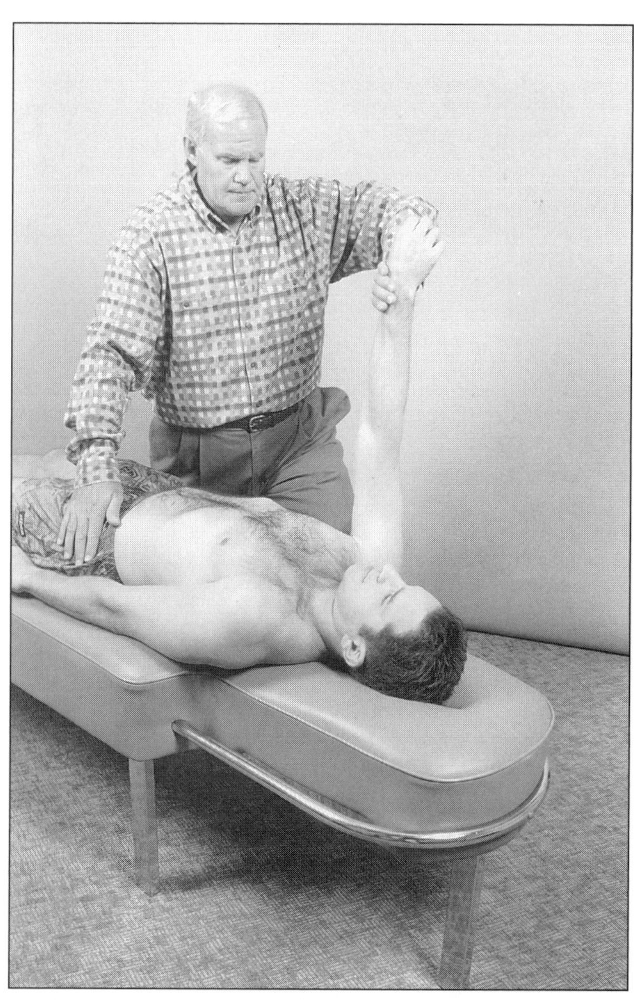

Serratus Anterior Muscle

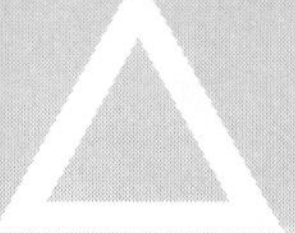

The serratus anterior muscle is important in pushing-type actions (such as contact sports and push-ups) and assists in forced inspiration.

Action

Abducts and rotates the scapula and holds it against the rib cage; depresses and elevates the scapula

Origin

Outer portion of ribs 1-8 (sometimes 9)

Insertion

Medial border of the scapula on the costal side

Nerve

C5-8

Therapeutic Reflexes

Chapman's—Anterior: third through fifth intercostal spaces at the sternal junction; posterior: laminae of T3-5

Acupuncture meridian—lung

Common acupuncture point—LU 9

Testing Position

Supine

Testing

In the supine position, the arm is flexed to about 120° and medially rotated 180° (palm is pronated). The scapula is stabilized by the patient's weight on the table (or if testing is being done in a sitting or standing position, the practitioner stabilizes the inferior border of the scapula with one hand). Contact is made proximal to the wrist with pressure in a caudal direction (into extension). Because of the difficulty of isolating and testing this muscle, slightly different tests are described in the literature.

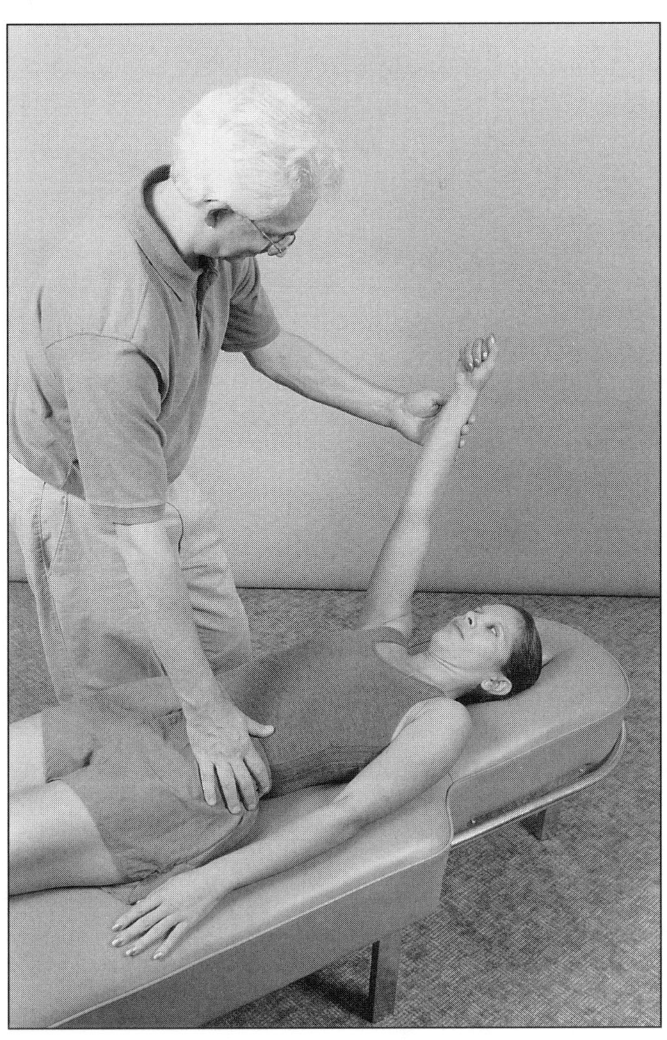

Biceps Brachii Muscle

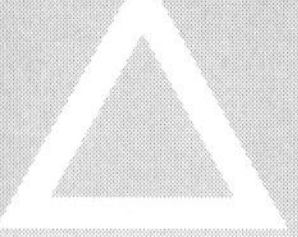

The two heads (origins) of this muscle give it diverse activity since it crosses two joints, the shoulder and the elbow, providing stability for both. This muscle is commonly used in weightlifting.

Action

Flexes the elbow and supinates the forearm; flexes the shoulder

Origin

Short head, coracoid process of scapula; long head, supraglenoid tubercle of scapula

Insertion

Radial tuberosity and aponeurosis (lacertus fibrosus)

Nerve

C5, 6

Therapeutic Reflexes

Chapman's—Anterior: intercostal space of fourth and fifth ribs, 1-2 cm from edge of sternum; posterior: laminae of C2

Acupuncture meridian—stomach

Common acupuncture points—ST 1, 41

Testing Position

Supine

Testing

Elbow is slightly flexed to about 45° with forearm supinated. Practitioner stabilizes the elbow with one hand, and the other hand contacts just proximal to wrist and applies force into elbow extension.

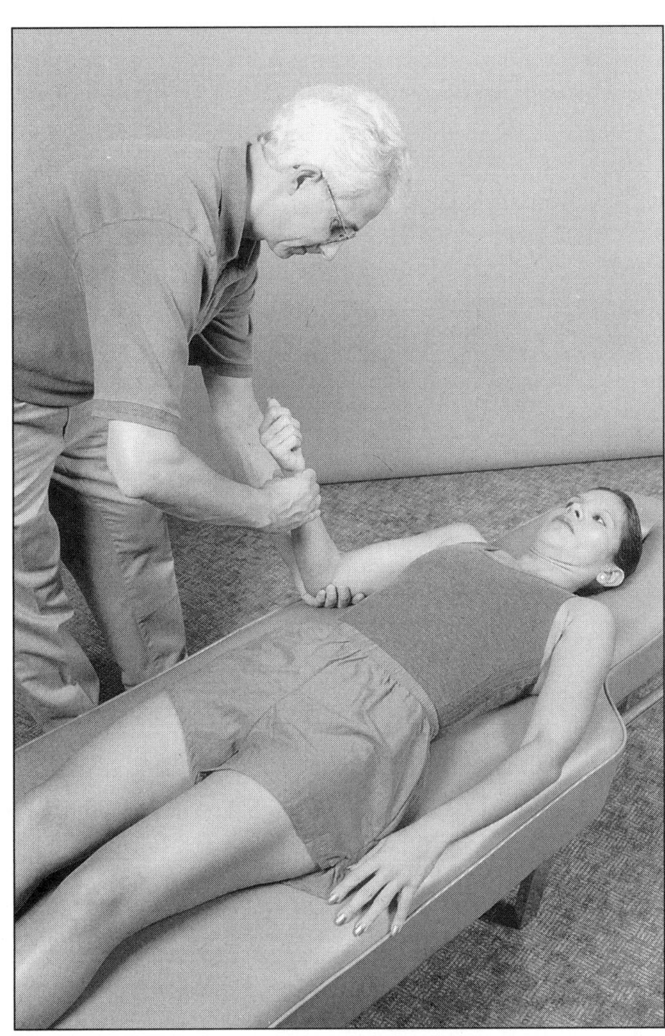

Triceps Brachii Muscle

Inhibition results in the inability to fully extend the elbow, often without pain. This muscle is especially important during pushing and throwing and in activities such as swimming, backhand racket sports, and baseball. Please note: As indicated in the following test and other tests in this chapter, spinal nerves are listed as C7, 8 with those in parentheses being spinal levels that are "sometimes" or "occasionally" found, as noted in the literature.

Action

Extends elbow; some adduction and extension of shoulder from the long head

Origin

Long head, infraglenoid tubercle of scapula; lateral head, posterior and lateral surface of the proximal half of the humerus, intermuscular septum; medial head, lower posterior humerus

Insertion

Olecranon process of ulnar and antebrachial fascia

Nerve

C(6), 7, 8, (T1)

Therapeutic Reflexes

Chapman's—Anterior: seventh intercostal space on medial end, left side only; posterior: between T7 and 8 laminae on left only

Acupuncture meridian—spleen

Common acupuncture points—SP 2, 3

Testing Position

Supine

Testing

Shoulder is slightly flexed, abducted, and laterally rotated; elbow is slightly flexed to approximately 45°. The practitioner stabilizes the arm with one hand and contacts the forearm just proximal to the wrist and applies pressure in the direction of elbow flexion.

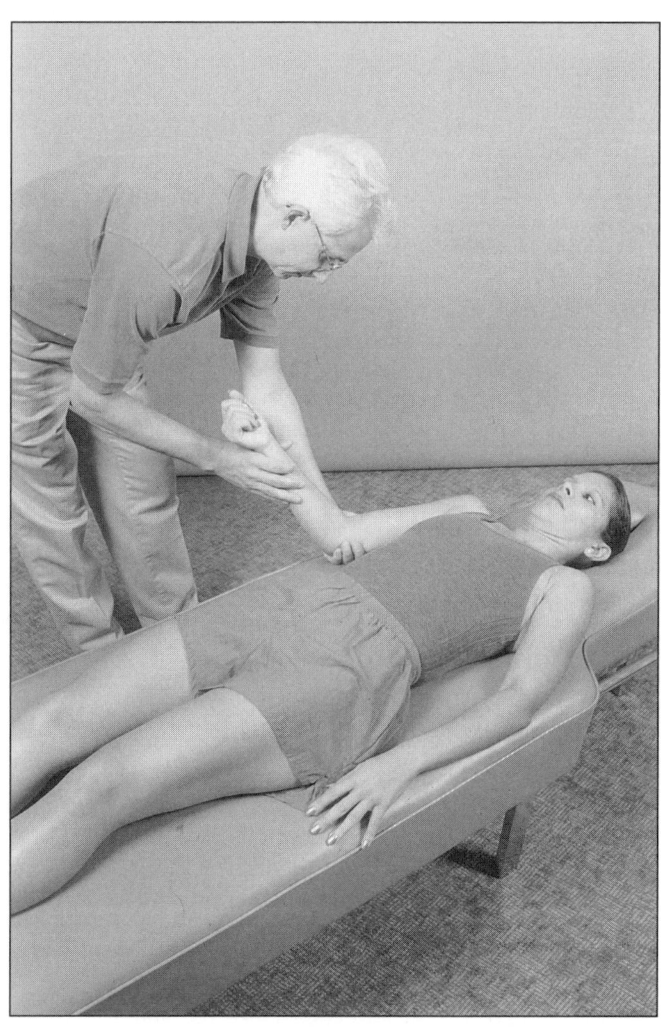

Opponens Pollicis Muscle

The opponens pollicis and opponens digiti minimi are grasping muscles of the hand; they can be tested separately or together. They are frequently inhibited when there is wrist dysfunction. Grasping a ball, baseball bat, racket, or other equipment that requires function of the thumb and fifth finger is difficult when these muscles are inhibited. When inhibited, the wrist extensors, evaluated here with a nonspecific muscle test, may also be associated with wrist dysfunction and are often the reason for secondary elbow pain. Note: The only significant reflexes for this muscle are those related to the acupuncture system.

Action

Flexes and abducts the thumb

Origin

Trapezium bone and flexor retinaculum of the wrist

Insertion

Full length of first metacarpal bone on the radial side

Nerve

C6, 7, (8, T1)

Therapeutic Reflexes

Acupuncture meridian—stomach

Common acupuncture points—ST 1, 41

Testing Position

Supine

Testing

The patient's hand is supinated and the thumb is flexed so the nail is facing the anterior. The practitioner stabilizes the posterior wrist and hand with one hand, and the fingers of the other hand apply pressure against the anterior metacarpal in the direction of extension and abduction.

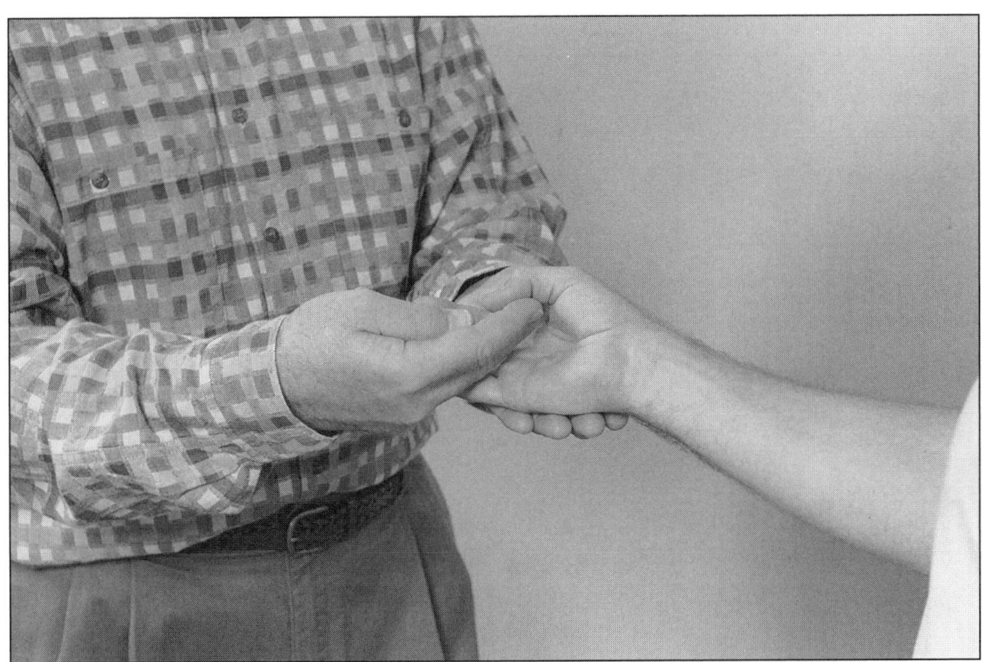

Opponens Digiti Minimi Muscle

Along with the opponens pollicis muscle, the opponens digiti minimi is frequently inhibited when there is wrist dysfunction. The grasping motion (requiring proper function of the thumb and fifth finger) is difficult when these muscles are inhibited. Note: The only significant reflexes for this muscle are those related to the acupuncture system.

Action

Flexes the fifth metacarpal joint

Origin

Hamate bone and flexor retinaculum of wrist

Insertion

Full length of fifth metacarpal bone on the ulnar side

Nerve

C(7), 8, T1

Therapeutic Reflexes

Acupuncture meridian—stomach

Common acupuncture points—ST 1, 41

Testing Position

Supine

Testing

The patient's open hand is stabilized by one of the practitioner's hands. The thumb from the practitioner's other hand contacts the distal end of the flexed fifth metacarpal bone and applies pressure into extension. Note that the opponens pollicis and opponens digiti minimi can be tested simultaneously as depicted here. In this case, the thumb and fifth metacarpal are approximated with both fingers straight and the pads of the two fingers coming into contact. The practitioner uses the thumb and index finger from each of his or her hands to grasp around the patient's thumb and fifth finger and applies pressure by pulling the two fingers apart. These muscles can be evaluated when muscle testing is being used for assessment as described in chapter 11, and the need is for a general muscle test, especially in the situation in which the practitioner or patient does not want to exert much force. If the patient is in great pain other than in the wrist or arm, these muscles are often the most practical ones to use.

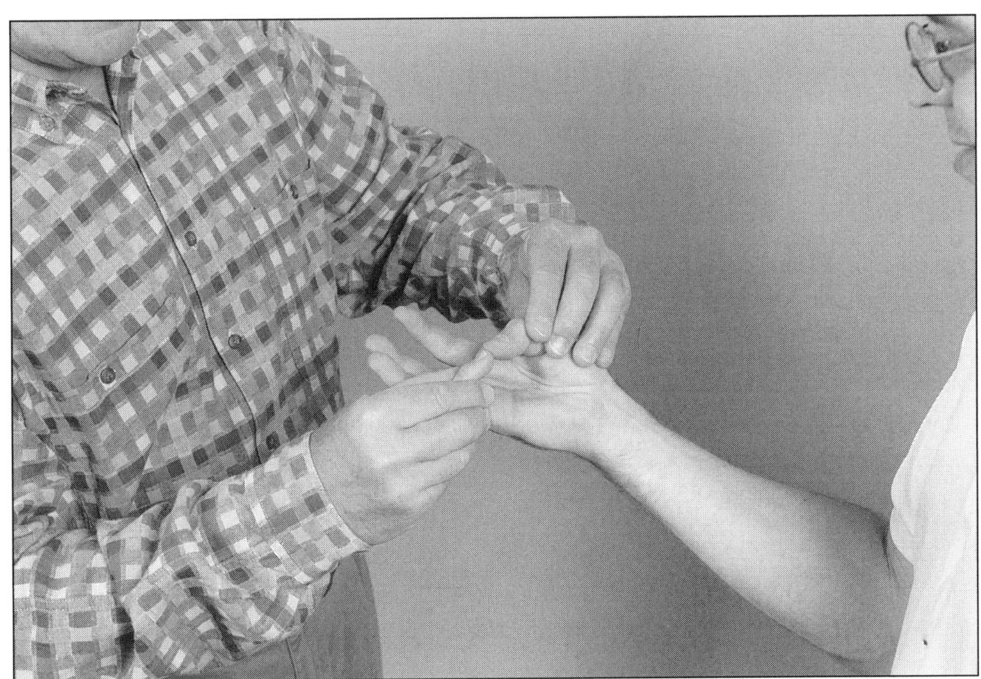

Wrist Extensor Muscles

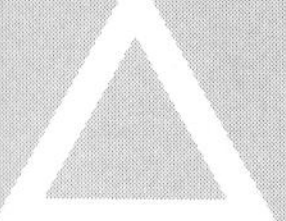

The wrist extensor and flexor tests are outlined here very generally, with the more commonly dysfunctional muscles listed. Those practitioners who find it necessary to test the isolated wrist muscles are directed to Kendall et al. (1993). These muscles are frequently inhibited due to local trauma and also to microtrauma with excess wrist action, as occurs in many racket sports. There are no commonly used reflexes, but the wrist muscles often require Golgi tendon organ/spindle cell therapy as described in chapter 16. The extensor muscles of the wrist include the extensor digitorum, extensor indicis, and extensor digiti minimi. When these are tested as a group, other muscles may also become active, including the extensor carpi ulnaris and extensor radialis longus and brevis.

Action

Extend the wrist

Origin

Extensor digitorum, lateral epicondyle of humerus and deep antibrachial fascia; extensor indicis, posterior distal ulna; extensor digiti minimi, lateral epicondyle of the humerus and deep antibrachial fascia

Insertion

Extensor digitorum: into extensor tendons proximal to the wrist joint with the tendons inserting into the second through fifth digit; extensor indicis: into extensor tendon at the wrist joint with the tendon inserting into the extensor expansion of index finger; extensor digiti minimi: into extensor tendon proximal to the wrist joint with the tendon inserting into extensor expansion of fifth digit.

Nerve

C6-8

Testing Position

Supine

Testing

The patient's elbow is placed on the exam table with slight flexion, with the hand pronated, relaxed, and fully extended. The practitioner grasps the dorsum of the hand and applies pressure in the direction of flexion.

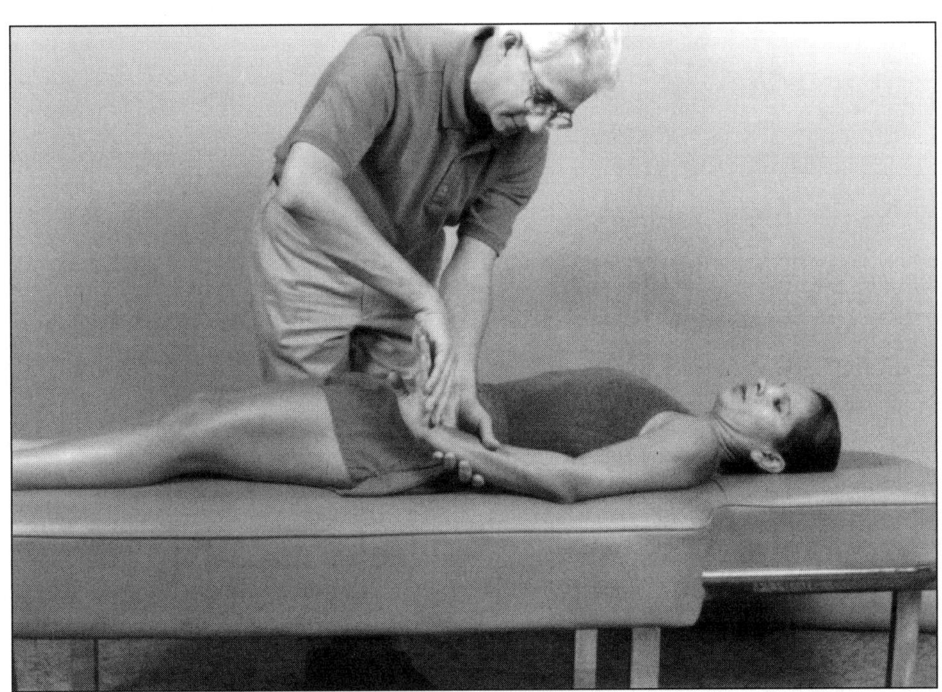

Wrist Flexor Muscles

This test is provided within a very general format. For testing of the isolated wrist muscles, see Kendall et al. (1993). Wrist muscles are commonly inhibited due to local trauma and also to microtrauma with excess wrist action, as occurs in many racket sports. There are no commonly used reflexes, but these muscles often require Golgi tendon organ/spindle cell therapy. The flexors of the wrist include the palmaris longus and flexor carpi radialis and flexor carpi ulnaris.

Action

Flex the wrist

Origin

All three muscles: common flexor tendon from medial epicondyle of humerus and deep fascia

Insertion

All insert into the visible tendons one-half to two-thirds distally down forearm. The palmaris tendon inserts into the flexor retinaculum, the flexor carpi radialis tendon into the second (and by ligaments to the third) metacarpal bone, and the flexor carpi ulnaris tendon into the pisiform bone (and by ligaments to the hamate and fifth metacarpal bones).

Nerve

C6-8, T1

Testing

The patient's forearm is placed on the exam table with the hand supinated and relaxed and the wrist fully flexed with fingers extended. The practitioner grasps the palm and applies pressure in the direction of extension.

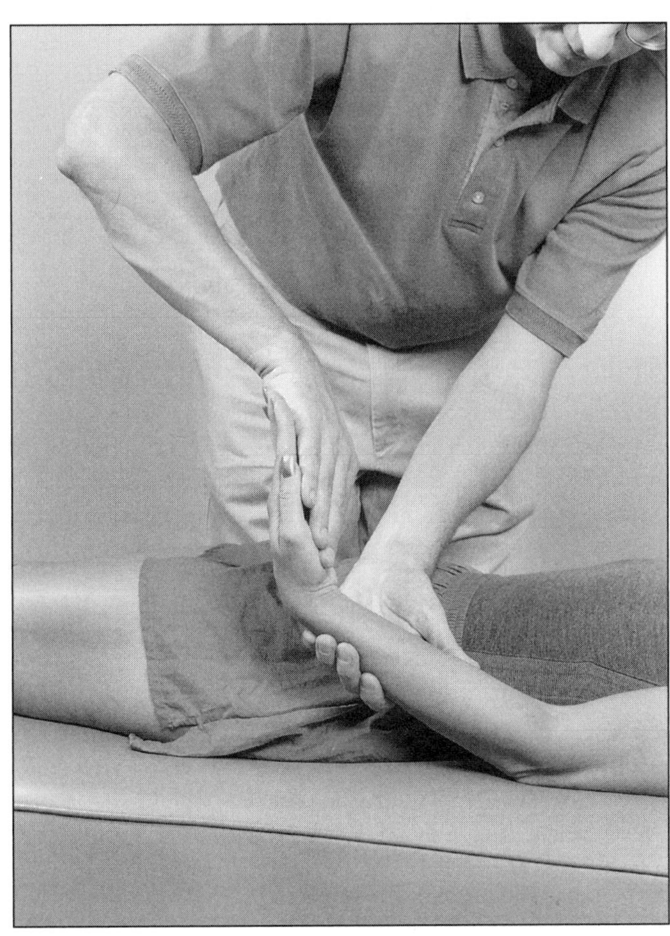

Rectus Abdominis

There are four different abdominal muscles: the rectus abdominis, transverse abdominal, external oblique abdominal, and internal oblique abdominal. They are important for many functions, including breathing; abdominal, rib, and low back stability during activity; and trunk rotation. They are also important in stabilizing and protecting the abdominal viscera. General tests for the rectus muscles and the oblique muscles are described. All abdominal muscles have the same therapeutic reflexes.

Action

Flexes the trunk, pelvis, and spine; stabilizes the thorax, allowing the neck flexors to raise the head when the person is supine (inhibited or weak rectus muscles will not allow neck flexors to function effectively even when facilitated). Weakness increases lumbar spine lordosis.

Origin

Pubic crest and symphysis pubis

Insertion

Costal cartilage of ribs 5-7, xiphoid process

Nerve

T5-12

Therapeutic Reflexes

Chapman's—Anterior: anteromedial thigh along the medial edge of the vastus medialis, from approximately 5-6 cm (2-3 in.) below the inguinal area to just above the knee joint; posterior: L5 transverse process

Acupuncture meridian—small intestine

Common acupuncture points—SI 3, 19

Testing Position

Supine

Testing

Patient sits at 60° with arms crossed (hands on opposite shoulders) and legs extended. The practitioner places one hand or forearm on the thigh to stabilize and one on the patient's outermost posterior forearm and applies pressure into extension. Isolation of left or right rectus may be accomplished by contacting the patient's left or right anterior shoulder, respectively, and applying pressure into extension.

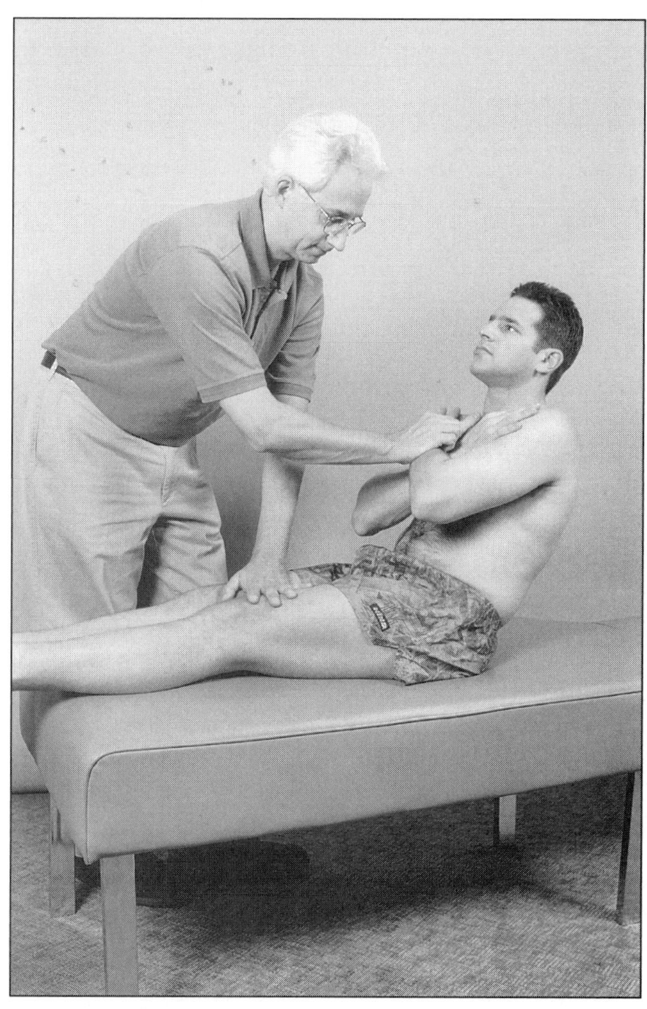

External Oblique Muscles

(Contains Anterior and Lateral Fibers)

There are four different abdominal muscles: the rectus abdominis, transverse abdominal, external oblique abdominal, and internal oblique abdominal. They are important for many functions, including breathing; abdominal, rib, and low back stability during activity; and trunk rotation. They are also important in stabilizing and protecting the abdominal viscera. General tests for the rectus muscles and the oblique muscles are described. All abdominal muscles have the same therapeutic reflexes.

Action

Bilaterally, the anterior fibers flex the spine, depress the thorax, and play a vital role in the breathing mechanism. When acting unilaterally, they rotate the trunk.

Origin

Anterior fibers, ribs 5-8; lateral fibers, ribs 9-12. Both interdigitate with the serratus anterior muscle, and the lateral fibers interdigitate with the latissimus dorsi.

Insertion

The anterior fibers blend into a broad flat aponeurosis extending from the xiphoid to the pubis, extending into the inguinal area between the anterior superior iliac spine and the pubic tubercle. Some fascial layers are attached to the fascia from the thigh, with some of the more posterior fibers attaching on the iliac crest.

Nerve

T5-12

Therapeutic Reflexes

Chapman's—Anterior: anteromedial thigh along the medial edge of the vastus medialis, from approximately 5-6 cm (2-3 in.) below the inguinal area to just above the knee joint; posterior: L5 transverse process

Acupuncture meridian—small intestine

Common acupuncture points—SI 3, 19

Testing Position

Sitting

Testing

Patient sits at 60° with arms crossed (hands on opposite shoulders), legs extended, and trunk fully rotated. The practitioner places one hand on the patient's thigh to stabilize and one on the forward shoulder and applies pressure in extension. With the patient rotated to the left, for example, the right external oblique and left internal oblique are tested.

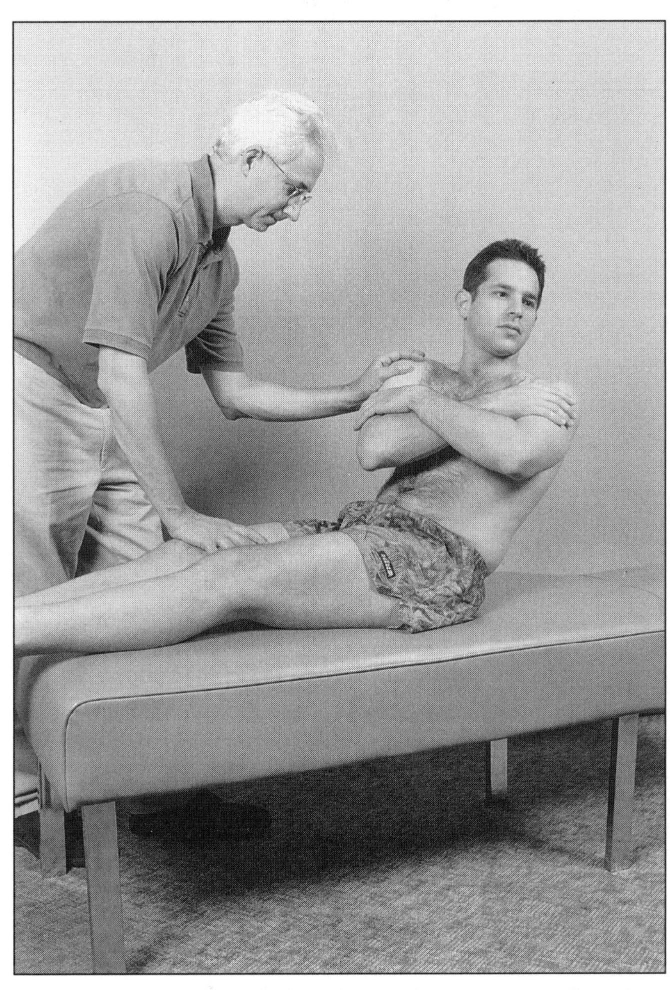

Psoas Major Muscle

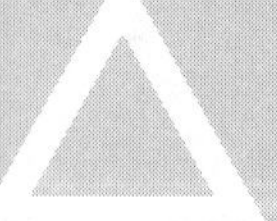

Because of its attachments and actions, the psoas major is a muscle with great significance in sport activity. It is often associated with so-called groin pulls and similar problems. The function of this muscle is sometimes combined with that of the iliacus but is treated separately in this text. The psoas minor muscle exists in less than half the population and is a very small and less important muscle.

Action

Flexes the hip with some lateral rotation and abduction of the femur; laterally flexes the trunk. Acting bilaterally, it flexes the trunk on the femur and increases lumbar spine lordosis.

Origin

Anterior aspect of transverse processes, bodies, and discs of all lumbar vertebrae; body of T12

Insertion

Lesser trochanter of the femur

Nerve

L1-4

Therapeutic Reflexes

Chapman's—Anterior: 2.5 cm lateral and 2.5 cm superior to the umbilicus; posterior: T12-L1 between spinous and transverse process

Acupuncture meridian—kidney

Common acupuncture point—KI 7

Testing Position

Supine

Testing

The hip is flexed, laterally rotated, and abducted with the knee fully extended. Practitioner applies pressure just inferior to the medial knee joint while stabilizing the contralateral anterior superior iliac spine with the other hand. Pressure is directed in line with the muscle fibers into extension and slight abduction. The patient should not be allowed to flex the knee, medially rotate the femur, or rotate the trunk.

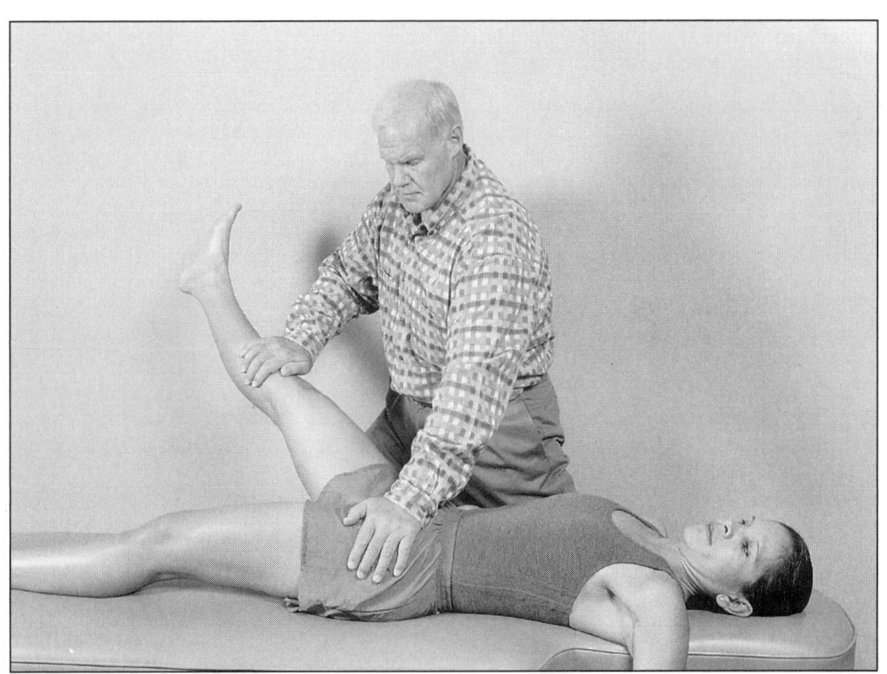

Iliacus Muscle

This muscle is very similar to the psoas major with the exceptions noted, including the slightly changed testing position because of its more lateral origin. The iliacus and psoas are often considered as one unit, referred to as the iliopsoas.

Action

Similar to that of psoas

Origin

Upper iliac fossa

Insertion

With the psoas major on the lesser trochanter

Nerve

L1, 2

Therapeutic Reflexes

Same reflexes as for psoas major

Testing Position

Supine

Testing

Same as for psoas major (see pages 134-135) except with near-maximum hip flexion and slightly more abduction.

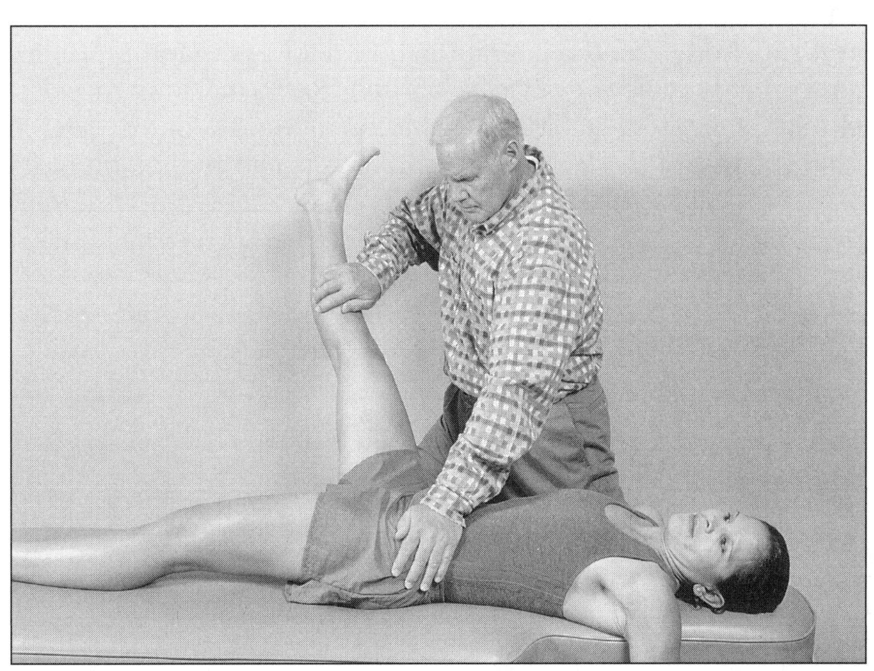

Tensor Fascia Lata Muscle

Chronic weakness or inhibition of this muscle presents the classic genu varum (bowleg) position. The tensor fascia lata is sometimes associated with the so-called iliotibial band syndrome, often as a secondary overfacilitation, but also when inhibited. The tensor fascia lata (along with the gluteus medius and maximus) attaches to a dense fascia called the fascia lata, which wraps the entire thigh and has connections to the linea aspera of the femur. The fascia lata also attaches to the inguinal ligament, pubic ramus, ischium, and iliac crest superiorly. On the lateral thigh, it thickens to form the iliotibial band, made partly of the tensor fascia lata and gluteus maximus muscles. In the lower thigh, the fascia lata blends with the retinacula of the patella, helps form the capsule of the knee joint, and attaches to the lateral tibial condyle.

Action

Abducts, flexes, and medially rotates the hip

Origin

Anterior part of external iliac crest, anterior superior iliac spine, and fascia lata

Insertion

Upper anterior portion of iliotibial band

Nerve

L4, 5, S1

Therapeutic Reflexes

- Chapman's—Anterior: along the iliotibial band on the anterior portion; posterior: transverse process of lumbar vertebrae 2-4
- Acupuncture meridian—large intestine
- Common acupuncture points—LI 11, 20

Testing Position

Supine

Testing

Patient is supine with practitioner standing by the patient's feet. Hip is flexed and abducted about 20° with moderate medial rotation, and the knee maintains maximal extension. One of the practitioner's hands stabilizes the contralateral distal leg, and the other holds under the distal end of the leg with the force toward adduction and extension (as if placing the test foot next to the contralateral foot).

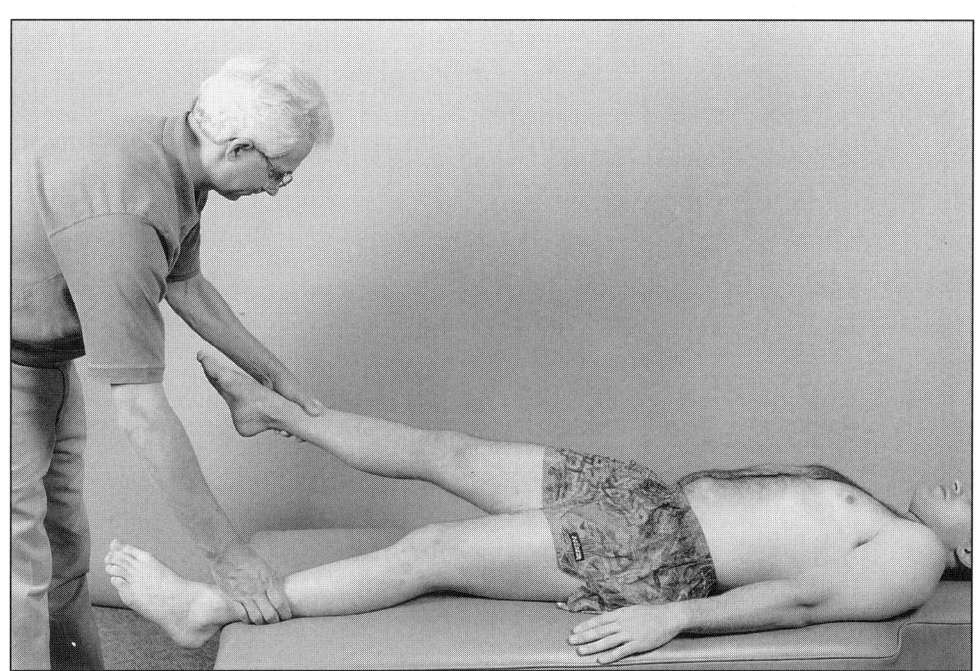

Sartorius Muscle

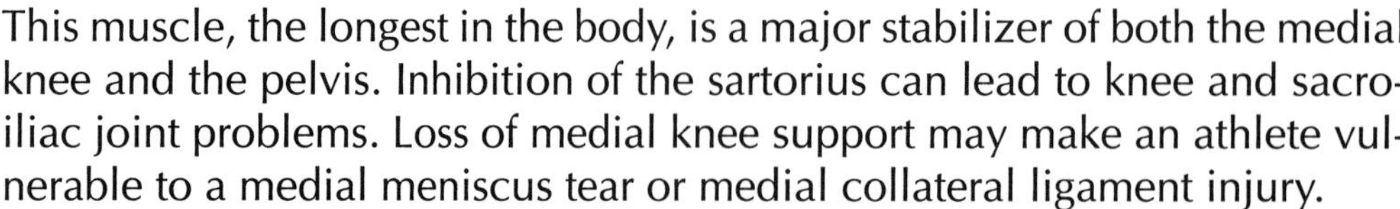

This muscle, the longest in the body, is a major stabilizer of both the medial knee and the pelvis. Inhibition of the sartorius can lead to knee and sacroiliac joint problems. Loss of medial knee support may make an athlete vulnerable to a medial meniscus tear or medial collateral ligament injury.

Action

Flexes, laterally rotates, and abducts the femur; medially rotates the tibia

Origin

Anterior superior iliac spine

Insertion

Upper medial surface of the tibia

Nerve

L2, 3, (4)

Therapeutic Reflexes

Chapman's—Anterior: approximately 2 cm lateral and 5 cm superior to the umbilicus; posterior: laminae of T11

Acupuncture meridian—circulation sex

Common acupuncture points—CX 9, TH 23

Testing Position

Supine

Testing

The hip is flexed, laterally rotated, and abducted with the knee flexed so that the Achilles approaches a point on the contralateral proximal tibia. In testing the right sartorius, the practitioner (either at the foot end of the exam table or on the side being tested) places the left hand on the lateral knee joint and the right hand on the posterior portion of the distal leg. Most of the force is directed into knee extension using the right hand, with some pressure directed medially with the left hand.

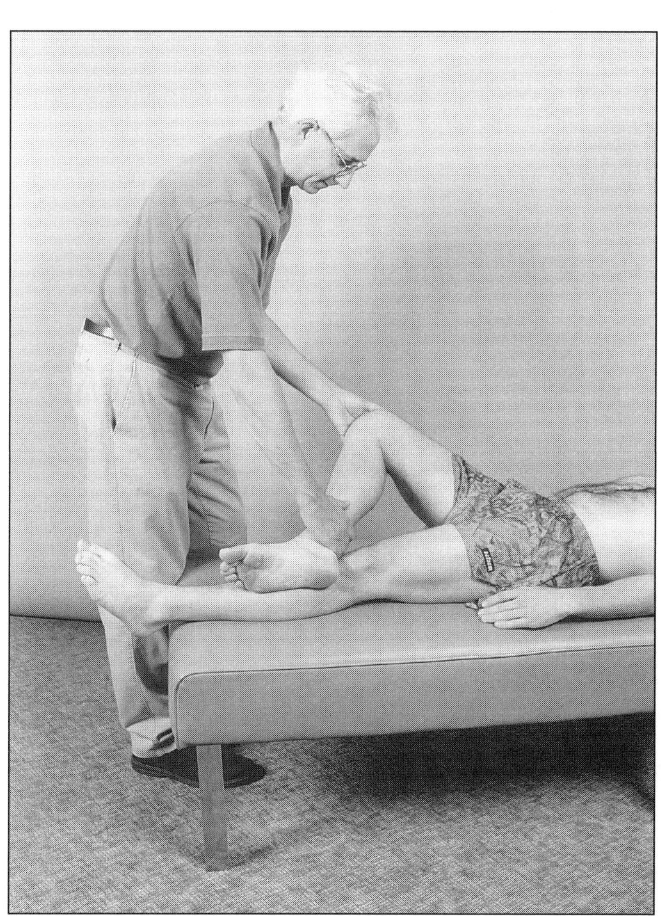

Quadriceps Femoris Muscles: Rectus Femoris

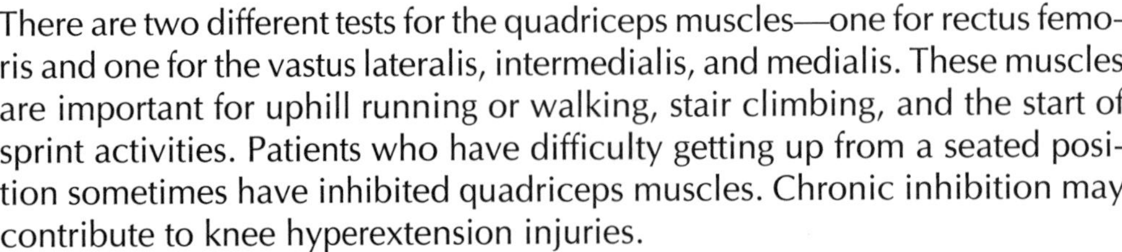

There are two different tests for the quadriceps muscles—one for rectus femoris and one for the vastus lateralis, intermedialis, and medialis. These muscles are important for uphill running or walking, stair climbing, and the start of sprint activities. Patients who have difficulty getting up from a seated position sometimes have inhibited quadriceps muscles. Chronic inhibition may contribute to knee hyperextension injuries.

Action

Flexes the hip joint

Origin

Has two heads: the straight head from the anterior inferior iliac spine and the reflected head from the superior rim of the acetabulum

Insertion

Inserts on the proximal border of the patella and patellar ligament to the tubercle of the tibia

Nerve

L2-4

Therapeutic Reflexes

Chapman's—Anterior: lower border of rib cage extending from xiphoid laterally along costal cartilages 8-11 (lower edge of rib cage); posterior: laminae of T8-11

Acupuncture meridian—small intestine

Common acupuncture points—SI 3, 19

Testing Position

Supine

Testing

The rectus femoris is tested with the patient supine; the hip is flexed to about 80° and knee flexed to 90°. The practitioner places one hand on the anterior distal thigh just superior to the patella, and force is in direction of hip extension. It is important to maintain knee position and not allow any thigh rotation. The rectus femoris can also be tested with the patient sitting. In this case, the position of the hip is flexed more than 90°, with the knee also flexed at 90°, as the patient sits at the edge of the examination table. The practitioner contacts the distal thigh and applies force downward, in the direction of the hip extension. Note: In both test positions, the rectus femoris muscle may be very powerful and difficult to test for some practitioners. Care must be taken to maintain an optimal test position.

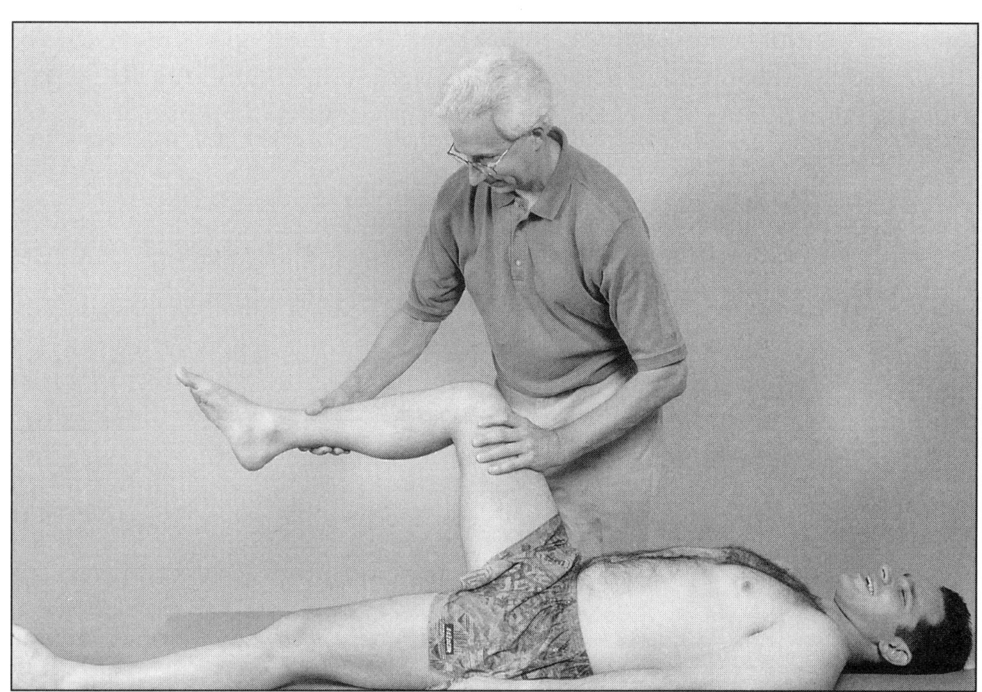

Quadriceps Femoris Muscles

(Includes Vastus Lateralis, Intermedialis, and Medialis)

There are two different tests for the quadriceps muscles—one for rectus femoris and one for the vastus lateralis, intermedialis, and medialis. These muscles are important for uphill running or walking, stair climbing, and the start of sprint activities. Patients who have difficulty getting up from a seated position sometimes have inhibited quadriceps muscles. Chronic inhibition may contribute to knee hyperextension injuries.

Action

Extends the knee

Origin

Vastus lateralis originates anterior and laterally on the proximal femur and the proximal linea aspera; vastus intermedialis originates on the anterior and lateral proximal two-thirds of the femur, the distal half of linea aspera, and lateral intermuscular septum; vastus medialis attaches on the medial lip of linea aspera, distal half of intertrochanteric line, proximal medial supracondylar line, and tendons of the adductor longus and magnus.

Insertion

The vastus lateralis, intermedialis, and medialis insert on the proximal border of the patella and patellar ligament to the tubercle of the tibia.

Nerve

L2-4

Therapeutic Reflexes

Chapman's—Anterior: lower border of rib cage extending from para xiphoid laterally along costal cartilages 8-11 (lower edge of rib cage); posterior: laminae of T8-11

Acupuncture meridian—small intestine

Common acupuncture points—SI 3, 19

Testing Position

Supine

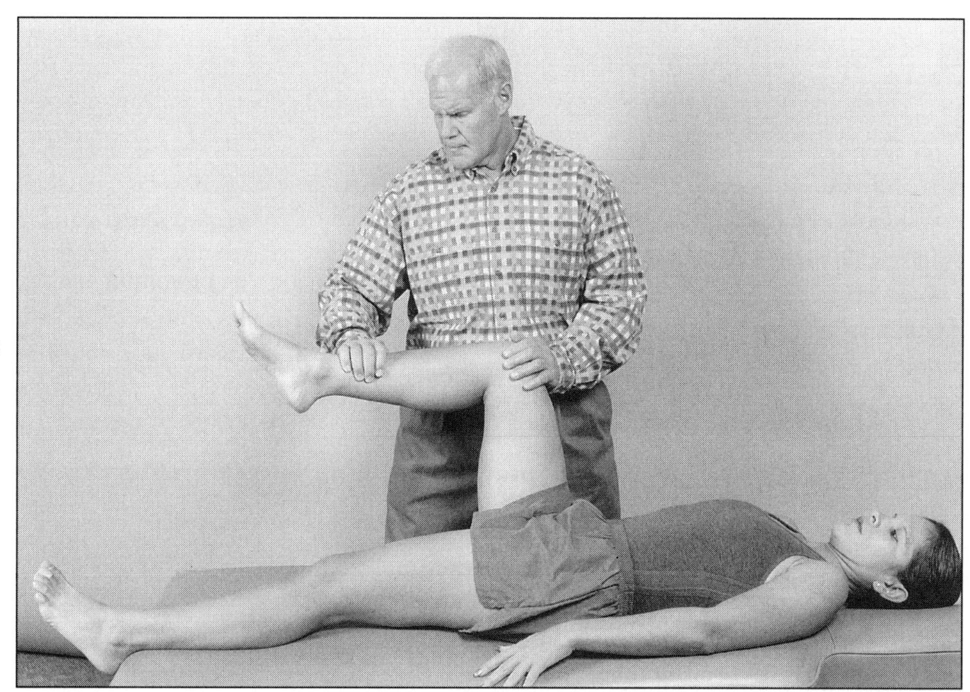

a

Testing

The vastus lateralis, intermedialis, and medialis muscles are tested with the patient supine; the hip is flexed to about 90° and knee flexed to 90°. The practitioner stabilizes the knee with one hand, and the other is placed on the distal end of the leg. Force is applied in the direction of the knee flexion. In the seated position, the legs are hanging off the table, and the test leg is extended to about 45° from full extension. One hand is placed on or under the posterior distal thigh and the other on the distal leg anteriorly with force into knee flexion. Note: These muscles may be very powerful and difficult to test for some practitioners. Care must be taken to maintain an optimal test position.

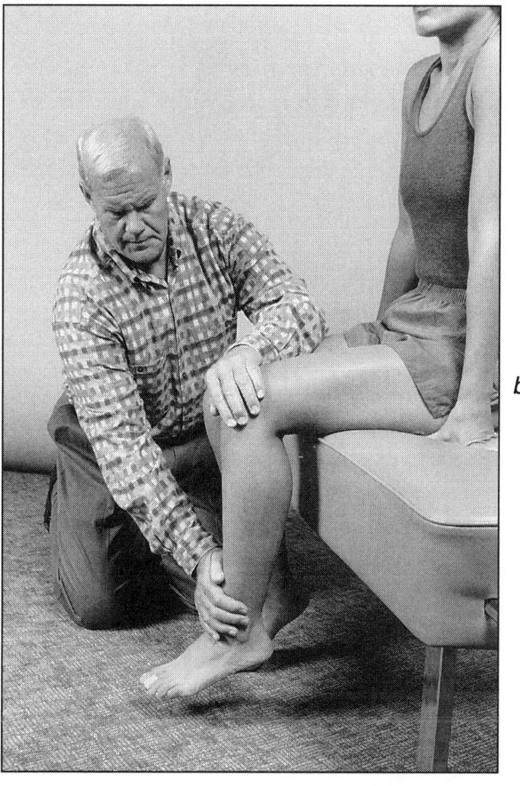

b

Tibialis Posterior Muscle

This may be the most important muscle associated with many types of knee, leg, foot, and ankle dysfunction. Inhibition of this muscle results in excess (abnormal) pronation that is associated with diminished longitudinal arch support. Function of this muscle is vital for sports requiring athletes to rise on their toes. Tibialis posterior inhibition may be followed by secondary tightness of the gastrocnemius and soleus and may be involved in "posterior shinsplints." Because of this muscle's numerous insertions, dysfunction may also predispose an athlete to many potential problems in a variety of joints and bones in the foot.

Action

Inverts and plantar flexes the ankle joint; stabilizes the joints of the medial ankle

Origin

Medial portion of the proximal posterior tibia, medial two-thirds of the posterior fibula, most of the interosseous membrane, and deep fascia

Insertion

Tuberosity of the navicular bone; plantar surfaces of the three cuneiform bones; the bases of the second, third, and fourth metatarsal bones; and the cuboid bone

Nerve

L(4), 5, S1

Therapeutic Reflexes

Chapman's—Anterior: approximately 2.5 cm lateral and 5 cm superior to the umbilicus; posterior: laminae of T11

Acupuncture meridian—circulation sex

Common acupuncture points—CX 9, TH 23

Testing Position

Supine

Testing

Foot and ankle are placed into maximum inversion and plantar flexion. Practitioner places stabilizing hand on posterolateral distal leg and one hand under anterior medial arch (i.e., the patient's right foot is tested by the practitioner's right hand). Pressure is directed into dorsiflexion and eversion. On contraction of the muscle, the tibialis posterior tendon should become prominent (just medial to the anterior tibialis tendon and just posterior to the medial malleolus).

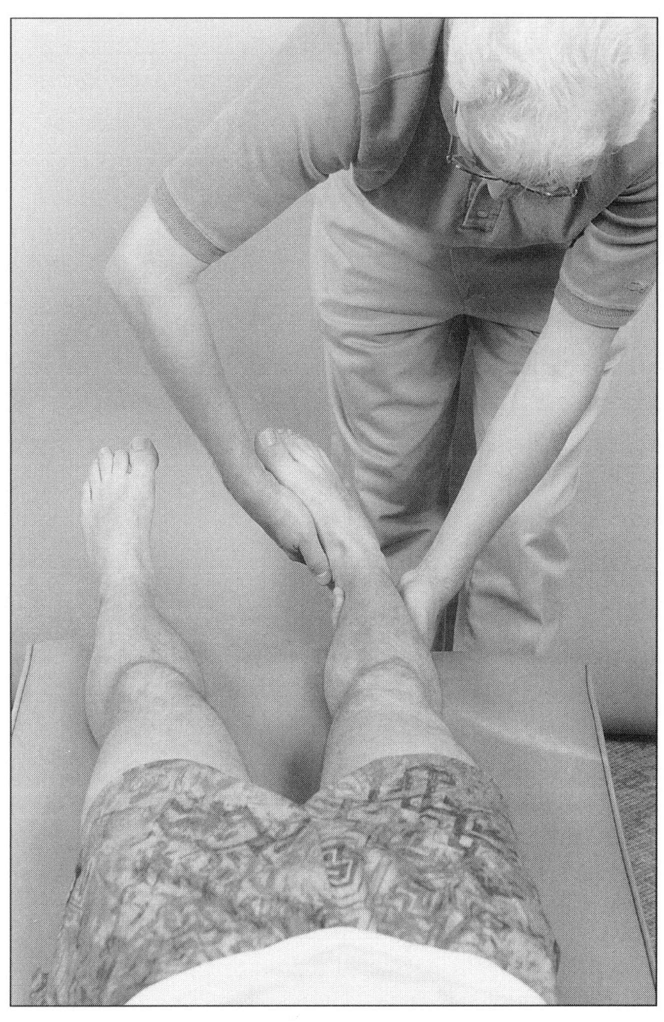

Tibialis Anterior Muscle

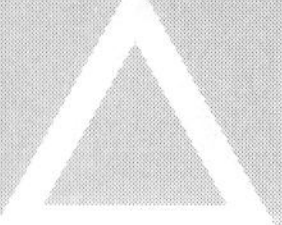

This is an important muscle for the lateral stability of the ankle joint. Inhibition may also be associated with first metatarsal problems and so-called shinsplints. The tibialis anterior, along with its posterior counterpart, is important for athletes in getting up on their toes and provides the "spring" in one's step.

Action

Dorsiflexes the ankle and inverts the foot

Origin

Proximal one-half of the lateral tibia from the lateral condyle, interosseous membrane, lateral intermuscular septum, and deep fascia; forms a tendon above the ankle joint

Insertion

Base of the first metatarsal bone and medial and plantar surface of medial cuneiform bone

Nerve

L4, 5, S1

Therapeutic Reflexes

Chapman's—Anterior: 1-2 cm above the anterior pubic bone, bilaterally; posterior: transverse process of L2

Acupuncture meridian—bladder

Common acupuncture points—BL 1, 67

Testing Position

Supine or sitting

Testing

With the patient supine or sitting, foot is inverted and ankle dorsiflexed. The practitioner stabilizes the heel; the other hand contacts the medial dorsal surface of the foot in the direction of eversion and ankle plantar flexion.

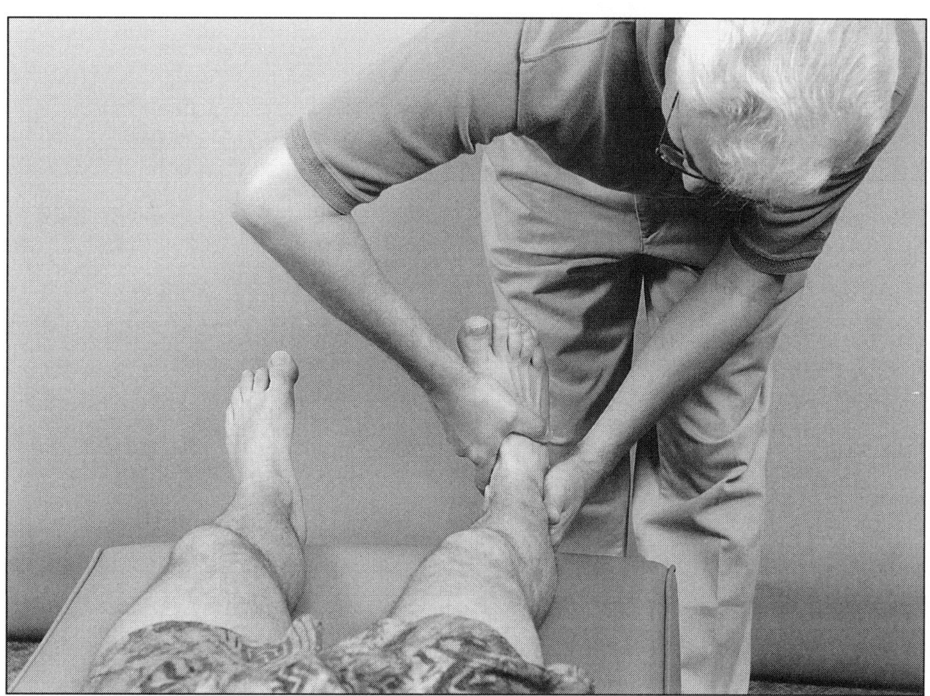

Peroneus Longus and Brevis Muscles

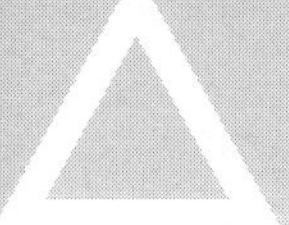

Tests for these two muscles are combined into one, although the primary action is from the peroneus brevis. The peroneus longus and brevis are lateral ankle stabilizers and also assist in rising on the toes.

Action

Assist in eversion of foot and plantar flexion of ankle joint

Origin

The peroneus longus attaches from the lateral condyle of the tibia, deep fascia, and head and proximal two-thirds of fibula; the brevis arises from the distal half of the lateral fibula and intermuscular septa.

Insertion

The peroneus longus inserts into the lateral medial cuneiform and the lateral side of the base of the first metatarsal bone; the brevis inserts on the lateral surface of the base of the fifth metatarsal.

Nerve

L4, 5, S1

Therapeutic Reflexes

Chapman's—Anterior: lower anterior pubic bone; posterior: transverse process of L5

Acupuncture meridian—bladder

Common acupuncture points—BL 1, 67

Testing Position

Supine

Testing

Foot is everted and ankle is plantar flexed. The practitioner supports the posterior leg distally and contacts the lateral border and plantar aspect of foot with force applied in the direction of inversion and dorsiflexion. During testing, the practitioner notes the tendon as it passes just posterior to the lateral malleolus.

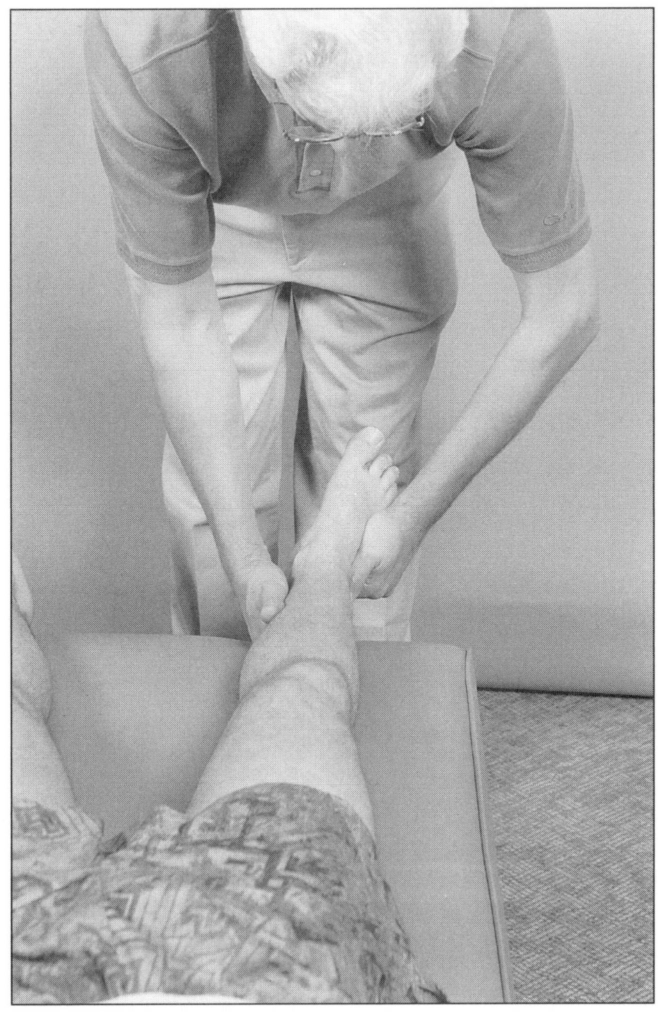

Peroneus Tertius Muscle

This lateral ankle stabilizer is assisted by the extensor digitorum longus and, when traumatized, is often what makes sprained ankles chronically disabling.

Action

Everts the foot and dorsiflexes the ankle

Origin

Distal anterior fibula, interosseous membrane, and intermuscular septum

Insertion

Proximal base of fifth metatarsal on dorsal surface

Nerve

L4, 5, S1

Therapeutic Reflexes

Chapman's—Anterior: upper anterior pubic bone; posterior: transverse process of L5

Acupuncture meridian—bladder

Common acupuncture points—BL 1, 67

Testing Position

Supine

Testing

Ankle is dorsiflexed and foot everted. Practitioner stabilizes posterior calf distally, and force is directed against the lateral dorsal foot near the muscle's insertion in the direction of plantar flexion and inversion. The peroneus tertius tendon should be noted during testing as it inserts into the fifth metatarsal.

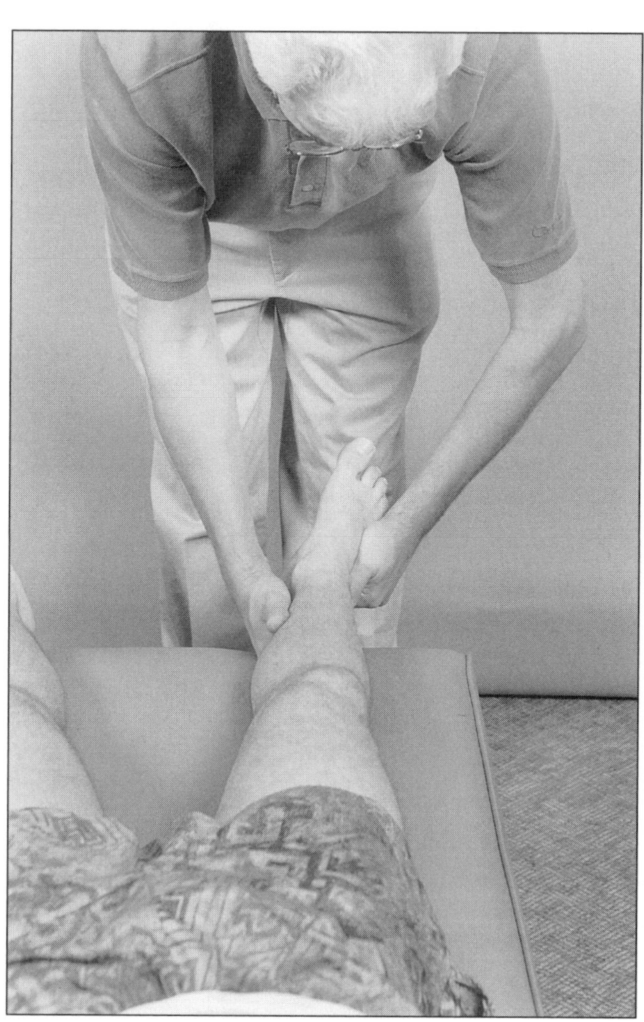

Hip Adductor Muscles

There are four separate adductor muscles of the hip: the pectineus, adductor magnus, adductor brevis, and adductor longus. These are tested together. This group is frequently associated with groin problems.

Action

The adductor muscles are hip adductors and provide some flexion. In addition, the posterior fibers of the adductor magnus extend the hip.

Origin

Pectineus: superior pubic ramus

Adductor Magnus: inferior pubic ramus, ischiopubic ramus, and ischial tuberosity

Adductor Brevis: inferior pubic ramus

Adductor Longus: anterior pubic ramus between crest and symphysis

Insertion

Pectineus: pectineal line of the femur beginning from the lesser trochanter

Adductor Magnus: linea aspera of femur from lesser trochanter superiorly to the adductor tubercle of the femur

Adductor Brevis: upper half of linea aspera and middle third of pectineal line

Adductor Longus: middle third of medial linea aspera

Nerve

Pectineus: L2-4

Adductor Magnus: L2-5, S1

Adductor Brevis: L2-4

Adductor Longus: L2-4

Therapeutic Reflexes

Chapman's—Anterior: sixth intercostal at a point between the midline and midaxillary line; posterior: inferior angle of the scapula

Acupuncture meridian—circulation sex

Common acupuncture point—CX 9, TH 23

Testing Position

Side-lying

Testing

The patient is side-lying on the muscle being tested; both knees are maximally extended with the whole-body alignment straight. The practitioner stands behind the patient and abducts the opposite (upper) limb, holding it with one hand at about 30°. The other hand applies pressure distal to the medial knee joint in the direction of abduction. The pelvis should not be allowed to tilt or the trunk to flex or extend.

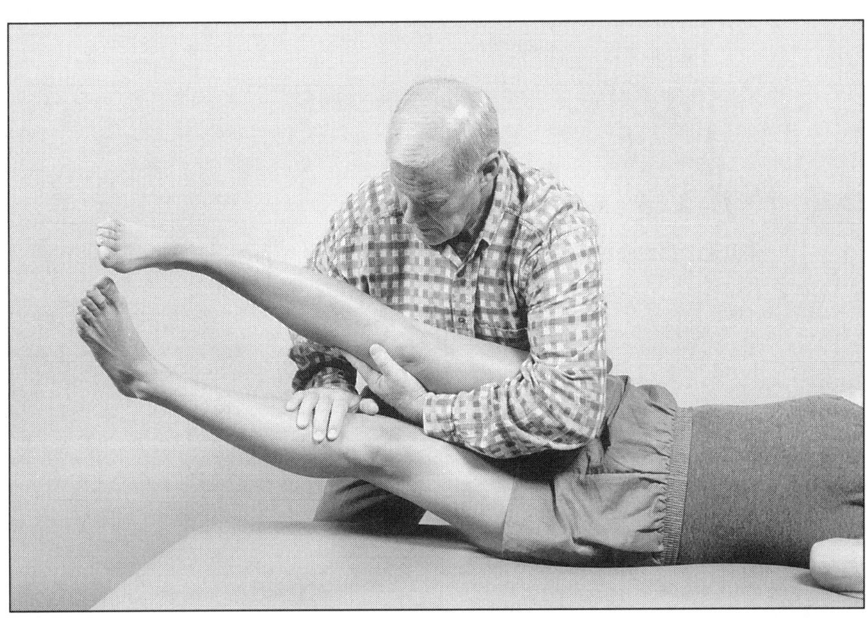

Gluteus Medius

Differentiating the gluteus medius and minimus in manual testing may present great difficulty and requires careful attention to test positions and possible recruitment. These muscles are important in stabilizing the pelvis and weight-bearing leg during walking, running, and other movements. Trendelenburg sign (pelvis drops down instead of up on the opposite side of weakness) may be seen in some patients with inhibited muscles. Problems in the hip joint are sometimes associated with dysfunction of one or both of these muscles.

Action

The gluteus medius abducts the hip, slightly medially rotates the hip, and flexes the hip. Some lateral rotation and extension takes place with the posterior fibers.

Origin

External ilium laterally, gluteal aponeurosis/fascia lata

Insertion

Laterally on the greater trochanter of femur

Nerve

L4, 5, S1

Therapeutic Reflexes

- Chapman's—Anterior: upper symphysis pubis; posterior: transverse process of L5 vertebra
- Acupuncture meridian—circulation sex
- Common acupuncture point—CX 9, TH 23

Testing Position

Side-lying

Testing

Patient is side-lying with the muscle to be tested facing up. Bottom hip and knee are slightly flexed for support. Test leg is aligned in slight extension, knee in maximal extension, and limb abducted to about 40° with slight external rotation. Practitioner stands behind patient and stabilizes lateral pelvis with one hand. Force is applied to the lateral leg distally into adduction and slight flexion. Inability to hold proper test position or cramping in test position usually indicates inhibition. The patient should not be allowed to flex the hip or rotate the pelvis.

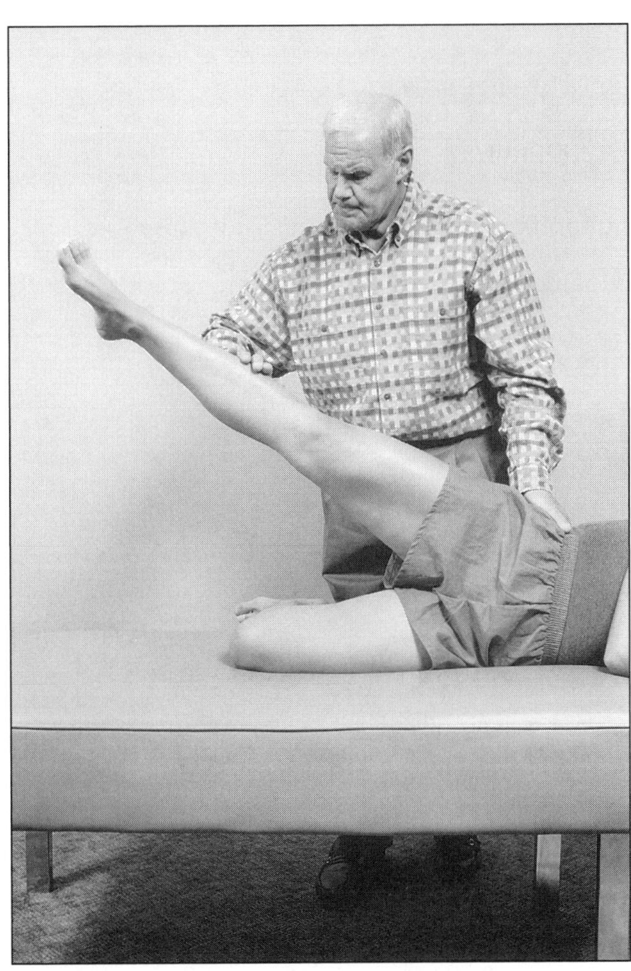

Gluteus Minimus

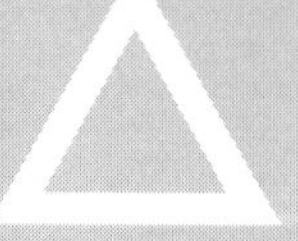

Differentiating the gluteus medius and minimus in manual testing may be very difficult and requires careful attention to test positions and possible recruitment. These muscles are important in stabilizing the pelvis and weight-bearing leg during walking, running, and other movements. Trendelenburg sign (pelvis drops down instead of up on the opposite side of weakness) may be seen in some patients with inhibited muscles. Problems in the hip joint are sometimes associated with dysfunction of one or both of these muscles.

Action

Abducts the hip, with some medial rotation of hip

Origin

External ilium laterally, margin of greater sciatic notch

Insertion

Anterior portion of greater trochanter of femur and hip joint capsule

Nerve

L4, 5, S1

Therapeutic Reflexes

Chapman's—Anterior: upper symphysis pubis; posterior: transverse process of L5 vertebra

Acupuncture meridian—circulation sex

Common acupuncture point—CX 9, TH 23

Testing Position

Side-lying

Testing

Patient is similar to the position for the gluteus medius except that the test limb is in neutral position (no flexion or extension, no rotation), and there is slightly less abduction. Direction of force is into adduction with slight extension.

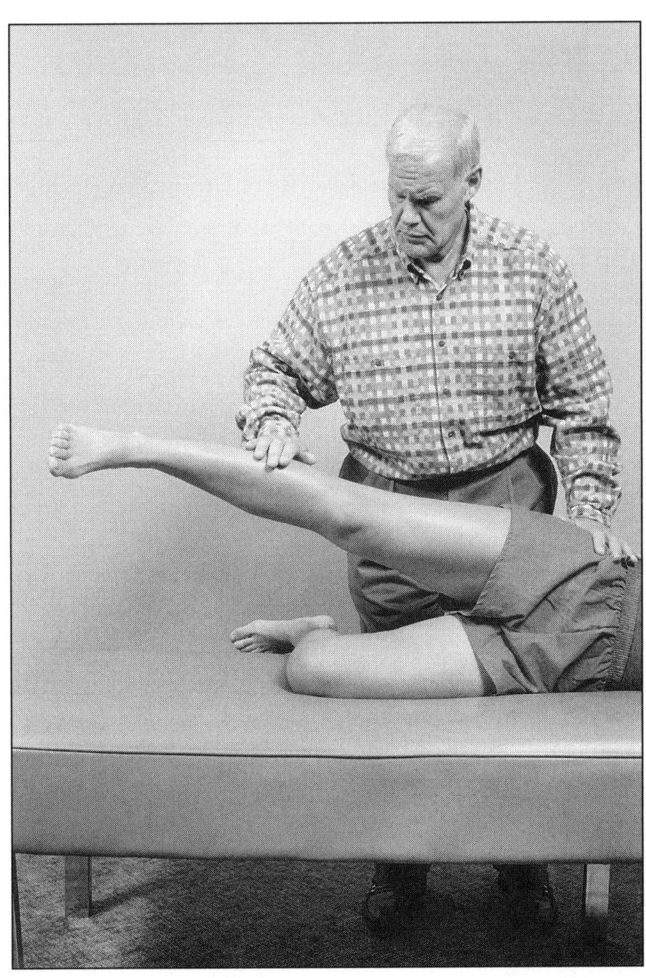

Upper Trapezius Muscles

There are separate tests for the three divisions of the trapezius muscle: upper, middle, and lower. The upper trapezius is illustrated here; the other two divisions are tested in the prone position. The upper trapezius is important for shoulder, neck, and head stability, especially in contact sports.

Action

Assists in rotation and adduction of the scapula, laterally flexes head to ipsilateral side, rotates head to contralateral side, and extends the head when acting bilaterally

Origin

Occiput bone from the external occipital protuberance and medial one-third of superior nuchal line; the ligamentum nuchae to the spinous process of C7. In a few individuals, the fibers do not reach to occiput bone.

Insertion

Lateral one-third of superior surface of the clavicle and acromion process

Nerve

C(2), 3, 4

Therapeutic Reflexes

Chapman's—Anterior: a 6 cm vertical line on the anterior proximal humerus; posterior: on posterior arch of first cervical vertebra

Acupuncture meridian—kidney

Common acupuncture point—KI 7

Testing Position

Sitting

Testing

Head is rotated 45° to contralateral side and slightly flexed; the shoulder is elevated to approximate ear. Practitioner stands behind patient and places one hand on the lateral cranium and one on the shoulder with force directed to separate shoulder and ear.

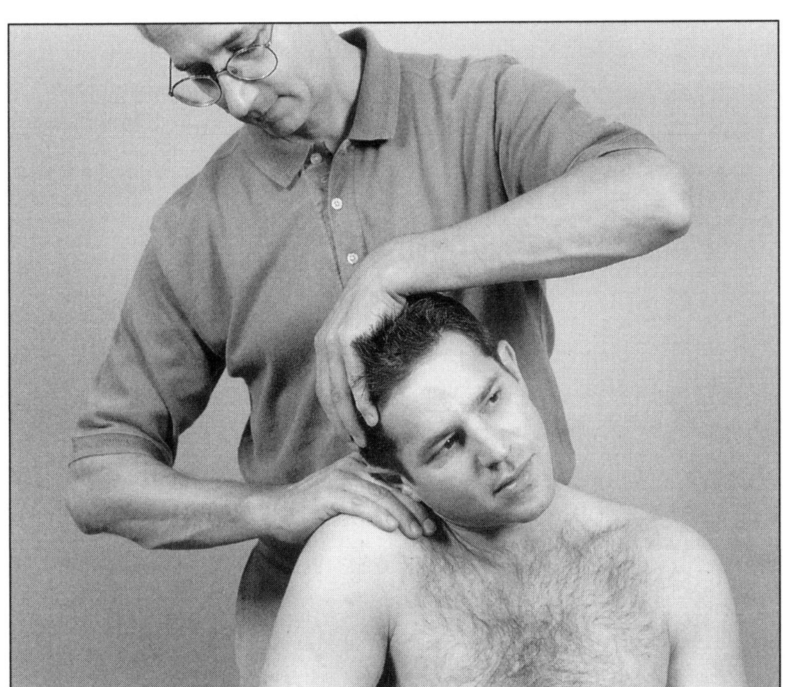

Levator Scapulae Muscle

This muscle is often associated with neck pain that radiates into the posterior neck and shoulder area; the contralateral levator is usually inhibited and the symptomatic one overfacilitated.

Action

Elevates and rotates scapula; laterally flexes and rotates cervical spine. It may extend cervical spine when acting bilaterally.

Origin

Transverse process of first four cervical vertebrae

Insertion

Superior medial border of scapula

Nerve

C3-5

Therapeutic Reflexes

Chapman's—Belly of teres minor muscle
Acupuncture meridian—lung
Common acupuncture point—LU 9

Test Position

Sitting

Testing

Elbow is flexed and humerus fully adducted with slight extension; shoulder is depressed, and head is slightly flexed and laterally rotated to contralateral side. Practitioner stabilizes shoulder with one hand and with the other hand contacts the medial elbow; force is directed into abduction.

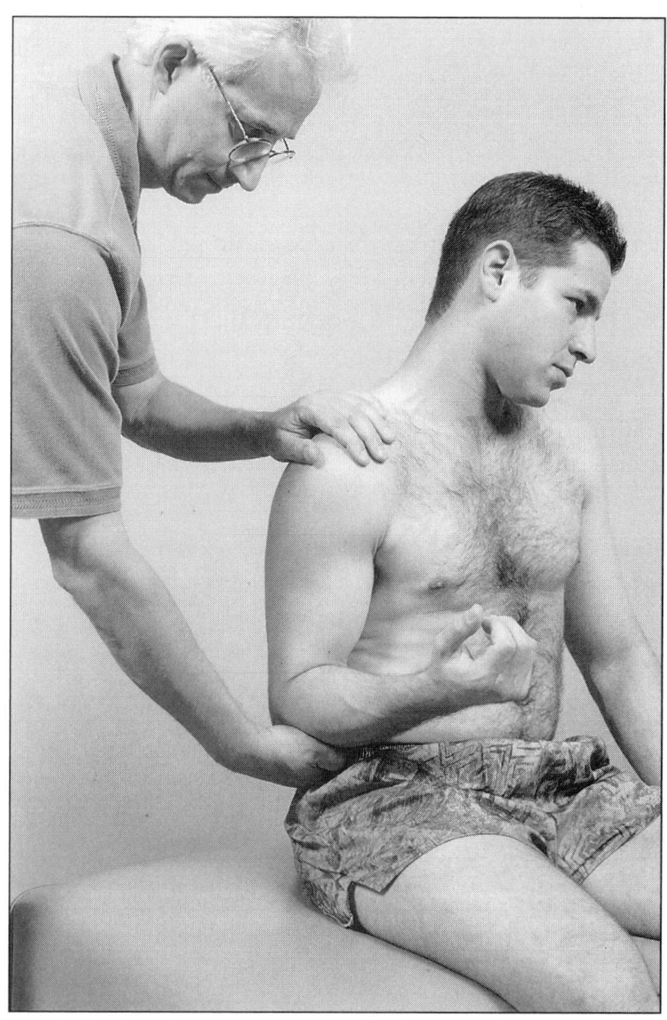

Deltoid Muscles

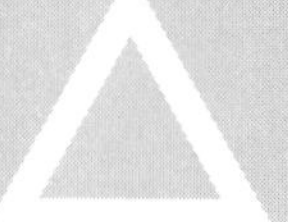

Three muscle tests differentiate the anterior, middle, and posterior deltoid muscles. These muscles provide major support for the shoulder. They are important for all throwing actions and are sometimes inhibited from trauma in athletes who participate in contact sports; they are also important in swimming and racket sports.

Action

These muscles abduct the shoulder. The anterior fibers provide some shoulder flexion and medial rotation, and the posterior fibers some extension and lateral rotation. The posterior fibers work with the supraspinatus to stabilize the glenohumeral joint.

Origin

The anterior fibers attach on the superior surface of the anterior distal one-third of the clavicle; the middle fibers attach on the lateral margins of the superior surface of the acromion; the posterior fibers attach on the posterior border of the spine of the scapula.

Insertion

All fibers insert into deltoid tuberosity of the humerus.

Nerve

C5, 6

Therapeutic Reflexes

Chapman's—Anterior: second through fourth intercostal spaces at junction of sternum; posterior: laminae of T3 and 4

Acupuncture meridian—lung

Common acupuncture point—LU 9

Test Position

Sitting

Testing

Shoulder is abducted to 90°; elbow is flexed to 90°. Practitioner stands behind the patient, stabilizes the contralateral shoulder with one hand, and contacts the distal humerus and elbow with the other. This is the position for the medial deltoid test, with force directed into adduction. For the posterior deltoid, the beginning position is the same; then the practitioner medially rotates the humerus approximately 45° and slightly extends it, with the force directed into adduction and slight flexion. For the anterior deltoid, the starting point is the same. The practitioner stands in front of the patient and laterally rotates the humerus approximately 45° with slight flexion, then contacts the anterosuperior distal humerus with the force directed into adduction and slight extension.

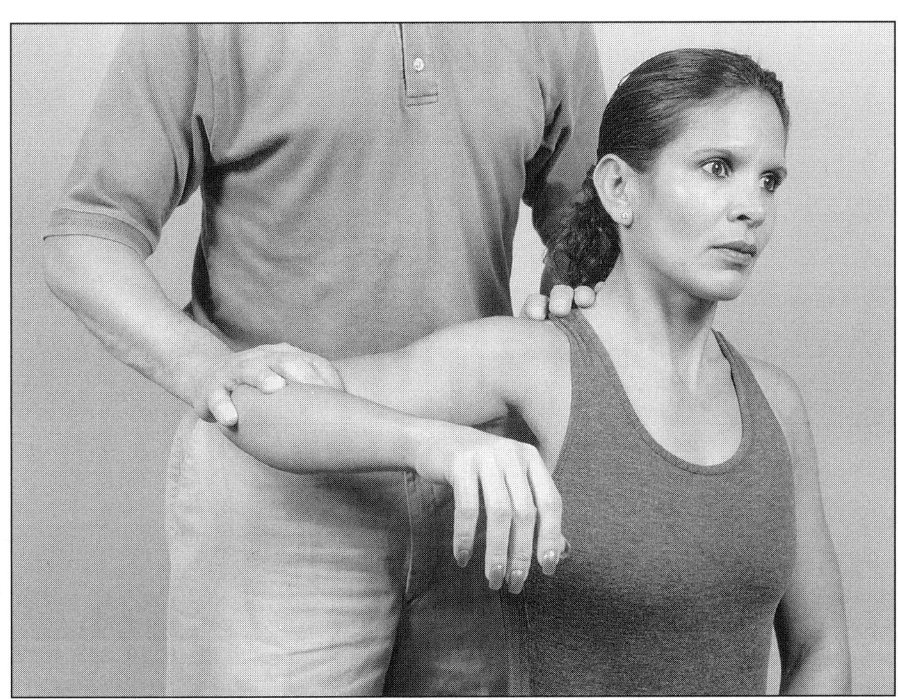

Supraspinatus

The tendon of this muscle stabilizes the capsule of the shoulder joint. Inhibition of this muscle can produce shoulder problems that are debilitating, although correction of the muscle resolves the problem very quickly. It may be difficult to separate this test from that for the deltoid muscles, but the supraspinatus is more active in the first 10-15° of abduction.

Action

Adducts the shoulder joint and stabilizes the head of the humerus during movement

Origin

Medial two-thirds of the supraspinous fossa of the scapula

Insertion

Great tubercle of the humerus and shoulder joint capsule

Nerve

C(4), 5, (6)

Therapeutic Reflexes

Chapman's—Anterior: in the PMC just below the coracoid process; posterior: on the posterior aspect of the transverse process of C1

Acupuncture meridian—conception vessel

Common acupuncture point—CV 24 (in the depression between the lower lip and chin)

Testing Position

Sitting

Testing

Arm is abducted to 15° maximum with 90° medial rotation (palm facing the patient). Practitioner makes contact proximal to the wrist and applies force into adduction with slight extension.

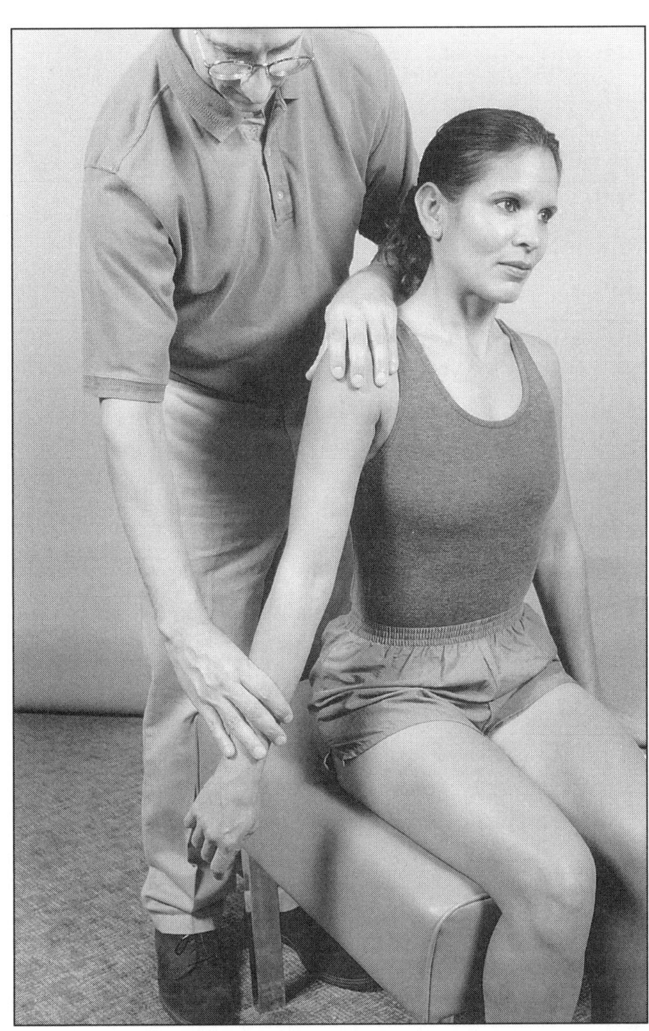

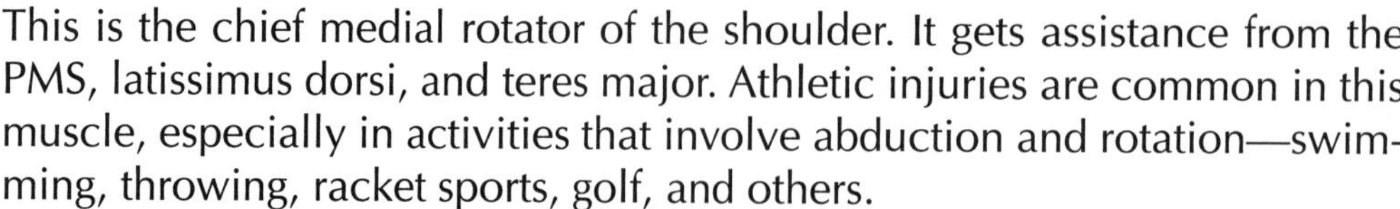

Subscapularis Muscle

This is the chief medial rotator of the shoulder. It gets assistance from the PMS, latissimus dorsi, and teres major. Athletic injuries are common in this muscle, especially in activities that involve abduction and rotation—swimming, throwing, racket sports, golf, and others.

Action

Medially rotates the shoulder and stabilizes the head of the humerus in the glenoid cavity during shoulder movement

Origin

Subscapular fossa of the scapula

Insertion

Lesser tubercle of the humerus and shoulder joint capsule

Nerve

C5, 6, (7)

Therapeutic Reflexes

Chapman's—Anterior: second and third intercostal spaces at sternum; posterior: laminae of T2 and 3

Acupuncture meridian—heart

Common acupuncture point—HT 9

Testing Position

Sitting

Testing

The shoulder is abducted 90° with medial rotation, and the elbow is flexed to 90°. Practitioner stabilizes the anterior elbow at the medial epicondyle area with one hand, and the other hand applies force proximal to the wrist in the direction of lateral rotation. All movements of the humerus except rotation should be avoided. Note: The three chief rotators of the shoulder are the subscapularis muscle (a medial rotator) and the teres minor and infraspinatus muscles (lateral rotators). Note that many other muscles described in this chapter, and some not listed, also have rotation capabilities. These are sometimes generally referred to as the "rotator cuff"; "rotator cuff syndrome" or "impingement syndrome" are terms commonly used to describe general dysfunction of the shoulder (Hall 1995). This is also called "swimmer's shoulder" in swimmers. Richardson et al. (1980) report that up to 50% of competitive swimmers complain of shoulder pain. The present author contends that the majority of swimmers have muscle inhibition of one, two, or occasionally all three of these rotator muscles as the primary cause of their pain, with successful correction requiring the therapies described here and in other chapters.

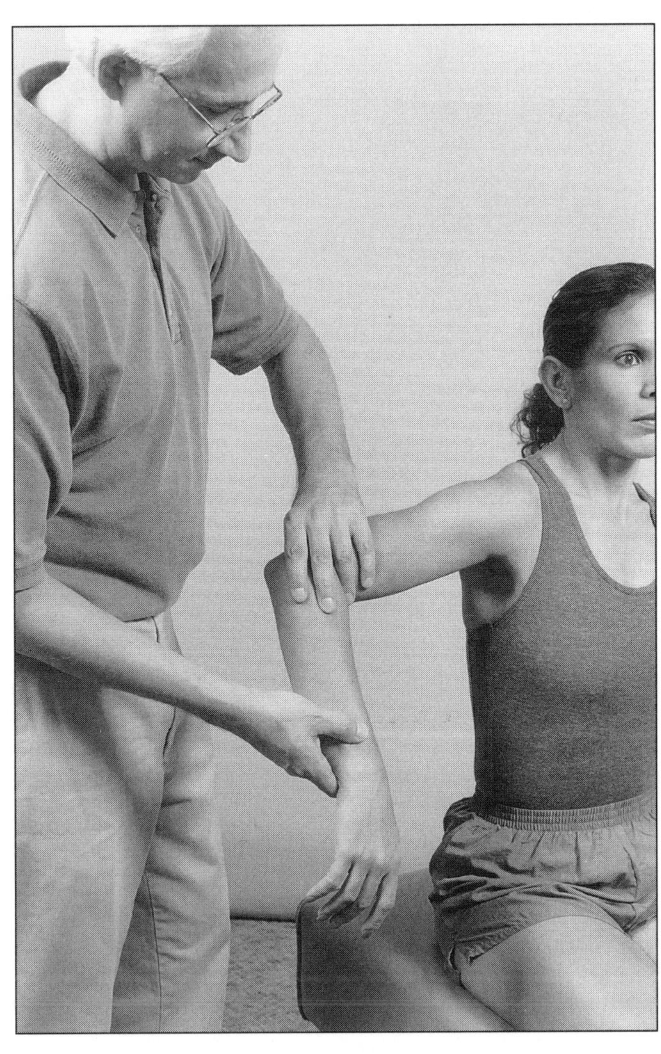

Teres Minor Muscle

Action

Laterally rotates the humerus and stabilizes the head of the humerus in the glenoid cavity during shoulder motion. Athletic injuries are common in this muscle, especially in activities that involve abduction and rotation—swimming, throwing, racket sports, golf, and others.

Origin

Middle to lower third of the axillary border of scapula

Insertion

Lowest facet of the greater tubercle of the humerus

Nerve

C5, 6

Therapeutic Reflexes

Chapman's—Anterior: second and third intercostal spaces approximately 1 cm from the sternum; posterior: laminae of T2 and 3

Acupuncture meridian—triple heater

Common acupuncture points—TH 3, 23

Testing Position

Sitting

Testing

The shoulder is adducted and laterally rotated; elbow is flexed to 90°. Practitioner stabilizes the medial elbow with one hand; the other hand makes contact just proximal to the posterior wrist and applies force into medial rotation. All movements of the humerus except rotation should be avoided during the test.

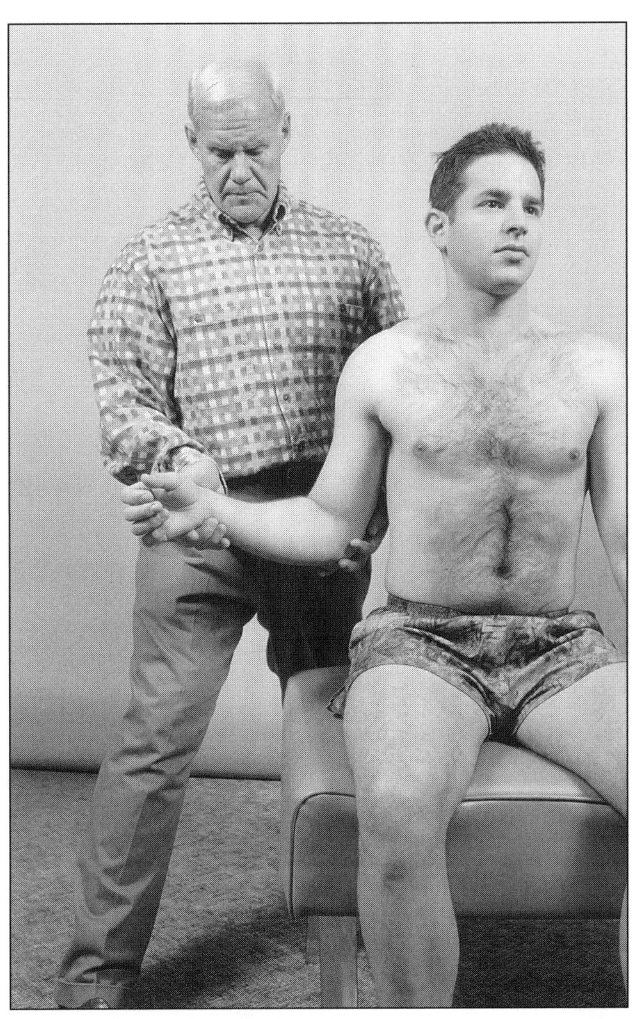

Infraspinatus Muscle

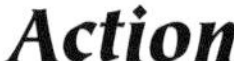

Action

Laterally rotates humerus and stabilizes head of humerus in the glenoid cavity during shoulder movement. Athletic injuries are common in this muscle, especially in activities that involve abduction and rotation—swimming, throwing, racket sports, golf, and others.

Origin

Medial two-thirds of infraspinous fossa of scapula

Insertion

Greater tubercle of humerus (middle facet) and shoulder joint capsule

Nerve

C(4), 5, 6

Therapeutic Reflexes

Chapman's—Anterior: fifth intercostal space beginning from midmammillary line to midaxillary line on right side only; posterior: laminae of T12 (bilateral)

Acupuncture meridian—triple heater

Common acupuncture points—TH 3, 23

Testing Position

Sitting

Testing

The shoulder is abducted to 90°; elbow is flexed to 90° with slight lateral shoulder rotation. Practitioner stabilizes the elbow and makes contact posterior and proximal to wrist, applying force into medial rotation. All movements of the humerus except rotation should be avoided during the test.

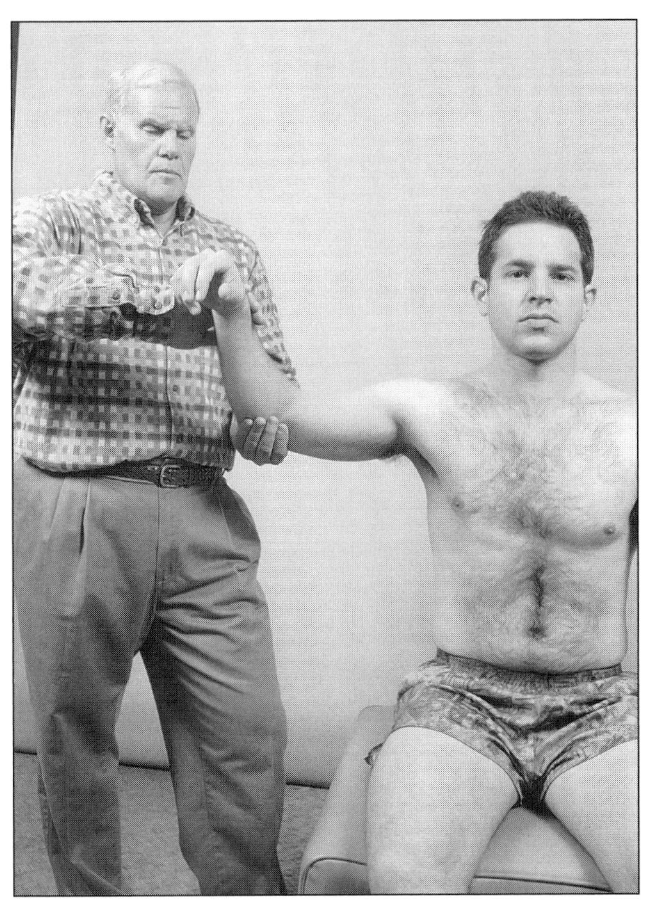

Gluteus Maximus Muscle

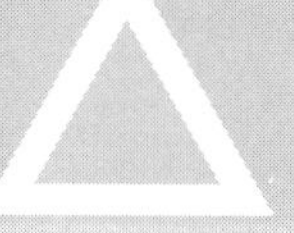

This large muscle is a major stabilizer of the pelvis and low back and is especially important for sacral and coccygeal stability. It has various actions. It is often involved in knee problems because of its stabilizing effect in knee extension through its insertion into the iliotibial tract. The smooth gait observed during running and other activities is, in great part, due to gluteus maximus function. Bilateral inhibition may be associated with a primary sagittal suture cranial fault and secondary spinal dysfunction.

Action

Predominantly extends hip; laterally rotates and adducts the hip. The upper fibers assist in hip abduction.

Origin

Posterior surface of sacrum and coccyx, outer portion of ilium (posterior gluteal line), sacrotuberous ligament, and aponeurosis of erector spinae muscle

Insertion

Iliotibial tract and gluteal tuberosity of femur

Nerve

L5, S1-2

Therapeutic Reflexes

Chapman's—Anterior: full length of anterolateral thigh; posterior: between posterior superior iliac spine and L5

Acupuncture meridian—circulation sex

Common acupuncture point—CX 9

Testing Position

Prone

Testing

The patient's knee is flexed more than 90° and the hip extended. The practitioner applies pressure at the posterior distal end of the thigh in the direction of flexion. The patient's head should be flexed more than normal in a face-down position.

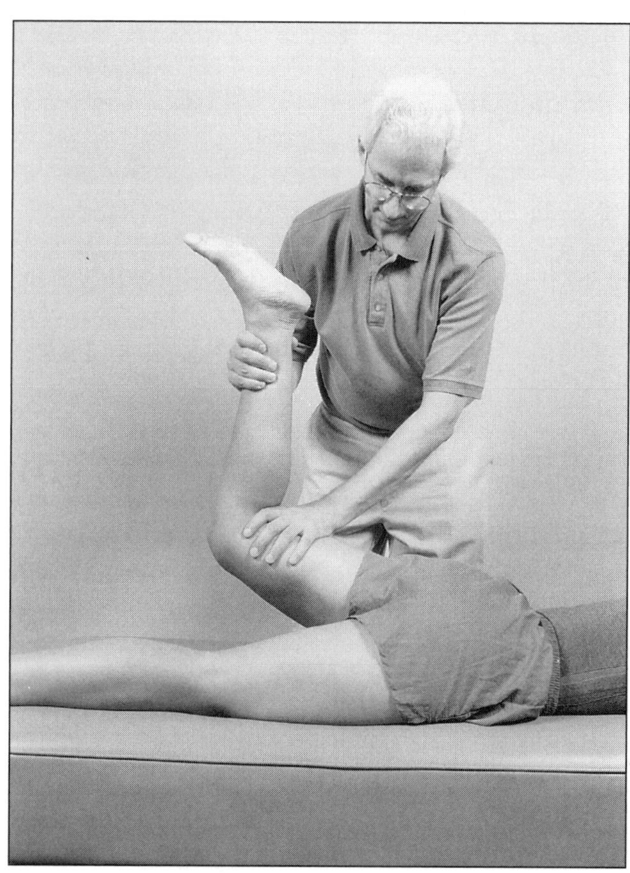

Hamstrings

Three muscles make up the hamstring group: the medial hamstring includes the semitendious and semimembranosus, and the lateral hamstring includes the biceps femoris (with a long and short head at the origin). Poor hamstring function can affect the knee, hip, pelvic, and low back stability. For example, hyperextension injuries of the knee and excess pelvic rotation are common. Bilateral inhibition can allow an excess anterior tilt of the pelvis and an excess lumbar lordosis. Hamstring inhibition is often associated with cranial respiratory faults.

Action

The medial hamstring flexes and medially rotates the knee, with some extension and lateral rotation of the hip.

Origin

Medial hamstrings: tuberosity of the ishium. Lateral hamstrings: the long head attaches to the sacrotuberous ligament and tuberosity of the ischium; the short head attaches on the lateral lip of lineas aspera, proximal two-thirds of the supracondyle line, and lateral intermuscular septum.

Insertion

Semitendinosus: proximal medial tibia and deep fascia of the leg; semimembranosus: medial condyle of the tibia, and deep fascia of the lateral leg

Nerve

L(4), 5, S1, 2, (3)

Therapeutic Reflexes

Chapman's —Anterior: over the area of the lesser trochanter of the femur; posterior: sacroiliac area near the posterior superior iliac spine

Acupuncture meridian—large intestine

Common acupuncture points—LI 11, 20

Testing Position

Prone

Testing

The knee is flexed 70°. The practitioner stabilizes the posterior thigh with one hand, contacts the posterior distal end of the leg or heel with the other, and applies force into the knee extension. Do not allow the patient to flex their hip by lifting the pelvis during the test. To further isolate the medial hamstring, begin with the same position then rotate the thigh slightly medial and in the direction of the force into the knee extension. To further isolate the lateral hamstrings, rotate the thigh slightly lateral and in the direction of the force into the knee extension.

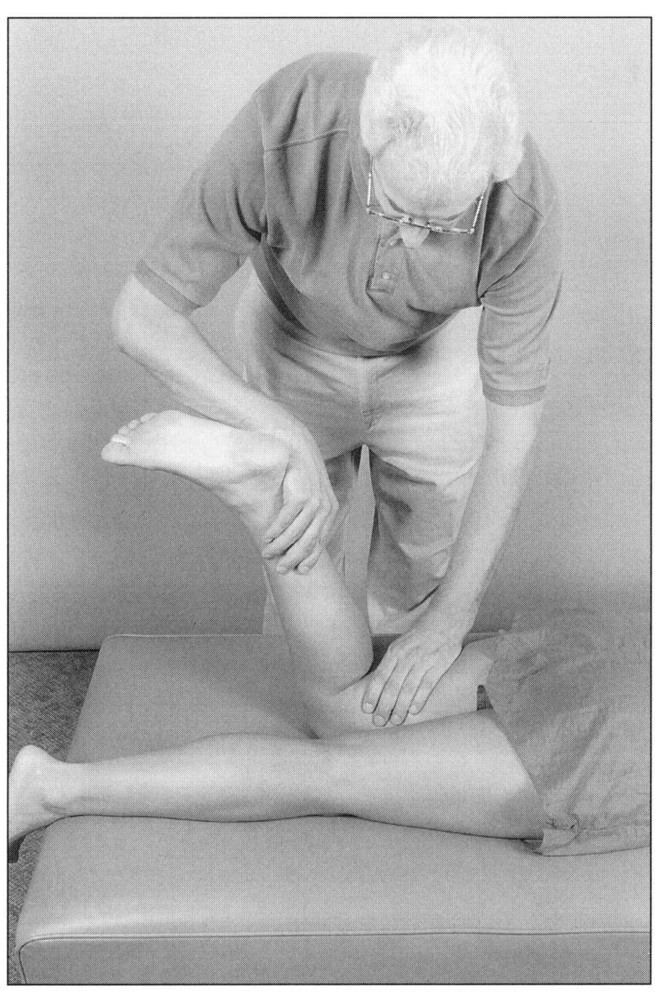

Gracilis Muscle

It may be possible to isolate the gracilis muscle from the medial hamstrings. This muscle helps stabilize the knee and pelvis.

Action

Flexes the knee; medially rotates and adducts the thigh

Origin

Body and inferior ramus of pubis symphysis

Insertion

Medial surface of the upper end of tibia distal to medial condyle

Nerve

L(2), 3, 4

Therapeutic Reflexes

Chapman's—Anterior: approximately 2.5 cm lateral and 5 cm superior to the umbilicus; posterior: laminae of T11

Acupuncture meridian—circulation sex

Common acupuncture point—CX 9, TH 23

Testing Position

Prone

Testing

Knee is flexed 45° and medially rotated. The practitioner extends the hip slightly by elevating the knee with one hand while the other hand applies pressure against the posteromedial aspect of the distal leg in the direction of medial rotation and knee extension.

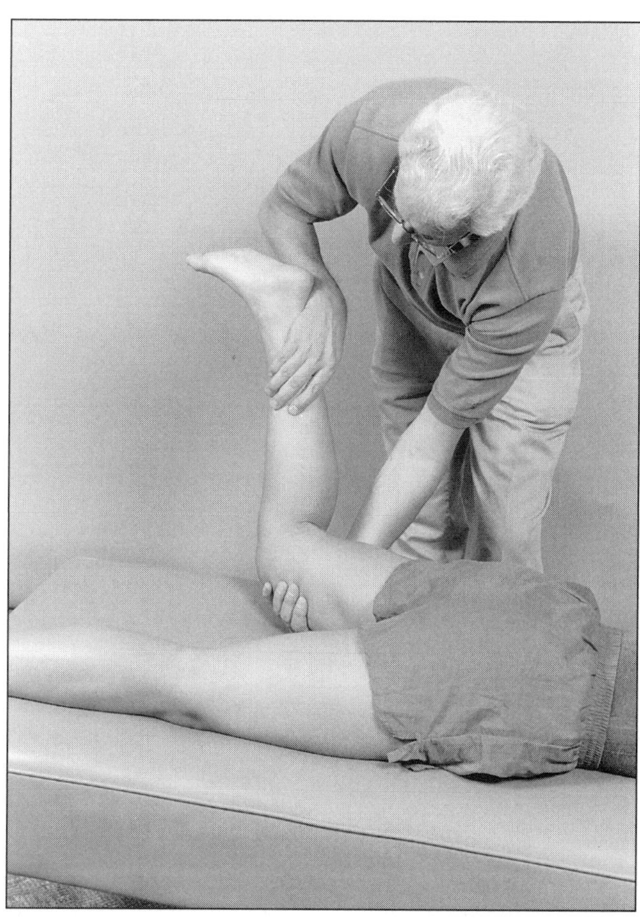

Middle Trapezius Muscle

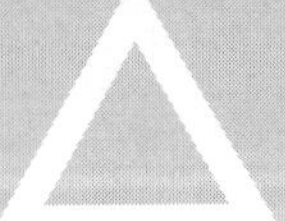

The middle fibers of the trapezius muscle help support the scapula and shoulder and the first five thoracic vertebrae during activity. This muscle also helps stabilize the shoulder during throwing motions and swimming and is an accessory muscle during respiration.

Action

Adducts and stabilizes the scapula

Origin

Spinous processes of the first five thoracic vertebrae

Insertion

Superior border of scapula and medial aspect of acromion

Nerve

C(2), 3, 4

Therapeutic Reflexes

Chapman's—Anterior: seventh intercostal space 8-15 cm from the costal cartilage near the sternum, on the left side only; posterior: between T7 and 8 near laminae on left side only

Acupuncture meridian—spleen

Common acupuncture points—SP 2, 3

Testing Position

Prone

Testing

The patient's shoulder is abducted to 90° and fully rotated laterally. (The arm is in line with the muscle fibers.) The elbow is fully extended. The practitioner contacts the distal arm and applies pressure in the direction of flexion (i.e., downward). In patients who are very powerful, it may be necessary to contact more distally (i.e., the distal forearm).

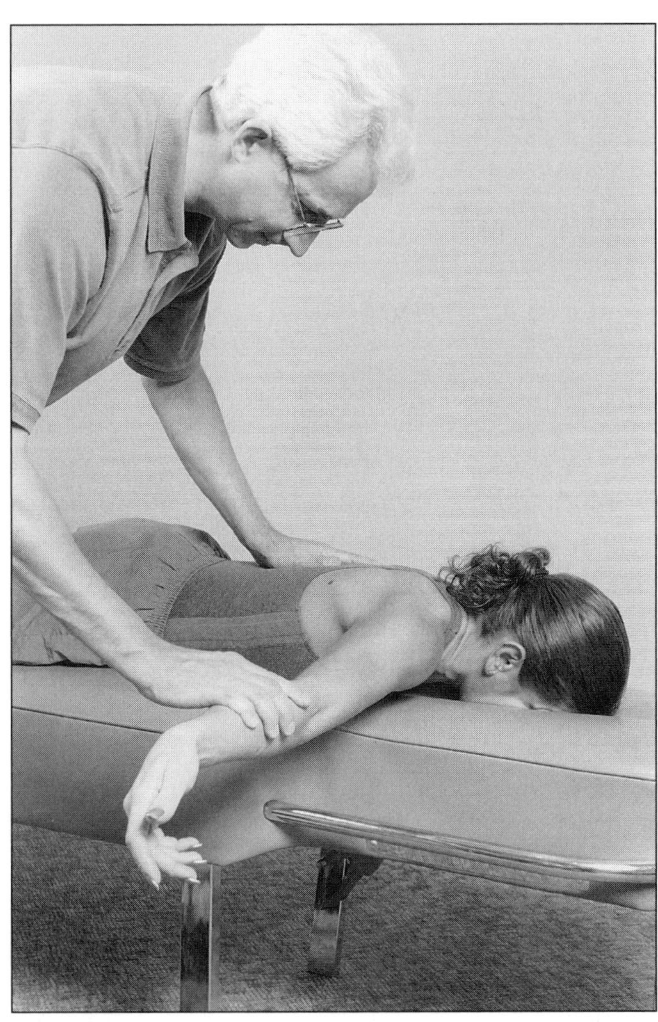

Lower Trapezius Muscle

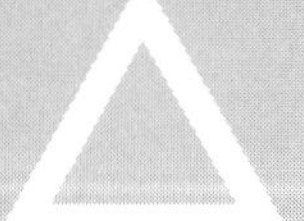

This muscle is an important mid and low thoracic spine stabilizer; it is important in arm extension in racket sports, baseball, and other activities with similar motions—especially those that require over-the-head motions using the arms, such as swimming.

Action

Rotates and stabilizes the scapula

Origin

Spinous processes of T6-12

Insertion

Medial one-third of the spine of the scapula

Nerve

C(2), 3, 4

Therapeutic Reflexes

Chapman's—Anterior: seventh intercostal space 8-15 cm from the costal cartilage near the sternum, on the left side only; posterior: between T7 and 8 near laminae on left side only

Acupuncture meridian—spleen

Common acupuncture points—SP 2, 3

Testing Position

Prone

Testing

The shoulder is abducted about 135° and fully rotated laterally. (The arm is in line with the muscle fibers.) The elbow is fully extended. The practitioner contacts the distal arm and applies pressure in the direction of flexion (i.e., downward). In patients who are very powerful, it may be necessary to contact more distally (i.e., the distal forearm).

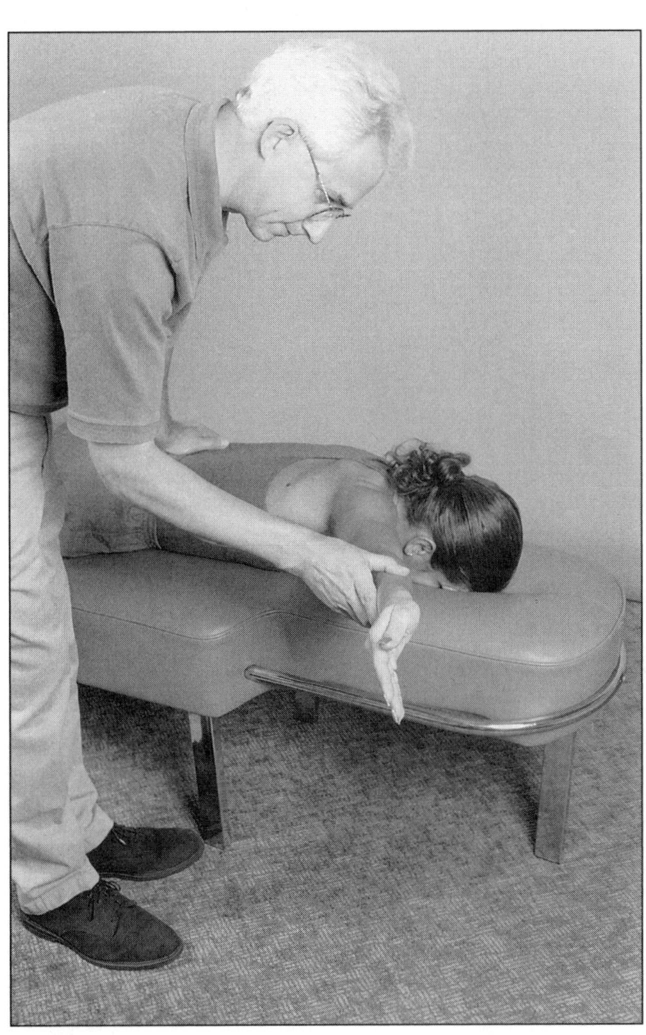

Latissimus Dorsi

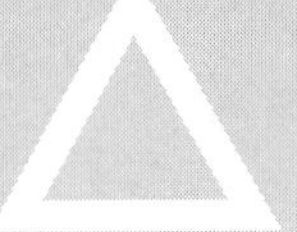

This muscle is important for proper arm movement during swimming, rowing, climbing, walking, and running, as well as for low back flexion and extension motion, and is a middle and low back stabilizer. It may be inhibited in patients who have pain or difficulty when placing their hand on their lumbar region and in patients with low back pain.

Action

Medially rotates, adducts, and extends the shoulder; depresses the shoulder joint. Also assists in anterior and lateral pelvic flexion and in hyperextension of the spine.

Origin

Spinous processes of T6-12, L1-5, and the upper sacral vertebrae; the thoracolumbar fascia of ribs 9-12 (and with connections to slips of origin of the external oblique muscle); the posterior third of the medial iliac crest; and occasionally the inferior angle of the scapula

Insertion

The muscle forms a tendon that passes through the axillary region (with the teres minor tendon) to attach on the intertubercular groove of the humerus.

Nerve

C6-8

Therapeutic Reflexes

Chapman's—Anterior: seventh intercostal space just lateral to sternal junction (left side only); posterior: T7-8 laminae on left only. These reflexes are for both left and right latissimus dorsi.

Acupuncture meridian—spleen

Common acupuncture points—SP 2, 3

Testing Position

Prone

Testing

The patient is prone or standing with the elbow locked in extension; the arm is in full adduction and in medial rotation with slight extension. Contact is made proximal to the wrist joint and pressure is applied in the direction of abduction and slight flexion.

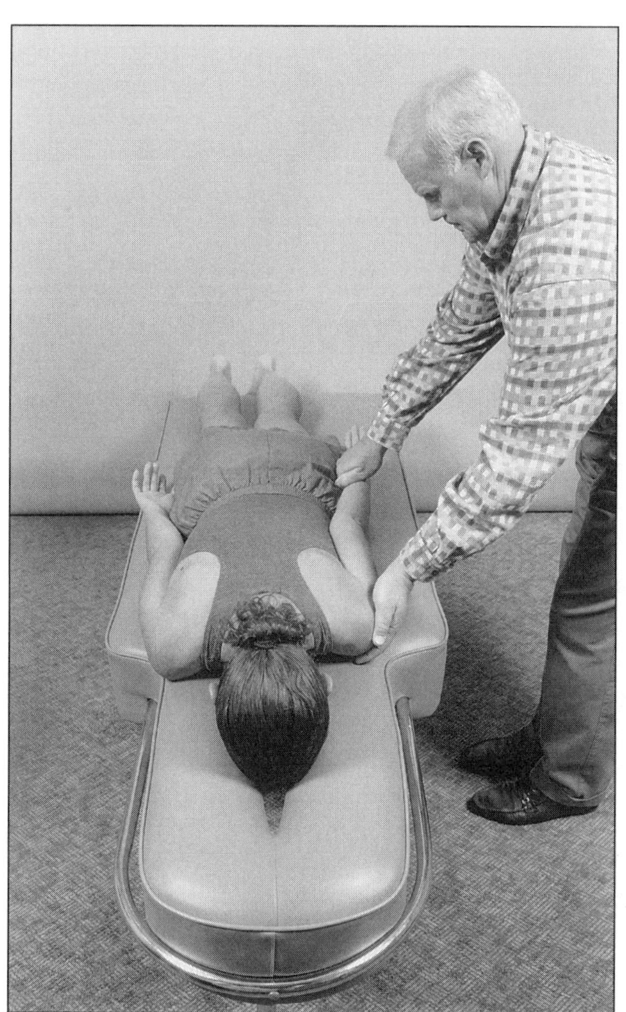

Piriformis Muscle

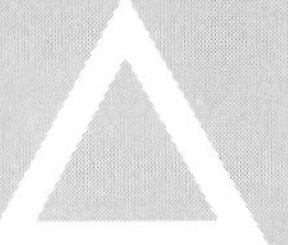

Dysfunction in this muscle is sometimes associated with numerous mechanical problems causing pain in and around the pelvis (i.e., the "piriformis syndrome") and sometimes with conditions diagnosed as "sciatica." The muscle is often inhibited in these conditions, but occasionally is secondarily overfacilitated.

Action

The piriformis is a primary lateral rotator of the hip. (Muscles that may have synergistic actions include the quadratus femoris, internal and external obturator, and superior and inferior gemellus.)

Origin

Anterior surface of sacrum, greater sciatic foramen, sacroiliac articulation, and sacrotuberous ligament

Insertion

Superior border of greater trochanter of femur

Nerve

(L5), S1, 2

Therapeutic Reflexes

Chapman's—Anterior: upper pubic bone; posterior: transverse process of L5 vertebra

Acupuncture meridian—circulation sex

Common acupuncture point—CX 9

Testing Position

Prone

Testing

The knee is flexed to 90°, and the hip is slightly rotated laterally (sometimes testing in the neutral or slight medial rotation position is best). Practitioner stabilizes the knee through lateral support and applies pressure on the distal end of the medial leg in the direction of medial hip rotation. This muscle can be tested in the sitting position in the same way.

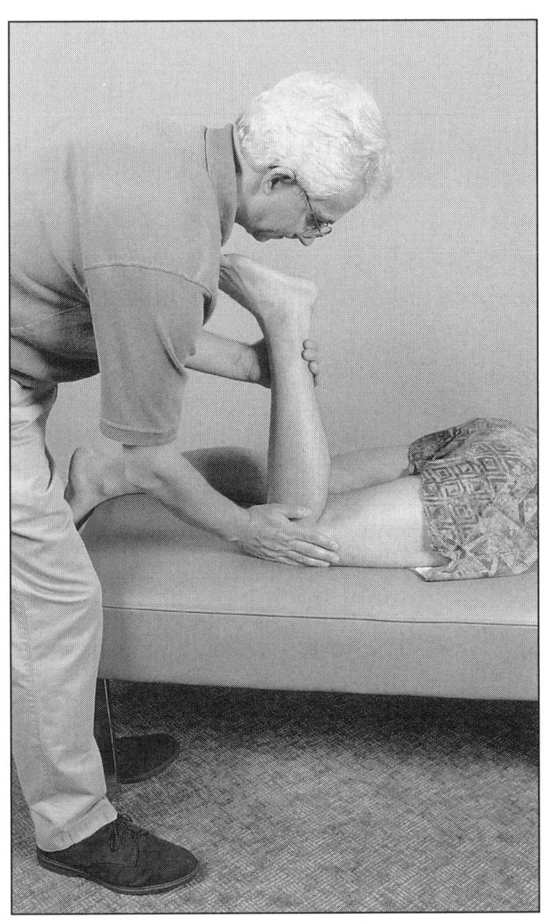

a

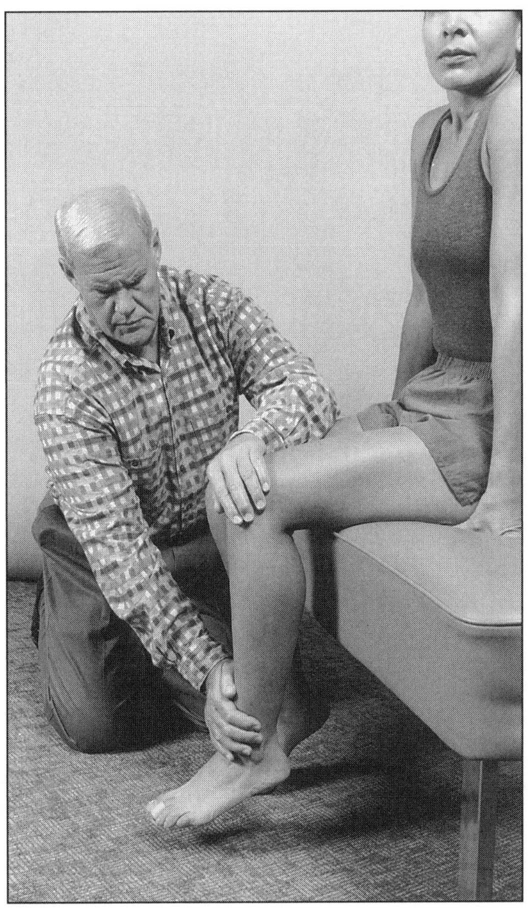

b

Neck Extensor Muscles

Injuries to the neck extensor muscles are common in sport often due to physical trauma such as that resulting from being hit in the front. Athletes most vulnerable are those who wear helmets since these add a component of weight to the head, potentially producing more stress in these delicate muscles. The neck extensor muscles are important for quick movements and balance, and they help stabilize the head for efficient eye-hand coordination. Four individual neck extensors are described here: the splenius cervicis, semispinalis cervicis, splenius capitis, and semispinalis capitis. They are tested generally as a group, either bilaterally or left and right.

Action

These muscles primarily extend the head and neck; lateral flexion and some rotation.

Origin

C7-T6

Insertion

On the occiput and C1-5

Nerve

C1-8

Therapeutic Reflexes

Chapman's—Anterior: a point just below the middle of the clavicle where the PMC attaches; posterior: over the laminae of second cervical vertebrae

Acupuncture meridian—stomach

Common acupuncture points—ST 1, 41

Testing Position

Prone

Testing

The patient's shoulders are abducted to 90°. To test bilaterally, the head is extended with no rotation. The practitioner applies pressure on the back of the head into flexion. To test left and right extensor function, the head is rotated as far as possible to the side being tested. Practitioner contacts the posterolateral side of the head and applies pressure anterior and slightly lateral. It is important to make sure the patient's face is protected from the table surface in case of significant dysfunction.

a

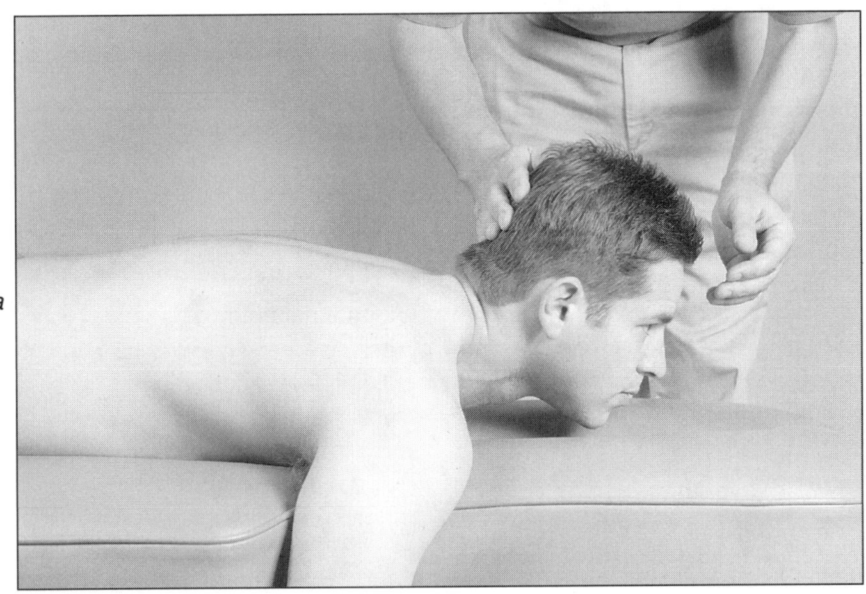

b

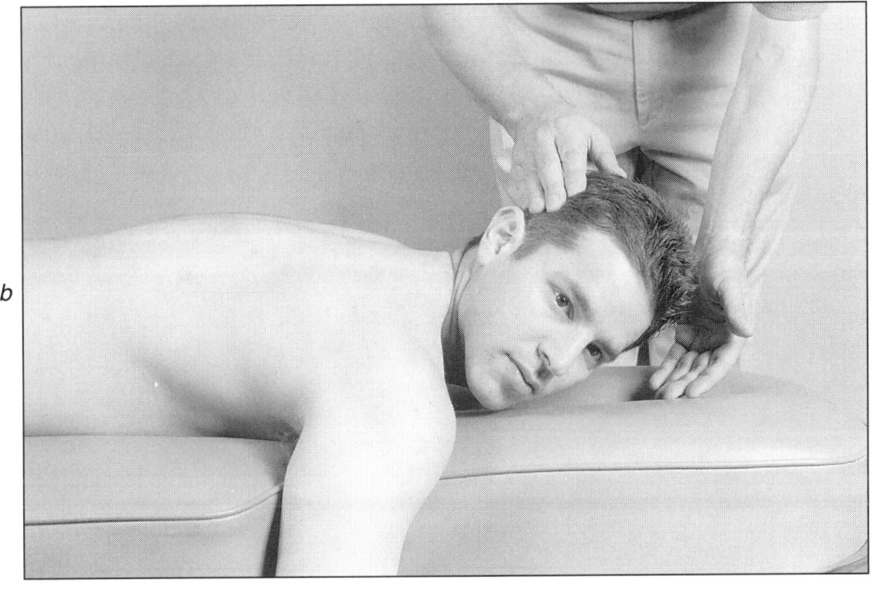

MUSCLES THAT ARE TESTED INDIRECTLY

The temporomandibular joint muscles and the diaphragm are not tested directly. But their function can be assessed using other muscle tests. They are best evaluated in the lying, sitting, or standing position.

Temporomandibular Joint Muscles

The temporomandibular joint muscles are the muscles that close (masseter and temporalis) and open (external pterygoid) the jaw joint. The masseter originates at the zygomatic process of the maxilla and zygomatic arch and is inserted on the mandible (angle of ramus and coronoid process). The temporalis originates at the temporal fossa and fascia and is inserted on the coronoid process and anterior border of the ramus of the mandible. The external pterygoid originates at the greater wing of the sphenoid and lateral surface of the lateral pterygoid plate. It is inserted on the anterior condyle of the mandible and the anterior portion of the articular disc of the temporomandibular joint articulation. All these muscles share the same therapeutic reflexes:

- Chapman's—Anterior: second through fourth intercostal spaces at sternum; posterior: T2-4 near laminae
- Acupuncture meridian—stomach
- Common acupuncture points—ST 1, 41
- Nerve—Cranial nerve V

Diaphragm Muscle

Breathing is an action that is clearly vital in all sport. Assessment of other breathing factors was discussed in chapter 8. The diaphragm muscle can be treated like any other except that it cannot be physically tested. The reflexes listed may be useful when vital capacity or breath-holding is low. Diaphragm dysfunction is sometimes associated with cranial problems or rib dysfunction and is also seen in cases in which many acupuncture problems are evident. In addition to causing breathing dysfunction, diaphragm muscle imbalance can adversely affect numerous structures because of its attachments.

The diaphragm creates a downward, "flattening" action on inspiration and helps expand the rib cage with continued contraction; this reverses on expiration (relaxation). As to origin, at the sternal part this muscle attaches to the dorsum of the xiphoid process; the costal part attaches on the inner surface of the lower six costal cartilages and ribs bilaterally with connections with the transverse abdominis; the lumbar part attaches to the upper lumbar vertebrae and 12th rib. The diaphragm inserts into a central tendon on top of the muscle with no bony attachments.

Therapeutic reflexes:

- Chapman's—Anterior only: entire full length of sternum
- Acupuncture meridian—conception vessel
- Common acupuncture point—CV 24 (in depression between lower lip and chin)
- Nerve—C(3), 4, (5) (phrenic nerve)

CONCLUSION

This chapter has addressed muscles that in a clinical setting are commonly found to be inhibited and has outlined manual testing of these muscles, their clinical relevance, their origin and insertion, their nerve supply, and certain therapeutic reflexes commonly used in complementary sports medicine. For a more extensive review of manual muscle testing, the reader is referred to Kendall et al. (1993) and Walther (1988) and for anatomical information to *Gray's Anatomy* (1995).

11

Applied Kinesiology Assessment

Part of the interactive neuromuscular assessment used in complementary sports medicine is referred to as applied kinesiology (AK). This is a functional assessment of the structural, chemical, and mental/emotional aspects of the patient; it is an interactive evaluation using manual muscle testing. During an examination, dozens of pieces of vital information enable the practitioner to chronicle the patient's normal and abnormal function. This process includes analysis of many movements of the patient and monitoring of a variety of neuromuscular activities. In addition to revealing neuromuscular imbalances, muscle testing is useful for measuring other types of body function and dysfunction, all of which are reflected in the nervous system. The outcome of the assessment process also helps the practitioner address lifestyle factors such as exercise, training, and diet.

APPLIED KINESIOLOGY MUSCLE TESTING

Applied kinesiology muscle testing is used to help the practitioner during an assessment process to (1) evaluate and differentiate normal function from dysfunction and (2) find the therapies that best match the specific needs of the patient during that particular treatment session. The treatment session involves interpreting muscle testing outcomes and, on the basis of this and additional information from other assessments, such as the history and other evaluations (blood tests, physical exam, and other tests), applying a specific therapy. More muscle tests then follow—a reevaluation process—to immediately appraise the efficacy of that treatment; the session continues in this manner for a period of time until, ideally, all dysfunction is normalized. This one session could take 30 to 60 min or longer (and the initial session 90 min or more).

Applied kinesiology should not be confused with general muscle testing. The general term kinesiology refers only to the movement of the human body (*Dorland's Illustrated Medical Dictionary* 1994). Applied kinesiology is a clinical approach to patient care that blends key features based on art and science—combining acupuncture and other reflex techniques, manipulation, nutrition, and other complementary therapies with neurology, biochemistry, and physiology. Applied kinesiology is currently practiced worldwide by chiropractors, medical doctors, osteopaths, and other professionals.

Although Goodheart developed AK beginning in 1964 and its clinical efficacy has been demonstrated through patient outcomes, most of its basic ideas—as in the parallel field of Chinese medicine—are still theoretical (like most forms of therapy). Motyka and Yanuck (1998) and Schmitt and Yanuck (1998) have described manual assessment of muscular function in relation to AK. In addition, however, the work of Leisman et al. (1989, 1995), Perot et al. (1991), Lawson and Calderon (1997), and others as described in this text has begun to demonstrate the scientific merits of AK when used properly. Research of this kind has led to more acceptance of AK, the funding of more studies, and increased use by a more diverse population of practitioners. It seems that AK is following the way of Chinese medicine in this regard—there are now many published studies on the use of various clinical aspects of Chinese medicine, especially acupuncture. In 1997, the National Institutes of Health officially accepted acupuncture for the treatment of a variety of problems. Today, the majority of health insurance companies reimburse for many complementary therapies that include AK.

MUSCLE RELATIONSHIPS

Many details of assessment, therapeutic, and lifestyle-improvement methods have evolved within AK since its inception. Use of muscle testing to observe reactions by the body to various stimuli is an important aspect of assessment of patients. When a muscle is not functioning or responding properly, the practitioner considers a variety of possible faults that may affect that muscle directly or indirectly through the nervous system. These potential problems may come from the muscle itself (Golgi tendon organ or muscle spindle cells), the acupuncture system, the nervous system, an organ or gland, the nutritional state, or mental/emotional or other sources (including the potential of pathology). Another important avenue within AK is the use of neurological sensory receptor inputs (referred to as a "challenge") and sensory receptor stimuli (called "therapy localization") to aid the practitioner further in determining the most successful treatments. These are discussed in this chapter from the standpoint of their clinical application rather than their theoretical basis.

Still another important concept in AK is that of muscle dysfunction secondary to dysfunction in other areas of the body. Other similar relationships have been discussed in the literature. Newsholme (1994) examines a relationship between muscles and the immune system, describing L-glutamine as the "metabolic link." Parry-Billings et al. (1990) characterize a similar relationship between the muscles, the immune system, and the brain. Weidner et al. (1997) demonstrated secondary gait changes in stride length and frequency in athletes who had colds. Essentially, any change in a patient's physiologic state will ultimately be reflected in the cortex, cerebellum, brainstem, and spinal cord, and these changes can be monitored at the level of the anterior horn motoneurons in the spinal cord through muscle testing.

In chapter 10, each muscle was reviewed and its relationship to three therapeutic factors was described: spinal nerve innervation, the related acupuncture meridian with some key acupuncture points, and Chapman's reflexes. These associations may have potentially great therapeutic benefits for the related inhibited muscle. In AK there are two other important associations: the relationship between a specific muscle inhibition and a specific organ or gland, and the relationship between a specific muscle inhibition and a specific nutrient.

The muscle and organ/gland association was identified by Goodheart, who found that when Chapman's reflexes (which are thought to be related to organs and glands) were stimulated, certain muscles improved their function. In addition, Chinese medicine had long ago theorized relationships between the acupuncture meridians and all the organs and glands, along with everything in the body including the musculoskeletal system. Goodheart also observed muscle relationships with acupuncture meridians similar to those with Chapman's reflexes (table 11.1).

It has generally been agreed in AK that if an organ or gland is dysfunctioning, the related muscle will also dysfunction, most commonly by becoming inhibited. The organ or gland dysfunction does not necessarily mean disease or other pathology, but more often a functional problem. This dysfunction in the organ or gland, followed by muscle inhibition, may

Table 11.1 Some Relationships Between Muscles, Nutrients, Organs and Glands, Nerves, and Acupuncture Points

Muscle	Nutrient	Organ/Gland	Spine	Acupuncture
Abdominal (all)	L-glutamine	Small intestine	T5-12	SI 3,19
Adductors	Vitamin E	Reproductive	L2-4	CX 9
Biceps brachii	Vitamin B1 or B2	Stomach	C5, 6	ST 1, 41
Deltoids (all)	Vitamin C	Lungs	C5, 6	LU 9
Gastrocnemius	Vitamin C, pantothenic acid	Adrenal	S1, 2	CX 9
Gluteus muscles (all)	Vitamin E	Reproductive	L1-S1	CX 9
Gracilis	Vitamin C, pantothenic acid	Adrenal	L3, 4	CX 9
Hamstrings	Vitamin E	Rectum	L5-S	LI 11, 20
Iliacus, psoas	Vitamins A and E	Kidney	L1-3	KI 7
Infraspinatus	Antioxidants	Thymus	C5, 6	TH 3, 23
Latissimus dorsi	Vitamin A, fatty acids	Pancreas	C6-8	SP 2, 3
Neck flexors and extensors	Vitamin B6 and niacinamide	Sinus	C1-7	ST 1, 41
PMC	Vitamin B1 or B2	Stomach	C5-7	ST 1, 41
PMS	Vitamin A	Liver	C6-8	LV 3, 8
Peroneus (all)	Vitamin B1, calcium	Bladder	L4-S1	BL 1, 67
Piriformis	Vitamin E	Reproductive	S1, 2	CX 9
Quadriceps (all)	L-glutamine	Small intestine	L2-4	SI 3, 19
Sartorius	Vitamin C, pantothenic acid	Adrenal	L2, 3	CX 9
Soleus	Vitamin C, pantothenic acid	Adrenal	S1, 2	CX 9
Subscapularis	Vitamin E, B1, or B2	Heart	C5, 6	HT 9
Tensor fascia lata	L-glutamine, iron when bilateral	Large intestine	L4, 5, S1	LI 11, 20
Teres minor	Iodine, fatty acids, calcium	Thyroid	C5	TH 3, 23
Tibialis anterior	Vitamin A	Bladder	L4, 5	BL 1, 67
Tibialis posterior	Vitamin C, pantothenic acid	Adrenal	L5, S1	CX 9
Trapezius, upper	Calcium, fatty acids	Eyes/ears	C3, 4	KI 7
Trapezius, middle and lower	Vitamin C, calcium	Spleen	C3, 4	SP 2, 3
Triceps brachii	Vitamin A, chromium	Pancreas	C7, 8	SP 2, 3

even be transient. For example, the adrenal gland may have normal function in the morning but by afternoon become abnormal when cortisol levels fall to below normal. This observation may be confirmed by testing salivary cortisol levels several times throughout the day and evening. It may also be evident from the results of the symptom survey completed by the patient (e.g., afternoon fatigue may have been noted) or from other areas examined in the assessment process.

Although it is generally thought that if an organ or gland is dysfunctioning the related muscle will be inhibited, the converse is not necessarily true; if a muscle loses its normal function because of other problems, such as local trauma, it will not necessarily adversely affect the related organ or gland.

NEUROLOGICAL SENSORY RECEPTOR CHALLENGE

With so many different therapeutic techniques to choose from, how can a practitioner determine which ones are best for a given patient during a particular session? Through the use of AK, this is done in part via a neurological sensory receptor challenge mechanism. According to *Dorland's Illustrated Medical Dictionary* (1994), to challenge is "to administer a chemical substance to a patient for observation of whether the normal physiological response occurs." Provoking the body's sensory mechanism with a stimulus and measuring the outcome are essentially how a challenge works.

Challenges have been used in mainstream medicine for many years and are still used today. These include various types of challenges in addition to nutritional ones. For example, an exercise challenge test is useful to assess exercise-induced asthma (Vacek 1997). Oral challenge (Pichichero and Pichichero 1998), nasal challenge (Baumgarten et al. 1997), psychological challenge (Ruegg et al. 1997), and other types have been used, especially specific challenges for the immune system (Elmquist et al. 1997) and free radicals (Biasioli et al. 1997).

Potential allergens or irritants are most often used as challenge substances, including moldy hay (Schwaiblmair et al. 1997), cholecystokinin (Shlik et al. 1997), and cold air (Lombardi et al. 1997), to name a few. It is important to note that patients can react to very small amounts of substances. For example, Hourihane et al. (1997) found that some patients who are allergic to peanuts react to an oral challenge of only 100 micrograms of the offending substance and that some react to peanuts even through intact skin or through the odor of peanuts. This demonstrates how sensitive the body can be to noxious stimulants.

In mainstream medicine, most challenges are used to help diagnose a specific condition (e.g., exercise-induced asthma) or allergy (e.g., to peanuts) and are examples of the chemical challenge. In complementary sports medicine, chemical challenges are generally used to assist the practitioner in determining allergic or hypersensitive conditions (such as dietary excess or insufficiency), but most especially to help determine nutritional balance or imbalance leading to potential nutritional supplementation. In addition, the challenge is used to demonstrate potentially helpful substances and therapies.

Chemical challenges are commonly implemented in AK because they are clinically useful to the practitioner in the assessment process. The taste receptors on the tongue detect even extremely small concentrations of substances within a fraction of a second of stimulation (Guyton 1986). Exposure to taste elicits a variety of immediate responses throughout the body, including neurological, digestive, endocrine, cardiovascular, thermogenic, and renal; such a response is referred to as a cephalic or preabsorptive response (Mattes 1997). The response to taste parallels that of olfactory, visual, cognitive, and other stimuli and may have been first proposed scientifically by Pavlov in the early 1900s (Pavlov 1910).

More importantly, studies of nutritional challenges have demonstrated the existence of functional nutritional imbalances. For example, Lukaski et al. (1991) reported that low iron levels in non-anemic women were associated with a significant reduction in oxygen uptake and aerobic energy production. Wada and King (1986) demonstrated that low zinc intakes were associated with significant decreases in metabolic rate and free thyroxin despite normal serum zinc levels. The use of chemical challenges in AK is of great help to the practitioner in assessing these functional nutritional problems. This type of challenge, along with physical and mental/emotional challenges, is described in subsequent sections of this chapter.

Since most therapies evoke sensory activity in the nervous system, it is possible to utilize most therapies described in this text through challenging the patient's neuromuscular system. In mainstream medicine, the response of the patient to a challenge is assessed through such measures as auscultation, verbal response, and antibody levels. In AK, the response is measured by the neurological reaction of the muscle (i.e., muscle testing). Three outcomes are possible:

- An inhibited muscle that normalizes on a challenge may suggest that the therapy will be compatible with the patient's needs.
- A normal muscle that becomes inhibited on a challenge suggests a negative effect of the therapy or substance.
- A lack of response by the muscle may suggest a benign therapy (i.e., no therapy may be necessary).

By using muscle testing before and after inducing a challenge, the practitioner can gain vital information about the specific aspects of a given therapy and the way in which it may apply to the needs of the patient. Through this approach, the patient is not treated in a "cookbook" fashion; the ineffective therapies are rejected and only those that elicit a positive muscle response are used. However, a therapy that is ineffective in the current session may be helpful during a future session, or an ineffective therapy for one patient might benefit another with similar imbalances. It must be emphasized again that the use of a challenge is only one part of the assessment process and that challenge does not replace other assessment tools. For example, Armentia (1997) found a challenge test more useful when combined with history. The practitioner can evaluate various potential therapies as part of the assessment process before applying the most useful ones. Three groups of therapeutic tools can be considered in the assessment process. These are outlined in more detailed explanations in the next section.

Structural or Physical Challenges

Structural or physical challenges include physical evaluation of acupuncture points, Chapman's reflexes, and local muscle areas (Golgi tendon organs and spindle cells). The locations of these areas have been previously described. With the assistance of the patient, who stimulates potential therapeutic points, the practitioner makes assessments using a technique called "therapy localization." This approach helps determine which therapy, or specific point, is best for the patient during the current session. In addition, joint dysfunction or cranial-sacral dysfunction can be assessed to determine whether there is a problem that requires correction and precisely how the correction should be made. In both situations, the practitioner observes for changes in muscle function before and after a challenge.

Chemical Challenges

Chemical challenges relate to nutritional, dietary, and other chemical factors that may be required by the patient. This type of challenge may also involve determining whether certain substances (foods, supplements, allergens, etc.) may be harmful for the patient. These assessments are made by stimulating the patient's gustatory (taste) or olfactory (smell) sensory areas with specific test substances (nutrients, potential allergens, foods, etc.) and observing for changes in muscle function.

Mental or Emotional Challenges

A mental or emotional challenge consists of imagery and relies on muscle function changes to show whether certain thoughts influence the patient's function. Mental images may have a negative effect on the patient, as indicated by muscle inhibition, or may have positive effects such as those that negate existing muscle inhibition. Thoughts about working out, fears relating to competition, and images of certain actions or persons in their sport may sometimes provoke negative stress or provide benefits.

These structural, chemical, and mental/emotional challenges may function simply through the normal neurologic mechanisms. An afferent stimulation—a specific challenge—travels from the skin, joint, or taste bud, for example, to the spinal cord, cerebellum, and cortex. This challenge evokes a change in the nervous system with specific efferent actions that can affect the body—physically through the muscles, chemically through the organs and glands—and the mental/emotional state. Muscle testing is an important tool that one can use in deciding what to do for a patient when a number of different alternatives are possible.

STRUCTURAL (PHYSICAL) CHALLENGE

The two types of structural or physical challenge described here are therapy localization and mechanical challenges. Therapy localization is a method that helps the practitioner determine which therapy point(s) will be most successful. This is accomplished through the patient's temporary stimulation of a specific reflex or therapy area. By touching a specific point on the skin the patient is stimulating mechanoreceptors, resulting in specific sensory input into the nervous system; the practitioner measures the results of the motor output through muscle testing. For example, if the patient has an abnormally inhibited sartorius muscle, there are several potential therapies (such as those described in chapter 10) that may help improve that muscle. These include two acupuncture points (CX 9, TH 23) and two different Chapman's reflexes. In therapy localization, the patient touches each of these areas, one at a time, and the practitioner retests the inhibited sartorius each time while the patient maintains contact with the reflex. For example, if the patient with an inhibited sartorius muscle touches the anterior Chapman's reflex and the muscle's function temporarily improves (to normal), the practitioner presumes that stimulating this reflex would help the dysfunction in that muscle. If the posterior Chapman's reflex causes the muscle to normalize while the patient touches it, the practitioner now has two therapeutic areas to treat. The next step is for the patient to touch each of the two acupuncture points. If neither acupuncture point causes the muscle to improve, these areas can be disregarded as useful therapy for this patient at this time. (These same acupuncture points may, however, be useful during a future session as indicated by therapy localization.) The practitioner now can stimulate both anterior and posterior Chapman's reflexes as previously described. When the stimulation is completed, the sartorius muscle is retested; if it is now normal, the therapy was successful. But if the muscle is still inhibited, the practitioner must assume there are other areas that require treatment.

Before stimulating Chapman's reflexes, one may also assess whether the spinal areas have an influence on the inhibited sartorius. In this case, the patient therapy-localizes the related spinal nerve areas (L2 and 3). If localization of these areas does not improve the muscle's function, these can be disregarded in terms of potential therapy. But if therapy localization to this spinal area improves muscle function, there may be a need to apply a therapy. Therapy to the spinal areas may involve the use of non-force techniques. After the therapy, the muscle should again be retested. If it is now normal, the therapy was successful, but if it is still inhibited, the practitioner knows that other therapies are required.

When therapy localization changes muscle function, it is referred to as a positive therapy localization; if it does not change muscle function, it is referred to as a negative therapy localization. A positive therapy localization only provides a clue that there is some dysfunction at that site and does not indicate what the precise problem may be. For example, if a patient has spinal pain at the area of T1 and therapy localization is positive to that area, the problem may be a spinal joint dysfunction, dislocation, an acupuncture or trigger point that requires stimulation, a fractured vertebra, or some other problem that must be determined by other assessments.

Therapy Localization Procedure

1. A psoas major muscle is inhibited.
2. The patient touches (therapy-localizes) each related therapy area, one at a time:
   - Chapman's reflexes
   - Acupuncture points
   - Spinal areas
3. As each area is therapy-localized, the psoas is retested. One set of outcomes could be the following:
   - Chapman's reflexes are negative (psoas remains inhibited).

- Acupuncture points are both positive (psoas becomes normal).
- Spinal areas are negative (psoas remains inhibited).

4. In this case, the acupuncture points are treated.
5. The other two areas that did not therapy-localize will not be treated.

A normally functioning muscle can also be used for therapy localization. A normal muscle will become inhibited with a positive therapy localization. For example, if a normal psoas muscle is used for testing and the patient therapy-localizes on an acupuncture point that requires treatment, the psoas muscle will become inhibited. Following successful therapy of that area, the psoas muscle will no longer become inhibited when the patient therapy-localizes it.

An alternative method for assessing whether an acupuncture point or Chapman's reflex would benefit the inhibited muscle is as follows. After finding an inhibited muscle, the practitioner stimulates the point in question for 1 or 2 sec and retests the muscle. If the muscle now functions normally, the practitioner completely stimulates that reflex for about 15 sec. Typically, a 1- or 2-sec stimulation of a reflex, if it is one that will improve muscle function, will only temporarily normalize the muscle; longer stimulation will be necessary to complete the correction. This method is useful in patients who cannot physically reach a particular reflex or have too much pain when attempting to do so.

Mechanical challenges are another form of structural challenge. This mechanism may function similarly to the common stretch or tendon reflex, or withdrawal reflexes: challenging a sensory receptor area sends messages to the spinal cord leading to a specific neurologic response that is measured in the muscle. For example, after a positive therapy localization to L2, the practitioner can "challenge" the vertebra to determine how it should be treated (after ruling out pathology). If the practitioner feels the vertebra requires physical correction (traditional chiropractic or osteopathic manipulation, or the non-force type described in chapter 16), the challenge can help determine on which side and in which direction the vertebra should be manipulated.

In this case, a normal muscle can be used for the challenge. For example, with the patient lying prone, the practitioner uses a normal latissimus dorsi, and the vertebra is challenged; the right transverse process of the vertebra is gently pushed anterior, with light pressure, and then released. The muscle is retested. If the muscle is still normal, the challenge was negative. If the muscle becomes inhibited, the challenge was positive. The inhibition of a challenge lasts only a few seconds. A positive challenge of a vertebra indicates a need for some type of manipulation in the same direction as the challenge. This is more fully described in chapter 16.

It has been observed in AK that when a gentle force is applied to a vertebra and then removed, the vertebra first moves with the direction of the force, then rebounds in the opposite direction when the force is removed. In the example just given, if challenging (pushing and releasing) the right side of the vertebra anteriorly produces a muscle inhibition, the vertebra can be described as abnormally rotated with the right transverse process posterior (and the left transverse process anterior).

In addition to the challenge, it is recommended that practitioners use palpatory skills, postural analysis, and other evaluations in determining the need for any type of correction.

Cranial and pelvic bones, when challenged, also have a rebound effect. However, this does not hold true for extravertebral joints such as those in the wrist, elbow, knee, and ankle. One might implement this type of challenge in a patient who trains in shoes that are too small, resulting in a posterior trauma of the proximal phalanx into the first metatarsal joint. With the patient lying supine, a normal psoas muscle is used as an indicator for the challenge. The practitioner gently pushes the first phalanx posteriorly, mimicking the stress produced from wearing a shoe that is too short. The psoas muscle is immediately retested and is now inhibited. This confirms the dysfunction in the first metatarsal joint and provides information about the possible direction of correction of that metatarsal (i.e., proximal to distal).

It is important to remember that after any treatment procedure, the joint should be retested to ensure that it was properly corrected. In many cases, the patient's lifestyle stress—for example, improperly fitting shoes—must also be addressed.

Mechanical Challenge Procedure: Spinal Vertebrae

1. The patient therapy-localizes, for example, T4, and it is positive.
2. The vertebra is challenged, using a normal muscle, by pushing in various directions:
   - Transverse process on right is pushed anterior.
   - Transverse process on left is pushed anterior.
   - Transverse process on right is pushed anterior and superior.
   - Transverse process on left is pushed anterior and superior.
   - Transverse process on right is pushed anterior and inferior.
   - Transverse process on left is pushed anterior and inferior.
   - Challenge is performed in other directions as necessary.
3. The normal muscle is retested each time the vertebra is challenged until a positive challenge is found.
4. If challenging the left transverse process anterior and superior (as in the second step above) causes muscle inhibition, therapy (i.e., manipulation or traction) is applied in the anterior and superior direction (vertebrae have a rebound action).

It should be noted that artful muscle testing becomes important in this type of situation in which a number of muscle tests are being performed using one muscle. Excessive pressure during the multiple tests may result in muscle fatigue. With proper testing, however, muscle fatigue should not occur.

Mechanical Challenge Procedure: Extravertebral Challenge

1. Therapy localization is positive to the head of the fibula.
2. The head of the fibula is challenged by pushing in various directions:
   - Head of fibula is pushed from anterior to posterior.
   - Head of fibula is pushed from posterior to anterior.
   - Occasionally, for example after trauma, a slight lateral, medial, superior, or inferior component may be necessary during the challenge.
3. The normal muscle is retested each time the fibula is challenged.
4. In one possible scenario, challenging the head of the fibula anterior to posterior causes muscle inhibition.
5. Therapy (i.e., manipulation or traction) is applied in the opposite direction (extravertebral joints do not rebound), that is, from posterior to anterior.

CHEMICAL CHALLENGES

In addition to acupuncture points, Chapman's reflexes, spinal areas, and the local muscle, another potential cause of muscle inhibition may be nutritional imbalance. A specific nutrient may improve muscle function for many reasons. It may supply the muscle itself with a needed nutrient (for example, calcium, which is important in contraction, or iron, for myoglobin), or it may be a nutritional support for whatever is causing the muscle to dysfunction, such as the related organ or gland. In these scenarios, applied kinesiologists use muscle testing to obtain information about potential nutritional needs of the patient. In general, one should use nutritional assessment after implementing other evaluation and treatment procedures instead of relying on nutritional therapy as a first line of treatment (although sometimes nutritional factors are primary causes of imbalance).

To test for a nutritional imbalance, two forms of chemical challenges have been developed in AK: oral and olfactory. These rely on sensory stimulation of the taste (oral challenge) or smell (olfactory challenge) centers that relay information to the central nervous system, followed by assessment of the efferent response through changes measured by muscle testing.

Observing for improved muscle function during an oral challenge—the change from an abnormally inhibited muscle to a normal one—is one way to utilize the oral challenge. Another approach involves stimulating the sensory mechanism with a potentially noxious substance—one that causes a negative stress in the patient, such as an allergic or toxic substance—and observing for an inhibiting effect on a normal muscle. For example, if the pectoralis major clavicular (PMC) muscle is normal and the patient is allergic to wheat, placing a small amount of wheat in the patient's mouth would typically cause inhibition of the PMC. Foods, nutrients, chemicals, and other substances can be evaluated using this approach. Some substances are better tested through the olfactory mechanism than by placing them on the tongue.

The olfactory challenge involves stimulating the patient's olfactory mechanism by having the person smell the substance being tested. It works the same way as the oral challenge. When the patient smells a substance, the result will be either a change in a muscle's function or no change. Olfactory stimulation by noxious substances in some patients is so significant that it is followed by an increase in heart rate or blood pressure (Bell et al. 1997).

A chemical challenge for nutrition can use the following process. After an inhibited muscle has been found, and other therapies (such as acupuncture, Chapman's reflexes, or spinal areas) either are not required or have already been tried without success, nutrition should be considered. If a certain nutrient is suspected, the patient should taste the nutritional substance. Then the muscle can be reevaluated. (If the substance is in a capsule or a coated tablet, it should be opened so the patient can taste the actual nutrient.) If the inhibited muscle normalizes after insalivation of the nutritional substance, supplementation with this nutrient may be beneficial to the patient. It must be emphasized that this is only one form of assessment for nutritional needs and that others should be considered, including the history, exam, blood tests, and dietary assessment. In addition, this type of assessment cannot determine the dose the patient requires. This must be up to the clinical judgment of the practitioner, perhaps in accordance with the commonly recommended doses published in the literature or those provided by the manufacturer. When testing more than one nutrient, it is important to be sure that the previously tested substance and its taste have been eliminated from the patient's mouth, since any remainder will maintain the challenge, including any muscle reaction. Once the taste is eliminated from the patient's mouth, the muscle should return to its previous state if the challenge was positive.

The particular nutrient the practitioner chooses for a given muscle dysfunction is based on the assessment data, including at least a diet survey, symptoms, blood tests, and perhaps the muscle-nutrient relationships developed in AK. These are much like the relationships between the muscles and the organs and glands. In reality, the patient's general health, absorptive ability, and other issues have significant influence on any nutritional relationship with a muscle. Macronutrient status also has a significant influence on the nutritional state and its relationship to a particular muscle. More importantly, it is vital to treat each patient as an individual; this may require that two patients receive very different nutrients despite having the same muscle inhibitions. For example, evaluation of two patients with knee pain, both having inhibition of the sartorius muscle, may show that there are different reasons why the sartorius muscle dysfunctioned. In one person, the adrenal gland hormones may be imbalanced, with cortisol being too high and dehydroepiandrosterone [DHEA(S)] too low. In the other person, cortisol may be too low and DHEA(S) normal. If both patients were given the same nutritional recommendations, it is unlikely that both would benefit since their needs would most likely be very different.

In addition to nutrients, other substances including homeopathic remedies and herbs can be evaluated using the same process, as long as the substance is tasted by the patient. Muscle-nutrient relationships have been developed in AK (see table 11.1).

Oral Chemical Challenge Procedure: Nutrient Remedies

1. The patient has a PMS muscle inhibition, for example.
2. The patient tastes the substance to be tested.
3. Retesting the inhibited muscle results in one of the following:
   - The muscle normalizes; the substance is considered a potential therapy.
   - The muscle does not change; the substance is removed and another is tested.
4. It is possible that multiple therapeutic remedies may be required, or none at all.

Oral Chemical Challenge Procedure: Allergic Substances

1. A normal latissimus dorsi muscle is used.
2. The patient tastes the substance to be tested.
3. Retesting the muscle results in one of the following:
   - The muscle remains normal; that substance may not be offensive to the patient.
   - The muscle becomes inhibited; the substance is removed, as it may be offensive to the patient, and appropriate dietary or lifestyle recommendations are made.
4. It is possible that many substances are offensive to the patient, or none at all.

Chemical Challenge Procedure: Noxious Substances

1. The patient has a normal latissimus dorsi, for example.
2. The patient smells the substance to be tested (i.e., perfume).
3. Retesting the latissimus dorsi results in one of the following:
   - The muscle remains normal; that substance may be considered nontoxic.
   - The muscle becomes inhibited; the patient may wish to avoid using this substance.

MENTAL/EMOTIONAL CHALLENGE

In AK, imaging is sometimes used as part of the assessment process, with muscle function changes acting as indicators. Mental imagery is also an option during therapy.

Much is known about the various aspects of mental imagery:

- Mental imagery correlates with specific autonomic nervous system actions, that is, sympathetic and parasympathetic activity (Deschaumes-Molinaro et al. 1992).
- Imagery can affect body chemistry. Hall et al. (1996) showed that test subjects could effectively change neutrophil counts using mental imagery.
- Szabo (1993) showed that responses to mental stress depend on body posture.
- Warner and McNeill (1988) described the use of mental imagery for improving physical skills by physical therapists.
- In competitive athletes, mental imagery has a positive relationship with performance improvement (Deschaumes-Molinaro et al. 1991).

Using muscle testing, mental/emotional challenges can assess the need for mental imagery or evaluate for existing mental/emotional stress. In the case of mental imagery, for example, the practitioner can ask the patient to think of a specific image related to competition or training. This may produce one of two possible outcomes. In the presence of muscle inhibition, the patient may be able to think of a mental image that normalizes the muscle. This thought can be used by the patient during training or competition. Or, a specific image may cause a normal muscle to become inhibited, which may give the practitioner and the patient a clue about mental/emotional stress. This is especially helpful with use of a muscle that was initially inhibited, then was corrected with certain reflexes as described earlier, and is now normal—a specific thought may cause a return of muscle inhibition.

In addition to these techniques, one can work with specific reflexes that are associated with mental/emotional stress, with certain muscle inhibition indicative of this type of stress. The indicator most commonly used in AK is bilateral inhibition of the PMC. Abnormal inhibition of both PMC muscles may be an indication that specific mental/emotional reflexes require stimulation. Most commonly these are two points on each frontal bone eminence (halfway between the eyebrow and the normal hairline), called the mental/emotional stress points or reflexes. These areas are stimulated differently from acupuncture points or Chapman's reflexes—with light touch rather than hard pressure. The practitioner lightly applies the fingertips of each hand on each frontal eminence and holds the points for 30-60 sec (see figure 11.1). This therapy is applied while the patient thinks about the same stress that caused a positive challenge. The inhibited PMC muscles are

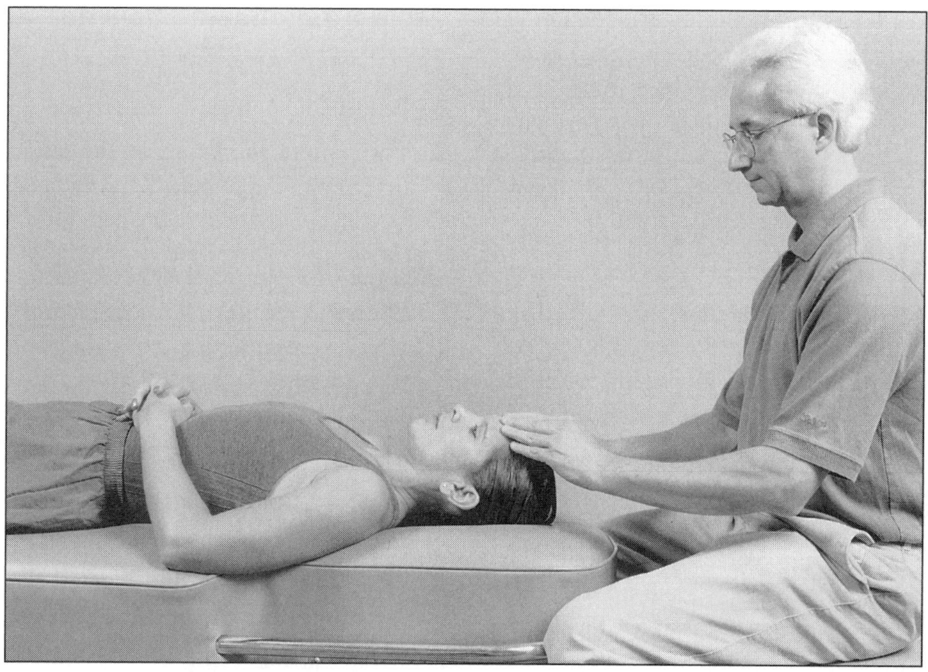

Figure 11.1 Practitioner stimulating the light touch reflexes for mental/emotional therapy.

retested following this treatment. In some cases, the muscle may still be inhibited and the points may need to be held for several minutes.

If the practitioner suspects a mental/emotional stress but the PMC muscles are normal, one can "challenge" patients by asking them to think about a particular stress (e.g., a very stressful event; patients do not need to vocalize the stress, but only to think about it). The PMC muscles are retested. If thinking about a stressful event causes the PMC muscles to become inhibited, the practitioner stimulates the mental/emotional stress points. (These points can also be therapy-localized; a positive therapy localization indicates a need for stimulation.) The process should be repeated to ensure that thinking about a particular stress no longer causes muscle inhibition. Athletes sometimes have mental/emotional stress reactions to certain types of competitions, certain competitors, or other factors. When mental/emotional stress is a problem, there may be several thoughts that could separately cause PMC inhibition. In the case of mental/emotional stress (and phobia, discussed further on), the types of problems described here are not the serious disturbances sometimes seen in patients, which may require medication, but the functional or subclinical mental/emotional problems common in sport. However, people who are already taking medication may still benefit from this procedure.

General Mental/Emotional Challenge Procedure

1. The patient has normal function of both PMC muscles.
2. The patient thinks of a particular stress.
3. The muscles are retested after each stressful thought (if more than one).
4. If a specific thought causes inhibition, the emotional stress points are treated with light touch while the patient thinks of that stress.
5. The PMC muscles are retested with the patient thinking about the same stress.
6. If the muscle still becomes inhibited, treatment of the emotional stress points is continued.

Some mental/emotional stress may be different, taking the form of fears or phobias that require one or more different therapy points. These fears may be treated similarly to less severe stresses, but the practitioner also may find that treatment is more successful with other reflexes as described by Callahan

(1985). In these cases, the acupuncture beginning and end points on the face (refer to chapter 17 and figure 17.2 for their locations) are often used, most frequently the stomach meridian point ST 1. The assessment procedure is the same as that described earlier. The PMC muscles are tested bilaterally. If they are normal, the practitioner asks the patient to think about the object or situation that is feared, such as a particular competitive event, crossing the finish line, or being injured and then retests the muscles. If the PMCs become inhibited from this mental/emotional challenge, the next step is to determine which acupuncture points on the face normalize the PMC inhibition. The practitioner taps this point for 20-30 sec at the rate of approximately four taps per second while the patient thinks about the object of the phobia. The same mental/emotional challenge is used to retest. If the muscles are initially abnormally inhibited, the patient can therapy-localize each acupuncture point ST 1 separately (one with each hand) to see if either one normalizes the inhibited PMC muscle, indicating a need for this treatment.

Mental/Emotional Challenge Procedure: Phobias, Fears, Stress

1. Both PMC muscles are normal.
2. The patient thinks about the situation or event that elicits the phobia.
3. The PMC muscles are retested.
4. If the PMC muscles become inhibited, the practitioner determines (through therapy localization) which acupuncture point or points normalize this inhibition (one or both, ST 1 being the most common).
5. The point or points are treated by tapping (20-30 sec) while the patient thinks of the object of the phobia.
6. The same muscles are retested with the patient thinking about the object of the phobia.
7. If the muscle still becomes inhibited, treatment of the points is continued, with the patient again thinking of the object of the phobia.
8. In some cases, the emotional stress points may also require stimulation.

Case History

After a couple of treatment sessions, Jack mentioned his fear about the upcoming marathon, a fear that he stated was unreasonable considering the great improvements he had made over the previous two months; specifically, this was the first time in four years that he was training without pain. His experience in his last three marathon attempts at qualifying for the Olympic trials had resulted in his having to drop out of the race due to severe leg pain. While he was talking about this mental/emotional stress, his previously normal PMC muscles became inhibited. He was asked to touch the left ST 1 point with one hand while the other PMC was tested. This was negative. He did the same for the opposite ST 1 point, which normalized the inhibited PMC. During this process, Jack had to be reminded on two occasions to continue thinking about that which he feared so that the inhibition of the PMC could be maintained. Jack was asked to continue thinking about what he feared while ST 1 was tapped for about 30 sec. While he maintained his fearful thoughts, the PMC muscles were retested. They were still inhibited, and when he therapy-localized to ST 1 it was still positive. ST 1 was tapped again for 30 sec. After Jack once again thought about the same stress, his PMC muscle remained normal. Jack was also asked to think about more of the details about his past races, but no other thoughts appeared to cause PMC inhibition. (Jack ran a personal best and qualified for the Olympic trials.)

ASSESSMENT OF AUTONOMIC FUNCTION

Sympathetic and parasympathetic imbalance may be observed in overtrained athletes and in those with high body fat, nutritional imbalance, and other problems noted throughout this text. In chapters 8 and 9, we considered assessment methods used in connection with autonomic dysfunction. In addition to these, other testing procedures have been traditionally used to evaluate autonomic balance. These include (1) postural decreases in systolic and diastolic blood pressures, as well as the systolic blood pressure decrease during phase II of a Valsalva maneuver, which reflect sympathetic function, and (2) the expiratory/inspiratory ratio and the difference between the maximum and minimum heart rate, both reflecting parasympathetic function (Freeman and Komaroff 1997). In addition, Groups One and Two of the Symptom Survey pertain to autonomic imbalance.

Manual muscle testing to challenge autonomic function has also been used as discussed by Schmitt (1997) and is briefly reviewed here. This challenge functions in the same way as those described above: if a muscle is inhibited and sympathetic (or parasympathetic) activity is stimulated, producing a normalization of muscle function, the person may benefit from increased sympathetic (or parasympathetic) activity. But if a muscle is normal and sympathetic (or parasympathetic) activity is stimulated, producing an inhibition of muscle function, the person may have increased sympathetic (or parasympathetic) tone.

Autonomic Function Challenge Procedure

1. To stimulate sympathetic activity, the patient should perform one or more of the following:
   - focus the eyes on the ceiling or other distal point,
   - follow a finger from near to far,
   - retrude the jaw, and
   - tense the intrinsic spinal muscles.
2. The practitioner then retests a muscle.
3. To stimulate parasympathetic activity, the patient should perform one or more of the following:
   - focus the eyes on the tip of the nose,
   - follow a finger from far to near,
   - protrude the jaw, and
   - relax the intrinsic spinal muscles.
4. The practitioner then retests a muscle.

A muscle is tested before and after one or more of the preceding steps.The results of these challenges should be noted with others obtained during the assessment process and should correlate with other findings regarding autonomic function as described throughout this text.

DIFFERENTIATING PRIMARY AND SECONDARY PROBLEMS

One important aspect of AK enables the practitioner to evaluate more complex clinical situations. Patients usually have several imbalances at one time, and it is not uncommon to find several structural, chemical, and mental/emotional imbalances that require attention. In this situation the practitioner must differentiate primary problems from those that evolved secondarily as a result of the initial problems. The secondary problems are frequently associated with symptoms, whereas the primary problems are often asymptomatic. Since patients may complain more about the secondary problem than the primary one, they often tend to conceal the more important primary problems. For example, in a patient with nontraumatic knee pain, which may be secondary, the tendency is to treat the knee. The knee may have some structural or chemical imbalance associated with the local discomfort, such as inflammation; the quadriceps muscles may be inhibited and the knee joint mechanically unstable. Correction of these muscles using Chapman's reflexes may improve muscle function, which may improve the pain symptoms. However, any relief obtained with this approach may not last more than a day or two, or even a few minutes, and the pain and muscle dysfunction may recur. If, for example, the ankle stability is poor because an inhibition of the tibialis posterior muscle is causing a problem in the talus bone, the ankle stress and instability could be a primary problem causing the knee problem. In many cases, the ankle would be asymptomatic. If the tibialis posterior muscle were the primary problem, correcting this muscle could enable the body to correct the ankle problem, and the quadriceps inhibition, resulting in more normal function of the knee joint. Potentially, the knee could be functioning normally after one treatment (although factors such as inflammation may take longer to dissipate). This example shows how important it can be to find the primary problem(s) and avoid treating the secondary imbalances.

Through the use of therapy localization, the practitioner may be able to determine which areas of dysfunction are primary and which are secondary. In the example just cited, the quadriceps muscles were inhibited and the related Chapman's reflexes produce a positive therapy localization. Likewise, the tibialis posterior was inhibited, and this muscle is positive to therapy-localizing to the related Chapman's reflex. However, if therapy localization to the tibialis posterior reflexes also normalizes the quadriceps but the reflex for the quadriceps does not normalize the tibialis posterior muscle, the practitioner can assume that stimulating the reflex for the tibialis posterior will improve both muscles. This same method can be used for any number of muscles and reflexes. In many cases, stimulation of one reflex could improve several unrelated muscles.

A similar scenario may exist with a primary reflex for a muscle, for example, with a joint problem being secondary. Suppose, for instance, that therapy localization to the spinal area L1 is positive. The abdominal muscles are inhibited and there is positive therapy localization to Chapman's reflex. The practitioner may find that therapy-localizing to Chapman's reflex negates the positive therapy localization of L1 (in this case, a tensor fascia lata muscle is used since the patient needs both hands to therapy-localize two different areas). Correction of the reflex will then negate the positive therapy localization to L1. In this case, it may be theorized that the normalization of the abdominal muscles improved spinal function, correcting the L1 problem. If spinal pain accompanied the problem at L1, it would not be unusual for the spinal pain to be significantly reduced or more often eliminated, after stimulation of Chapman's reflexes for the abdominal muscles.

Primary problems may stem from any structural, chemical, or mental/emotional source. They could relate to any type of reflex or therapy area that has been described, including spinal or extravertebral areas, the cranial bones, acupuncture points, Chapman's reflexes, the muscle itself, or even to nutrients or foods. For example, a patient may have a variety of imbalances—inhibition of the left PMC and upper trapezius, the right latissimus dorsi, tibialis anterior, and tensor fascia lata, all having positive therapy localization to the corresponding Chapman's reflexes, acupuncture points, or spinal areas—but have the primary problem as a need for calcium. The practitioner may determine this through an oral challenge using calcium, which would normalize all the muscles and negate other abnormal findings. The practitioner may have considered the potential need for calcium for a number of reasons: calcium is associated with the upper trapezius, the patient has muscle cramps during certain workouts, the patient's diet analysis showed very low calcium, adrenal gland function (which helps regulate minerals) was poor, and the patient drinks large amounts of diet soda (containing phosphorus, which can increase calcium loss from the body).

After all the problems in the patient are corrected, the practitioner may wish to assess potential harmful substances. In the example just cited, an oral challenge with phosphorus may cause all the patient's problems to temporarily recur, after having been corrected, while phosphorus is in the mouth. Removing the phosphorus from the mouth restores the normal function. Through the results of this challenge, the practitioner can emphasize to the patient the need to avoid excess phosphorus, such as is contained in most soda. (Phosphorus is not always bad; it may be required by other patients, especially to increase sympathetic activity.)

Case History

Joe was a weight lifter who had developed chronic right knee pain during the previous six months. There was no history of trauma. Joe could not squat more than halfway without pain, even without any weights. Examination was negative for all orthopedic tests but revealed inhibition of several muscles: the right rectus femoris, psoas, and tibialis posterior, and the left gluteus maximus and rectus abdominis. The following areas were positive for their respective muscles during therapy localization: rectus femoris—Chapman's reflex and SI 19; psoas—L2; tibialis posterior—Chapman's reflex; gluteus maximus—L5; rectus abdominis—Chapman's reflex. Through the process of therapy-localizing, only the Chapman's reflex for the abdominal muscles proved to normalize all other muscle function. This reflex was stimulated and the muscles were retested, but without change. The Chapman's reflex still therapy-localized and was stimulated for a longer period of time (about 45 sec). The muscles were retested and all were normal, and none of the reflexes or spinal areas now therapy-localized. Joe was able to squat normally without pain. On Joe's forms, he had noted potential stress associated with competition. I asked him to think about this potential stress and retested several muscles that had been previously inhibited but were now normal. Two of these muscles, the rectus femoris and abdominis, became inhibited again. Joe was asked to squat again, which caused pain. The ST 1 points therapy-localized bilaterally, and both were treated (by tapping for about 30 sec) while Joe thought about the potential stress. After this therapy, Joe was asked to think about the potential stress again. No inhibition was found. Squatting was not painful. I asked Joe to think about various other stresses, but none caused any dysfunction. Joe returned for a follow-up visit two weeks later, with no recurrence of the initial problems, and had no recurrence of the knee pain.

CONCLUSION

Applied kinesiology helps guide the practitioner through the potential maze of structural, chemical, and mental/emotional imbalances that the patient may manifest. This chapter has reviewed only a few of the many procedures that have been developed in AK. The predominant feature is the concept that the muscles have relationships with a number of other areas: organs, glands, spinal vertebrae, acupuncture meridians and specific points, and nutrition. Any dysfunction in these areas may be reflected through muscle inhibition and assessed through muscle testing.

Assessments of Aerobic and Anaerobic Function

A dysfunction of the aerobic and anaerobic systems may be reflected in their neuromuscular components; these include the so-called slow and fast muscle fibers and their neurological elements, which transmit impulses from the fiber at relatively slow or fast speeds. A physical test has been developed that assesses these components through muscle testing, as an effective way to help evaluate aerobic and anaerobic function (Maffetone 1996). In addition, a variety of signs and symptoms are sometimes associated with aerobic and anaerobic imbalance and are outlined here.

The aerobic and anaerobic challenges can be utilized as an assessment tool to help the practitioner differentiate six potential conditions: normal aerobic or anaerobic function, deficient aerobic or anaerobic function, and excess aerobic or anaerobic function.

THE AEROBIC CHALLENGE

The basis of this challenge is the theory that easy aerobic activity has an important therapeutic component, as demonstrated in those who begin an exercise program and obtain benefits of various kinds. (The concept that training has an important therapeutic aspect is part of the complementary sports medicine approach and is discussed in chapter 21.) These changes can be demonstrated immediately in a patient with good aerobic function: any muscle inhibition is temporarily facilitated, or normalized, following slow repetitive movements that stimulate aerobic fiber activity as occurs during aerobic exercise. This is referred to as the aerobic challenge, and is outlined next.

Aerobic Challenge Procedure

1. The patient is supine (although any position can be used) and has a pectoralis major sternal (PMS) muscle inhibition, for example, and a normal latissimus dorsi.
2. The patient slowly and alternately raises and lowers the lower limbs 8 to 10 times, as in a walking movement.
3. The muscles are retested.
4. In a normal response, the PMS normalizes and the latissimus dorsi remains normal.
5. In an abnormal response, the PMS remains inhibited; this is referred to as an aerobic deficiency. The latissimus dorsi remains normal.
6. On rare occasions, the latissimus dorsi may become inhibited. The significance of this is discussed in the next section.
7. Any changes in muscle function last only 10-20 sec.

Following aerobic movement, if any muscle inhibition fails to normalize, as in step 5, the aerobic system may be termed deficient, implying that it is in a state of underactivity. This dysfunction is usually accompanied by a number of clinical features associated with aerobic deficiency. Secondary signs and symptoms may include elevated respiratory quotient (RQ), lower oral pH, declining endurance performance, fatigue, increased body fat content, excess hunger, depression, insomnia, and hormonal imbalance. Aerobic deficiency is often associated with adrenal dysfunction, and the relationships of each are further discussed in chapter 27.

Diminished aerobic function may be due to increased structural, chemical, or mental/emotional stress and is often a result of excess anaerobic training. For example, Colliander et al. (1988) showed that overdevelopment of the anaerobic system is associated with lower content of aerobic muscle fiber enzymes. In addition, excess high-intensity training diminishes the availability of fat for use by the aerobic muscle fiber (Hodgetts et al. 1991). A classical secondary symptom associated with aerobic deficiency is the so-called chronic fatigue syndrome. Patients with this condition have reduced aerobic function (Sisto et al. 1996). Improper dietary and nutritional factors can often contribute to aerobic deficiency. Essentially, any stress that adversely affects the aerobic system can contribute to its dysfunction, including a lack of training of the aerobic system as seen in inactive patients or in those involved strictly in anaerobic training, such as weight lifters. Common signs, symptoms, and causes of the aerobic deficiency syndrome include the following:

- Fatigue
- Recurrent injuries
- Increased body fat
- Increased hunger
- Hormonal imbalance
- Diminished performance
- Increased RQ
- Decreased oral pH
- Insomnia

Treatments for the patient with aerobic deficiency include those that address the causes. These are among the causes:

- Diminished quality or quantity of aerobic muscle activity (reduced aerobic training)
- Excess anaerobic training
- Dietary and nutritional excess or deficiency
- Any other physical, chemical, or mental stress

For example, if the patient is iron deficient, myoglobin content may also be low and aerobic fiber function diminished, leading to aerobic deficiency. Treatment is directed at finding the cause of the iron deficiency. Or, if carbohydrate intake is too high, the utilization of fats for energy may be low and aerobic function diminished. Treatment is directed at balancing the diet. In most cases, a combination of causes exists. A common single cause is excessive anaerobic training as part of overtraining.

THE ANAEROBIC CHALLENGE

Anaerobic dysfunction may also occur, and can be assessed through the anaerobic challenge. In this test, the anaerobic system is stimulated; the neuromuscular components that perform fast, powerful activity are activated, and the results are observed in muscle-testing outcomes. A frequent finding is an overactivity of this system, referred to as an anaerobic excess.

Anerobic Challenge Procedure

1. The patient is supine (although any position can be used) and has a pectoralis major clavicular (PMC) muscle inhibition, for example, and a normal psoas muscle.
2. The patient stimulates anaerobic activity by clenching the fists, and rapidly and powerfully flexing and extending (alternating left and right arms) the elbows for approximately 6 to 8 sec.
3. The muscles are retested.
4. In a normal response, the muscles remain the same; the PMC remains inhibited and the psoas remains normal.
5. In an abnormal response, the psoas muscle becomes inhibited. The PMC remains inhibited. This is termed anaerobic excess and is the most common imbalance.
6. On rare occasions, the PMC may normalize (and the psoas remain normal).

When a normal muscle becomes inhibited following anaerobic stimulation, the condition is termed an anaerobic excess. This condition may occur by itself, or it may occur in conjunction with, or be the cause of, aerobic deficiency. In the case of aerobic deficiency and anaerobic excess, the treatment consists of removing all anaerobic training for a time period that will allow rebuilding of the aerobic system (and recovery of the anaerobic system).

OTHER AEROBIC AND ANAEROBIC IMBALANCES

Occasionally, the anaerobic challenge may result in an inhibited muscle's becoming normal. The condition is referred to as anaerobic deficiency. In this case, the condition may be due to the body's need for anaerobic training as a means to balance the aerobic and anaerobic systems. As described in chapter 21, performing light anaerobic work three times per week, during a period of one to three weeks, may suffice to correct the problem. The condition is usually associated with an aerobic excess.

Only on rare occasions will there be an aerobic excess, as seen when the aerobic challenge causes a normal muscle to become inhibited. Many of these cases are due to neurological disorganization. In some instances, the person has developed too much aerobic function relative to anaerobic function and requires some anaerobic stimulation in the form of training to restore balance.

As indicated, the conditions of anaerobic deficiency and aerobic excess may occur together. Likewise, aerobic deficiency and anaerobic excess often occur together. Any other pattern, such as aerobic deficiency and excess, or anaerobic excess and deficiency, is not likely to occur.

It should be emphasized that a good history, as discussed later in this chapter, may reveal imbalances of the aerobic and anaerobic systems.

It may be easiest to view the balance of aerobic and anaerobic function, and its assessment with muscle testing, from the perspective of Chinese medicine and qi. If too little aerobic or anaerobic energy exists, adding more improves muscle function (an inhibited muscle becomes normal). If too much aerobic or anaerobic energy exists, adding more will cause decreased muscle function (a normal muscle becomes inhibited). The exception is the scenario in which a muscle inhibition is normalized by aerobic activity, which is normal—this is an example of the therapeutic action of aerobic activity.

Case History

Bob had chronic low back pain of four years' duration. Examinations ruled out pathology. Bob had just ended his fall racing season and wanted to prepare for the spring season without pain. His biggest concern was his low back, so he did not complain of other problems or note anything about other issues on his patient history forms. When asked about other problems during the consultation, he stated that his main concern was his low back problem. After an explanation of the holistic approach and the importance of looking at all systems, Bob admitted to fatigue, insomnia, increased weight gain (body fat) and constant hunger, shoulder and neck pain, and a significant loss in his cycling performance. Aerobic challenge did not change the muscle inhibition of the psoas major, indicating an aerobic deficiency which correlated well with his history. The anaerobic challenge caused a normal PMC to become inhibited, indicating an anaerobic excess. A significant part of Bob's treatment was adjusting his training schedule—increasing easy aerobic work while eliminating all anaerobic training and competition for the next three months. Bob completely recovered, and his performances also significantly improved during the spring season.

THE AEROBIC DEFICIENCY SYNDROME

The most common imbalance between the aerobic and anaerobic systems is a dysfunction of the aerobic system and a relative excess of anaerobic function. The chronic state of poor aerobic function, with its many signs and symptoms, has been termed the aerobic deficiency syndrome (Maffetone 1997).

The primary problems contributing to this syndrome are (1) an aerobic deficiency as previously described, often accompanied by an anaerobic excess, and (2) adrenal dysfunction, which is often associated with aerobic deficiency. These two conditions are most often inseparable, as they have common signs and symptoms. A third contributing problem is overtraining resulting in diminished aerobic and excess anaerobic muscle fibers.

During the history-taking process, patients may indicate a variety of seemingly unrelated complaints that are actually all part of the aerobic deficiency syndrome. These include fatigue, increased body fat, structural injuries, hormonal imbalance, reduced endurance capacity and overtraining, stress, and dietary or nutritional factors, among other symptoms that we will note.

Fatigue is a common complaint. This may also be related to blood sugar-handling stress and is often associated with numerous complaints on the Symptoms Survey described in chapter 7, especially carbohydrate intolerance. Mental and emotional stress is a frequent association; feelings of depression, anxiety, or clinical depression are the most common symptoms.

Increased body fat (relative to diet and training levels) may result from diminished utilization of fat. Dietary imbalance is often associated with aerobic deficiency. Patients often consume excess carbohydrates and have low fat and protein intakes. Nutritional imbalance may occur. For example, iron levels that appear normal in traditional blood tests may be functionally low, adversely affecting aerobic muscle fiber activity (Lukaski et al. 1991). These may be associated with a high RQ or increasing RQ relative to results of previous tests.

Patients with this syndrome may also have structural injuries, sometimes as a result of the lack of aerobic muscle fiber function around joints. In addition, specific muscle inhibition of the sartorius, tibialis posterior, and gracilis is common due to adrenal dysfunction, making the low back, knee, ankle, and foot areas the most vulnerable to structural injury.

Hormonal imbalance may be associated with aerobic deficiency syndrome, especially in the form of high levels of cortisol and low dehydroepiandrosterone [DHEA(S)]. High cortisol may be associated with insomnia. In more chronic conditions, especially in late-stage overtraining, low cortisol may be evident. In women, premenstrual syndrome and menopausal symptoms may be secondary complaints. Sexual dysfunction may also accompany the aerobic deficiency syndrome as a result of secondary diminished DHEA(S) and sex hormones.

Reduced endurance capacity and overtraining are often associated with the aerobic deficiency syndrome. This is usually reflected in the Maximum Aerobic Function test described in the next chapter.

Other clues may be seen on the Symptom Survey (chapter 7), specifically in Groups Three and Seven. Other common examination findings include orthostatic hypotension (sometimes in the functional stage), lowered body temperature, abnormal cold pressor test, low oral pH, low vital capacity, and high salivary cortisol with low DHEA(S).

CONCLUSION

Correction of aerobic and anaerobic imbalance involves properly assessing the whole patient, treating all primary problems, and addressing the appropriate lifestyle factors. The aerobic and anaerobic challenges can greatly assist the practitioner in making decisions about various therapies and training issues. Reduced aerobic function may be a very common problem in athletes, presenting various structural, chemical, and mental/emotional aspects to consider.

13

Heart Rate Monitor Assessments

Heart rate monitors are commonly used in complementary sports medicine as a biofeedback device and assessment tool. Biofeedback is the process of furnishing information in an auditory or visual form from a physiological variable such as heart rate (*Dorland's Illustrated Medical Dictionary* 1994). This may be useful for assessing a number of important factors during training, including aerobic progression and aerobic speed and, most importantly, the potential of structural, chemical, or mental/emotional stress as a prelude to overtraining. These factors are evaluated through the Maximum Aerobic Function test using the 180-formula (Maffetone 1996).

THE USE OF MONITORS

Modern heart rate monitors are accurate for use in many exercise activities and at many intensities (Seaward et al. 1990; Moore et al. 1997) and may be particularly valuable in both assessment and training situations.

Lee et al. (1996) found that a significant number of male coronary heart patients failed to achieve target heart rates. Heart rate monitors can be used to motivate certain individuals who may not normally exercise with enough intensity to gain optimal benefits. In most cases, however, the heart rate monitor can help limit exercise intensity in individuals who may otherwise train at too high a heart rate resulting in potential stress or overtraining (Lehmann et al. 1997). Remember, higher intensities and longer-duration workouts can suppress the immune system (Newsholme 1994; Keast et al. 1988).

Heart monitors also can help regulate high-intensity training and are more accurate than measures of blood lactate, which can fluctuate significantly during hard workouts (Boulay et al. 1997). Moreover, the use of heart monitors is more practical and cost effective than measuring blood lactate.

In addition, heart monitors have value as an assessment tool. These devices are important for objective feedback for both practitioner and patient, providing information on another form of body language.

MANUAL VERSUS ELECTRONIC HEART RATE EVALUATION

A heart rate monitor can improve the accuracy of calculating the heart rate during any exercise as compared to manual evaluation (Ring and Brener

1996). In general, monitors are obviously more sensitive and accurate than manual pulse counting (see figure 13.1). Bell and Bassey (1996) showed that manual palpation to determine heart rate leads to errors—specifically, to results that are significantly lower than actual values. Deriving accurate heart rate counts is vital if the patient is on a specific program that has therapeutic applications. In addition, accurate determination of the maximum exercise heart rate is very important in that low maximum exercise heart rates, and especially low differences between resting and maximum exercise heart rates, are strong predictors of cardiovascular mortality (Sandvik et al. 1995).

In addition, in some individuals, manual evaluations of heart rate via the carotid pulse may be inaccurate for physiological reasons. External pressure on the carotid sinus may increase parasympathetic activity, lowering the heart rate. Boone et al. (1985) reported significantly lower postexercise pulse readings as compared to electrocardiogram values when subjects obtained their heart rates by manually palpating the carotid pulse. Results of earlier studies (Oldridge et al. 1981), however, were not consistent with these findings. These differences may reflect the errors obtained with manual pulse taking in general.

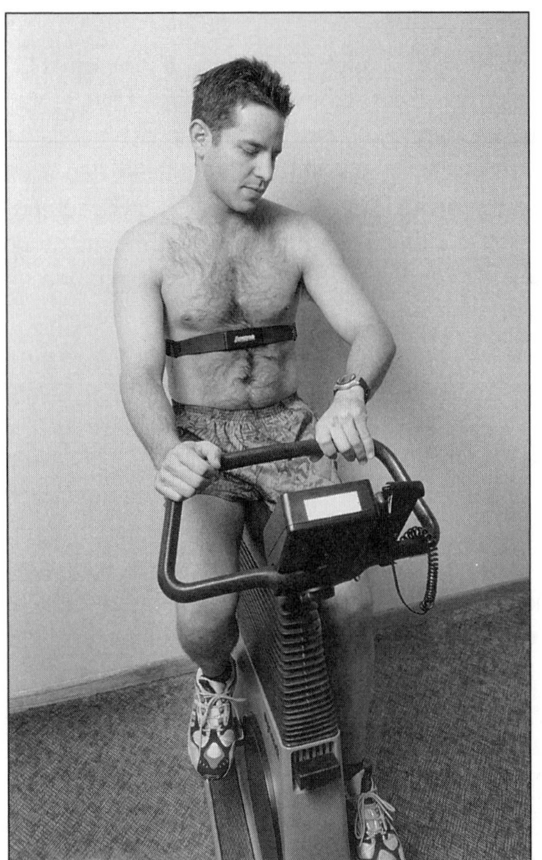

Figure 13.1 A patient monitors his heart rate during exercise. Heart rate monitors are considered more accurate than manual pulse counting.

NEUROLOGICAL ASPECTS OF HEART RATE

The heart rate is controlled by both intrinsic and extrinsic factors. Intrinsically, the heart muscle contains four main components that control the heartbeat. These include the sinoatrial node, the atrioventricular node, the atrioventricular bundle, and the Purkinje fibers. These components affect the cardiac muscle through nerves within the heart.

The heart rate is also influenced by factors extrinsic to the heart itself, including the autonomic nervous system and hormonal function. Both of these factors can be influenced by various therapies, training techniques, and lifestyle. The autonomic nervous system affects the components within the heart, with parasympathetic stimulation slowing the heart rate. During endurance training, lowered resting heart rates reflect parasympathetic activity. Sympathetic activity increases the heart rate at other times, such as during training and competition. This activity results from increased catecholamine release.

Autonomic imbalance may be reflected through the heart rate. With the help of a heart monitor, athletes may become more aware of warning signs. For example, the resting heart rate may be too low in some overtrained athletes due to excessive parasympathetic activity (Kuipers and Keizer 1988). Likewise, high resting heart rates may indicate excessive sympathetic activity during overtraining (Wilmore and Costill 1994). As described later, the training heart rate can also indicate overtraining; and, more importantly, subtle changes in training heart rates may predict an impending overtraining syndrome (see also chapter 23).

OTHER HEART RATE RELATIONSHIPS

Accurately recording the heart rate is useful for obtaining other information. The heart rate can be used to estimate energy expenditure (McArdle et al. 1991). If an individual's heart rate is known, the oxygen (O_2) consumption can be estimated (the heart rate is linearly related to O_2 consumption). Traditionally, training heart rate intensities are related to specific levels of O_2 uptake. The approach used by the author, however, focuses as much on the heart rate's relationship to the neurological and hormonal aspects of the patient as on its relationship to O_2. Training the patient with a focus on improving all these factors, rather than only on improving O_2 uptake (sometimes at the expense of these factors), contributes a therapeutic component to training as discussed in later chapters. It should be noted that the heart rate is identical to the pulse rates obtained from the radial artery and other pulses (McArdle et al. 1991).

THE MAXIMUM AEROBIC FUNCTION TEST

By regularly measuring the duration of a particular activity with a given heart rate and distance (or other measure such as watts), athletes can monitor themselves to check on their progress and to assess potential over- or undertraining. This assessment, referred to as the Maximum Aerobic Function (MAF) test, may be implemented with almost any training activity such as running, walking, biking, or use of stationary apparatus. It is not applicable for use with weight lifting or similar power equipment (i.e., a heart monitor may be useful during power workouts, but not for MAF testing during power workouts). The MAF test can also be used for noncompetitive patients, such as those on weight-loss or cardiac rehabilitation programs in which improved metabolism (i.e., increased utilization of fats) is important. It is also valuable in athletes in sports, such as basketball, baseball, and football that rely on endurance and aerobic speed (defined in chapter 2). In any of these cases, the MAF test can be performed on an ergometer, treadmill, track, and so on.

When compared to results of previous tests, MAF test results may indicate progress, a loss of progress seen as a plateau, or a regression. This test does not, however, provide information about the cause of a plateau or regression in function. During MAF testing, the athlete must use the same heart rate for each test and wear a heart monitor to ensure accuracy. The person must constantly observe the heart rate and must increase, decrease, or maintain the indicated intensity of activity. For someone who has never used a heart monitor, there may be only slightly less accuracy, since maintaining a pace at or near the desired heart rate is sometimes difficult for novices. People who have some experience with heart monitors can often maintain a pace that keeps their heart rate almost precisely at the desired level. In addition, a number of other factors described later may affect the heart rate during the MAF test.

Performing a Maximum Aerobic Function Test

An example of performance of a MAF test by a runner will be useful. After an easy walking or jogging warm-up, the athlete runs a predetermined distance, such as 5 km (3.1 miles), at a predetermined heart rate such as 150 beats per minute (bpm). The time of each kilometer (or mile) is recorded, as is the total time. A beginner might have a total time of 36 min, for example. The MAF test for this individual on that date is 36 min. If the test at the same heart rate is completed a month later, the expected result would be a faster time, perhaps 34 min; after six months, perhaps the runner will have progressed to 31 min (see figure 13.2).

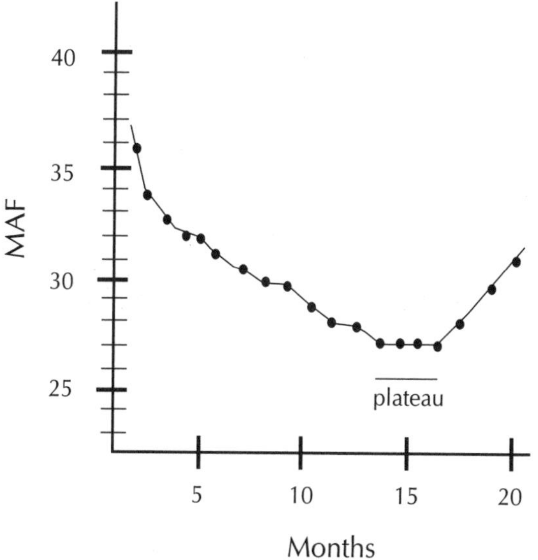

Figure 13.2 Maximum Aerobic Function test results (total time) of a runner during a 12-month training period using a 5-km course.

As already mentioned, it is important to measure each kilometer (or mile) when performing the MAF test by running. It is normal to obtain slightly slower times during the test period as each successive kilometer or mile is run. The faster the initial kilometer or mile, the more the time will slow between the first and last segments of the run. For example, if the first kilometer is 5 min 20 sec, the fifth kilometer may be 7 min; if the first kilometer is 3 min 44 sec, the fifth may be 4 min 21 sec. If this slowing is not seen, for example if the first kilometer is 6 min 46 sec and the second is 6 min 29 sec, the athlete may not have warmed up enough.

Table 13.1 presents data for an actual case of a runner who used a heart rate of 145 bpm and a 5-mile MAF test.

Table 13.1 An Actual Case of a Runner's 5-Mile Maximum Aerobic Function Test in Minutes Per Mile

	April	May	June	July
Mile 1	8:21	8:11	7:57	7:44
Mile 2	8:27	8:18	8:05	7:52
Mile 3	8:38	8:26	8:10	7:59
Mile 4	8:44	8:33	8:17	8:09
Mile 5	8:49	8:39	8:24	8:15

Looking at Maximum Aerobic Function Test Results

If autonomic or hormonal imbalance, neuromuscular dysfunction, or other problems develop during the training period, they will usually be revealed in the MAF test results. For example, if the runner of figure 13.1, who has progressed for the first 12 months of training, develops imbalances such as adrenal dysfunction and neuromuscular imbalance, these problems may be reflected in the MAF test as a slower time or by a plateau. That is, months 14 through 17 may show times of 27 min; month 18, a test of 28 min; month 18, a test of 29 min; and month 19, a test of 31 min.

Potential imbalances that may cause a lack of progression, or a regression, may come from excess training volume, excess training intensity, nutritional or dietary problems, or any other type of stress. Most often, however, a combination of factors is involved. It is up to the practitioner and patient to determine together which factors are the cause of the problem and what therapies and lifestyle modifications are necessary to correct it. Proper correction usually results in a rapid return to improved MAF test times, although in some difficult cases, such as chronic overtraining, restoration to healthy progress may take several weeks or months.

Case History

Sarah began a training program of walking that progressed to jogging and running. Her MAF test initially showed about 18.5 min/mile. After about 10 months she improved to faster than 13.5 min/mile, but it was difficult for her to walk at that rapid pace, so she began jogging. After about a year, her MAF test was just under 11 min/mile, and six months later it was 9 min 30 sec. At that time she began participating in local 5-km and 10-km road races and increased her training. Her MAF improved to 8 min 45 sec and remained there for three months. The next month's test was 9 min 15 sec. After not having consulted with me for over a year, Sarah arrived at my office with bilateral knee pain, increased fatigue, and for the first time a declining MAF test. She was assessed and treated; she showed a number of overtraining signs and symptoms including orthostatic hypotension, a variety of neuromuscular inhibitions (including both sartorius muscles), and other problems. After three office visits, including modifications of diet and training, Sarah began to feel better. During this time her MAF test remained at 9 min 15 sec. Two weeks later it improved to about 9 min. In another month she was nearly symptom free, and her MAF test improved to about 8 min 20 sec and continued to reflect slow improvements. As the MAF test improves, the overall rate of improvement for each kilometer or mile will diminish; initially, especially with a patient who has never trained, the improvements may be dramatic. In time, as the pace improves significantly, further improvement rates are decreased.

Adjusting Time and Distance

The factors of time, heart rate, and distance can also be adjusted and used in other ways. In the examples already cited, heart rate and distance were constant and time was the variable. In swimming, heart rate and time can be the constants, with the number of laps covered being the variable. For example, after an easy warm-up, a swimmer maintains a 145-bpm heart rate and swims for 30 min, counting the number of laps covered in that time period. After several weeks, the swimmer will complete more laps during the 30-min period (assuming proper aerobic progress).

One can perform a MAF test on a bike by choosing a road course that takes about 30 to 45 min to complete. After an easy cycling warm-up, the person rides at a specified heart rate and records the total time. With progress, the time to complete the course should get faster. For example, it may at first take 36 min 50 sec to complete a specific course. A month later, it may take 35 min 30 sec at the same constant heart rate, and in another month 34 min 15 sec.

Frequency of Maximum Aerobic Function Tests

The MAF test is best performed regularly throughout the year, every three to four weeks, and the results should be recorded in both the athlete's diary and the office records. Performing the test more often than this may contribute to mental/emotional stress. Daily or weekly changes may be more difficult to measure objectively, especially since on certain days a temporary worsening may be evident as a result of variables to be described later. In addition, focusing on the test too frequently can foster an obsession much like that of athletes who are addicted to weighing themselves on the scale daily or even more often.

One of the great benefits of the MAF test is that it can objectively inform both practitioner and patient of a structural, chemical, or mental/emotional obstacle to further progress long before the condition manifests as an injury or as declining athletic performance. Performing the test irregularly or not often enough defeats this purpose. The MAF test parallels other assessment measures described in previous chapters, including respiratory quotient (RQ), postural blood pressures, oral pH, breath-holding, vital capacity, and other indicators related to functional health. As the MAF test improves, the RQ decreases. This correlates with an increase in the utilization of fats and a decrease in reliance on glucose. Since most patients do not have access to a gas analyzer for RQ testing, the MAF test becomes even more useful. As defined in chapter 2, an increased utilization of fat is one source of improved endurance and aerobic speed.

A significant relationship has been found by the author between improved MAF tests and diminished structural, chemical, and mental/emotional injuries. In general, athletes whose MAF test was improving could almost be assured of being injury free. Those who became injured usually had a plateaued or regressing MAF test.

Maximum Aerobic Function Test Plateau

At some stage, the MAF test will normally plateau for a brief period. In other instances, though, the plateau is not normal and is a result of some structural, chemical, or mental/emotional stress—often a combination of stresses. It is important for the practitioner to distinguish between a normal and an abnormal plateau in MAF test results. This differentiation is not always very clear, and practitioner and patient must work together to assess the plateau. The following information provides only general guidelines.

A normal plateau typically occurs after approximately six months of progress. In some cases, for example in a patient just beginning a training program, progress can continue for a year or more before a plateau is observed. This plateau may last for several weeks but generally lasts no more than one to three months. Any continued plateau might be considered abnormal and could be the start of a period of overtraining. In some cases, any plateau may be abnormal as various imbalances can cause a halt in progress. Therefore any plateau should be looked at very carefully, with the idea that there might be a problem causing the loss of progress. If the plateau turns into a regression, then it is certain it is an abnormal plateau.

FACTORS THAT AFFECT THE MAXIMUM AEROBIC FUNCTION TEST RESULTS

A number of external factors may cause errors in the MAF test. In running, for example, the type of track surface may have a slight influence on pace. Modern high-tech track surfaces result in a slightly faster pace at the same heart rate as compared to cinder or dirt tracks, which will slow the pace. For testing on a bike, a velodrome—though not available for most athletes—is ideal, allowing the greatest speed. The roughness or smoothness of a road surface, the varying grades, and automobile traffic will all affect the MAF test. The net result of hills usually is a slowing of pace as compared to that on flat surfaces unless there are significantly more downhills. A good option is to use a wind trainer or rollers for the MAF test on a bike, especially in climates in which weather factors may be significant.

Usually these factors, and the others to be described, will make a relatively insignificant difference. But to ensure that the MAF test is most accurate, it is best to use the same course or method each time one performs the test. In the event that the test course is changed, it is important that this be noted in the patient's diary and the office records.

Other factors that potentially interfere with the MAF test include weather, altitude, equipment, hydration, and food. Some of these factors work against the athlete by increasing physical effort, which increases the heart rate, forcing the athlete to slow the pace.

The weather can influence the MAF test in several ways:

- A head wind may physically counter the forward motion, raising the heart rate. A tailwind will have the opposite effect; the athlete will go faster at the same heart rate.
- Temperature may be a factor; extremes of heat and cold can raise the heart rate, slowing the pace.
- High humidity can act much like a head wind. It is a physical barrier of water that requires increased effort on the part of the athlete to work through. The increased effort raises the heart rate, causing the pace to slow.
- Rain and snow are similar to humidity and head winds in their effects. Testing in the rain (and to a lesser extent snow) requires more effort. In addition, if the road or track surface is wet, with water or snow, additional physical effort may be required, raising the heart rate and slowing the pace.
- A very low barometric pressure may adversely affect the MAF test, possibly as a result of a slightly lowered O_2 uptake.

Often, weather stress is not the result of a single factor. A combination of cold and wind, for example, can elevate the heart rate significantly. The combination of summer heat, humidity, and low pressure may also be a significant stress that results in higher heart rates. For these reasons, the MAF test should not be performed when the weather is extreme.

Altitude can have a significant effect on the test results, especially if the athlete has not adapted to the new altitude. If an athlete is visiting a high-altitude location, the MAF test results will not be consistent with results of tests performed at lower altitudes; generally the time will be much slower. When traveling to lower altitudes, athletes usually show improved MAF tests within the first three weeks.

Equipment—including the bicycle and its components, other pieces of exercise equipment, and running shoes—can also affect the outcome of the MAF test. The bike setup and positioning, the pressure and wear on the tires, and any other factors that change drag, such as clothing, will affect the test. Athletes should note in their diary when they have performed the test using a different bike setup or wearing more clothing, or when any other factor has changed.

Running shoes may also affect the results of the MAF test. In general, shoes with more cushioning and more support, and shoes that are heavier, will result in slower times. Lighter shoes, including racing styles, generally allow faster MAF tests. These issues are discussed in chapter 24.

Running stride length can influence the MAF test as well. A runner who maintains a constant heart rate on a track can determine the optimal stride length by experimenting with increasing and decreasing stride length. If stride length becomes inefficient, that is, too short or too long, heart rate will rise. Heinert (1988) showed that stride-length variation could significantly affect O_2 uptake. This occurs because of increases and decreases in mechanical stress, which affect the running gait (Cavanagh and Kram 1985). Runners may increase their stride length when fatigued; this is also the case during a fever or cold (Weidner et al. 1997). Both of these examples result in increased stress. If athletes can move at their most comfortable pace, this pace may correlate with the optimal stride length and lowest heart rate.

Other equipment, such as treadmills, stationary bikes, and steppers, can be used for the MAF test, but the results cannot be compared with those from tests using other equipment or test locations. For example, the treadmill MAF test cannot directly be compared to a running test done on a track, and a MAF test on a stationary bike is not comparable to one done on a bike on a road course. Equipment maintenance may also affect the MAF test; poorly lubricated gears, improperly aligned wheels, or other structural stress may be a factor.

Hydration and preexercise food influence body function and can significantly impact the MAF test. In general, even slight dehydration will have a negative effect. This problem is discussed in chapter 20. Preexercise food can also influence exercise heart rate (Bird and Hay 1987) and the MAF test. It may be possible with the use of a heart rate monitor to determine in a specific individual which foods can improve and which can hinder performance. These issues are discussed in chapter 18.

Finally, a variety of health problems will worsen the MAF test results. These include fever, cold and flu, allergies, and anemia. More importantly, a MAF test that is unexpectedly poor may be an indicator of an oncoming illness.

MAXIMUM AEROBIC FUNCTION TEST AND COMPETITION

A relationship is seen in competitive endurance runners between the MAF test results (first kilometer or mile) and competitive times for all road-race distances between 5 km (3.1 miles) and 10 km (6.2 miles), excluding cross-country races and road races on very uneven terrain. This relationship was observed after compilation of several hundred MAF times as compared to race results in healthy and fit runners over a five-year period. On the basis of these data, if a runner's MAF test is 8 min/mile, he or she would be expected to complete an average 5-km race in just over 20 min, averaging about 6 min 30 sec/mile. This relationship can be considered one between aerobic maximum function (i.e., 8 min/mile) and all-out effect or anaerobic maximum function (i.e., 6 min 30 sec/mile). Table 13.2 presents a compilation of times from healthy runners; first-mile MAF test times are compared with 5-km average mile times for road races.

If the expected results are not found in a patient, the possibility of a structural, chemical, or mental/emotional imbalance in the athlete should be considered. An example might be a runner whose MAF test is 9 min/mile and who runs a 5-km race in 19 min, averaging just over 6 min/mile. This MAF test

Table 13.2 Comparison of Average First-Mile Maximum Aerobic Function Test Times With 5-km Average Mile Times for Road Races in Healthy and Fit Athletes

MAF (minutes per mile, 1st mile)	5-km race pace (average mile time)	5-km time (total race time)
10:00	7:30	23:18
9:00	7:00	21:45
8:30	6:45	20:58
8:00	6:30	20:12
7:30	6:00	18:38
7:00	5:30	17:05
6:30	5:15	16:19
6:00	5:00	15:32
5:45	4:45	14:45
5:30	4:30	13:59
5:15	4:20	13:28
5:00	4:15	13:12

time of 9 min is expected to produce an average 5-km race time of about 21 min 45 sec, which averages to about 7 min/mile. Instead, the athlete averages nearly a minute faster than expected. While this may appear to be a positive result, it is at the expense of some significant stress. This imbalance is not an uncommon one; it often precedes a structural, chemical, or mental/emotional injury and represents a functional overtraining state. This state may signify excess sympathetic activity, often an early sign of overtraining (Fry and Kraemer 1997).

Likewise, a runner whose first-mile MAF test is 6 min 30 sec is expected to average 5 km in 16 min 19 sec. If the actual time is 18 min, it represents some imbalance. Perhaps the runner is undergoing some structural, chemical, or mental/emotional stress; a number of neuromuscular imbalances could cause the slower time, as could a metabolic problem disturbing energy production. Or perhaps the runner was not mentally capable of "pushing" his or her body to its maximum potential.

Data such as these have not been collected for other sports. But it can be expected that the same relationships exist in triathlons, cycling, swimming, and even sports such as tennis, basketball, hockey, and those that involve endurance. Improvements in performances almost always accompany improvement in the MAF test.

The MAF test can be used to measure any type of training program, and any submaximal heart rate can be used during training and for the MAF test. However, the author has developed a formula that helps individualize the heart rate for each patient for use during training and the MAF test.

THE 180-FORMULA

The author proposes a simplified, clinical method, referred to as the 180-formula, for determining a more effective individualized heart rate for use during assessment (such as the MAF test) and aerobic training. This replaces the commonly used 220-formulas. Heart rates obtained from the new formula are generally lower than those obtained with the formulas previously described in the literature. The predominant differences are that the older formulas are very general and that they are based on oxygen-consumption tables and estimated maximum heart rates, whereas the 180-formula is based on each individual's general health and fitness level as evidenced by clinical trials and RQ studies.

Changes in heart rate that accompany exercise intensity are not just related to O_2 uptake; heart rate changes also reflect coronary artery blood flow, autonomic nervous system function, hormonal function, individual muscle recruitment, and other factors including the mental/emotional state. For example, autonomic tone influences heart rate; sympathetic activity increases and parasympathetic activity diminishes heart rate (Guyton 1986). In various conditions of physiologic imbalance including adrenal dysfunction, carbohydrate intolerance, and overtraining, autonomic function can also become imbalanced as described throughout this text. These patients may have differences from normal subjects in their heart rate responses to exercise. For example, Cordero et al. (1996) demonstrated a subtle abnormality with reduced parasympathetic activity to the heart of patients with the chronic fatigue syndrome. Early stages of overtraining may be associated with increased sympathetic activity resulting in higher resting and training heart rates (Lehmann et al. 1997). Chronic overtraining, however, may result in excess parasympathetic function associated with lower resting and training heart rates (Stone et al. 1991). These variabilities must be considered with the use of any heart rate–based training program. They are also considered in the 180-formula because it is adjusted to each patient's state of health and fitness.

Using the 180-Formula to Calculate Heart Rate

The 180-formula is based on the theory that training allows aerobic progress while establishing or maintaining balance in all other systems of the body. As such, use of the formula not only is an effective training approach but also adds a therapeutic component to the patient's program.

180-Formula

1. Subtract the age from 180 (180 − age).
2. Modify this number by selecting among the following categories the one that best matches the patient's health and fitness profile:
   - If the patient has or is recovering from a major illness (heart disease, any operation, any hospital stay, etc.) or is on any regular medication (discussed later), subtract an additional 10.
   - If the patient has not exercised before, has been inconsistent with exercise, has been exercising with injury, has regressed in training or competition, gets more than two colds or bouts of flu per year, or has allergies, subtract an additional 5.
   - If the patient has been exercising regularly (at least four times weekly) for up to two years without any of the problems just mentioned, keep the number (180 − age) the same.
   - If the patient is a competitive athlete who has been training for more than two years without any of the problems listed and has made progress in competition without injury, add 5.

For example, if the patient is 30 years old and fits into the second category, we have the following:

180 − 30 = 150. Then 150 − 5 = 145 bpm.

If it is difficult to decide which of two groups the patient best fits into, choose the group or outcome that results in the lowest heart rate. In patients who are taking medication that may affect the heart rate, those who wear a pacemaker, or those who have special circumstances not discussed in this text, further individualization by the practitioner or specialist may be necessary.

The heart rate obtained with this formula is referred to as the maximum aerobic heart rate and is used for the MAF test described in this chapter and for training as described in chapters 21 and 22. This heart rate is usually lower, sometimes significantly lower, than when the traditional 220-formulas are used.

The 180-formula may need to be further individualized for people over the age of 65. For these patients, up to 10 beats may have to be added, depending on individual levels of health and fitness, according to the clinical judgment of the practitioner. For those 16 years of age and under, the formula is not applicable; rather, a heart rate of 165 bpm has been used by the author for this group. A lower heart rate based on the individual's health and fitness may occasionally be appropriate.

Once a maximum aerobic heart rate is found, a range from that number to 10 beats below that number should be used. For example, if an athlete's maximum aerobic heart rate is determined to be 155, that person's aerobic training zone would be 145 to 155 bpm. For the MAF test, the maximum aerobic heart rate is usually applied.

THE TRADITIONAL 220-FORMULA

The traditional 220-formula relies on two very general indicators: an estimated maximum heart rate and training at a specified percentage of that number based on very subjective evidence. The maximum heart rate is estimated traditionally by subtracting the individual's age from 220. However, this estimation of an individual's maximum heart rate can vary considerably, and is referred to by McArdle et al. (1991) as "a rough approximation." Wilmore and Costill (1994) state that only 68% of 40-year-olds have actual maximum heart rates between 168 and 192; the 220-formula would imply that a 40-year-old should have a maximum heart rate of 180 bpm. The author has observed that only about 35% of individuals fit this equation. The individual variations seen may be due to age, resting heart rate, body weight, and even smoking status (Whaley et al. 1992). Miller et al. (1993) hold that when one is calculating exercise heart rates for obese patients, 200 − 0.5 × age is more appropriate for maximum heart rate estimation than the traditional formula. Individualizing training heart rates using only chronological age may not be the best approach, as a patient's physiological age may be more of a consideration.

After the chronological age is subtracted from 220, this number is multiplied by either a percentage of VO_2max or a percentage of estimated maximum heart rate. This percentage ranges from 65% to 85%. These two percentage levels are very different, and patients sometimes interchange them.

The percentage most athletes choose is the higher option rather than a lower one. When deciding to calculate a training heart rate, many athletes use 85% most often, followed by 80%. Some may use 75%, with few using 70% or 65%. The reason may be that most athletes feel the need to train with more intensity to obtain benefits—the "more is better" attitude.

If both the 220- and 180-formulas were applied to the same individual (a 36-year-old male who has a chronic injury and shows reduced performance), the 220-formula would give 156 bpm and the 180-formula 139 bpm. A level of 85% of maximum heart rate is used (75% VO_2max) for the 220-formula since this level correlates with the upper limit for sustained power output and is a level for which ventilation, acid-base balance, and blood lactate can be stabilized (Gaesser and Wilson 1988).

220-Formula

220 − 36 = 184. Then 184 × 85% = 156 bpm.

180-Formula

180 − 36 = 144. Then subtract an additional 5 beats:
144 − 5 = 139 bpm.

Other Versions of the 220-Formula

The Karvonen method (Karvonen et al. 1957) is another version of the 220-formula and considers the maximum heart rate reserve, which is the difference between the maximum and the resting heart rate. The results of this method correlate with VO_2max but may not be appropriate for all athletes. Goldberg et al. (1988) found through the use of ventilatory threshold that individuals of average fitness, and those of low fitness levels (i.e., those beginning an exercise program), did not match formulas derived from the Karvonen method.

Still other methods of finding a training heart rate include correlation to perceived exertion, which uses the Borg scale, and the metabolic equivalent (MET) system. However, these are based on subjective feelings of the patient and on estimates. They are more easily influenced than other formulas by structural, chemical, and mental/emotional factors (especially when one is training with others) and may not be sufficiently precise and objective.

Karvonen and Vuorimaa (1988) state that an individual's training heart rate is best determined in the laboratory through measurement of O_2 uptake and lactic acid concentration. While this approach may be useful, these assessments are not practical for most practitioners and patients.

TRAINING RELATIONSHIPS AND THE 180-FORMULA

Leaf and Allen (1988) demonstrated important relationships between RQ and training levels. The 180-formula was developed in part from RQ tests performed on trained and untrained individuals; it takes into account the patient's overall health and fitness and is outcome oriented. Finding an effective heart rate will enable the athlete to progress (in terms of the MAF test and other long-term training and performance outcomes) and avoid overtraining even when that same heart rate is used for long periods of time. While the 220-formula approaches can result in initial and short-term improvements in O_2 uptake and other measurable factors, long-term effects are not always positive and are often typical of the overtraining syndrome. In research, improvements that are measured only by short-term performance changes can be misleading.

It is important to note that athletes using the 180-formula for the first time usually find the new training intensity too easy. This may be the case because many athletes are training at such high intensities or are overtraining. In time, however, as their aerobic system improves and pace or speed increases with the same heart rate, they no longer complain that workouts feel too easy. In many cases, the required effort increases and becomes more difficult to maintain. Details about this therapeutic and training approach are provided in chapters 21 and 22.

The recommendation is to continue to use the same maximum aerobic heart rate for the MAF test and aerobic training for about three to five years if health and fitness continue to progress. At this time,

Case History

John's running ability had improved during the past year, but his list of symptoms had grown, too: the onset of hip pain, worsening of allergies, colds every five to six weeks, and gastrointestinal bloating. His family medical doctor ruled out serious problems and offered medication to ease some of the symptoms, which John elected not to take. Then he was assessed with a heart rate monitor, and his training heart rate at his normal training level averaged about 168 bpm. For a 28-year-old athlete with the problems listed, the training heart rate range should be between 137 and 147 bpm. John's MAF test at 147 was almost 8 min/mile. With the proper care and lifestyle changes, after about 15 months, John improved his 10-km race time by a full minute (to under 33 min), performed his MAF test in 6 min 25 sec, and had no hip pain, allergies, colds, or gastrointestinal stress.

the training rate should be decreased by about 3 beats. At this stage, the training heart rate may not necessarily match the 180-formula, since the athlete is in better overall health and fitness. Thus, use of this formula is most beneficial at the start of a program. However, if training progress is halted, the reason could be that the individual's training heart rate is too high, sometimes because the 180-formula was not calculated properly. It is important to be honest and objective in determining the maximum aerobic heart rate using this formula.

CONCLUSION

Heart rate monitors, devices that accurately provide the athlete with a continual measurement of heart rate, can be used for assessment. By comparing the time over a constant distance and the heart rate, using the MAF test, both practitioner and athlete can plot training progress; doing so makes prevention of training regression possible.

Heart rate monitors are also useful for regulating the intensity of training and for helping the athlete avoid overtraining, thereby preventing structural, chemical, and mental/emotional injuries. Specifically, these devices are important in building the aerobic system during training, helping athletes reach their potential.

14

Treatment of Muscle and Neurological Dysfunction

Trauma is a very obvious and common problem in sport. It includes not only the hits taken during contact events, but also the more subtle shock of microtrauma that evolves over an extended period of time. In many sports including football, basketball, soccer, squash, track and field, and gymnastics, almost half the injuries are muscular (Safran et al. 1988). Muscle injuries usually occur at the origin and insertion at the musculotendinous junction, with fewer injuries occurring in the muscle belly. Complementary sports medicine uses a method referred to as Golgi tendon organ/spindle cell therapy; in applied kinesiology, this is referred to as origin and insertion therapy. Golgi tendon organ/spindle cell therapy is most valuable for conditions of muscle inhibition or overfacilitation brought about by micro- or macrotrauma.

GOLGI TENDON ORGAN/ SPINDLE CELL THERAPY

A significant number of physical injuries in athletes occur at the musculotendinous junction or at the muscle's origin or insertion, with some injury also occurring in the muscle belly. Such injuries have a high incidence of recurrence (Safran et al. 1989). Much less injury occurs in the tendon. Such trauma to the muscle, theoretically, may cause dysfunction of either the Golgi tendon organ (GTO) or the spindle cell, or sometimes both. This trauma may be the result of competition, overtraining, or the onset of new training. Golgi tendon organ/spindle cell therapy helps restore normal function to these neuromuscular components. This problem may also account for delayed-onset muscle soreness.

Recall that the GTOs and spindle cells respond to specific pressure, with the result of either facilitating or inhibiting the muscle. Either of these actions can be reproduced by the practitioner at will when the muscle is stimulated in a precise way. Stimulating the GTOs or spindle cells with physical pressure in one direction creates facilitation; stimulating in the opposite way creates inhibition. Also, recall that skeletal muscles have a rebound-type action when pressed, so that when a certain action is desired, the muscle is pushed in the opposite direction. This process is described further on.

One assesses the need for GTO/spindle cell therapy through a history, although sometimes this is difficult especially in cases of microtrauma, where the problem is not so obvious. Therapy localization to the origin, insertion, or the muscle belly may be the most useful assessment tool.

Golgi Tendon Organ/Spindle Cell Therapy (General Procedure)

1. The muscle in question is tested to determine whether it is inhibited.
2. The GTO/spindle cell therapy is applied as indicated to an inhibited muscle.
3. The muscle is retested to ensure that the therapy was successful.
4. The muscle is put through a normal range of motion or weight bearing; it is then retested to ensure that the therapy will be maintained.

Sometimes a muscle requires more than one therapy. In performing step 4, practitioners may find that the muscle tests normal as in step 3 but that when the patient attempts normal function (such as walking, in the case of the quadriceps, or moving the shoulder through a throwing motion, in the case of a pectoralis major clavicular [PMC]), the muscle returns to its previously inhibited state. This usually indicates a need for other types of therapy, such as acupuncture, stimulation of Chapman's reflexes, or other methods described later in this chapter. In some cases, having athletes actually utilize the muscle as they normally would in their sport and then retesting is an ideal approach. For example, in a baseball player with an inhibited PMC requiring GTO/spindle cell therapy, after correction, one would further test the muscle by having the patient throw a ball several times and then retest the muscle. Also, note that it is not physically possible to contact the origin, insertion, or belly of every muscle. In these instances, using only one contact point may be sufficient.

The four possible uses of the GTO/spindle cell therapy are described next. The two most common uses are for muscle inhibition and are described first; two other methods are used to treat overfacilitated muscles or spasms.

Golgi Tendon Organ Therapy for Inhibition

1. The muscle is manually tested to ensure that it is inhibited.
2. The practitioner contacts the origin and insertion of the muscle with the fingers from each hand and pushes these areas toward each other (away from the attachment) six to eight times with moderate, deep pressure. If the attachment is more than a centimeter in width (such as the origin of the PMS), all areas of the attachment must be pushed (see figure 14.1).
3. The muscle is retested to ensure that it is now normal.
4. Range of motion or other stresses, if applicable, are applied; the muscle is then retested.

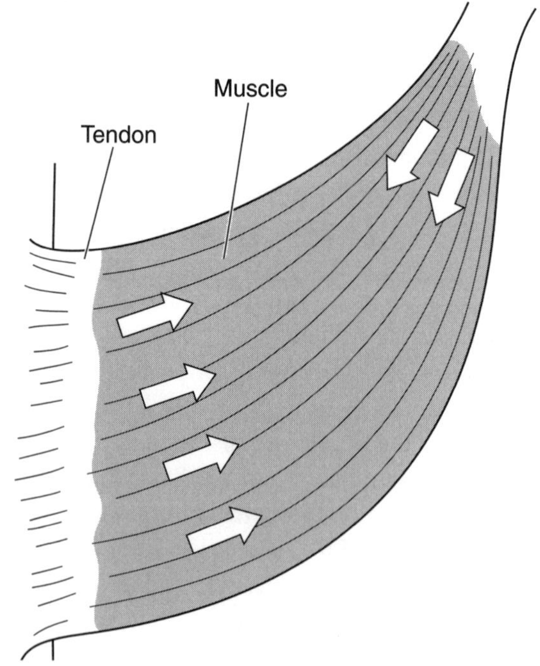

Figure 14.1 Treating an inhibited muscle to create facilitation (normalize) using Golgi tendon organs. The arrows indicate the direction of pressure.

Muscle Spindle Cell Therapy for Inhibition

1. The muscle is manually tested to ensure that it is inhibited.
2. The practitioner contacts the belly (center) of the muscle with fingers from each hand and pushes these areas away from each other along the muscle fibers six to eight times, with moderate, deep pressure. If the muscle belly is broad (such as that of the latissimus dorsi), all areas of the belly must be pushed (see figure 14.2).
3. The muscle is retested to ensure that it is now normal.
4. Range of motion or other stresses, if applicable, are used; the muscle is retested.

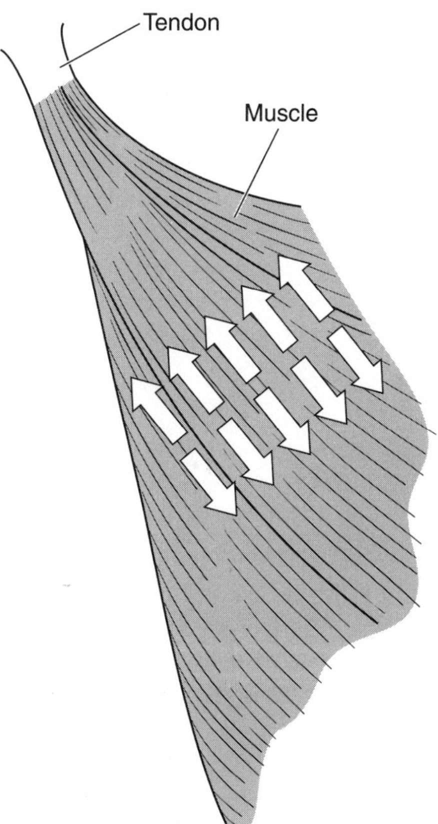

Figure 14.2 Treating an inhibited muscle to create facilitation (normalize) using muscle spindle cells. The arrows indicate the direction of pressure.

The methods described next are sometimes employed to treat overfacilitated muscles, or muscle spasms. This is the treatment of choice in most cases of temporomandibular (TMJ) dysfunction due to muscle dysfunction.

Golgi Tendon Organ Therapy for Overfacilitated Muscles or Muscle Spasms

1. The practitioner determines that the muscle is overfacilitated or in spasm (through muscle testing, range of motion, pain, or palpation).
2. The origin and insertion of the muscle are contacted with one or more fingers and pushed toward the muscle's attachments (i.e., away from each other) six to eight times with moderate, deep pressure (see figure 14.3).
3. If the attachment is more than a centimeter in width (such as the origin of the PMC), all areas of the attachment must be pushed.
4. The muscle is reevaluated to ensure that it functions normally.
5. Range of motion or other stresses, if applicable, are used; the muscle is retested.

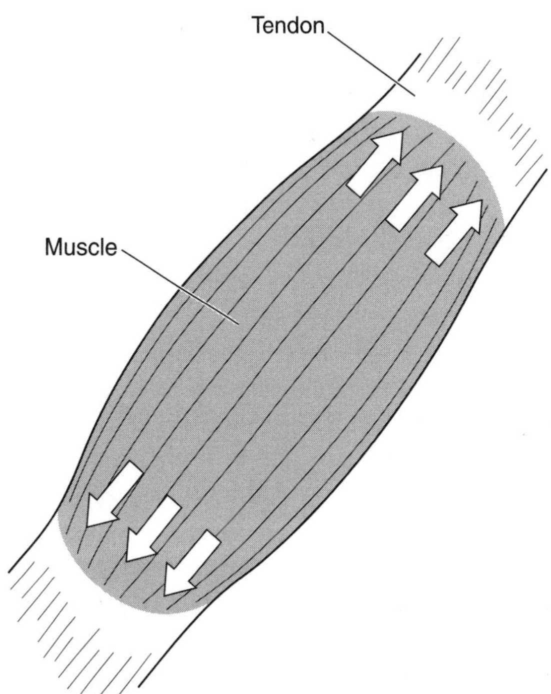

Figure 14.3 Treating an overfacilitated muscle (tightness or spasm) using the Golgi tendon organs. The arrows indicate the direction of pressure.

Muscle Spindle Cell Therapy for Overfacilitated Muscles or Muscle Spasms

1. The practitioner determines that the muscle is overfacilitated or in spasm.
2. The belly (center) of the muscle is contacted with two fingers (i.e., as if pinching), and these areas are pushed toward each other six to eight times with moderate, deep pressure. If the muscle belly is broad (such as that of the latissimus dorsi), all areas of it must be pushed (see figure 14.4).
3. The muscle is reevaluated to ensure that it is now normal.
4. Range of motion or other stresses, if applicable, are used; the muscle is retested.

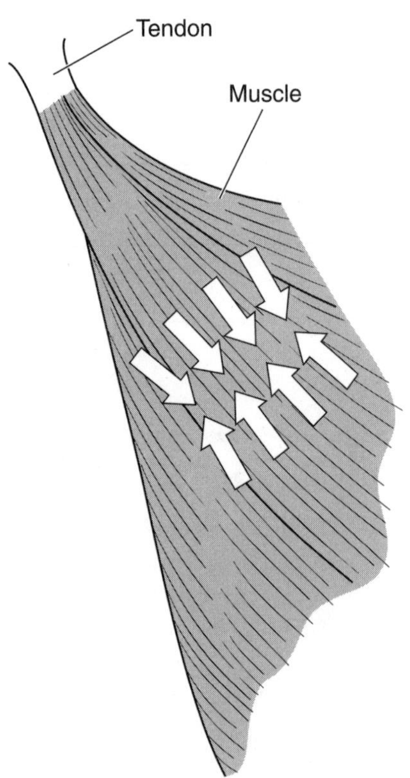

Figure 14.4 Treating an overfacilitated muscle (tightness or spasm) using muscle spindle cells. The arrows indicate the direction of pressure.

In some patients, an inhibited muscle requiring GTO/spindle cell therapy may be well compensated such that testing does not reveal the inhibition. In many of these cases, slightly stressing the muscle by having the patient put it through its range of motion will often enable the practitioner to observe the inhibition. For example, in a patient who complains of calf and ankle problems, it is common to find an inhibited tibialis posterior muscle that requires GTO/spindle cell therapy. However, initially testing the muscle sometimes reveals normal function. The patient then puts the tibialis posterior muscle through its range of motion (plantar flexion and inversion), repeating the action approximately 10 times. The practitioner immediately retests the muscle and may now find that it is inhibited. (Like any challenge, this inhibition may last for only 30 sec until the body compensates.) In any muscle, if testing does not reveal inhibition and the practitioner feels the problem may exist but is well compensated, having the patient move the muscle through its normal range of motion several times will frequently reveal the inhibition.

It is also possible to specifically determine which precise areas of each muscle require therapy. For example, one uses therapy localization on the GTOs and spindle cells of a muscle that requires GTO/spindle cell therapy. The precise location of therapy can be determined using this approach.

TEMPOROMANDIBULAR JOINT DYSFUNCTION

Golgi tendon organ/spindle cell therapy may be effective for treatment of neuromuscular dysfunction of the jaw muscles. Temporomandibular joint dysfunction is a common problem. An associated problem is the lack of symptoms that come from the jaw itself. More often, the dysfunction is an asymptomatic primary problem causing other, secondary imbalances. The use of applied kinesiology methods, especially therapy localization, greatly assists the practitioner in finding concealed or hidden TMJ problems.

The TMJ is part of a complex system including the bones of the skull and cervical spine, the mandible and hyoid bone, the related muscle attachments and other soft tissues, and neurologic and vascular components. This complex is often referred to as the stomatognathic system (Walther 1983). Any dysfunction in this system can have adverse effects throughout the body. For example, Westling (1992) showed that patients with TMJ dysfunction had more musculoskeletal problems than controls, as well as significantly more systemic hypermobile joints—which was more important as an etiology for TMJ dysfunction than bruxism (grinding of the teeth). Still other conclusions of Westling were a positive relationship between TMJ dysfunction and insufficient mitral valve function and a positive relationship between TMJ patients and lower values of total collagen. Ishii (1990) showed significant relationships between imbalance of stomatognathic function and the center of gravity of the upright posture; Aragao (1991) found the same in children—an important relationship between the stomatognathic system and whole-body posture. According to de Wijer et al. (1996), TMJ problems caused by muscle dysfunction should not be considered only a local disorder of the stomatognathic system; rather the whole area including the shoulder girdle should be considered during assessment and treatment.

While many patients with TMJ problems do not have localized pain, they sometimes report various sounds coming from their jaw joint. Wabeke and Spruijt (1993) concluded that TMJ sounds are a fairly common sign associated with mild deviations in certain morphologic and functional aspects of the stomatognathic system. Other information obtained from a history is very helpful, especially regarding bruxism—the grinding of teeth, usually at night. Many patients are unaware of this activity but are told of it by a spouse. Sometimes the patient's dentist observes excess wear on the biting surface of the teeth that indicates bruxism.

Two steps are required to assess TMJ dysfunction. The first is to determine whether there is a problem and which joint requires treatment. If the patient has an inhibited muscle (anywhere in the body) and therapy-localizes the TMJ by lightly touching the joint, normalization of the muscle indicates the need to treat that joint. (A normally functioning muscle is not useful for therapy-localizing the TMJ in this part of the assessment, but useful in other aspects of TMJ assessment described below.)

The next step is to diagnose the type of TMJ problem, specifically to determine which muscles are not functioning properly. These may be the muscles that close the jaw, predominantly the masseter and temporalis (and to a lesser extent the internal pterygoid and buccinator); this is referred to as a closed TMJ problem. This is a more common problem than dysfunction of the muscle that opens the jaw, usually the external pterygoid muscles, which is referred to as an open TMJ problem. In most cases of TMJ dysfunction due to muscle imbalance, either the jaw openers or closers are overfacilitated.

Differentiating between a closed and an open TMJ problem is accomplished by therapy-localizing the TMJ in a closed and open position using a normal muscle, such as the psoas. While the patient therapy-localizes the TMJ, the patient clenches the jaw to contract the masseter and temporalis (and internal pterygoid and buccinator) muscles, and the psoas is tested again. If the psoas becomes inhibited, the practitioner assumes that the jaw-closing muscles are overfacilitated. If this test is normal, the patient opens the jaw wide and the psoas muscle is tested. If this causes psoas inhibition, the problem is assumed to be with the jaw-opening muscles.

Assessment of Temporomandibular Joint Dysfunction

In patients who have TMJ dysfunction, it is important to determine two important clinical facts: which TMJ (left or right) is not functioning, and which group of muscles—the jaw openers or closers—is not functioning. We look next at an example of this process.

Temporomandibular Joint Dysfunction Assessment

1. An inhibited muscle normalizes while the patient therapy-localizes the right TMJ. This assumes a right TMJ dysfunction.
2. Using a normally functioning muscle, such as the psoas, the patient therapy-localizes the right TMJ.
3. The patient clenches the teeth and the muscle is retested.
4. If this creates muscle inhibition, the dysfunction is a closed TMJ problem, and the masseter and temporalis (and internal pterygoid and buccinator) may be overfacilitated.
5. If step 4 is negative, the patient opens the jaw wide and the psoas (or whichever normal muscle was tested in step 2) is retested.
6. If this creates muscle inhibition, the dysfunction is an open TMJ problem, and the external pterygoid may be overfacilitated.

Treatment of both opened and closed TMJ problems includes the use of GTO/spindle cell therapy to normalize the overfacilitated muscles. In addition, trigger points are frequently encountered in these muscles, especially in the masseter and temporalis.

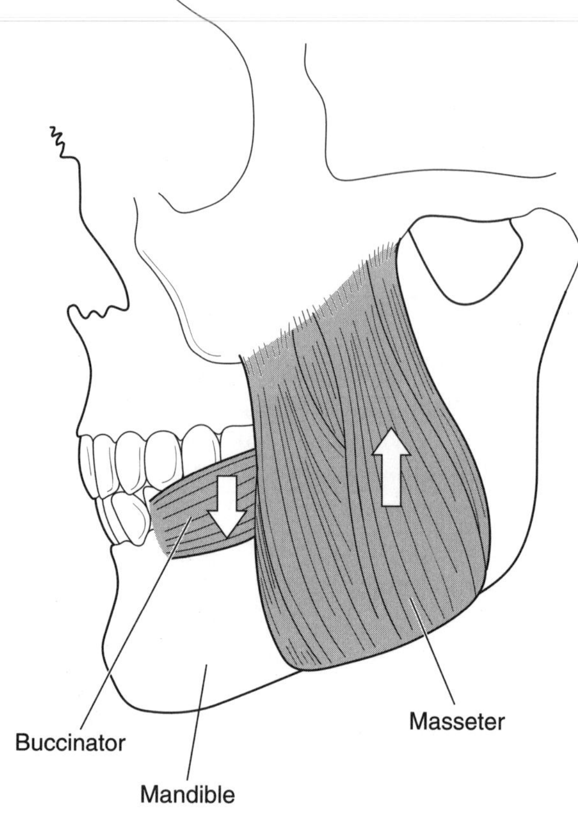

Figure 14.5 Treatment of buccinator and masseter concurrently. The arrows indicate the direction of pressure.

Treatment of a Closed Temporomandibular Joint Problem

Treatment for a closed TMJ problem involves the methods just described: treatment of the overfacilitated muscles using both the GTOs and spindle cells. The masseter and temporalis (and sometimes the internal pterygoid and buccinator) are frequently all part of a closed TMJ problem. Each muscle's GTOs and spindle cells are treated. Goodheart (1976) first described treating the buccinator and masseter at the same time (see figure 14.5). Whichever approach is used, the TMJ should be retested as in steps 1-5 to ensure that the problem has been corrected.

Treatment of an Open Temporomandibular Joint Problem

Palpation of the external pterygoid muscle may appear to be a very difficult task. However, if the muscle has been palpated, very little stimulation on the muscle is required to correct this muscle and the associated open TMJ problem.

The best way to learn how to find the external pterygoid is first to palpate your own muscle. With an index finger, follow the line of the outside upper teeth and continue posterior until soft tissue is palpated (to the external pterygoid plate). Opening the jaw wide to feel the contraction of the muscle ensures that the proper muscle is being palpated (see figure 14.6). Note that in cases of TMJ dysfunction, this muscle is usually very tender on palpation. Treatment consists of pressure on the muscle for 2 to 3 sec, which should be applied according to the patient's tolerance. (It is not unusual to stimulate tear duct activity via a reflex mechanism, with

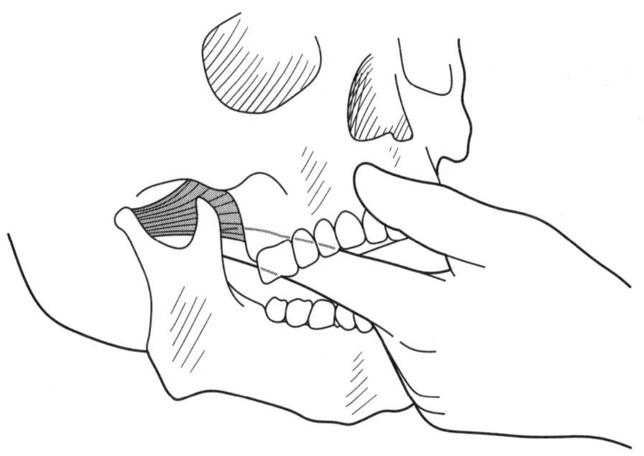

Figure 14.6 View of the external pterygoid muscle.

the patient producing some tearing.) It is difficult to say what aspects of the muscle are being stimulated (i.e., GTOs, trigger points), but the most clinically effective approach is to locate the muscle and apply pressure into it as best as possible. If the treatment was successful, the reassessment will be negative.

It is obvious that certain sports produce higher numbers of dental injuries than others (Lee-Knight et al. 1992). These problems can have an adverse effect on the function of the stomatognathic system. Salonen et al. (1993) showed that persons wearing poorly fitting dentures had dysfunction of the cervical spine. The work of Westrum (Westrum and Canfield 1977; Johnson and Westrum 1980; Westrum et al. 1980, 1984) showed that each individual tooth has specific projections to the brain and can influence the nervous system during normal eruption and tooth loss. This research showed that the neurological distribution from the teeth indicated a wider central representation than had been previously reported. Clinically, Walther (1988) discussed the relationships developed in applied kinesiology between individual teeth and related muscles throughout the body. For this reason, it is vital to include a complete history of any previous dental trauma and other pertinent dental history during the initial exam and on follow-up visits.

MYOFASCIAL TRIGGER POINTS

Most practitioners are familiar with myofascial trigger points. Borg-Stein and Stein (1996) describe trigger points as areas in muscles, tendons, bursae, or fat pads that are painful to palpation, characterized by the presence of taut bands, and refer pain on pressure. According to Hong (1996), trigger points may be activated by acute or chronic injury to a muscle, tendon, ligament, joint, disc, or nerve.

Gerwin (1997) states, "Treatment is directed toward inactivating the myofascial trigger point, correcting underlying perpetuating factors, and restoring the normal relationships between the muscles of the affected functional motor units" (p. 130). These three elements are the basis for the therapeutic aspect of trigger-point therapy and are critical for both practitioner and patient: correcting the local trigger point, finding and correcting related factors that may have contributed to the problem, and correcting the neuromuscular dysfunction associated with the problem. Gerwin (1994) makes an important comment: "The clinical phenomenon of the [trigger point] is accessible to any clinician who takes the time to learn to palpate skeletal muscle gently and carefully, and who is willing to learn the functional anatomy necessary to understand the regional spread of [trigger points] through functional muscle units" (p. 747). For more detailed information on the clinical aspects of trigger points, the reader is referred to Travell and Simons (1983).

The two most popular treatment approaches include pressure on the trigger point and cooling of the area, usually with a gentle stretch to the muscle (referred to as "spray and stretch"). Pressure directly on the trigger point, held for a prolonged period (up to 2 min if necessary, or occasionally more), is an effective treatment for most trigger points. This is accomplished with the practitioner's thumb or a blunt instrument designed for muscle therapy. This pressure will typically produce a referred pain and should be exerted to the patient's tolerance. Cold is best applied with a spray, such as Fluori-Methane. The muscle, and frequently the area of pain, are quickly sprayed; they are then gently stretched until an increased range of motion is obtained.

Therapy localization can also make trigger points easier to find.

ASSESSMENT AND TREATMENT OF NEUROLOGIC DYSFUNCTION

Two general types of neuromuscular dysfunction may be observed in patients. We have already considered the first type, typically an abnormal inhibition of a muscle that may be corrected with various methods, including stimulation of acupuncture points or Chapman's reflexes and GTO/spindle cell therapy. The other general dysfunction observed in patients is the neurologic type, which may involve improper signals sent to the muscles. If a patient is tested in a walking gait position as if taking a step forward with the left leg and with the right shoulder flexed, the left PMC and the right latissimus should be inhibited. But testing of both these muscles may show that they are both facilitated while the right PMC and left latissimus are inhibited; this pattern or any other unexpected result is not normal. The problem is usually one of neurological disorganization as described by Walther (1988). Neurological disorganization is a functional problem in the neuromuscular system that results in specific patterns of abnormal muscle function. For example, in a normal walking or running gait pattern, when the arm is flexed, the PMC muscle is facilitated and the latissimus dorsi is inhibited. In the patient with neurological disorganization, the same gait results in an abnormally inhibited PMC muscle and an abnormally facilitated latissimus dorsi. It is a problem that has obvious disadvantages for those who are active, especially in competitive circumstances, for several reasons: it can predispose the person to injury, it can be a direct cause of an injury, it can prevent an injury from being corrected even when the proper therapy is applied, and it may cause a continual recurrence of another injury or imbalance.

The possibility of neurological disorganization also should be considered when other muscle testing results are unlikely or not logical. It is unlikely, for example, for the aerobic and anaerobic challenges described in chapter 12 to show a pattern of aerobic deficiency and anaerobic deficiency. It is also unlikely, in a patient who has an elevated right shoulder and an inhibited left latissimus dorsi, for the right latissimus dorsi to be normal. Correcting neurological disorganization will immediately result in a change in these improbable patterns. After correction, for example, the patient's right latissimus dorsi will test as inhibited, as expected, and the left one will test normal.

Since neurological disorganization occurs in a high percentage of patients, many practitioners routinely treat the reflexes associated with this problem. However, it is best to know when the problem of neurological disorganization exists and to record this observation in the patient's records. Sometimes certain exercise and lifestyle factors can cause a recurrence of neurological disorganization: poor swimming mechanics, improper footwear, and possibly even the traditional "jumping jacks."

The correction of neurological disorganization entails a variety of possible treatments. The three most common corrections for neurological disorganization are the following:

- Treatment of acupuncture points KI 27 (bilaterally) and CV 8
- Treatment of the gait reflexes
- Correction of improperly functioning labyrinthine reflexes

KI 27 and CV 8

The two most effective acupuncture points for the treatment of neurological disorganization are KI 27 and CV 8. KI 27 points are the end points of the kidney meridian, and each one is located in an indentation at the junction of the clavicle, first rib, and sternum. CV 8 is a single point found in the umbilicus. These three points can be successfully stimulated with finger pressure. In this situation, the

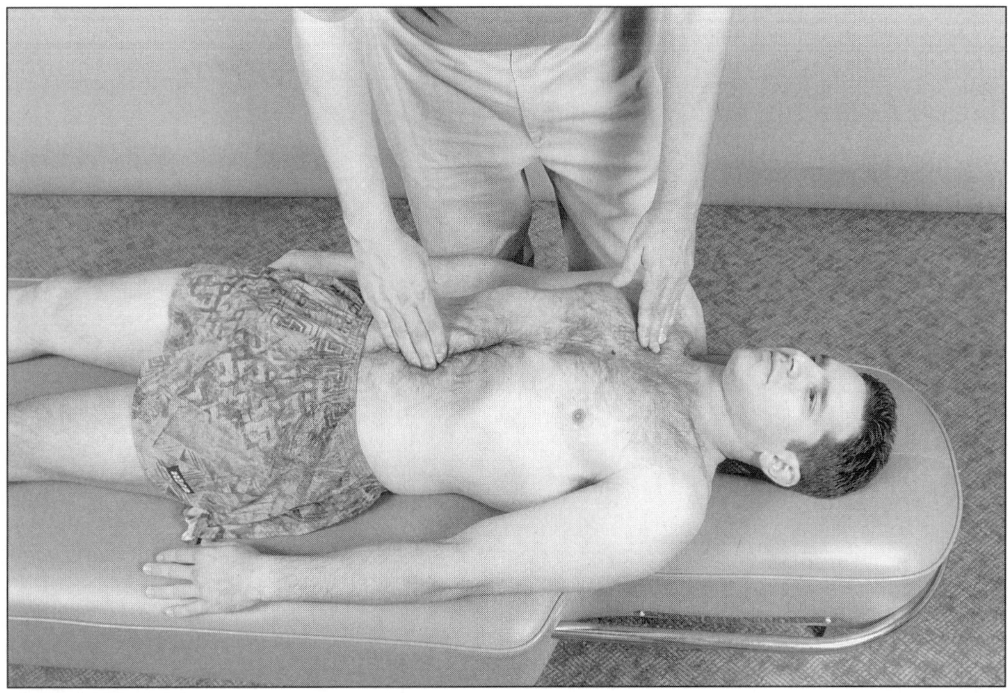

Figure 14.7 A practitioner treating KI 27 and CV 8.

practitioner stimulates one KI 27 point and the CV 8 point simultaneously by applying moderate pressure for approximately 10 sec (see figure 14.7), then contacts the other KI 27 point and stimulates it for the same amount of time while maintaining the stimulation on CV 8.

Gait Reflexes

A group of acupuncture points on the foot collectively referred to as gait reflexes may also require stimulation to correct neurological disorganization. As the name implies, these points are related to the gait—specifically, the neuromuscular activity that occurs during gait. Recall that specific reflexes are related to specific muscles (i.e., acupuncture points, Chapman's reflexes). In this discussion, a specific acupuncture point will be linked to a pair of muscles or to muscle groups that function during gait. During normal gait activity, the following muscles or muscle groups and their specific acupuncture point relationships are as follows:

- Muscles that extend the shoulder and contralateral hip/SP 3—medial side of foot just proximal to first metatarsal head
- Muscles that flex the shoulder and contralateral hip/LV 2—dorsum of foot where the skin joins the first two toes
- Muscles that abduct the shoulder and contralateral hip/ST 44—lateral to LV 2 between first two tendons of extensor digitorum longus
- Muscles that abduct the gluteus medius and flex the contralateral abdominals/GB 42—just proximal to fifth toe between extensor digitorum longus tendons
- Muscles that adduct the shoulder and contralateral hip/BL 65—lateral aspect of foot proximal to the fifth metatarsal head
- Muscles that flex the psoas major and contralateral pectoralis major sternal/KI 1—plantar aspect of foot between second and third metatarsal bones

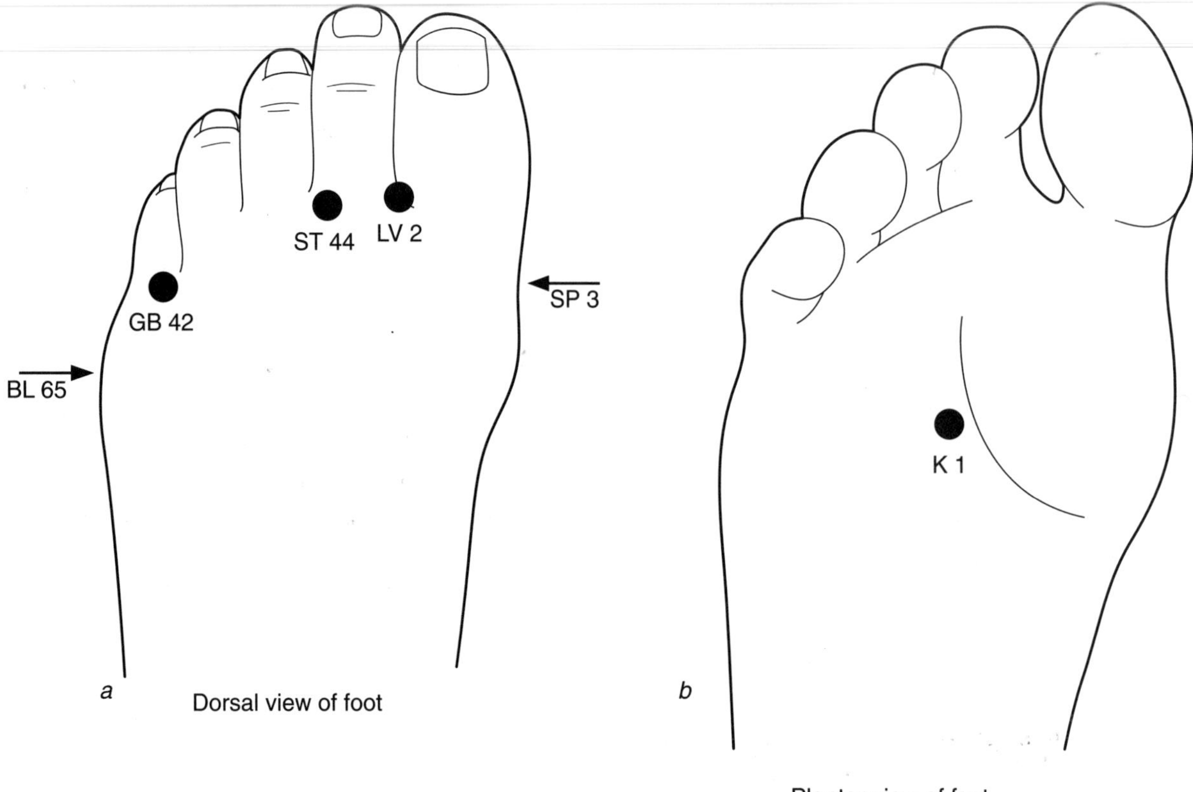

Figure 14.8a–b Gait reflexes (acupuncture points) on the foot: (*a*) dorsum of foot; (*b*) plantar view.

Figure 14.8a–b shows the locations of these acupuncture points.

There are three ways to assess the need to treat gait reflexes. First, each point can be therapy-localized separately. If positive, the point is treated and reevaluated. Second, the muscle groups associated with each point can be manually tested, but each one needs to be tested at the same time. Testing two muscles or muscle groups at the same time is somewhat cumbersome but usually not too difficult in athletes. Except for the psoas muscle and contralateral pectoralis major sternal, these are general manual muscle tests. Abnormal muscle inhibition is found when these muscle groups are tested together but each muscle tested separately functions normally. It is important to first test the muscle groups separately to ensure that there is no individual inhibition (if this is the case, it is corrected as discussed previously). Testing the gluteus medius and contralateral abdominals is best done with the patient holding a partial "sit-up" position, which suffices for the abdominal test while testing the gluteus medius in the supine position. The third and simplest approach in the assessment of gait reflexes is to test the patient in the standing position while mechanically stressing the gait reflexes. This can be done by placing the foot in a particular gait position as described below.

Assessment of Gait Reflexes

1. With the patient standing in a neutral position (feet together and flat on the ground), a PMC is tested to ensure that it is normal.
2. The patient positions the contralateral foot by slightly flexing the knee and lifting the heel while keeping the toes on the ground and maintaining some weight bearing through the front of the feet where the gait reflexes are located.
3. The PMC is retested. If it becomes inhibited, the inhibition may be due to the need to stimulate some or all of the gait reflexes.

4. After treatment, a retest (steps 1-3) is performed to ensure correction.

Labyrinthine Reflexes

In chapter 9, we considered the importance of the labyrinthine reflexes in relation to posture and gait. In the normal function of labyrinthine reflexes, certain types of muscle inhibition should never occur in specific postures. For example, the latissimus dorsi has significant extensor muscle activity. When abnormally inhibited, this state should make itself evident in all positions except when the head is facing upward, such as when the patient is supine, since this position (face up) normally causes extensor facilitation. The following list is a review of the normal facilitation and inhibition during specific head positions.

Head facing down (prone position)	All flexors facilitated
Head facing up (supine position)	All extensors facilitated
Head sideways with the right ear down	Right extensors and left flexors facilitated Left extensors and right flexors inhibited
Head sideways with the left ear down	Left extensors and right flexors facilitated Right extensors and left flexors inhibited

If an abnormally inhibited latissimus dorsi remains in that state when the patient is supine, this usually indicates neurological dysfunction. Likewise, if a flexor, such as the PMC, is found to be abnormally inhibited when the patient is in the prone position, or when the head is facing down, neurological dysfunction is the usual indication.

Correction of the problem begins with finding which of three potential Chapman's reflexes requires stimulation:

- Teres minor muscle (anterior—second and third intercostal space approximately one centimeter from the sternum; posterior—laminae of T2 and 3)
- Sartorius muscle (anterior—approximately 2.5 cm lateral and 5 cm superior to the umbilicus; posterior—laminae of T11)
- Gluteus medius muscle (anterior—lateral pubic bone areas; posterior—transverse process of L5 vertebra).

The next step is to use therapy localization or stimulate one reflex at a time and retest the related dysfunctional muscle. The potential reflexes should be found on the ipsilateral side of muscle dysfunction.

CONCLUSION

Treatment of muscle inhibition is often relatively easy once the assessment of dysfunction is made through manual muscle testing. The use of related acupuncture point(s), Chapman's reflexes, or both is a common requirement. In cases of trauma, including microtrauma, treatment of the local muscle components is often necessary to restore function immediately. This may be with either GTO or spindle cell therapy, and sometimes both. Throughout the assessment process, it is important to ensure that the patient does not have a neurological disorganization, which can distort the testing process and make assessment difficult. If this is the case, the neurological disorganization should be treated first.

Treatment of Cranial and Pelvic Dysfunction

This chapter addresses cranial and pelvic dysfunction and treatments of these problems using conservative methods. The dysfunction of the cranium and pelvis is often referred to as a "fault." Cranial and pelvic faults are usually primary problems, and their correction can have a significant impact on other, secondary problems. Cranial and pelvic dysfunction can also have a significant negative impact in all types of patients involved in sport, and correction of this type of dysfunction can offer dramatic relief for many types of problems. The types of imbalances described in this chapter are commonly seen in a complementary sports medicine practice.

CRANIAL DYSFUNCTION

As described in chapter 3, cranial-sacral therapy was first introduced in modern times by William Garner Sutherland, DO, as a subspecialty of osteopathic manipulative medicine. Cranial-sacral therapy focuses on the movements of the cranial bones and their relationship with the sacrum. Assessment and therapeutic aspects of this cranial-sacral mechanism were expanded upon by others as they were shown clinically to have a significant effect on the physical, chemical, and mental status of the patient (DeJarnette 1981; Upledger and Vredevoogd 1983; Upledger 1987; Walther 1988). Cranial dysfunction is typically reflected in any muscle imbalance in the body rather than as cranial pain. This can have obvious adverse effects on training efficiency and sport performance. In addition, cranial-sacral function has a close relationship to the diaphragmatic breathing mechanism, also a key factor in all athletic activity.

The most important aspect of cranial-sacral therapy is assessing the need to make a specific correction. Unfortunately, many practitioners apply cranial-sacral therapy without assessing the need for it. Proper assessment and therapy are best accomplished by muscle testing; a normal or inhibited muscle, anywhere in the body, can be used, since cranial dysfunction can affect all areas of the body.

Cranial faults are frequently primary problems, with muscle inhibition, acupuncture imbalances, and spinal problems developing secondarily. The most common cranial problem, and the easiest one to assess and correct, is the cranial-sacral respiratory fault.

CRANIAL-SACRAL RESPIRATORY FAULTS

There are two very common types of cranial-sacral respiratory faults that correspond to the movement of the cranial bones during diaphragmatic breathing: the inspiration-assisted fault (IAF) and the expiration-assisted fault (EAF). They are named by the phase of respiration—inhalation or exhalation—used to assist in their correction.

These types of cranial-sacral respiratory faults, as is the case with most cranial faults, can be either unilateral or bilateral. The fault will correspond to muscle inhibition on the same side of the body; a cranial respiratory fault on the right will correspond to a muscle inhibition on the right.

A cranial-sacral respiratory fault is one in which, hypothetically, the cranial bones and sacrum do not move through their normal range of motion during respiration. The mastoid processes of the temporal bone, for example, are thought to move posterior on inspiration and anterior on expiration. This is only part of the whole cranial movement with respiration, as all the bones move in a specific direction with inspiration and expiration. The apex of the sacrum also moves anterior on inspiration and posterior on expiration, rotating around a fulcrum at or about the second sacral segment (i.e., the sacral base moves anterior on expiration). Cranial-sacral respiratory faults may have a variety of consequences, but one measurable one is muscle dysfunction. Any inhibited muscle may be dysfunctional because of a cranial-sacral respiratory fault. If this is the case, the inhibited muscle will become facilitated, or normal, when the patient either inhales or exhales deeply. For example, if the pectoralis major clavicular (PMC) is inhibited, the practitioner asks the patient to take a deep breath in and hold the breath, and then retests the PMC. If the PMC is now normal, this is an indication of a cranial-sacral IAF. The correction, as described further on, will be made during inspiration.

If the PMC continues to be inhibited after inhalation, the problem may be an EAF. For example, if the PMC is inhibited and the patient exhales completely, normalizing the PMC, the problem is an EAF. The correction will be made on expiration.

Assessment of Cranial-Sacral Respiratory Faults With Muscle Inhibition

1. The patient has an inhibited right PMC.
2. The patient breathes in deeply and maintains inhalation.
3. The PMC is retested.
4. If the PMC becomes facilitated, the patient has an IAF on the right.
5. If the PMC remains inhibited, the patient does not have an IAF on the right.
6. The patient then fully exhales and maintains exhalation.
7. If the PMC is facilitated, the patient has an EAF on the right.
8. If the PMC has not changed and is still inhibited, the patient does not have an EAF on the right.

As an alternative to an inhibited muscle, a normal muscle can be used to assess respiratory faults. In this case, the opposite of what has just been described will occur. If the patient has a normal latissimus dorsi, he or she inhales deeply and maintains inhalation, and the latissimus dorsi is immediately tested. If there is an EAF, the muscle will become inhibited, or if the patient exhales deeply and maintains the breath and the latissimus dorsi becomes inhibited, the patient has an IAF.

Assessment of Cranial-Sacral Respiratory Faults With Normal Muscle Function

1. The patient has a normally functioning right latissimus dorsi.
2. The patient breathes in deeply and maintains inhalation.
3. The right latissimus dorsi is retested.
4. If the muscle is still normal, the patient does not have an EAF. In this case, the patient then fully exhales and maintains exhalation.

5. If the right latissimus dorsi is now inhibited, the patient has a right IAF.
6. If the muscle is still normal, the patient does not have a respiratory fault on the right.

An additional means of assessing these problems is to therapy-localize the mastoid process and sacrum. When a cranial-sacral respiratory fault exists, this therapy localization will be positive (a normal muscle will become inhibited), and either inspiration or expiration will negate the muscle inhibition. To correct the fault, the practitioner uses the phase of respiration that negated the inhibition.

Correction of an IAF, the more common problem of the two, is accomplished most easily with the patient prone (although any positions can be used). For correction of a bilateral IAF, the practitioner uses one hand for the cranium and one for the sacrum. On the cranium, the thumb and index finger are placed on the posterior aspect of the mastoid process, and the fingertips of the other hand are placed on the lower half of the sacrum. The correction is done while the patient inhales deeply; the mastoid process and the sacral apex are gently pushed anterior during inhalation. (The pressure applied is moderate but not uncomfortable for the patient.) The patient then exhales and the pressure is removed. This pressure is applied four to six times during full inhalation only, as the patient breathes in and out. The muscle(s) and respiratory phases originally used to assess the fault are retested to ensure that the problem has been corrected.

Occasionally, the pressure on the mastoid process and sacrum needs to be applied more than 6 times; some difficult cases require up to 15 times or more. This will be evident in the reassessment phase. For example, when the muscle originally used is retested, if it is still inhibited and still responds positively (i.e., normalizes or facilitates) to inhalation, this usually indicates the need for prolonged correction.

Correction of an Inspiration-Assisted Fault

1. The patient is prone with the practitioner's thumb and index finger on the posterior mastoid process and sacral apex.
2. The patient inhales deeply and the practitioner pushes the mastoid process and sacral apex anterior.
3. The patient exhales and at the same time the practitioner removes the force.
4. The patient inhales deeply again while the same pressure is applied to the mastoid process and sacrum.
5. This cycle is repeated four to six times.
6. The muscle or muscles used in the assessment process are retested.

Correction of an EAF is similar, although the cranium and sacrum are moved in the opposite direction on exhalation. The patient is in the prone position and the practitioner uses two hands for each location, as the cranial and sacral faults are corrected separately. The index fingers contact the anterior aspect of each mastoid process, and pressure is applied posteriorly as the patient exhales. The pressure is removed on inhalation, then reapplied on exhalation. This cycle is repeated four to six times.

The sacrum is contacted on its most superior aspect on either side of the midline. Through the application of pressure in the anterior direction, the sacral apex can be moved in a posterior direction, around the S2 fulcrum. This is done four to six times during the exhalation phase.

The muscle or muscles originally used to assess the EAF are retested to ensure that the problem has been corrected. As with the IAF, the pressure exerted on the mastoid process and sacrum may need to be applied up to 15 times, or more, in difficult cases.

Correction of an Expiration-Assisted Fault

1. The patient is prone with practitioner's index fingers on the anterior portion of each mastoid process.
2. The patient exhales deeply and the practitioner pulls the mastoid process posterior.
3. The patient inhales and the practitioner removes the force.
4. The patient exhales deeply again, and the same pressure is applied to the mastoid process.
5. This cycle is repeated four to six times.
6. Steps 2-5 are repeated except that contacts are on the superior-most portion of the sacrum, applying pressure anteriorly.
7. The muscle or muscles originally used in the assessment process are retested.

To check that the cranial-sacral respiratory fault has been corrected, the practitioner uses a normal muscle and evaluates it for potential inhibition during inspiration and expiration. For example, a normal pectoralis major sternal (PMS) is tested. The patient is asked to exhale and the PMS is retested; then the patient is asked to inhale and it is tested again. If none of these actions causes muscle inhibition, correction of the respiratory fault was successful.

Cranial respiratory faults are typically bilateral, although they may also be unilateral—on the same side as muscle inhibition normalized by inhalation or exhalation. Occasionally, one side may have an IAF and the opposite side an EAF. In addition, a cranial respiratory fault may sometimes exist without a sacral fault, but usually the reverse does not occur.

SPHENOBASILAR RESPIRATORY FAULTS

A similar type of fault, not nearly as common as the IAF and EAF, is the sphenobasilar respiratory fault, classified into the sphenobasilar inspiration-assisted fault (SIAF) and the sphenobasilar expiration-assisted fault (SEAF). Theoretically, these faults are reflected in the improper movements of the sphenoid and occiput bones, with the focus of the fault being the relationship between these two bones at the sphenobasilar junction. These faults also may cause muscle inhibition anywhere in the body, and can occur without sacral faults.

Any inhibited muscle may be dysfunctional as a result of a sphenobasilar respiratory fault. If this is the case, the inhibited muscle will become facilitated, or normalize, when the patient either inhales or exhales deeply followed by additional exaggerated inhalation or exhalation. For example, if the tensor fascia lata is inhibited, the patient is asked to take a deep breath in and hold the breath and then is asked to inhale more, as much as possible. Then the tensor fascia lata is retested. If it is now normal, this is an indication of a SIAF. The correction, as described further on, will be made during deep inspiration.

If the tensor fascia lata continues to be inhibited after exaggerated inhalation, the problem may be a SEAF. For example, if the tensor fascia lata is inhibited and the patient exhales completely and then forces out more breath, and this normalizes the tensor fascia lata, a SEAF is present. The correction will be made on expiration.

Assessment of Sphenobasilar Respiratory Faults With Muscle Inhibition

1. The patient has an inhibited right tensor fascia lata.
2. The patient breathes in deeply, then adds additional forced inspiration and maintains it.
3. The tensor fascia lata is retested.
4. If the tensor fascia lata becomes facilitated, the patient has a SIAF.
5. If the tensor fascia lata remains inhibited, the patient does not have this fault.
6. The patient fully exhales, then forcibly exhales more.
7. If the tensor fascia lata is facilitated, the patient has a SEAF.
8. If the tensor fascia lata has not changed and is still inhibited, the patient does not have this type of cranial respiratory fault.

In addition to an inhibited muscle, a normal muscle can be used to assess sphenobasilar respiratory faults. If the patient has a normal PMS, he or she inhales deeply, then adds more forced inhalation and maintains it, and the PMS is immediately tested. If there is a SEAF, the muscle will become inhibited. If the patient exhales deeply and forces out more of the breath and the PMS becomes inhibited, the patient has a SIAF.

Assessment of Sphenobasilar Respiratory Faults With Normal Muscle Function

1. The patient has a normally functioning PMS.
2. The patient breathes in deeply and then forces in more breath.
3. The PMS is retested.
4. If the muscle is still normal, the patient does not have a SEAF. In this case, the patient fully exhales and then adds more forced exhalation.
5. If the PMS is now inhibited, the patient has a SIAF.
6. If the muscle is still normal, the patient does not have a sphenobasilar respiratory fault.

An additional means of assessing sphenobasilar respiratory faults is to therapy-localize one of the areas where treatment will be directed—to the roof of the mouth at the junction of the maxillary and palatine bones. When a sphenobasilar respiratory fault exists, this therapy localization will be positive, and either forced inspiration or expiration will negate the muscle inhibition.

Correction of a SIAF is accomplished most easily with the patient supine. Two contacts are required: one at the area of the maxillary and palatine bones and the other on the posterior mastoid process. Using a glove or finger cot, the practitioner places one index finger inside the mouth and contacts the roof of the mouth. The thumb and index finger of the other hand are placed on the posterior aspect of the mastoid process. The correction is done while the patient inhales deeply with an additional forced inspiration; the maxillary and palatine bones are gently pushed superiorly, and the mastoid process is gently pushed anterior. (The pressure applied is moderate but not uncomfortable for the patient.) The patient then exhales and the pressure is removed. This cycle is repeated four to six times during forced inhalation as the patient breathes in and out. The muscle(s) originally used to assess the fault is retested to ensure that the problem has been corrected.

Occasionally it may be necessary to apply the pressure more than 6 times; in some difficult cases, up to 15 or more times may be required. This will be evident in the retesting phase. If, for example, the muscle originally used is retested and is still inhibited and still responds positively (i.e., normalizes or facilitates) to forced inhalation, this may indicate the need for prolonged correction.

Correction of a Sphenobasilar Inspiration-Assisted Fault

1. The patient is supine with the practitioner's gloved index finger on the roof of the mouth and the thumb and index finger of the other hand on the posterior mastoid process.
2. The patient inhales very deeply; the practitioner pushes the roof of the mouth superiorly and the mastoid process anterior.
3. Patient exhales and the practitioner removes the force.
4. Patient inhales very deeply again and the same pressure is applied.
5. This cycle is repeated four to six times.
6. The muscle used in the assessment process is retested.

Correction of a SEAF is accomplished similarly, although the cranium is moved in the opposite direction on exhalation. In this correction, the index finger from the gloved hand contacts the maxilla just above the posterior aspect of the central incisor left or right (if the fault is only on either the left or right), or both (if the fault is bilateral), and the pressure is directed anterior (this action hypothetically pulls the sphenobasilar junction downward). The other hand contacts the anterior portion of each mastoid process, and pressure is applied posteriorly. Both areas are treated as the patient exhales forcibly. The pressure is removed on inhalation, then reapplied on exhalation. This cycle is repeated four to six times. If the practitioner is unable to contact both mastoid processes with one hand, these two maneuvers can be done separately, with the incisor contact performed first.

The muscle or muscles originally used to assess the SEAF should be retested to check that the problem has been corrected. The pressure may need to be applied to the incisors and mastoid process up to 15 times or more in difficult cases.

Correction of a Sphenobasilar Expiration-Assisted Fault

1. The patient is supine with practitioner's index finger on the maxilla just above the posterior incisor(s) and the other index finger on the anterior portion of the mastoid process.
2. The patient exhales very deeply and the practitioner pulls the maxilla below the incisor(s) anteriorly and pushes the mastoid process posteriorly.
3. The patient inhales and the practitioner removes the force.
4. The patient exhales very deeply again, and the same pressure is applied.
5. This cycle is repeated four to six times.
6. The muscle(s) originally used in the assessment process should be retested.

To ensure correction of the sphenobasilar respiratory fault, a normal muscle is used and evaluated for potential muscle inhibition during forced inspiration and forced expiration. For example, a normal PMS is tested. The patient is asked to forcibly exhale and the PMS is retested. Then the patient is asked to forcibly inhale, and the PMS is retested. If none of these actions has caused muscle inhibition, there is no sphenobasilar respiratory fault.

Sphenobasilar respiratory faults are typically bilateral, although they may also be unilateral—on the same side as muscle inhibition normalized by forced inhalation or exhalation. Occasionally, one side may have a SIAF and the opposite side a SEAF.

SAGITTAL SUTURE CRANIAL FAULT

A common cranial problem known as the sagittal suture cranial fault is usually associated with an inhibition of any or all of the abdominal muscles or with the bilateral inhibition of the gluteus maximus muscles. Inhibition of any of these muscles may be due to a primary cranial problem with the sagittal suture.

When a sagittal suture cranial fault is present, it is almost always in a state in which the medial borders of the two parietal bones are approximating each other; this is referred to by Walther (1988) as a "jammed" sagittal suture. Correction involves contacting the medial-most portion of the parietal bone with the fingertips of each hand and pulling the bones away from each other with moderate pressure.

Any normal muscle can also be used to assess the possibility of a sagittal cranial suture fault. For example, when a normal hamstring muscle is tested, if there is a sagittal suture fault, the muscle will become inhibited when the parietal bones are pushed together (as a challenge). Also, if an inhibited muscle is used, it will normalize if the parietal bones are pulled apart.

When present, a sagittal suture cranial fault will also therapy-localize. For example, if the gluteus maximus muscles are inhibited and the patient touches the sagittal cranial suture, this will normalize the inhibited muscles.

To correct the sagittal suture fault, the practitioner pulls the parietal bones away from the midline with the fingertips, five or six times with moderate pressure. Figure 15.1 shows this treatment. The procedure can be done with the patient in any position. The general consensus is that there is no breathing pattern associated with this fault. Most importantly, if a sagittal suture cranial fault is present and is associated with specific muscle inhibition, correction of the fault will result in normal function of that muscle.

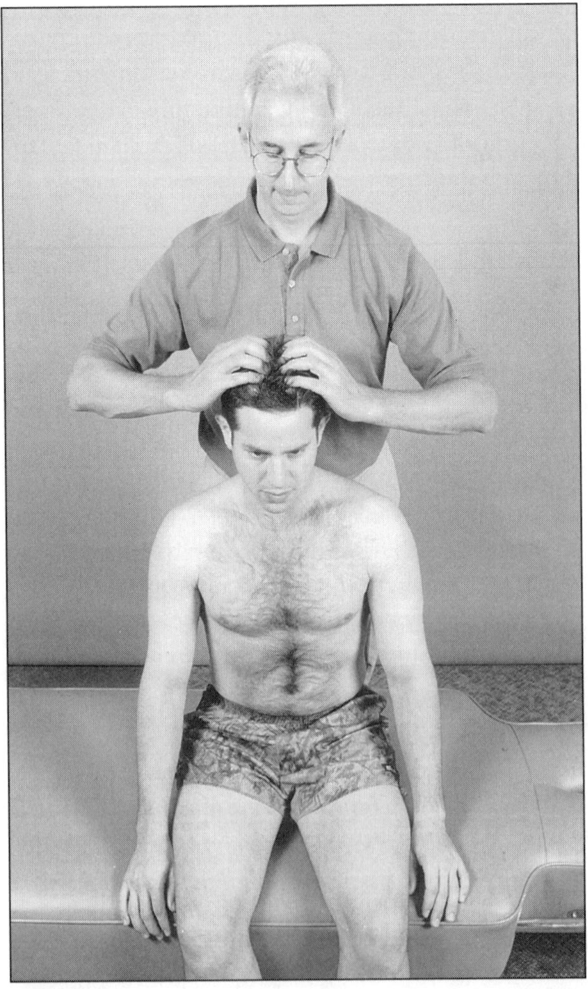

Figure 15.1 Correction of a sagittal suture cranial fault

Case History

Steve, 17 years old, had been injured in his high school football game six days earlier. He had been tackled head-on by two opponents while running at high speed and was immediately taken to the local hospital. All tests were negative for serious problems except what the doctor described as a "slight concussion." Another series of X-rays three days later was also negative. Steve had severe pain in the neck, shoulders, and arms; had headaches; and had restricted ranges of motion in almost all joints. Examination revealed neuromuscular inhibition of the sternocleidomastoid (bilateral), right PMC, right latissimus dorsi, middle deltoids (bilateral), middle and lower trapezius (bilateral), gluteus maximus (bilateral), right piriformis, and right psoas. Neurological disorganization was evident. Cranial dysfunction included an IAF bilateral and a sagittal suture fault. Correction of the neurological disorganization required digital stimulation of KI 27 (bilateral) and CV 8 and of the gait reflexes. After this correction, the muscle inhibition pattern changed; the PMC was now normal on the right and inhibited on the left, and the psoas was now normal on the right and inhibited on the left. The inhibited latissimus dorsi was evident in the supine position (altered labyrinthine reflex pattern), and Chapman's reflexes for the sartorius muscle required stimulation (this eliminated the inhibition in the supine position, but the muscle was still inhibited in the prone position). Correction of the IAF eliminated the inhibition of the sternocleidomastoid, PMC, latissimus dorsi, piriformis, and psoas muscles. (A pelvic fault was also corrected as described later.) The remaining pattern of bilateral inhibition was normalized after the correction of the sagittal suture fault. This office visit eliminated about 90% of Steve's pain and dramatically improved his ranges of motion. He was seen one week later; there had been minimal recurrences and continued improvement.

PELVIC DYSFUNCTION

This section addresses two pelvic imbalances that are very common in complementary sports medicine. They are referred to as Category I and Category II pelvic faults. These problems are usually primary imbalances; proper treatment typically allows the body to correct many other, secondary problems. For example, correcting a Category I pelvic fault will often allow the body to correct secondary joint dysfunction in the cervical, thoracic, or lumbar spine. Occasionally, however, the Category I or II pelvic fault is a secondary problem, usually to a major primary problem such as a temporomandibular joint imbalance or cranial respiratory fault, or some dysfunction in the foot or ankle.

Category I Pelvic Fault

The Category I pelvic fault is usually found in conjunction with the cranial-sacral respiratory faults described earlier. Theoretically, it is related to the movement of the pelvic bones—the two iliac bones and sacrum—that occurs with normal diaphragmatic respiration; the problem arises when the normal movement does not occur. The exact position of the problem is an opposite rotation of each ilium around the sacrum, as if the pelvis were being maintained in a gait position when the patient is actually in a neutral position. A Category I pelvic fault is often asymptomatic and usually causes many secondary problems, especially structural ones. This imbalance is best treated at the same time as the cranial-sacral respiratory fault associated with it.

Assessment of a Category I Pelvic Fault

Assessment of a Category I pelvic fault can be achieved through therapy localization and challenge. Correction takes place with orthopedic wedges, or DeJarnette blocks, that are used to support specific areas of the pelvis while mild pressure is applied to other areas as described in the following sections.

Evaluation of a Category I pelvic fault is done with the patient in the prone position and requires three steps.

Step One: To determine whether a Category I pelvic fault exists, the patient therapy-localizes with each hand palm down on each sacroiliac joint (see figure 15.2a). If a Category I pelvic fault is present, this therapy localization will be positive; either a normal muscle will become inhibited or an inhibited muscle will normalize during this process. If therapy localization is negative, most likely the patient does not have a Category I pelvic fault.

Step Two: If Step One is positive, the patient therapy-localizes each sacroiliac joint separately with two hands as in figure 15.2b while either an inhibited or a normal muscle is tested. One sacroiliac joint will be positive. The patients' hands are then moved away.

Step Three: The final step is to challenge each posterior superior iliac spine (PSIS) and opposite ischium, in the anterior direction, using a normal muscle. One of these two challenges will be positive.

a

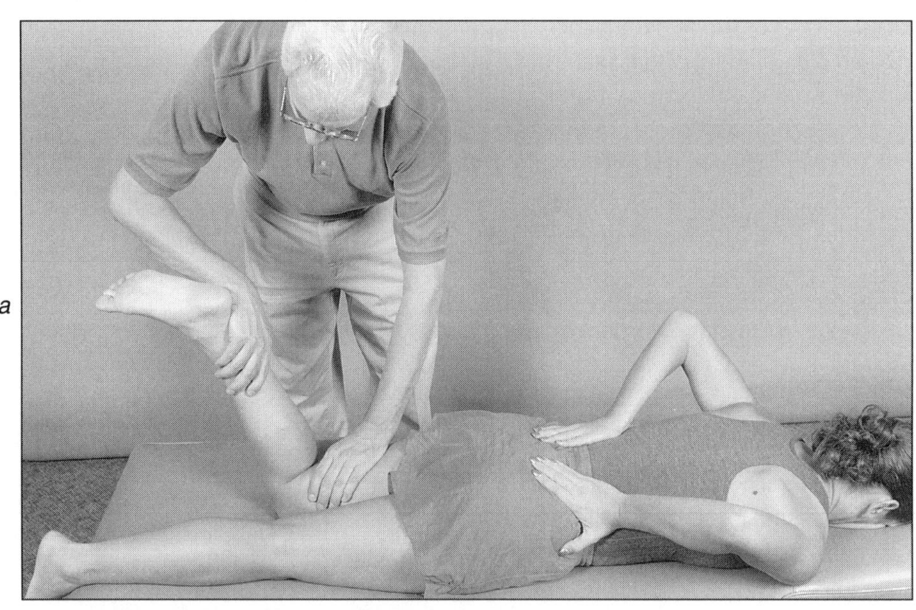

b

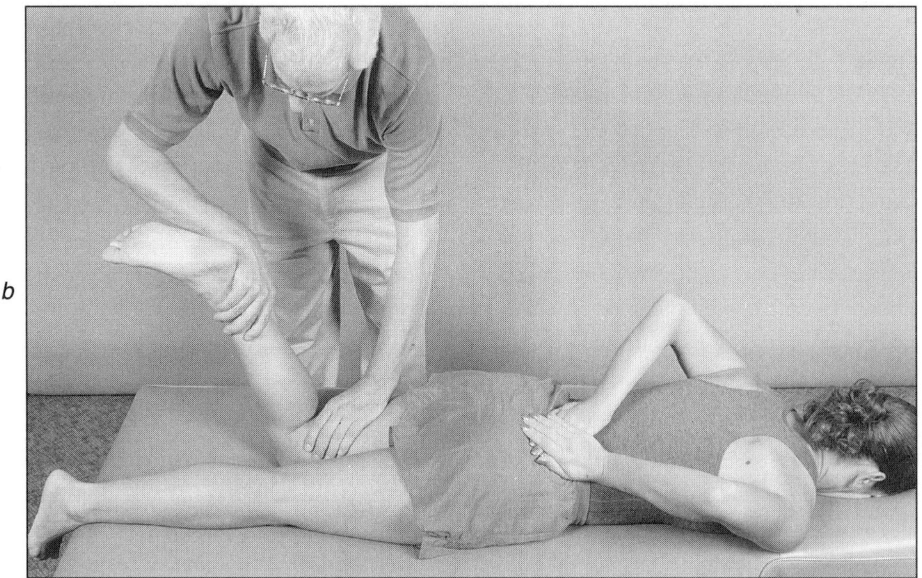

Figure 15.2a–b (*a*) The first step in assessing for a Category I pelvic fault—determining whether the fault exists. (*b*) The second step in assessing for a Category I pelvic fault—finding the side of irritation.

Correction of a Category I Pelvic Fault

Correction of a Category I pelvic fault is a two-step process. The first step is placement of the orthopedic wedges, or DeJarnette blocks, under the patient's pelvis. When one is making an on-the-field correction, an effective substitute for blocks is a pair of shoes placed upside down with the heels facing outward. Place one block under the ischium and one under the anterior superior iliac spine (ASIS) depending on the challenge in Step Three of the evaluation. If anterior pressure to the right PSIS and left ischium was a positive challenge, one block is placed under the right femur at the level of the ischium and one block under the left ASIS, as shown in figure 15.3. If anterior pressure to the left PSIS and right ischium was a positive challenge, one block is placed under the left femur at the level of the ischium and one block under the right ASIS.

The second step in the correction process is to allow the pelvis to correct itself with its weight on the orthopedic wedges. This may take about 3-5 min with the patient relaxing. Some professionals, such as chiropractors and osteopaths or others licensed to manipulate, apply four to six very light thrusts directed anteriorly on the side of the pelvis opposite the one that had the positive therapy localization in Step Two of the evaluation.

In most cases of a Category I pelvic fault, there is a specific accompanying muscle inhibition. This is either in the piriformis or the sacrospinalis muscle. (The sacrospinalis muscle, not listed in chapter 10 because it is not possible to manually test with accuracy, is usually corrected by stimulating Chapman's reflexes—the anterior being approximately 2 in. (5 cm) lateral to the umbilicus and the posterior at the level of L2 just lateral to the spinous process.) It is important also to correct this muscle inhibition; typically correction requires stimulation of Chapman's reflexes. In addition, correction of a cranial sacral respiratory fault can be made while the patient is resting on the orthopedic wedges, since the two problems, Category I pelvic fault and cranial respiratory fault, often occur together. If the muscle inhibition or the cranial respiratory fault is a primary problem, correcting it will also correct the Category I pelvic fault spontaneously.

The following is an example of specific correction of a Category I pelvic fault, cranial respiratory fault, and piriformis inhibition. A hamstring muscle is used for the challenge.

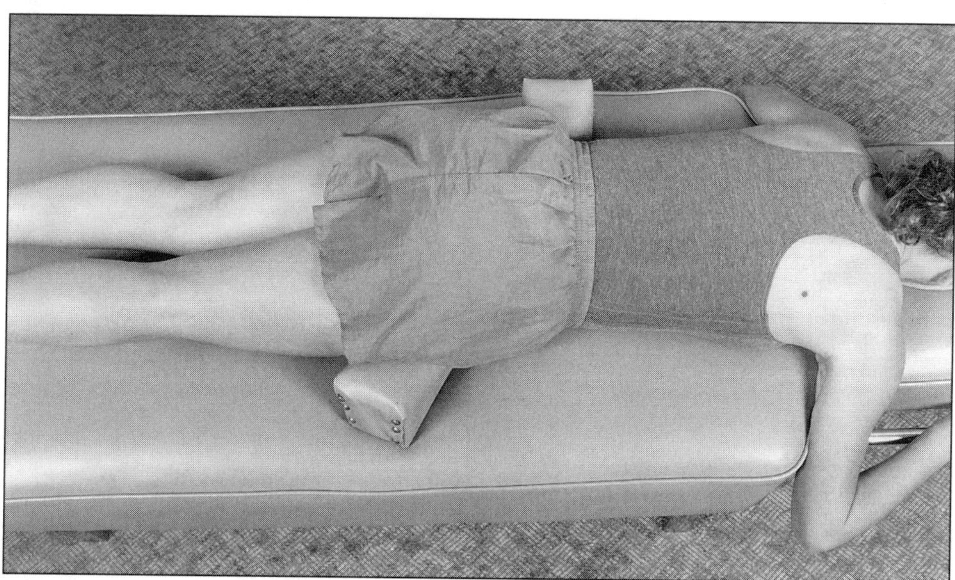

Figure 15.3 Placement of blocks when the right posterior superior iliac spine and left ischium are challenged

Correction of Category I Pelvic Fault, Cranial Respiratory Fault, and Piriformis Inhibition

1. The patient is prone and has a normal right hamstring muscle.
2. The patient therapy-localizes with one palm-down hand on each sacroiliac joint, which results in an inhibition of the hamstring muscle. This is positive for a Category I pelvic fault.
3. The patient then therapy-localizes first to the right, then to the left sacroiliac joint with two hands. Therapy localization to the left one causes hamstring muscle inhibition. The patient removes his or her hands.
4. Using the hamstring, the right PSIS and left ischium are challenged anteriorly and are negative. The left PSIS and right ischium are challenged and are positive.
5. The left piriformis muscle is tested and found to be inhibited.
6. The inhibited piriformis normalizes on inhalation, indicating an IAF; the muscle also normalizes when the patient therapy-localizes to the left Chapman's reflexes on the lateral pubic bone.
7. Therapy is applied as follows:
   - The orthopedic wedges are placed under the left femur at the level of the ischium and the right ASIS.
   - The left mastoid process and sacrum are treated for correction of inspiration-assisted cranial respiratory fault.
   - Chapman's reflexes are stimulated for the piriformis.
8. The orthopedic wedges are removed and the Category I pelvic fault, cranial respiratory fault, and piriformis function are reevaluated.

Category II Pelvic Fault

The Category II pelvic fault is often found following trauma, especially in the acute phase before the body has compensated. This is a structural problem of one ilium that has abnormally distorted, causing sacroiliac joint dysfunction. It is often symptomatic, and in the acute phase the pain can be debilitating. In some patients, an acute, painful Category II pelvic fault may compensate by changing to a less painful but equally dysfunctional Category I pelvic fault.

Category II pelvic faults are treated by some professionals (chiropractors and osteopaths) by manual manipulation. An alternative, and sometimes more effective, non-force approach is to use orthopedic wedges and to find and correct the muscle inhibition that is either causing or maintaining the dysfunctional ilium.

The mechanical problem associated with a Category II pelvic fault is a unilateral one; the ilium has abnormally distorted either anteriorly, or more commonly, posteriorly. A common related muscle inhibition is in the sartorius, in part because of its attachment on the ASIS. Inhibition of the sartorius contributes to a loss of muscular support from the front of the pelvis, allowing the ilium to move more easily posterior. Other muscles, including the quadriceps and gracilis, can cause the same vulnerability. An ilium that moves more easily anteriorly may be associated with inhibition of the hamstrings, gluteus maximus, or tensor fascia lata (see figure 15.4).

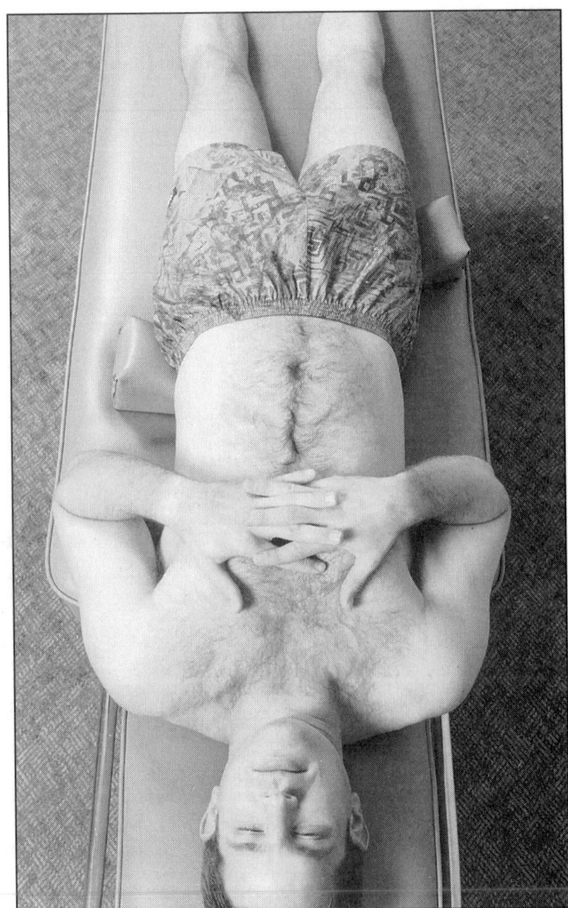

Figure 15.4 Placement of blocks for a Category II pelvic fault, posterior on the left

In many patients, the muscle inhibition is a primary problem, with the Category II pelvic fault being secondary. In this case, correction of the muscle inhibition can eliminate the Category II pelvic fault.

Assessment of a Category II Pelvic Fault

Assessment of a Category II pelvic fault can be made by therapy localization and challenge. The patient is supine, since this is the position used for the correction. The patient therapy-localizes one sacroiliac joint with one hand while a normal muscle is tested. If the muscle becomes inhibited, there is most likely a Category II pelvic fault on that side. For example, a normal psoas muscle is tested. The patient touches the right sacroiliac joint, and the psoas is retested and is now inhibited. This implies a Category II pelvic fault in the right sacroiliac joint.

The challenge is used to determine which direction the ilium has rotated—anterior or posterior. Recall from chapter 11 that the bones of the pelvis will rebound when challenged. With the patient supine, the practitioner uses a normal muscle for the challenge, such as a PMC. The practitioner challenges each ilium by gently pushing the ASIS posterior, then retests the PMC, then gently pulls up anteriorly on the PSIS and retests the PMC. If pulling the right PSIS anterior causes the PMC to become inhibited, the Category II pelvic fault is posterior on the right. If pushing the ASIS posterior is positive, the Category II pelvic fault is anterior on the right.

Correction of a Category II Pelvic Fault

Correction of the Category II pelvic fault is made by first determining which muscles are inhibited. Correction of this muscle inhibition may result in elimination of the Category II pelvic fault. If this does not occur, the practitioner places orthopedic wedges under the patient's pelvis. In the case of a posterior ilium, one wedge is placed under the PSIS on the posterior side and one under the ischium on the opposite side (see figure 15.3). In the case of an anterior ilium, one wedge is placed under the ischium on the anterior ilium side and one under the opposite PSIS. The patient remains on the orthopedic wedges for about 1-2 min. The placement of the orthopedic wedges makes sense anatomically; the wedges are used simply to allow gravity to realign the ilium. The blocks are removed, and the Category II pelvic fault is reevaluated.

Assessment and Treatment for Category II Pelvic Fault

1. The practitioner evaluates the function of the muscles outlined in figure 15.4.
   - Sartorius
   - Gracilis
   - Quadriceps
   - Hamstring
   - Tensor fascia lata
   - Gluteus maximus
2. The patient is supine, with the practitioner testing a normal psoas or other normal muscle.
3. The patient therapy-localizes the right sacroiliac joint; the practitioner retests the psoas, and it is negative.
4. The patient therapy-localizes the left sacroiliac joint, which causes psoas inhibition. The patient's hand is removed.
5. The practitioner challenges the left ilium by pushing the ASIS posterior; this does not change the normal psoas.
6. The practitioner then challenges the left ilium by pulling it up (anterior) from the PSIS, which causes psoas inhibition. This is a Category II pelvic fault, posterior on the left.
7. The practitioner corrects any muscle inhibition found in the preceding steps.
8. The practitioner reevaluates (through therapy localization or challenge) for the Category II pelvic fault. If the Category II pelvic fault has not been corrected by treatment of the inhibited muscles, orthopedic wedges are placed under the patient's pelvis:
   - In the case of a posterior ilium, one wedge is placed under the PSIS of the posterior ilium and one under the opposite ischium.
   - In the case of an anterior ilium, one wedge is placed under the ischium of the anterior ilium and one under the opposite PSIS.
   - The orthopedic wedges are removed after 1 to 2 min, and the Category II pelvic fault is reevaluated.

Case History

Karen was a triathlete whose training schedule was apparently causing undue stress. Her symptoms included extreme fatigue, difficulty waking in the morning, insomnia, low back pain, and knee pain. Her lying blood pressure was 118/70 and standing pressure was 96/66. The results of her salivary tests showed that cortisol was very high and dehydroepiandrosterone (DHEA[S]) very low. Karen had an inhibition of the sartorius and gracilis muscles, Category II pelvic fault, and a number of other mechanical and chemical imbalances. During the first office visit, the Category II pelvic fault and muscles related to adrenal dysfunction were corrected. Karen was instructed to diminish her coffee intake (which had been between 8 and 10 cups per day), reduce her training by half, and avoid competition until her mechanical and chemical problems could be ameliorated. A number of dietary recommendations were also made. Two weeks later Karen returned—and the sartorius muscle inhibition also returned with the Category II pelvic fault. A number of other problems that had been corrected on the first visit did not recur. A temporomandibular joint problem was found and treated, and correction of the sartorius muscle eliminated the Category II pelvic fault. Karen's lying blood pressure was now 112/72 and standing pressure 110/70. Her energy was much better (60% by her estimation), as was the low back and knee pain. Her sleeping problems were the same. Correction of a sagittal suture fault completely eliminated the low back pain. Karen returned two weeks later and manifested a Category I pelvic fault with a piriformis inhibition. This was corrected, eliminating the need to treat several other inhibited muscles. Blood pressure from lying to standing was 118/74 and 124/74. Karen was told she could compete in short events, but no more than one per month. She returned in five weeks with no low back or knee pain; she was sleeping through the night, felt rested when she woke for her 5:15 A.M. swim, and had very good energy. She had competed in a short triathlon the previous week and performed a personal best relative to her age group. There were no indications of excess stress in the pelvis and muscles. Her lying and standing blood pressures were 116/74 and 124/78.

Some professionals routinely stabilize the sacroiliac joint with a support or brace after correction of a Category II pelvic fault. In most cases, however, correcting all muscle inhibition provides sufficient and effective support. For some athletes who are in competition, especially those currently involved in contact sports, temporary support for the sacroiliac joint may be necessary, but only after the muscles and Category II pelvic fault are corrected, and only for a relatively short period of time depending on the individual.

Note that an inhibited sartorius and/or gracilis is often associated with a Category II pelvic fault. Adrenal dysfunction and the Category II pelvic fault are very frequently related in athletes. Any stress adversely affecting adrenal function may result in a chronic sartorius and/or gracilis inhibition and a chronic Category II pelvic fault. This is an added stress and can significantly affect performance. The scenario is common in overtrained athletes.

CONCLUSION

Assessment and treatment of cranial and pelvic structural problems are not difficult, although there are many factors involved. Correction of the most basic cranial-sacral respiratory faults—the inspiration- and expiration-assisted faults—and Category I and II pelvic faults can have an immediate and dramatic impact on the athlete's health and performance.

16

Treatment of Vertebral and Extravertebral Dysfunction

This chapter describes a non-force method of treating vertebral problems. In addition, extravertebral imbalances are discussed, including those of the foot and ankle, metatarsals, ribs, and wrist. The vast majority of these problems do not require first aid or surgical treatment and are not otherwise life threatening. In some patients these dysfunctions cause pain, restrict normal ranges of motion, and can adversely affect muscle function. In others, the same problems may not be symptomatic if they are well compensated by the body. In either case, vertebral and extravertebral dysfunctions may predispose the patient to further, more serious injury that may require more radical care. In addition, these dysfunctions may also have a significant and adverse affect on sport performance.

PRIMARY VERSUS SECONDARY STRUCTURAL PROBLEMS

Assessing and treating primary structural problems, such as muscle inhibition, often eliminates the need to address a secondary joint dysfunction. In no area is the concept of the body correcting its own problems most evident than in the spine. Joint complex dysfunction in the spine has been assessed and treated by chiropractors and osteopaths for more than a hundred years. Since the advent in applied kinesiology of assessment methods such as therapy localization and challenge, it has become evident that many spinal dysfunctions are secondary mechanical problems. They may be secondary to muscle imbalance, cranial or pelvic faults, or even other spinal problems. They may also be secondary to chemical problems; adrenal dysfunction, for example, may cause a secondary joint complex dysfunction in the thoracic spine. Mental and emotional stress can also cause structural problems in the spine.

Many secondary problems are mechanical compensations for primary dysfunction. Primary structural problems that result in secondary spinal imbalances are easy for the mechanically oriented practitioner to understand. As an example, consider a patient with chronic back pain and diminished range of motion: a psoas muscle inhibition may have caused the pelvis to become posturally distorted. This pelvic tilt forced the lumbar spine to compensate by flexing and rotating laterally with the pelvis. Since the eyes try to maintain a horizontal position, the thoracic spine must compensate by laterally flexing and rotating in the opposite direction. This typically creates an abnormal curvature, or scoliosis, in the spine, along with a number of secondary spinal, pelvic, or cranial dysfunctions. These problems can then cause other secondary dysfunctions, including those that produce pain and diminished range of motion. In this example, improving the function of the psoas muscle may allow the pelvis to return to normal, remove the need for the spine to compensate, and eliminate the secondary problems and the symptoms they created.

A more common example is in the patient with acute low back pain; an inhibited right latissimus dorsi results in secondary overfacilitation of the left latissimus muscle. Since the latissimus dorsi attaches to the lower six thoracic vertebrae and all the lumbar vertebrae, these bones are literally being pulled by their spinous process toward the left, potentially causing vertebral dysfunction. In this case, the spinal problems can often be relieved by improving balance in the latissimus dorsi muscles by addressing the needs of the inhibited latissimus (such as treating the related Chapman's reflexes and stimulating related acupuncture points).

If a secondary spinal problem is treated by manipulation and the primary cause is not addressed, the spinal problem will most likely recur. Occasionally, secondary spinal corrections may even cause the patient to feel worse after treatment since the body's compensation has been removed. In either case, the recurring spinal distortions will require frequent symptomatic treatment.

NON-FORCE CORRECTION OF SPINAL DYSFUNCTION

Chapter 11 dealt with the challenge method used in applied kinesiology. This assessment tool allows the practitioner to precisely evaluate a particular vertebra's malposition, if present. Recall that vertebral challenging involves a rebound mechanism. For example, a particular vertebra may be rotated into dysfunction such that the right transverse process is more posterior and the left transverse process is more anterior. In this case, challenging the vertebra by gently pushing anteriorly on the right transverse process and removing the pressure will result in the vertebra's rebounding further into distortion. A normal muscle will temporarily become inhibited. This is the first step in correcting this problem using a non-force method.

The second step is to assess whether there is a relationship with respiration, similar to that for the cranial faults described in chapter 15. Since the spine is also thought to move with inspiration and expiration, like the cranium and pelvis, inhaling or exhaling may negate the inhibiting effect of the vertebral challenge. For example, repeating the vertebral challenge in the first step after the patient has inhaled may negate muscle inhibition. As with cranial and sacral faults, this inspiration-assisted fault is corrected during the inhalation phase of diaphragmatic breathing.

The third and final step in this process is making the correction. This is accomplished by gently pushing the vertebra in the direction that caused muscle inhibition during the patient's inhalation (i.e., the right transverse process anteriorly in the example just cited). The pressure is removed on exhalation. (The pressure is about what one would use to push a doorbell.) This should be done five to six times.

Non-Force Vertebral Assessment and Correction

1. The practitioner determines that a specific vertebra is not functioning properly (i.e., through therapy localization, palpation).
2. The vertebra is challenged through its various normal ranges of motion to determine which direction produces muscle inhibition. For example, pushing the left transverse process anterior and superior causes inhibition.
3. This anterior and superior direction is used to challenge the vertebra while the patient first inhales, then exhales, to determine whether there is an effect from respiration. For example, inhalation negates the muscle inhibition.

4. The practitioner corrects the vertebra by gently pushing it anterior and superior on the left during inhalation. It is released on exhalation, pushed on inhalation, and so on; the pushing is repeated five to six times.
5. The vertebra is reevaluated as in step 1.

All vertebrae can be assessed and treated in this manner. Different vertebrae may require challenge through different ranges of motion depending on their location. For example, because of the articulations with vertebrae above and below, thoracic vertebrae often require a superior direction as part of the challenge, (causing them to rebound posterior and inferior), as in the examples cited earlier. The atlas may require a lateral challenge or one that adds an anterior-to-posterior directional force.

Correction of vertebral problems using this method is relatively safe in patients who may have underlying pathology in the spine or local blood vessels, or in those who are already experiencing significant pain or muscle spasms making other forms of manipulation very difficult. It may also be important in on-the-field treatment, for example, before an athlete has been X-rayed to rule out fracture.

For those practitioners who are trained and licensed to manipulate the vertebrae using more traditional techniques, the challenge method with respiration can still be employed. This specificity may allow for an easier, less forceful correction and often eliminates patient discomfort.

EXTRAVERTEBRAL DYSFUNCTION

Recall that spinal vertebrae (and cranial and pelvic bones) have a rebound; gently pushing them in one direction causes them to react (through muscle action) by rebounding in the opposite direction. This is not the case with extravertebral articulations.

A variety of mechanical problems are due to dysfunction of extravertebral joints. Many traditionally named conditions, including the compartment syndromes, plantar fascitis, medial tibial stress syndrome, and others, have as their cause some of the problems described in this section on foot and ankle, metatarsal, wrist, and rib problems.

FOOT AND ANKLE PROBLEMS

Dysfunction of certain bones or joints in the foot and ankle often causes secondary muscle inhibition. For example, dysfunction of the talus bone may cause psoas muscle inhibition. This muscle problem may then cause a number of other secondary dysfunctions, possibly as high as the cervical spine.

Case History

Jim's low back gradually tightened to the point of pain during a long ride on his new bike. By the time he showered and laid down, his low back was in severe pain and it was very difficult for him to move in any direction. He was seen the next morning, still in severe pain and antalgic. It was not possible to perform testing on all muscles because of the pain, although some muscles, including the biceps, which tested normal, were not painful. Some of the muscles could be tested, and several were inhibited. They all demonstrated a positive therapy localization to the fifth lumbar vertebra. This was challenged and corrected gently with respiration. This produced an almost immediate improvement in Jim's pain, and he was able to move more freely and stand up straight. He was sent for X-rays, which were negative, and seen again the next morning. Jim was still in some pain but was much improved. It was now possible to do all the muscle testing necessary and make other corrections that resulted in complete recovery. In cases such as Jim's, if some effective therapy is not applied relatively soon after the injury, the patient may become much more difficult to treat as the body compensates and adapts.

Until the talus problem is corrected, these other secondary dysfunctions can maintain chronic injuries. Sometimes a foot and ankle problem on one side is due to a dysfunction in the contralateral foot—presumably because of the compensation of shifting weight bearing away from the original problem to the opposite side, which ultimately produces excess mechanical stress.

Four bones of the foot and ankle discussed here are the talus, calcaneus, navicular, and cuboid. Dysfunction of these bones has been clinically associated with specific secondary muscle inhibition; if there is joint dysfunction associated with one bone, the related muscle is usually inhibited. Specific proprioception from the foot causes certain muscles to be facilitated and inhibited, helping to control or reestablish normal posture. The exception is the calcaneus, which may cause muscle inhibition due to local stress affecting the neurological components innervating the muscle. A dysfunction in the calcaneus bone will typically inhibit the plantar muscles of the foot. The other three bones, when dysfunctional, usually have predictable relationships with specific muscle inhibitions away from the foot and ankle. The talus problem may cause inhibition in the psoas muscle; navicular dysfunction is often associated with adductor muscle inhibition; and cuboid problems are often linked to tensor fascia lata muscle inhibition.

These relationships imply that usually a secondary muscle inhibition exists that is associated with talus, navicular, and cuboid dysfunction. However, this does not mean that along with a psoas, adductor, or tensor fascia lata inhibition there is necessarily a dysfunction associated with the related bone. The practitioner should consider inhibition of one of these muscles as a clue to the possibility of dysfunction in one of these bones. (It is also possible that almost any muscle imbalance that can cause postural distortion can also increase the stress in the foot and ankle, producing a joint dysfunction associated with these bones.)

Although foot and ankle bone dysfunctions often result from trauma, they are also caused by a lack of local muscle support. For example, the tibialis posterior muscle helps support or attaches to many bony structures in the foot and ankle. Dysfunction of this muscle may have adverse effects on any of these bony areas. Inhibition of the tibialis posterior is a common muscle inhibition associated with foot and ankle dysfunction; correction often requires Golgi tendon organ (GTO)/spindle cell therapy, since the inhibition is frequently due to micro- or macrotrauma. If the tibialis posterior is a primary problem with other secondary foot and ankle imbalances, correction of this muscle will usually result in the elimination of the foot and ankle problems.

Dysfunctions of the joints in the foot and ankle can be assessed by therapy localization and challenge. Recall that specificity is important for accurate therapy localization, and that when the bones of the foot and ankle are challenged, they do not rebound like a spinal vertebra.

Talus Dysfunction

Talus dysfunction, very common in athletes, is often produced by ankle sprains and strains and muscle imbalance and is usually associated with excess pronation. Many times this injury is so painful that it mimics the symptoms of a fracture, but X-rays are negative. This leads some to assume that the undiagnosed problem is a "stress fracture," which can be a misdiagnosis in these patients. In some patients, however, talus dysfunction is asymptomatic. The related psoas dysfunction still exists, as do many other secondary imbalances that may cause pain or diminished ranges of motion away from the ankle. A common example is seen in the patient with knee pain. Assessment of the knee itself may produce few or no findings. The existence of an asymptomatic talus problem may cause dysfunction of the knee joint due to improper weight-bearing vectors from the ankle up the calf to the knee. In this situation, correction of the talus problem often relieves the knee pain and restores function very quickly.

Assessment of talus dysfunction can be made using the related psoas muscle inhibition, or any normal muscle. With use of the inhibited psoas, the talus is challenged so as to temporarily produce a normal psoas muscle; pushing the talus from lateral to medial will result in an inhibited muscle becoming normal. When a normal muscle is used, the talus is challenged with the result of producing an inhibited muscle; pushing the talus from medial to lateral will cause a normal muscle to become inhibited. Most often, talus dysfunction is the result of the bone's being too everted and is sometimes referred to as a "lateral" talus distortion. The fault most likely occurs at the subtalar joint. On rare occasions, usually as a result of trauma, the talus may become medially distorted.

Correction of the lateral talus problem is accomplished with the patient supine and the practitioner standing near the patient's foot (see figure 16.1). The practitioner grasps the patient's foot with one hand under the calcaneus (with the fingers around the Achilles tendon) and with the thumb under the lateral malleolus. The other hand is placed on the dorsum of the foot with the thumb on top of the other thumb. The foot and limb are tractioned and slightly medially rotated, and light traction is applied for about 30 sec, with the force medially through the thumbs and inferiorly toward the practitioner. Not only is the correct position important, but the patient's limb must be relaxed; otherwise the muscle tightness elicited will counter the practitioner's traction. In those trained and licensed to manipulate, a very light thrust can be applied instead of extended traction.

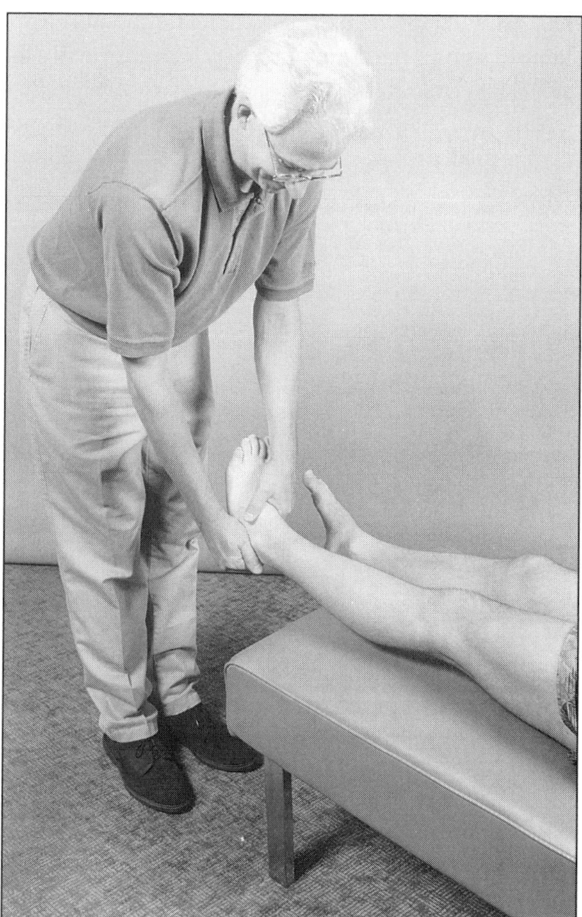

Figure 16.1 Positioning for the correction of a "lateral" talus joint dysfunction

After the correction, the related muscles are retested as previously described and the talus is rechallenged. Most importantly, to ensure that the correction will be maintained, the patient should walk or run in place for 20-30 sec, and the talus should be then reassessed. Sometimes this type of weight bearing will cause the problem to immediately recur. In some athletes, it is best to reproduce their normal activity and attempt to cause the problem to recur. If it does recur, the reason is usually some primary muscle inhibition that is causing the talus problem to return. On occasion, the ankle may require additional support, preferably via traditional taping for a pronated foot, for three to five days. The use of orthotic devices is usually not necessary. In most cases, correction of related muscle inhibition will support the foot and ankle sufficiently to maintain correction of the talus problem and allow complete healing. Supporting the ankle when it is not absolutely necessary may result in diminished muscle function and recurring muscle inhibition, hence incomplete healing and incomplete correction of the problem.

Lateral Talus Distortion

Many patients have improper shoe-wear patterns that will alert the practitioner to the possibility of a talus problem. Such a pattern takes the form of excess wear on the lateral edge of the heel portion of the shoe, also typical of excess pronation. It is due at least in part to the toe-out position of the foot, causing the heel strike to be more lateral. Postural analysis may indicate excess weight bearing more medially on the heels or a convexity of the Achilles tendon to the medial side. Inspection of the plantar surface of the foot may reveal more callusing on the medial heel.

An alternative test for lateral talus distortion can be done with the patient standing. The pectoralis major clavicular or another normal muscle is used. The patient is asked to exaggerate eversion while maintaining weight bearing through the ankle, and the muscle is retested. Muscle inhibition following this activity may be due to talus dysfunction. Confirmation with challenge should be performed before correction. It should be noted, however, that in patients with severe foot dysfunction (of any bone or joint), any weight bearing through the foot and ankle may cause inhibition of any or all muscles.

Calcaneal Dysfunction

Although the calcaneal dysfunction is not associated with predictable muscle inhibition, it frequently causes other secondary mechanical stress, including almost any mechanical problem if it is a primary problem. The calcaneal problem is similar to, although much less severe than, a compartment syndrome, and Walther (1988) refers to it as a "functional tarsal tunnel syndrome." As such, the calcaneal distortion may still cause inhibition of the plantar (flexor) muscles.

As with the talus, a calcaneal problem may cause pain or may be asymptomatic. In either case it can produce other, secondary problems often far from the heel. Calcaneal problems may cause local pain or paresthesia in the plantar surface of the foot and toes, and typically pain radiating up the posterior calf. As a result, the problem is sometimes misdiagnosed as "Achilles tendinitis." It is worsened by activities that force the calcaneus posterior and superior (the common direction of distortion), such as downhill running or walking, skiing, and jumping. Athletic shoes that have heels too thick for the patient's condition, or that increase pronation, often aggravate the symptoms. Eversion of the foot will also exaggerate or create local pain, as the calcaneal problem is frequently associated with pronation.

A problem with the calcaneus is often asymptomatic but can still cause many secondary problems: knee, hip, pelvic, spinal, and shoulder dysfunction is commonly associated with an asymptomatic calcaneal problem. Clinically, it is not unusual to find that the correction of a calcaneal problem eliminates a significant number of the functional problems found on an examination.

Calcaneal problems may be caused by micro- or macrotrauma, improper shoes, overtraining, pronation, and muscle inhibition. The most common muscle inhibition associated with this problem is in the tibialis posterior, which frequently requires GTO/spindle cell therapy for correction.

The calcaneus can be therapy-localized and challenged. It often develops an abnormal posterior and superior position, and challenging the bone in that direction will cause a normal muscle to become inhibited; challenging it anterior and inferior will cause an inhibited muscle to become normal.

When the calcaneus is in an abnormal posterior and superior position, correction is made with the patient prone, although some practitioners prefer patients in the supine position for correction. With the patient prone, the practitioner contacts the posterior and superior aspect of the calcaneus with the palm of the left hand. The right hand cradles the dorsum of the foot. The foot and leg are lightly tractioned and held for 30 sec. In those trained and appropriately licensed, a light thrust is applied by the left palm in an anterior and inferior direction (see figure 16.2).

It is important not only to retest the calcaneal bone, but also to ask patients to either run in place or reproduce their normal sport activity to ensure that the problem does not immediately recur. As with the talus, if this happens it is usually due to local muscle inhibition previously undiagnosed. Occasionally the calcaneus requires taping for added support for three to five days, with use of traditional taping techniques. Using heel lifts may be contraindicated, especially when there is a superior aspect to the distortion.

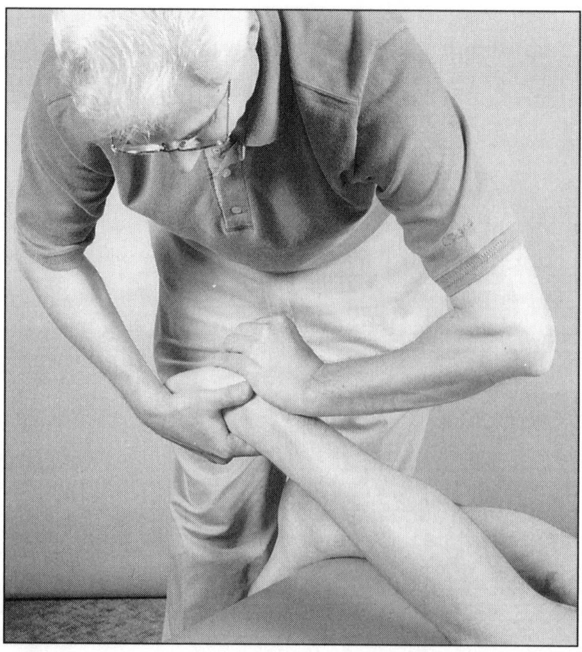

Figure 16.2 Positioning for the correction of calcaneal joint dysfunction

Case History

Janet had chronic medial knee pain, frequent groin pain, and recently, hip and shoulder pain that occurred after her swimming workout. Her running schedule included more hills to prepare for her fifth triathlon season. Examination revealed many mechanical faults, including cranial, spinal, and pelvic faults, and many muscle inhibitions that included the psoas, adductor, abdominals, tensor fascia lata, quadriceps, pectoralis major sternal, and sternocleidomastoid. Among the significant primary problems was a right calcaneal bone dysfunction, and this was the first correction made. Following this correction, most muscle dysfunction normalized, most mechanical faults normalized, and Janet had immediate improvement in knee and groin pain. After she ran in place the calcaneal problem returned, as did all the other problems, including the pain. Only after this activity did an inhibition of the tibialis posterior become evident. Correction was accomplished with GTO/spindle cell therapy. This treatment also corrected the calcaneal problem and all others that had originally improved. After an easy 5-min run on the treadmill, the calcaneal problem recurred again. At this time, the only other problem that became evident was a left talus distortion. This was corrected without recurrence following the treadmill run. Janet's next appointment one week later was to be preceded by a 30-min swim and a 30-min run. A few problems recurred that were secondary to neurological disorganization, possibly due to her swimming gait. Testing her immediately before and after swimming at the pool showed that even a 5-min swim caused the neurological disorganization to recur. The problem seemed to be her unilateral head turn. Her swim coach was contacted and asked to assess her swim stroke, which required improvement—including her habit of turning the head to only one side, which could cause neurological disorganization. Within two weeks, Janet was pain free, and her swimming times would improve significantly over the next two months.

Navicular Bone Dysfunction

Navicular bone problems may cause secondary adductor muscle inhibition. Patients may have a sense of tightness in the opposite adductor and complain of groin pain, and the problem may be misdiagnosed as a "groin pull." The navicular problem may sometimes be secondary to a primary talus or calcaneal problem. Assessment is made by therapy localization to the navicular and by challenge. When an adductor inhibition is used, a direction of challenge that typically results in a normal adductor is on the navicular from the dorsum of the foot in an inferior and slightly lateral direction. With use of a normal muscle, this same distortion produces a positive challenge when the practitioner's finger is hooked around the medial aspect of the foot, pulling superiorly on the navicular. A positive challenge in either of these directions means that the correction is made with traction or a thrust that is inferior on the navicular from the dorsum of the foot. The position of the correction is similar to that for the talus, except that the focus of the traction is slightly medial to the midline on the navicular with either the thumbs or the medial side of the hand.

The navicular may become distorted in other directions, and the direction of traction or thrust may need to be different depending on the challenge. Frequently, the navicular develops an abnormal inferior and medial position. In this case, the correction is made with the patient prone; the practitioner grasps the foot with the fingers around the dorsum and the thumbs contacting the inferior aspect of the navicular from the medial arch. The traction or thrust is through the thumbs following light traction of the

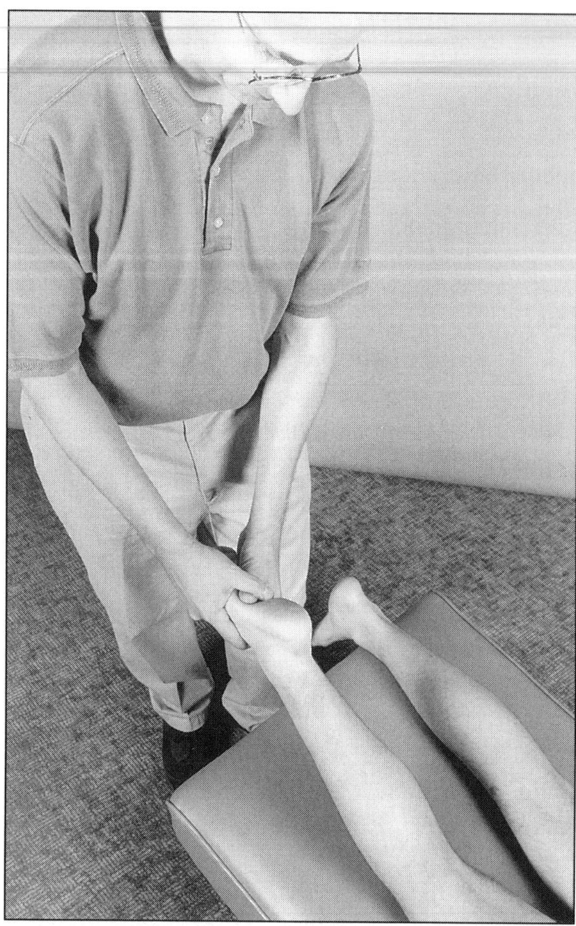

Figure 16.3 Position for the correction of an inferior navicular correction. A similar position is used for cuboid dysfunction.

foot (see figure 16.3). After correction, the practitioner retests the navicular; this includes asking the patient to run in place or reproduce his or her sport activity.

Cuboid Bone Dysfunction

The cuboid bone may also dysfunction and produce secondary inhibition of the tensor fascia lata. This is sometimes the cause of the pain in what is commonly misdiagnosed as the "iliotibial band syndrome." The cuboid typically develops an abnormal inferior and lateral position.

Challenging the cuboid involves pushing the bone through its normal ranges of motion, especially inferiorly and laterally. A normal muscle that becomes inhibited or an inhibited muscle that normalizes indicates the direction of distortion, as with the bones already described. For example, if pushing the cuboid inferiorly causes a normal muscle to become inhibited, the correction is made in the opposite direction.

Correction is made with the patient prone; the practitioner grasps the foot with the fingers around the dorsum and the thumbs contacting the inferior and/or lateral aspect of the cuboid bone (positioning is similar to that shown in figure 16.3). The foot is lightly tractioned and held for 30 sec. Those licensed can apply a light thrust made by the thumbs in a superior and medial direction. The practitioner reassesses the cuboid following correction, including asking the patient to run in place or reproduce his or her sport activity.

RESPIRATORY CORRECTION METHOD

Regarding any foot and ankle problem, it should also be noted that in cases in which pressure in the foot may be contraindicated, such as with a suspected fracture, or in cases in which manipulation is not within the professional's legal scope of practice, the bones can be treated with a non-force technique like that described earlier for the vertebrae. The same methods are used except that the bones and joints of the foot, like all other extravertebral areas, do not rebound when challenged. When using this non-force technique, the practitioner determines whether there is a respiratory relationship and incorporates this into the treatment. For example, one finds the direction of challenge that causes muscle inhibition and the phase of respiration that negates the positive challenge. The practitioner pushes the bone in the direction of correction with the appropriate respiratory phase. This is done four to six times, and the problem is reassessed. What follows is an outline of this procedure.

Non-Force Respiratory Correction of Foot Dysfunction

1. The bone or joint is challenged through its normal ranges of motion using a normal muscle.
2. The direction that causes the test muscle to become inhibited is noted.
3. The bone or joint is rechallenged in the same direction during inspiration, then with expiration.

4. If inspiration negates the positive challenge, the procedure is to push the bone in the direction of correction during inspiration and repeat four to six times.
5. The bone or joint is rechallenged as in step 1.

Below are some common names frequently used in undiagnosed problems, with the potential functional foot and ankle problems and their related muscle dysfunction in parentheses.

- "Stress fracture" (talus dysfunction/psoas inhibition)
- "Achilles tendinitis" (calcaneus dysfunction/tibialis posterior inhibition)
- "Groin pull" (navicular dysfunction/adductor inhibition)
- "Iliotibial band syndrome" (cuboid dysfunction/tensor fascia lata inhibition)

METATARSAL PROBLEMS

Metatarsal problems are very common in people who exercise and train, and especially those who compete. The problems in this area that practitioners most often encounter include hallux valgus, hammertoes, and bunions. Once these problems manifest themselves, however, dysfunction in the foot and toes has become chronic. Recognition of the dysfunction in its earliest stages, and correction of existing imbalances and primary causes, can prevent these common problems from developing. More importantly, these dysfunctions can cause secondary imbalances in the foot and ankle, knee, pelvis, and other areas. The first metatarsal joint is especially vulnerable because of improper or poorly fitting sport shoes.

A very common problem in athletes is a posterior distortion of the first metatarsal joint. This is most often the result of wearing shoes that are too short. A survey by the author (Maffetone 1996) showed that 52% of athletes wore training shoes that were too small. At any stage, this problem may be asymptomatic, but it can still cause secondary dysfunction in any of the bones of the foot and ankle as already described. The first metatarsal problem is sometimes painful, and when other findings are negative, it is often misdiagnosed as some type of sesamoid bone problem.

Assessment may initially be made by observation of both the patient's foot and the shoes being worn. The ends of the toes may show callusing, and the nail of the first toe is sometimes darkened ("black and blue") as a result of the trauma of being forced into the front of the shoe. The first metatarsal joint may be warm and slightly inflamed.

The shoe may show signs that the nail is pushing forward. By palpating the inside of the shoe on the area where the nail of the first toe would rest, one often feels a wear pattern—sometimes to the point that there is tearing through the anterior portion of the shoe. If the shoe has an insert, removing it to inspect the imprint made by the first toe may reveal that the shoe is too small.

Distortion of the first metatarsal joint usually involves the proximal phalanx jamming posteriorly into the first metatarsal bone. This can be challenged; if a muscle inhibition such as that in a psoas is used, gently pulling the first phalanx distally will result in a normalization of the psoas muscle. When a normal muscle is used, such as the tensor fascia lata, pushing the phalanx proximally to temporarily worsen the problem will cause tensor fascia lata inhibition.

Correction is twofold. The joint is tractioned anteriorly by grasping the proximal phalanx and lightly tractioning it distally, and the cause of the problem must be addressed so that the problem does not recur. Recurrence is usually the result of wearing shoes that are too small overall or too short.

FIBULA DYSFUNCTION

The fibula is another example of a bone that may require light traction. Like all extravertebral bones, the fibula can be challenged and does not produce a rebound. A problem with this bone is often at the proximal end, with the head distorted, or "jamming" posteriorly, most often due to trauma. (Occasionally the distal joint can become distorted.) This ordinarily produces localized pain, although when chronic, the pain may be more general and difficult for the patient to localize.

Challenging the head of the fibula posterior, causing a normal muscle to become inhibited, or challenging the head anterior, causing an inhibited muscle to normalize, means that the correction will be made from posterior to anterior. This is best done with the patient supine and the hip and knee flexed and the foot flat on the table. The practitioner sits in front of the foot and places one hand around the lateral side of the proximal leg so that the index finger contacts the posterior aspect of the head of the fibula, with the other hand around the medial leg placing it on top of the first hand. Traction is done anteriorly and held for about 30 sec. The practitioner rechallenges to ascertain that the correction has been made and asks the patient to run in place or perform other activities to ensure that the problem will not immediately return.

RIB JOINT DYSFUNCTION

Another common problem encountered in a complementary sports medicine practice is joint dysfunction of a rib articulation, resulting, in most cases, from trauma and producing localized pain. Occasionally, improper movement and distortion occur with several ribs. This may have adverse effects on breathing—usually reflected in a diminished vital capacity as described in chapter 8. When assessing using a challenge, one needs to remember that the anterior rib joints do not have a rebound effect whereas the posterior rib articulations do have a rebound effect. The reason for the difference may be that the posterior rib joints are located near the spine (whose joints rebound) and thus act similarly.

Rib joint dysfunction may occur anterior along the sternum, but it is often found posterior along the spine. Rib problems often occur as an individual joint dysfunction. When several ribs have problems, they can all be challenged as a group. For example, the practitioner places both hands against the posterior rib cage 2 or 3 cm lateral of the spine and challenges the ribs in a superior direction. If this causes a normal muscle to become inhibited, the next step is to determine whether a phase of respiration negates the inhibition (usually inhalation). Correction is made by gently pushing in the direction that caused inhibition, during inhalation, four to five times. The ribs are rechallenged to ensure that the proper correction was made. Measuring vital capacity before and after this treatment sometimes shows a significant improvement in the vital capacity.

WRIST JOINT DYSFUNCTION

Dysfunctions of the wrist joint, similar to those of the calcaneus, can be likened to a "functional carpal tunnel syndrome" and are often misdiagnosed as the more serious version. They are very common in athletes who play racket sports or in those who traumatize the wrist by hyperextension. There is frequently local pain or dysfunction, but sometimes the wrist is asymptomatic. In either case, secondary problems may occur, especially in the elbow. A tennis player, for example, may develop an asymptomatic wrist dysfunction that ultimately causes pain in the general area of the lateral elbow ("tennis elbow"). In some cases, a secondary trigger point is found in the extensor carpi radialis muscle, or there is a secondary dysfunction of the proximal ulna or radius. Correcting the primary wrist problem usually eliminates these secondary problems and their symptoms.

Assessment of the wrist dysfunction is made by testing the muscles that support the wrist as described in chapter 10, especially the general wrist extensors, and using a general muscle test of approximating the thumb and fifth finger. Inhibition of these muscles is often due to local micro- or macrotrauma and requires GTO/spindle cell therapy.

Dysfunction in the radioulnar joint is a common occurrence in wrist dysfunction. The action of wrist extension causes the distal end of the ulna and radius to separate, causing joint dysfunction. In this case, approximating the distal ends of these two bones will cause an inhibited muscle to normalize, or separating the joint further (by lightly extending the wrist) will cause inhibition in a normal muscle. To make the correction, the practitioner grasps the distal end of the radius with the thenar pad of the thumb with the fingers wrapped around the ulna; the other hand is then placed over the first as shown in figure 16.4. Light traction and a "squeezing" mild pressure are applied, approximating the two bones. The joint is challenged and put through its ranges of motion to ensure that there is no immediate re-

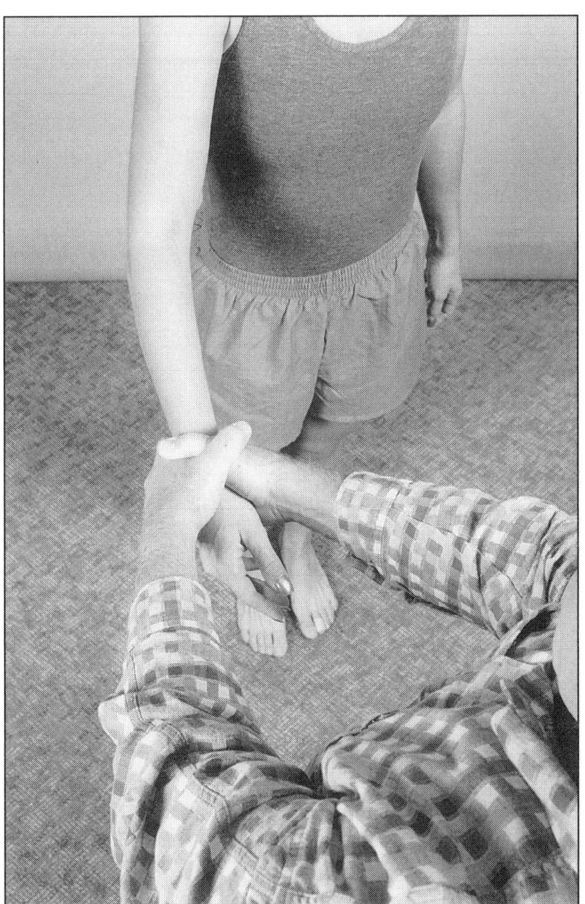

Figure 16.4 Position for the correction of a wrist joint dysfunction

currence. Occasionally the wrist requires additional support via taping or a wrist brace for three to five days. However, support should be provided only after all joint and muscle imbalances have been corrected.

CONCLUSION

Any vertebra or extravertebral bone or joint can be evaluated for dysfunction. Therapy localization informs the practitioner that a problem may exist in that location. The challenge, along with other evaluations, is useful for determining what type of problem exists. While the cranium, pelvis, vertebrae, and posterior rib joints have a rebound when challenged, all extravertebral bones and joints do not. After correction, it is equally important to perform a reassessment, including physically stressing the area, to ensure that the problem has been properly treated and will not recur too easily.

Pain and Pain Control

This chapter concerns the use of certain acupuncture points to control pain. In this connection, however, it is important for both practitioner and patient to understand the various aspects of pain, including its positive attributes. The chapter also includes a discussion of muscle pain, with specific directions for assessment and treatment possibilities.

Among the "benefits" of pain are that it informs the patient of a problem, provides the practitioner with important information, helps the body compensate (i.e., by shifting weight bearing), and often—but not always—prevents the patient from continuing the activity that caused the pain. But the lack of pain is meaningful also. As implied throughout this text, pain need not exist for there to be a problem. Significant dysfunction is possible without symptoms of pain.

ORIGINS OF PAIN

Pain originates in nerve endings or pain receptors called nociceptors, which are found predominantly in the skin, blood vessels, nerve fibers, joints, and periosteum and within the cranium (Guyton 1986). If the nervous system transmission from these nociceptors ends in the limbic system (within the cortex), it is interpreted by the person as pain. (Some transmissions from nociceptor stimulation do not end in the limbic system and therefore do not result in pain awareness.) Technically, pain is an emotion as opposed to a "sense", such as the sense of smell or taste. If the nervous system included pain in the same neurological sense as smell, taste, vision, and hearing, it would be much more difficult, if not practically impossible, to control pain by physical (e.g., acupuncture, cold), chemical (e.g., aspirin), or mental (e.g., hypnosis) measures.

Pain originates from one (or more) of three types of nociceptor stimulation:

- Mechanical stress, including physical micro- or macrotrauma or pressure, such as a swelling, may produce pain through the mechanical stimulation of nociceptors.
- Chemical stress may produce pain through the chemical stimulation of nociceptors. By-products of both inflammation (including prostaglandins and histamine) and muscle fatigue (such as lactic acid) are responsible for this effect.

- Thermal stress, such as cold or heat, may produce pain through the thermal stimulation of nociceptors. In some situations, cold pain may begin below 15 °C (59 °F) and heat pain at or above 45 °C (113 °F).

It is not unusual to develop pain from more than one source. Muscle spasm, for example, may cause pain from physical stress (mechanical stimulation of nociceptors) and through ischemia and the accumulation of metabolic by-products (chemical stimulation of nociceptors). Also, sunburn (thermal stimulation of nociceptors) causes physical tissue damage (mechanical stimulation of nociceptors) and inflammation (chemical stimulation of nociceptors).

Pain Quality

Pain quality may be associated with its source and is an essential part of assessment in all patients. Although patients may complain just of pain, this complaint is usually too general, and the practitioner must obtain more precise information. For example, patients should be asked to describe their pain. Those with mechanical pain may use words such as "stabbing" or "knife-like," "pressure," or "grabbing." If the pain is from mechanoreceptors around blood vessels, the words "pulsating," "throbbing," or "pounding" are often used. In these instances, physical problems may be found to be causing the pain. If chemical causes exist, the patient typically describes the pain as "hot," "searing," or "burning." When chemoreceptor-stimulated pain occurs, addressing the chemical needs of the patient is vital to a successful therapeutic outcome. Words typically used by patients to describe their pain, providing practitioners with clues about its source, are as follows:

- Mechanical pain—stabbing, pressure, knife-like, grabbing
- Mechanical pain around a blood vessel—pulsating, throbbing, pounding
- Chemical pain—burning, hot, searing

Unlike other bodily senses, the nociceptors become more sensitive as the pain stimulus becomes more chronic. A patient with chronic pain will generally become increasingly aware of the problem, sometimes to the point of becoming hyperalgesic.

PAIN AS AN ASSESSMENT TOOL

In addition to using pain as a general indicator of improvement over time, one can use pain as an assessment tool to furnish immediate information about how effective a particular therapy is during a treatment session. Although pain is relatively subjective, patient feedback still provides a good clinical indication of success or failure during the treatment process. In the majority of cases of dysfunction, the practitioner should look for significant improvements, such as a 50% or more reduction in pain, rather than a small change such as 10%. Following a particular treatment, it is important to ask the patient if the pain is the same, worse, or better. If the answer is either of the latter two, the patient should be asked to give a percentage change. For example, a patient may complain of "stabbing" shoulder pain that worsens during movement. The practitioner finds that the patient's attempt to touch the contralateral hip causes the most pain and uses this as one indication of treatment efficacy. If an inhibition of the middle deltoid is found and corrected, the patient is again asked to touch the same hip and states that now the movement produces only slightly less pain, about 10%. The practitioner then finds an inhibition of the pectoralis major clavicular and corrects it, and the patient is once more asked to touch the contralateral hip. This time the patient states that the pain is more than 50% improved. The practitioner then finds and corrects a closed temporomandibular joint problem, and this allows the patient to touch the hip with about a 95% pain reduction. Although this method puts the practitioner and/or the procedure "on the spot," it is most relevant in monitoring the success of the treatment.

Muscle testing that elicits pain from the muscle, ligaments, tendons, or joints may still be a valid method of assessment. Especially if the reason for the pain is a mechanical imbalance, correction of the primary problem(s) often results in a significant improvement as in the example just given. In addition, when there is a positive therapy localization, the painful muscle will not only have improved function, but often less pain occurs during retesting. A muscle test that causes excruciating pain may not be a useful assessment tool.

VISCERAL REFERRED PAIN

Practitioners are familiar with referred-pain patterns. For example, a patient with midthoracic spinal pain may actually have referred pain originating from the stomach. Differentiating the two is accomplished with an effective consultation and examination. Referred pain occurs because the sensory signals from the organ and those from a specific area of skin (the referred-pain area) synapse on the same cells in the spinal cord. These cells then transmit the message to the brain (via the ascending anterolateral spinal tracts), where it becomes impossible to differentiate between the origins of the signals. The most common referred-pain pattern is associated with a heart attack, which refers pain to the lower neck, shoulder, and arm—usually the left side, but occasionally the right.

NATURAL PAIN CONTROL

Some individuals are more tolerant of pain than others. The reason is probably the natural pain-control mechanisms of the nervous system. Two important neurotransmitters—serotonin and enkephalin—act to diminish pain at the level of the spinal cord. In addition, a number of naturally occurring endorphins and enkephalins in the brain have opiate-like qualities and play a part in pain reception.

In addition, tactile stimulation on the skin may block pain. This is accomplished by rubbing the skin at or near an area of pain. When people are injured, they typically, and usually subconsciously, rub the area of injury as a way to control pain; this stimulates large mechanoreceptor sensory fibers. This is the same mechanism as employed by transcutaneous electrical nerve stimulation devices, used in patients with extreme or continual pain.

NONSTEROIDAL ANTI-INFLAMMATORY DRUGS AND PAIN

Nonsteroidal anti-inflammatory drugs (NSAIDs), including aspirin (acetylsalicylic acid), are among the most commonly recommended and prescribed drugs in the world (Wright 1995). This includes significant use by athletes. The analgesic, anti-inflammatory, and antipyretic effects of these drugs are also accompanied by delayed tissue healing and other problems to be described later. Fatty acid manipulation used to improve the body's natural anti-inflammatory response and the pain-control techniques described in this chapter offer the complementary sports medicine practitioner potentially effective tools for patients who have pain and inflammation.

Nonsteroidal anti-inflammatory drugs have three main effects: analgesic, antipyretic, and anti-inflammatory. These effects, obtained through inhibition of the cyclooxygenase enzyme, result in not only inhibition of the pro-inflammatory prostaglandins but also, unfortunately, inhibition of natural anti-inflammatory prostaglandins. (Some inflammation continues through the lipoxygenase pathway that is not inhibited by NSAIDs.) However, the doses of over-the-counter NSAIDs primarily produce analgesic and anti-pyretic effects, and not anti-inflammatory (Amadio et al. 1993), although inflammation itself can contribute to edema and hyperalgesia (Portanova et al. 1996). Achieving anti-inflammatory effects from NSAIDs requires twice the dose needed to produce analgesic effects. The analgesic and antipyretic effects occur through actions in the central nervous system.

It has been theorized in complementary sports medicine that patients who improve their symptoms by taking NSAIDs have eicosanoid imbalance because NSAIDs "balance" eicosanoids. This concept has been applied to an oral challenge using aspirin. In this case, if an oral challenge with aspirin normalizes muscle inhibition, the practitioner considers eicosanoid imbalance and assesses this mechanism as discussed in chapters 18 and 19.

In addition to slowing inflammation through inhibition of the cyclooxygenase pathway, NSAIDs have other anti-inflammatory effects, including inhibition of neutrophil aggregations and migration to sites of injury, slowing of lysosomal enzyme release, reduction of oxygen free radicals by neutrophils and phagocytes, and inhibition of T-cell activity and histamine by mast cells (Hertel 1997). This may delay tissue healing and impair scar formation, resulting in diminished strength of the mature scar. Nonsteroidal anti-inflammatory drugs may also inhibit the repair process of fracture healing, since the first critical stage of this process involves inflammation (Khan 1997).

Nonsteroidal Anti-Inflammatory Drugs Side Effects

Nonsteroidal anti-inflammatory drugs are commonly associated with an increased incidence of gastric and duodenal ulcers, gastrointestinal (GI) bleeding, and increased morbidity and mortality (Dajani et al. 1991). The prevalence of GI ulcers in patients using NSAIDs for at least six months may be as much as 44% (Wright 1995). Interference by NSAIDs with prostaglandin activity in the GI tract, which is necessary for normal cytoprotective mucus formation, is the probable cause (Clyman 1986). In addition, GI blood flow may be reduced in patients taking NSAIDs (Taha et al. 1993). This could affect digestion and especially absorption of nutrients.

Other adverse side effects of NSAIDs have been reported. The use of NSAIDs can produce muscle dysfunction (Swaak 1997) due to biochemical alterations. Studies have not led to a consensus that NSAIDs adequately reduce delayed-onset muscle soreness (DOMS) (Hertel 1997).

Moreover, NSAIDs can adversely affect articular cartilage repair through inhibition of proteoglycan synthesis (David et al. 1992; Smith et al. 1995). The adverse effects of NSAIDs are greater on osteoarthritic cartilage than on normal cartilage (Brandt 1987).

Glucuronosyltransferase (an enzyme involved in chondroitin sulfate metabolism) activity was inhibited by sodium salicylate and aspirin in concentrations commonly reached in synovial fluid of patients treated with an anti-inflammatory dose of the drug, by 54% and 75%, respectively (Hugenberg et al. 1993). Nonsteroidal anti-inflammatory drugs may cause kidney damage, especially in those who are dehydrated (Hertel 1997).

Other side effects of NSAIDs can include headaches, skin rash (Wright 1995), tinnitus, and drowsiness (Hertel 1997). In addition, especially aspirin, acetaminophen, and ibuprofen can interfere with normal sleep patterns, including suppression of melatonin and changes in body temperature (Murphy et al. 1994, 1996). Reye's syndrome (a potentially fatal condition in children causing liver, neurological, and mitochondrial damage) has been associated with use of aspirin and other salicylates in conjunction with viral infections (Koester 1993).

Effectiveness of Nonsteroidal Anti-Inflammatory Drugs

An important question to ask all patients taking a NSAID is whether it helps their pain. Among patients who take aspirin for pain, some continue to take it despite the fact that they do not obtain significant relief. Dieppe et al. (1993) demonstrated that 20 of 44 patients who had osteoarthritis were able to stop their regular NSAID use without return of significant pain (and without other therapy). It is important to know which of these two categories a patient belongs to, since this information may provide vital clues about certain fatty acids that may improve or worsen pain through prostaglandin production. In patients who get pain relief from aspirin, the need for essential fatty acids and for balancing dietary fats may exist.

It should be noted that acetaminophen (sold as Tylenol and Anacin 3) also has analgesic and antipyretic effects but does not have anti-inflammatory actions (Koester 1993). Prolonged overuse or use with alcohol may result in liver damage. The NSAIDs can also cause liver damage.

OTHER DRUGS AND PAIN

Tranquilizers (benzodiazepines) such as Valium and Xanax may diminish pain through the action of reducing anxiety (Schmitt 1988). Anxiety may stimulate cortical arousal and increase pain awareness. Other drugs may also affect pain; alcohol depresses neurons in the central nervous system and can suppress pain, although small amounts may amplify pain. Caffeine may also increase pain sensation. A variety of other medications are often used for specific pain patterns in patients with migraine headaches, burns, and cancer as well as in other clinical situations. Discussion of these is beyond the scope of this text, as is the potential for addiction from longer-term use of certain pain medications. Any painkiller may cause an increased reliance on the part of the patient—all the more reason to find and eliminate the cause of the pain.

NATURALLY OCCURRING CHEMICALS IN PAIN CONTROL

Since chemoreceptor stimulation is a significant source of pain, other chemical relationships must be considered for pain control. In addition to balancing prostaglandin production with diet and supplementation, a number of other factors must be considered. According to Schmitt (1988), six chemicals may cause stimulation of chemoreceptors; in the order of their effectiveness to depolarize pain nerve endings, these are histamine, prostaglandins, leukotrienes, kinins, serotonin, and potassium ions. Lactic acid (by-product of muscle fatigue) does not cause pain directly but rather by creating an acid medium that can cause activation of kinins. In addition to creating their own nociceptor stimulation to produce pain, these chemicals can amplify existing mechanical stimulation of nociceptors, exaggerating pain.

Schmitt (1988) states, "Controlling pain must consider all aspects of the generation and transmission of the nerve impulses that create pain. This includes an evaluation of the patient's body chemistry to determine whether or not there is a chemical basis for part or all of the patient's pain" (pp. 3-4). In some patients, allergies may contribute significantly to their pain since histamine production may be high. In these cases, the source of potential allergens (foods, environmental chemicals, etc.) must be controlled and the related body dysfunction (such as adrenal, GI, or immune dysfunction) corrected. These patients will typically get relief from antihistamines and usually have a positive oral challenge to the amino acid histidine, the precursor to histamine, and to foods or other allergens. Products such as Antronex (Standard Process, Inc.), which may have natural antihistamine effects, may be useful not only as therapy but also as part of the assessment process. For example, if a patient's muscle inhibition normalizes with an oral challenge to Antronex or an over-the-counter antihistamine (e.g., diphenhydramine), this may indicate the patient's susceptibility to some allergy. It is then up to the patient and practitioner to find out which substance or substances may be allergy producing (i.e., elements of the diet, airborne substances, matter from animals).

Another chemical that can have significant effects on pain is oxygen free radicals when produced in excess. Significant relief from pain can be achieved through control of these free radicals with the correct antioxidants. This is especially important in athletes performing increased anaerobic work (because of increased lactic acid production); the condition is frequently associated with overtraining.

Another common source of pain is certain by-products of muscle activity, especially during muscle fatigue. These include potassium ions and, indirectly, lactic acid. Both increased sweating and hypoadrenia result in sodium loss and potassium excess; this problem is common in athletes. Lactic acid excess may exist in patients who perform too much anaerobic training as described earlier and in those who are unable to chemically break down lactic acid, a process that requires thiamin and other nutrients. In addition, increased dietary fat and reduced carbohydrates can reduce pain tolerance.

ACUPUNCTURE THERAPY FOR PAIN CONTROL

Traditionally, a variety of acupuncture points have been used for pain control, many times selected in a "cookbook" fashion. Unfortunately, there is no one point or set of points that is always successful in all patients. Each patient with pain is unique, and the successful control of pain is best accomplished through the assessment and treatment of specific acupuncture point(s) for a particular patient's need at that precise time. Finding the most successful point is the goal of an effective assessment process. It must also be emphasized that pain is often the result of—or is amplified by—some physical, chemical, or emotional imbalance and that the first step in pain control is to treat the cause of the pain. Therefore, it is important when one is using pain-control techniques to have corrected the patient's overall imbalances first. (In some instances, such as an on-the-field injury, this is not always immediately possible.) Indeed, if the cause of the pain is a mechanical dysfunction or one or more chemical problems that are not addressed, acupuncture pain control may not work. Even in the case of a bone fracture, there are typically functional problems; correction of these not only helps control pain, but also speeds the healing process.

Case History

Fred, who had been under my care for two years, had severely fractured his fibula as a result of a collision with an opponent during a soccer match. The orthopedist successfully tended to his immediate first-aid needs that day. The next day, Fred consulted me. His leg was very painful, and certain areas on his fibula elicited more pain on palpation. Fred had a number of inhibited muscles, all on the same side as the fibula fracture: the tensor fascia lata and piriformis (both requiring stimulation of Chapman's reflexes); peroneus longus, brevis, and tertius, assessed with therapy localization to the muscles rather than testing of the muscles (all requiring Golgi tendon organ [GTO]/spindle cell therapy); and psoas major (related to a lateral talus corrected by respiration). There was a pelvic Category I fault with a cranial-sacral inspiration assist that was corrected. Reevaluation of Fred's lateral leg for pain indicated an approximately 40% improvement. A specific acupuncture point on the left medial knee, KI 10, was stimulated for pain control. Immediately following this treatment, the lateral leg was again reevaluated for pain and showed more than 90% improvement, which was maintained and improved during the healing process.

In the next section, two separate techniques are described that are used to treat specific acupuncture points by tapping (various methods of treating acupuncture points were discussed in chapter 10). The most effective points are found through use of muscle testing as an assessment tool. The two techniques are stimulation of acupuncture tonification points on the arms and legs and stimulation of the so-called beginning and end points on the face.

PAIN CONTROL USING TONIFICATION POINTS

In Chinese medicine, tonification points are traditionally used when qi needs to be increased in a particular meridian. Each meridian has a tonification point. Goodheart (1977) first described these and other related points as a way to individualize pain-control techniques, and the clinical outcome continues to be successful, especially when inflammation is present. The following is a list of the tonification points with a brief description of the location of each. Figure 17.1, a–d, shows the locations of these points.

- LU 9: Anterior wrist at the most lateral end of the wrist crease
- LI 11: Lateral end of the elbow crease found during elbow flexion
- ST 41: Mid-dorsum of foot at anterior ankle flexure, lateral to the tibialis anterior tendon
- SP 2: Medial edge of big toe at base of the proximal phalanx (distal to the gait reflex SP 3)
- HT 9: Just proximal to the nail of the fifth finger on radial side
- SI 3: Medial side of hand just proximal to head of the fifth metacarpal
- BL 67: Just lateral to the fifth toenail
- KI 7: Three finger-widths above and slightly posterior to the medial malleolus
- CX 9: Just proximal to the nail of the third finger on the radial side
- TH 3: Posterior hand just proximal to the fourth metacarpal head on the ulnar side
- GB 43: Lateral to the proximal end of the fourth proximal phalanx (gait reflex is GB 42)
- LV 8: Medial knee just posterior to the medial meniscus (intertubercular space)

The first step in finding the best point for pain control is to determine which meridian is underactive. This is associated with a muscle inhibition. (The relationships between muscles and meridians and between muscles and organs were described in chapters 10 and 11, respectively.) For example, if the patient has an inhibition of the sartorius muscle only (related to the

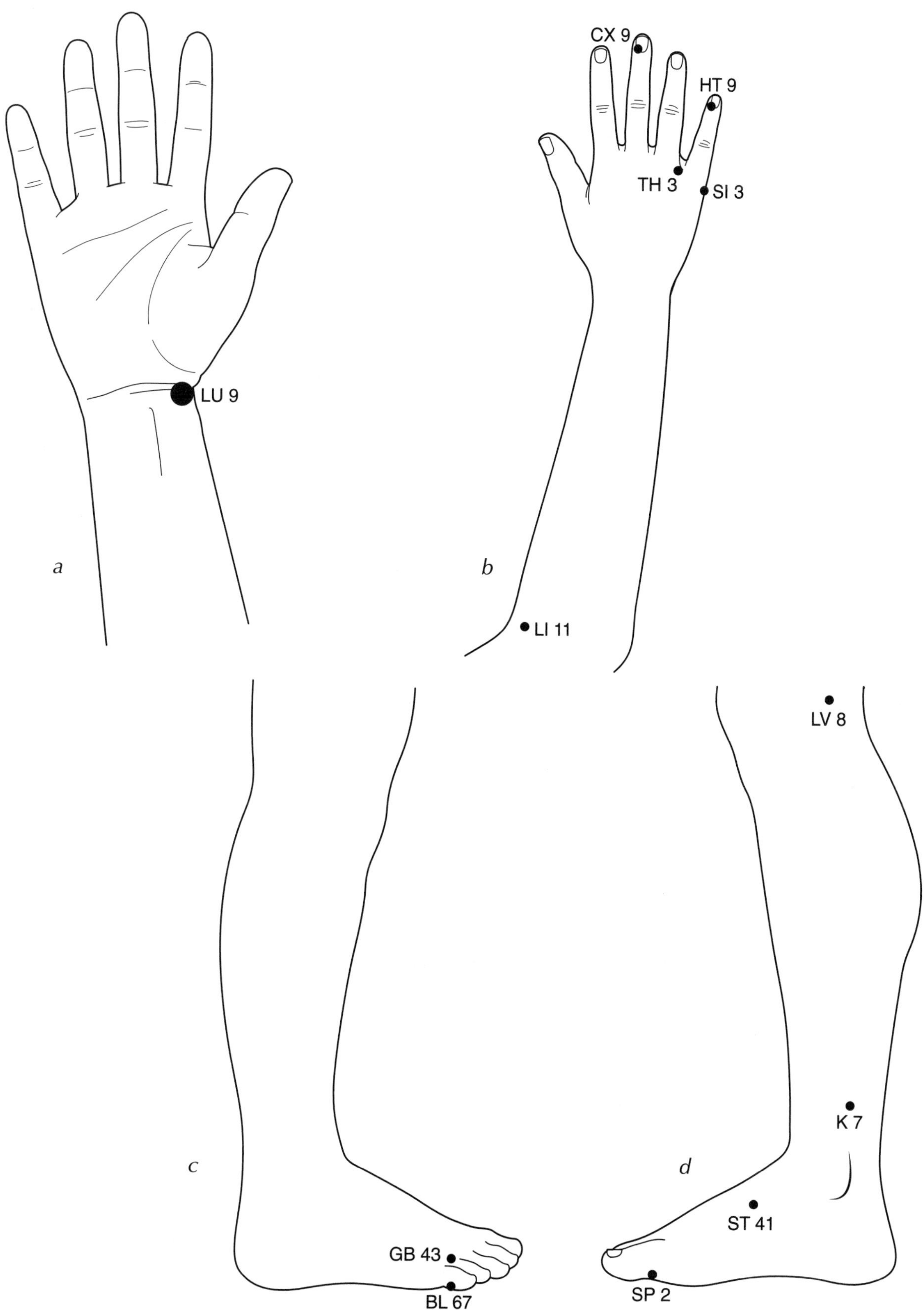

Figure 17.1a–d Location of acupuncture meridian tonification points: (*a*) palmar view; (*b*) dorsal view; (*c*) lateral view; (*d*) medial view.

CX meridian), the best point for pain control may be CX 9. If the patient has more than one muscle inhibition, therapy localization can help the practitioner find the most therapeutic point. If, for example, the sartorius, psoas (related to KI 7), and pectoralis major clavicular (ST 41) were inhibited, the practitioner would need to therapy-localize each of the three related tonification points (CX 9, KI 7, and ST 41) to discover which one was positive. Rarely will more than one positive tonification point be found.

An alternative approach is to stimulate each suspected point by tapping it several times and retesting the inhibited muscle. The most useful point for pain control (and the primary therapy point) will be the one that when stimulated normalizes the inhibited muscle (most likely, this will also normalize all inhibited muscles).

Once an acupuncture point is found, it is tapped rapidly at the rate of approximately four taps per second for about 20-30 sec. It is important to obtain feedback from the patient regarding the pain before and after stimulating the point. If the pain is not improved, more stimulation may be required. Sometimes the point requires stimulation for more than 1 min, and occasionally, pain reduction is maximized by tapping at a slower rate.

If the pain has not changed or is not improved by more than 50% after stimulation of the tonification point, stimulation of an additional corresponding point may be required. In Chinese medicine, this point is called the associated point. The associated points are on the bladder meridian just lateral to the spine on each side, located from the level of approximately the third thoracic vertebra to the second sacral foramen. Table 17.1 lists each associated point and its spinal location. For additional pain control, one treats the point associated with the tonification point (and meridian) that has already been treated. The best approach when treating the associated point is to tap it concurrently and simultaneously with the tonification point.

Note that when any of the associated points are successfully treated, the related inhibited muscles should normalize. Continued inhibition of the related muscle after treatment indicates that more therapy is required. This may mean more tapping on either acupuncture point or possibly the need to correct other problems. Occasionally, the spinal area related to the associated point may be dysfunctional, as a primary or secondary problem. If the dysfunction is primary, correction may result in additional improvement in pain. If it is secondary, the primary problem(s), typically other muscle imbalances, must be assessed and treated.

Table 17.1 Tonification and Associated Points and Corresponding Spinal Level

Tonification point	Associated point	Spinal level
LU 9	BL 13	Between T3 and 4 transverse processes
LI 11	BL 25	Between L4 and 5 transverse processes
ST 41	BL 21	Between T12 and L1 transverse processes
SP 2	BL 20	Between T11 and 12 transverse processes
HT 9	BL 15	Between T5 and 6 transverse processes
SI 3	BL 27	At first sacral foramen
BL 67	BL 28	At second sacral foramen
KI 7	BL 23	Between L2 and 3 transverse processes
CX 9	BL 14	Between T4 and 5 transverse processes
TH 3	BL 22	Between L1 and 2 transverse processes
GB 43	BL 19	Between T10 and 11 transverse processes
LV 8	BL 18	Between T9 and 10 transverse processes

Tonification Point Pain Control

1. The practitioner determines which meridian is the primary problem (by finding an inhibited muscle).
2. The practitioner locates and treats the tonification point on that meridian by tapping for 20-30 sec.
3. The patient's pain is monitored.
4. If there is no significant improvement, the practitioner continues tapping on the tonification point or changes to a slower rate of tapping.
5. If there is no significant improvement, the practitioner locates the related associated point on the spine and taps that concurrently and simultaneously with the tonification point.

If there is still no significant change, one should consider using the second approach to be described, which utilizes the beginning and end meridian points on the face.

Those who are more familiar with meridian therapy may find two other methods of finding the best tonification point helpful. Using the acupuncture meridian pulse points on the radial artery of each wrist (which represent the 12 meridians), therapy localization is employed to determine which of two paired pulse points is positive. The muscles related to these paired pulse points are both tested; the inhibited one is usually related to the "low-energy" meridian, and its tonification point is treated. For example, suppose a normal psoas muscle is used for testing. The patient therapy-localizes the three pulse points on the right wrist (representing 6 of the meridians), touching each one with a different finger. If this does not change the psoas muscle, the left wrist points are therapy-localized. If this causes inhibition of the psoas, each point is therapy-localized separately. If the SI/HT point causes the psoas to become inhibited, the related muscles are tested (quadriceps and subscapularis, respectively). If the subscapularis is inhibited, HT 9 is treated. The second alternative method of finding the best tonification point uses an inhibited muscle. The suspected tonification point is therapy-localized or tapped several times; if this normalizes an inhibited muscle, the test is positive, and that point requires stimulation.

PAIN CONTROL USING BEGINNING AND END POINTS

As an alternative to using tonification points as a method of pain control, or when this method is not effective, the meridian beginning and end points on the face may be helpful for pain control. These were originally described by Schmitt (1989). The locations of the points are described here and shown in figure 17.2. These points were also discussed in chapter 11 in relation to their use for certain psychological conditions.

- BL 1: Just lateral to the lateral canthus of the eye
- TH 23: Lateral edge of eyebrow
- BL 1: Medial eye between medial canthus and nasal bone
- ST 1: On infraorbital ridge directly below pupil
- LI 20: Just lateral and inferior to the nasal sulcus
- SI 19: Just anterior to the tragus of the ear in an indentation made when mouth is open (the best position for treatment)

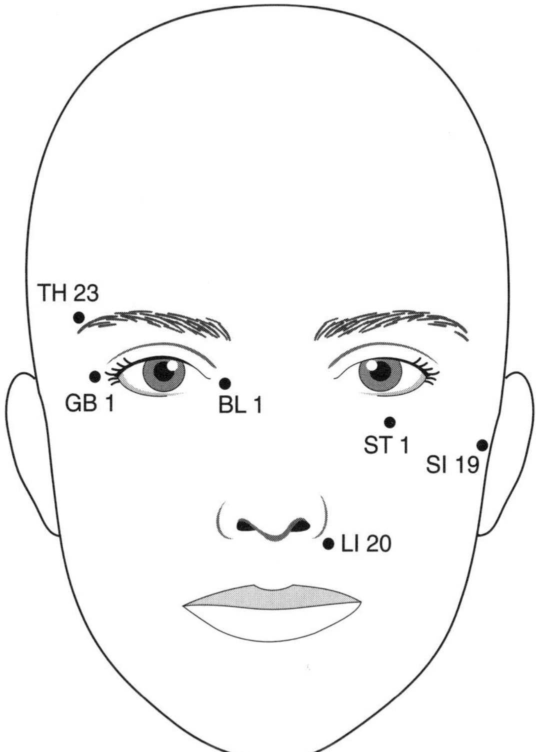

Figure 17.2 Location of the acupuncture meridian beginning and end points

The most useful point for pain control is found by using muscle testing. Testing a normal muscle, the practitioner carefully reproduces or slightly exaggerates the pain area. This can be done by pushing on a painful area such as a muscle or bone, or moving a painful joint. The test muscle is immediately retested. If it becomes inhibited, the process is repeated with the patient therapy-localizing the beginning and end points on the face; this can be done by touching more than one point at a time. In some cases the patient can touch several or all of the points on one side of the face with one hand. (If the test muscle does not become inhibited after the elicitation of pain, either the pain was not strong enough or the technique is not useful in this instance.) The goal is to find the one point that negates the muscle inhibition. For example, in a patient with a fractured clavicle, palpation on the point of fracture produces increased pain and also inhibition of a normal psoas muscle. The patient places one hand on the left side of the face with the practitioner making sure that all the acupuncture points are being touched. The clavicle is palpated again, and this time the pain does not cause psoas muscle inhibition. The patient then touches each acupuncture point; each time, the practitioner palpates the clavicle, causing psoas inhibition, until therapy-localizing one point does not cause the psoas to become inhibited. This is the acupuncture point used for treatment.

In patients who have intense pain or who have just been injured, all muscles may be inhibited. In this case, the practitioner uses any inhibited muscle and finds the point (by therapy-localizing or tapping each point a few times) that normalizes the muscle.

The acupuncture point is treated by tapping for 20-30 sec or until pain reduction is maximized. This can take up to one to two minutes or more in acute and on-the-field situations.

Beginning and End Point Pain Control

1. Using a normal muscle, the practitioner slightly exaggerates the pain in the patient to cause muscle inhibition.
2. The practitioner determines which acupuncture point on the face negates this inhibition.
3. An alternative is to use an inhibited muscle to determine which point (through therapy localization or by tapping each point a few times) normalizes muscle function.
4. The practitioner taps this acupuncture point for 20-30 sec at a rate of about four taps per second, or longer if required.
5. The pain is reevaluated.

When a point is found that significantly eliminates pain, patients can be shown how to stimulate that point themselves if the pain returns. The practitioner should show the patient exactly where the point is or can mark it on the skin. In some cases, however, that same point will lose effectiveness and it may be necessary to find another point.

In addition to using the tonification, associated, and beginning and end points for pain control, many practitioners consider these common acupuncture points routinely as a therapy for any imbalance. It is possible for any of these acupuncture points to be a primary problem in any patient, even those without pain. Correcting these points will result not only in improved muscle balance (in muscles corresponding to the respective meridians), but also potential improvements in organ and gland function, mental and emotional state, and other types of balance.

MUSCLE PAIN

Generally considered, there are three types of discomfort and pain related to exercise in athletes who are not injured:

- Pain experienced during or immediately after workouts
- Delayed-onset muscle soreness (DOMS)
- Pain induced by muscle cramps (Miles and Clarkson 1994)

The degree of pain is positively associated with the intensity and duration of the workout; the type of workout performed with eccentric muscle contractions produces the greatest pain (McArdle et al. 1991). Associated with this discomfort and pain is diminished performance that is due to factors other than pain (Cleak and Eston 1992). Although some information is available about these phenomena, many of the underlying mechanisms have not yet been discovered.

Pain experienced during or immediately after a workout usually has a chemical origin, perhaps including a hormonal component. Lactic acid does not cause pain directly, but may be responsible for pH changes or bradykinin production that may be associated with pain. Circulatory factors, specifically the occlusion of blood flow, may also be linked to this type of muscle pain. If this is the case, the pain will subside quickly once activity is stopped.

Delayed-onset muscle soreness usually develops within 24-48 hr after activity, with a peak in discomfort between 48 and 72 hr (and only occasionally longer). This pain is associated with structural stress, that is, damage to the muscle. Muscle dysfunction (inhibition) and diminished range of motion accompany discomfort and pain, although the muscle dysfunction may continue after pain has resolved (Cleak and Eston 1992). A common cause of DOMS may be localized at the origin and insertion of the muscle, in the area of the musculotendinous junction (Safran et al. 1988). These types of problems respond very well to GTO/spindle cell therapy. Chemical stress may also be associated with elevated blood creatine kinase and myoglobin levels and with inflammation. However, inflammation does not always parallel the pain, confirming that the pain comes from more than one source (Kuipers 1994). Another chemical stress may come in the form of free radical damage (Pyne 1994).

Muscle cramps may occur any time as a sudden onset of pain and in association with motor neuron hyperexcitability. The cause of muscle cramps is unknown, and it appears that this is somewhat individual. Cramping during activity may be associated with electrolyte imbalance, although most studies have not been able to support this the way empirical evidence has.

Clinically the three most successful responses to treatment are seen after correction of structural imbalances (within the muscle and other primary mechanical problems, especially in the foot, ankle, or pelvis), proper hydration, and the use of sodium (the latter two are discussed in chapter 20). According to Miles and Clarkson (1994), low magnesium may also be a factor. A common aspect of structural imbalance includes the need for GTO/spindle cell technique as previously described. Bentley (1996) holds that the GTOs and muscle spindles may dysfunction after exercise resulting in increased motor neuron activity and motor unit recruitment, stating, "Treatment of cramp is directed at reducing muscle spindle and motor neuron activity by reflex inhibition and afferent stimulation" (p. 409).

It is important for the practitioner to assess and treat each patient's problem individually rather than using a prescribed formula for muscle soreness or pain. Stretching is a typical example of a general recommendation, but static and ballistic stretching have both been shown to significantly increase DOMS and creatine kinase (Smith et al. 1993). In general, regular muscle soreness may not be normal; and muscle pain, with few exceptions (such as after a competition), may also be abnormal.

Not only do postexercise symptoms constitute important information, but the outcome of the follow-up treatment also provides critical information for future assessment and treatment sessions. This information is especially important for lifestyle recommendations on such issues as training and diet and nutrition, discussed in the next three chapters.

CONCLUSION

An understanding of the mechanisms of pain helps form the basis for taking a history from an athlete who has pain. Proper use of various aspects of the acupuncture system with tapping can significantly reduce pain. This is accomplished first through a complete assessment process to find the specific point or points that best match the patient's needs. Using a "cookbook" formula for pain control may sometimes be helpful for some patients but for the most part is overly general and not recommended.

Diet Therapy

The simplest but most important concept regarding the diet is the desirability of eating a variety of foods in as fresh, unprocessed, and whole a state as possible. Obtaining a balanced diet should be the focus of both the practitioner and patient. This is accomplished through proper assessment, correction of dietary imbalance, and reassessment of the patient's diet on a regular basis. As each patient is unique, learning to adjust to the body's needs is a priority and may best be considered as an ongoing food "trial."

THE THERAPEUTIC EFFECT OF FOOD

Fresh foods have a therapeutic effect. Potter and Steinmetz (1996) describe these effects of common dietary foods, with emphasis on vegetables and fruits. All levels of medical practices—both past and present—often involve the prescription of specific foods (almost always plants), or their potent derivatives, to treat a wide spectrum of illnesses. Some of these "prescribed" foods include the Cruciferae group (cabbages, broccoli, cauliflower, kale), the allium family foods (garlic and onion), legumes (beans, bean sprouts, peas), and others such as celery, cucumber, endive, and parsley. Plant foods also have preventive potential, especially raw and fresh fruits and vegetables. Consumption of these foods is lower in those who subsequently develop cancer.

Also, most soy products (such as soybeans and tofu), which contain isoflavones and affect estrogen activity, are associated with a lower risk of sex hormone-related cancers. Phytoestrogens (plant estrogens) are also derived from some vegetables and berries as well as from grains and seeds.

Unfortunately, a recent survey showed that only 1 in 11 Americans eats at least three servings of vegetables and two servings of fruit per day; 1 in 9 ate no vegetable or fruit on the survey day (Craig 1997). Consumption of more vegetables and fruits can not only improve health, but may also improve fitness levels and potentially performance, as part of the process of improving the body's overall balance.

ENERGY FROM FOOD

Another key function of the diet is to provide the nutrients that help generate the energy obtained from macronutrients. The energy used to power human movement and all other activity, even at rest, is derived from dietary macronutrients—carbohydrates, fats, and proteins. In addition, micronutrients and other important substances, such as many phytonutrients and fibers prevalent in nature, should be supplied by these macronutrients. When and if this is not possible, the diet must be supplemented.

The energy content of foods can be defined as either kilocalories (kcal) or kilojoules (kJ) and is measured by scientists from the complete combustion of food in a bomb calorimeter (1 kcal equals 4.128 kJ). One kilocalorie is the amount of heat required to raise the temperature of one liter of water 1 °C. Clinically, patients generally use the word calorie (a common term for kilocalorie). Foods are oxidized to CO_2, water, heat, and adenosine triphosphate, and the energy is used for three bodily functions:

- Basal metabolism maintains the body's basic metabolic functions at rest.
- Diet-induced thermogenesis provides energy to digest, absorb, distribute, and store food and its nutrients and to stimulate brown adipose tissue to produce heat.
- Physical activities require varying amounts of energy depending on work intensity. The adenosine triphosphate produced in the body is derived mostly from carbohydrates (as glucose) and fats (as fatty acids), with much smaller quantities derived from protein (certain amino acids).

Disordered eating is common in athletes, predominantly women, and often involves reduced intake of appropriate kilocalories in relation to energy expenditure. Female athletes have an incidence of eating disorders as high as 62% (Benson et al. 1996). This is a complex issue with a full spectrum of eating problems, from poor eating, dieting, and preoccupation with fat levels to anorexia nervosa and bulimia. Menstrual problems are frequently associated with disordered eating at all ranges of this spectrum. Vegetarianism is twice as high in amenorrheic runners as in eumenorrheic runners, possibly due to lower protein and/or higher carbohydrate intake.

MACRONUTRIENTS

A key concept in complementary sports medicine is that each patient's dietary requirements are unique, and an important part of therapy is finding the proper balance of carbohydrates, proteins, and fats. However, it would be extremely difficult, if not impossible, to determine each athlete's exact day-to-day nutritional needs. One goal of the practitioner is to work with the patient to help find the balance that best matches that individual's needs. An even higher priority is the education of patients regarding their dietary needs—not only from a scientific standpoint, but also in relation to the art of eating, or the instincts of diet selection—to help them avoid the marketing hype so prevalent in the sport community.

The Importance of Chewing Food

The taste receptors on the tongue detect extremely small concentrations of substances within a fraction of a second of stimulation by food (Guyton 1986). This stimulation elicits a variety of immediate responses throughout the body's systems, including the neurological, digestive, endocrine, cardiovascular, thermogenic, and renal systems; this type of response is referred to as a cephalic or preabsorptive response. It is vital that patients elicit this response by chewing their food. Mattes (1997) makes some important points on this subject:

- Mastication (chewing) involves many processes of action and produces the highest cephalic response, followed by taste, smell, sight, and thought of food. The cephalic-phase response improves or optimizes the digestion, absorption, and use of nutrients contained in ingested foods.
- Quality and quantity of the saliva, as well as the action of chewing, are important in the cephalic response and help regulate nutrient use through gastric (hydrochloric acid) and intestinal (pancreatic and other enzyme) phases of digestion.
- The cephalic response may affect nutritional status through enhanced nutrient absorption.
- Insulin and glucagon release begins with the cephalic response, especially with the chewing mechanism. This helps to control blood sugar.

• Thermogenesis is increased by the cephalic phase of eating.

• Cephalic stimulation may be involved in fluid and electrolyte balance (via a renal response).

• Infants with increased oral stimulation have enhanced growth and fewer medical complications.

Rather than counting each mouthful, patients should be encouraged to chew their food until it is crushed into very small pieces and thoroughly moistened with saliva. Learning to eat properly is the first step to good digestion and absorption of nutrients.

Macronutrient Self-Selection

Macronutrient self-selection is a topic of controversy, although many scientific studies, mostly of animals, demonstrate the phenomenon. Davis (1928) was one of the first to show the intuitive and instinctual aspects of self-selection of foods in human infants. Other researchers have reported on various aspects of self-selection in animals:

• Harper and Peters (1989) demonstrated self-selection between high- and low-protein diets to obtain adequate amounts of that macronutrient.

• Miller et al. (1994) provided evidence that rats on a self-selection diet ate most meals from a single macronutrient source.

• Cook et al. (1996) found that cats select appropriate diets to maintain acid-alkaline balance.

• Rieth and Larue-Achagiotis (1997) reported that exercising rats on a self-selection diet ate more fat but lost more body fat than those on regular feedings.

• Fromentin and Nicolaidis (1996) showed that rats were successful at self-selecting the proper combination of foods to balance amino acid needs.

• Larue-Achagiotis et al. (1992) found day-night patterns in self-selecting rats: during the day, carbohydrate intake was higher; during the night, protein and fat intakes were significantly higher.

In recent years, scientists have learned more about the possible mechanisms of self-selection. Tordoff and Friedman (1986) postulated that the relationship between food preference and intake is associated with glucoreceptors in the liver (which send messages to the central nervous system). According to Bernardis and Bellinger (1996), the lateral hypothalamic area is the location of dietary self-selection. Holder and DiBattista (1994) reported that protein intake following protein deprivation can be attributed in part to the oral-sensory properties of protein. Heinrichs and Koob (1992) showed that the action of the corticotropin-releasing factor was an important aspect in the control of dietary self-selection in rats. Thibault (1994) showed that the nature of the carbohydrate (i.e., glucose vs. fructose) was important in self-selection in rats.

Practitioners, or their staff, can help make patients more aware of their diets in several ways. First, it is important to have the patient keep a diet diary. The act of writing down one's weekly diet as meals are eaten rather than on recall (i.e., recalling all the food eaten over the past day or week) can have a significant impact. After going through this exercise, many patients report that they had been unaware of how much (or little) they consumed, how poorly they ate, or other factors regarding their eating habits.

Practitioners need to educate their patients about diet. Patients should also be made aware of any important relationships between their physical, chemical, or mental/emotional stress and diet. One can build such awareness by relating certain dietary habits to appropriate signs and symptoms (see chapter 7). For example, gastrointestinal discomfort may occur during a workout soon after breakfast but not during a workout 3 hr after lunch, or a Maximum Aerobic Function (MAF) test may be worse if it is performed after consumption of a sugared drink than if it is not.

Practitioners can also help patients perform their own food "trials"—with a pregame meal, for example—to help establish the optimal eating routine before events. Such trials can also be conducted with foods or drinks taken during and after competition. Patients should understand that their particular needs may be unique and often significantly different from those of their training companions, and their needs may change with time of year, training and competition, and aging.

Practitioners can also help athletes by reviewing the results of a computerized dietary analysis. Such a report often reinforces the importance of improving eating habits and of emphasizing the quality of carbohydrates (unprocessed vs. processed), proteins (amino acid balance), and fats (saturated vs. unsaturated).

Finally, the practitioner should periodically reassess the diet of the athlete. This can have an added value for patients, helping them to make progress with the diet itself and with their understanding of this important health and fitness component.

The Quality of Macronutrients

The quantity of food necessary for optimal health and fitness, in kilocalories, varies with each athlete. Grandjean (1997) demonstrated that the daily diets of elite athletes varied from 1865 kcal to over 6000 kcal, with percentages of energy from carbohydrate, protein, and fat ranging from 33% to 57%, 12% to 26%, and 29% to 49%, respectively.

Opinions vary regarding the ideal macronutrient makeup of the diet for an athlete. A traditional suggestion is a diet of predominantly carbohydrate, with 60-70% of food coming from carbohydrate, 12-15% from protein, and the remainder from fat (Williams 1995). Others have suggested that these high carbohydrate intakes, contrary to the beliefs of many athletes who follow this advice, may not provide additional performance benefits (Hawley et al. 1997). High-carbohydrate, low-fat diets may be favored partly because of a fear of eating too much fat and protein (Pendergast et al. 1996). The current U.S. Food Guide Pyramid suggests, for a 2800-kcal diet, 55% carbohydrate, 30% fat, and 15% protein

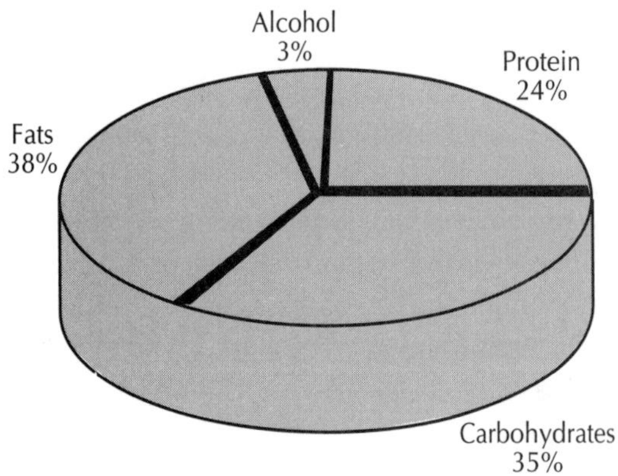

Figure 18.1 Example of determination of dietary macronutrients by computer analysis
Reprinted by permission of NutrAnalysis, Inc.

(Welsh 1996). In complementary sports medicine there is an understanding that each patient has his or her own specific requirements, and it is the goal of the practitioner to provide assistance in determining this balance. Figure 18.1 provides an example of dietary macronutrient determination via computer analysis.

CARBOHYDRATES

Dietary carbohydrates provide the body with glucose. This glucose is used in three ways: approximately 50% is used immediately for energy in the cells, approximately 40% is converted to fat, and up to 10% is converted to glycogen (Granner 1993). Insulin affects this utilization pattern. Insulin can increase fat stores and inhibit the utilization of fat for energy. Excess insulin (hyperinsulinemia) and high-carbohydrate diets have also been implicated in a number of disease states (Reaven 1997). In addition, Coulston et al. (1993) showed that a low-fat, high-carbohydrate diet increases insulin production in relatively healthy men and women. Recall that insulin also increases the activity of delta-5-desaturase, which converts gamma-linolenic acid to arachidonic acid to increase the production of the Series 2 eicosanoids, which is pro-inflammatory.

Many scientists believe that humans have no true requirement for concentrated carbohydrates (such as in grains, or sweeteners—natural or processed) (Szepesi 1996). But an important feature of concentrated carbohydrates is their fiber content. However, vegetables and fruits also offer significant amounts of fiber. Most individuals consume carbohydrates as the predominant macronutrient and source of glucose, typically from about 40% to 70% or more of their diet.

The quality of the carbohydrate food is an important factor and is related to the glycemic index (GI) (Wolever et al. 1994). The GI is a general measure of the ability of a carbohydrate food to raise blood sugar (and the production of insulin by the pancreas); many practitioners apply this measure to diets of athletes. In general, processed carbohydrate foods have a higher GI (raising blood sugar and insulin more quickly), and whole, unprocessed foods have a lower GI, although this is not always true. In addition, other factors in a meal can lower the GI of the meal, including its fat, protein, and fiber content (Joannic et al. 1997). The health of an individual also influences GI. The same meal may have a higher GI, for example, in a patient who is insulin-resistant compared to one who is not. Lower-glycemic foods produce greater satiety than high-glycemic foods (Holt et al. 1992). A number of studies have resulted in an extensive list of foods and their GIs. The most comprehensive of these studies was produced by combining all the others (Foster-Powell and Miller 1995). Table 18.1 lists some common foods and their GIs. Note that juices usually have a much higher GI than the whole fruit. For example, a grapefruit has a GI of 36 and the juice 69; an orange has an average GI of 62 and the juice 74.

Table 18.1 Some Common Foods and Food Groups and Their Average Glycemic Index Listing, Using White Bread as the Standard (GI = 100)

Food group/Food	Glycemic index
SUGAR	
Honey	104
Sucrose	92
Maltose	150
Glucose	138
Fructose	32
Soft drinks	97
GRAINS	
White bread	100
Whole-grain breads	52-73
Cakes and muffins	70-102
Bagel	103
Rolls	90-106
CEREALS	
All-Bran	45-75
Cheerios	106
Corn Flakes	110-130
Cream of Wheat	94-105
Crispix	124
Grapenuts	96
Nutri-Grain	94
Total	109
Oatmeal	77
1 Minute Oats	94
Puffed Wheat	96-114
Rice Krispies	117
Shredded Wheat	83-118
Special K	77
White rice	71-83
Instant rice	128
Brown rice	79
DAIRY FOODS	
Whole milk	39
Skim milk	46
Yogurt with fruit	47

Food group/Food	Glycemic index
FRESH FRUITS	
Apple	52
Apricot	44
Banana	76
Cherries	32
Grapefruit	36
Grapes	62
Orange	62
Peach	40
Pear	51
Pineapple	94
Plum	34
Raisins	91
Watermelon	103
BEANS	
Baked	69
Chick peas	47
Kidney	42
Green	42
Pinto	59
Soybeans	25
Lentils	41
Pasta	68 (average)
Peanuts	21
VEGETABLES	
Beets (root)	91
Carrots	101
Baked potato	121
Boiled potato	80
New potato	81
French fried potatoes	107
Sweet potato	77
Sweet corn	78
Peas	68
Yams	73

Reprinted by permission of NutrAnalysis, Inc.

Intake of high-quality (i.e., low glycemic) carbohydrates such as whole-grain foods and whole fruits, versus lower-quality (i.e., high glycemic) ones such as sucrose or white flour products (bagels, rolls, muffins) and fruit juice, may also affect athletic performance. Thomas et al. (1991, 1994) showed that low-glycemic foods resulted in higher concentrations of energy substrates, even after exercise, including more stable blood sugar levels.

The traditional concept from the '60s, '70s, and '80s, that muscle glycogen depletion is the factor associated with exercise fatigue, is being challenged in the '90s (Simi et al. 1991), although it has been known for many years that carbohydrate consumption 45 min before exercise may have a detrimental effect on performance (Foster et al. 1979). Bird and Hay (1987) showed that glucose taken 3 hr before exercise resulted in lower heart rates at the same intensity, whereas glucose consumed 1 hr before exercise had the opposite effect. In addition, carbohydrate "loading" prior to exercise does not necessarily result in sparing of muscle glycogen stores (Bosch et al. 1993, 1994). Excess carbohydrate may also inhibit the use of fats for energy (Nestel 1993), which do spare glycogen; and glucose and maltodextrin consumed before workouts raise the respiratory quotient (MacLaren et al. 1994), indicating diminished utilization of fats for energy.

Consuming large amounts of carbohydrates after exercise or competition, also a common routine for athletes, may help replace lost glycogen stores. But Tarnopolsky et al. (1997) found that a mixed meal of carbohydrate, protein, and fat will accomplish the same.

DIETARY FATS

As discussed in chapter 4, fats can provide significant amounts of potential energy not only for training and competition, but also for many other daily bodily functions. Grynberg and Demaison (1996) demonstrate that at times, the heart may derive 100% of its energy from fatty acids. The importance of fat as a nutrient for energy in endurance-type athletes is well established (Bjorntorp 1991). The use of higher-fat diets, but not excess fat (and reduced carbohydrate), to improve athletic performance in humans is also well supported in the literature (Muoio et al. 1994; Lambert et al. 1994; Griffiths et al. 1994; Pendergast et al. 1996). These studies demonstrated that increasing dietary fat above the traditionally recommended levels—or levels typically consumed by athletes—and reducing carbohydrate significantly improved $\dot{V}O_2$max, performance, endurance, carbohydrate sparing, and resistance to fatigue. Improved utilization of fats, which has been traditionally held to take place up to 60% $\dot{V}O_2$max, was shown by Pendergast et al. (1996) to take place up to 80% when athletes consumed higher-fat diets. In these same athletes, 90-95% of their $\dot{V}O_2$max could be maintained despite marked glycogen depletion. The athletes maintained anaerobic power in addition to endurance. These findings confirmed earlier results in animals (Miller et al. 1984) and observations made by those in the clinical field (Maffetone 1997). In addition, according to Arena et al. (1995), high-fat diets can improve the response of growth hormone to exercise.

The usual recommendation is that dietary fat should be limited to 30% or less of total consumption (National Cholesterol Education Program 1991). However, many patients attempt very low fat diets, often to reduce body fat. Regarding this approach, Grundy (1996) states, "One can question whether it is realistic, necessary, or strongly based on scientific data" (p. 44). Consuming a diet higher in fat, even in excess of 30% of the total kilocalories, can be accomplished without risk of cardiovascular (Pendergast et al. 1996) or immune stress (Venkatraman et al. 1997). In addition, the type of dietary fat does not seem to be a factor in whether or not one obtains the benefits of increased exercise energy (Vukovich et al. 1993). However, it is vital that proper essential fatty acid intakes are maintained and that the various dietary fats are balanced, for many other reasons to be discussed.

Increasing dietary fat intake can increase lipoprotein lipase, which hydrolyzes triglycerides, allowing their fatty acids to be released and available for energy use in muscles (Borensztajn 1979). Consuming a diet too high in carbohydrates may diminish lipoprotein lipase and may be associated with diminished ability to obtain fatty acids from triglycerides, resulting in less utilization of fats for energy, increased dependency on carbohydrate stores, and increased blood levels of triglycerides (Jacobs et al. 1982).

In general, female endurance athletes utilize more fats and less carbohydrates than men, and women store less glycogen from dietary carbohydrates than men (Tarnopolsky et al. 1995). This may make women more efficient in endurance sports than men.

In some situations, significant dysfunction may be associated with low levels of fat intake. For example, Deuster et al. (1986) showed that amenorrheic female athletes consumed less fat (and more carbohydrate) than their eumenorrheic counterparts. Nutter (1991) states, "The desire to be thin may influence dietary intakes of female athletes more than changes in exercise training" (p. 395). Low-fat diets have also been associated with significantly lower levels of testosterone in men (Reed et al. 1987). Dermatological problems may also be related to imbalances of fatty acids (Miller et al. 1991). Fat may also reduce pain tolerance. Zmarzty et al. (1997) showed that patients who ate high-fat (low-carbohydrate) meals significantly reduced their pain 1.5 hr after ingestion.

A point worth emphasizing is that fat intake must be balanced. Broadhurst (1997) states,

> "Natural whole foods contain fats as structural components, and have a balance of polyunsaturated fat, monounsaturated fat, and saturated fat. Since we are still a Paleolithic species, adapted to eating only wild foods, it is difficult to justify the consumption of anything other than an overall balance of [fats] in an evolutionary sense. No natural fats are intrinsically good or bad—it is the proportions that matter. Variety is recommended in dietary lipid structure, degree of saturation, and chain length. Pathological n-3/n-6 [omega-3/omega-6] polyunsaturated fat imbalance, obesity, and progressive glucose intolerance are consequences of adopting cereal grain based diets by both humans and livestock. Food processing and refining amplify these problems" (p. 247).

A number of important dietary studies have dealt with lipid profiles and the risk of disease. Jeppesen et al. (1997) and Dreon et al. (1997) showed that women developed higher risk for heart disease with a lower-fat, higher-carbohydrate diet versus a higher-fat, lower-carbohydrate diet. Golay et al. (1996) showed that the higher-fat, lower-carbohydrate diets, in addition to reducing triglyceride levels, improved fasting blood insulin and the glucose/insulin ratio. Liu et al. (1983) also showed that a high-carbohydrate, low-fat diet raised insulin and triglyceride levels.

CHOLESTEROL

Dietary and serum cholesterol may be a concern for patients and practitioners, especially when an increase in dietary fats is considered. Litchtenstein (1996) states, "Although a vast literature exists on the effect of dietary cholesterol on plasma lipids, the area remains somewhat controversial because of the inconsistent nature of the observations" (p. 435).

Cholesterol is an important substance for everyone, especially athletes. The production of steroid hormones by the adrenal glands depends on cholesterol. This includes the glucocorticoids and estrogen, progesterone, and testosterone. In addition, the production of bile and the formation of vitamin D in the skin are cholesterol dependent. Cholesterol is also an important component of the cell membranes, including the myelin sheath of neurons of the central nervous system.

Most individuals have effective feedback control mechanisms regarding cholesterol intake (McNamara et al. 1987), with consumption of high levels of cholesterol not necessarily affecting blood levels. The body requires about 1000 mg of cholesterol per day for normal function. Most of this is synthesized by the liver (and some in the small intestine), with only about 10%-20% coming from the diet. If less cholesterol is consumed through foods, more is synthesized by the liver, and if more is eaten, the liver produces less. Dysfunction in the liver may be the major reason for abnormal blood levels of cholesterol, since it is here that cholesterol is broken down into bile salts and eliminated into the gastrointestinal tract. In addition, low dietary fiber may allow reabsorption of more cholesterol from the lower gastrointestinal tract after biliary removal.

Most of the concerns about cholesterol relate to its association with cardiovascular heart disease (CHD). Current evidence indicates that this association involves the low-density lipoprotein (LDL)-cholesterol fraction (Expert Panel on Detection, Evaluation, and Treatment of High Blood Cholesterol in Adults 1994), with every 0.026 mmol/L (1 mg/dl) increase producing an increased risk for CHD of 1%-2%. It has also been shown that the oxidation of LDL-cholesterol is a key factor in this process, and that the use of antioxidants (discussed in the next chapter) may play a role in preventing this problem (Diaz et al. 1997; Mosca et al. 1997). (Oxidized LDL may also produce neuronal cell death [Sugawa et al. 1997].)

Some dietary fatty acids have been shown to increase LDL-cholesterol (Grundy 1996). For example, palmitic, myristic, and lauric acids, which are a significant component of foods high in saturated fat (Group B fats), raise LDL and total cholesterol. Foods high in these fatty acids include palm kernel oil (78%), coconut oil (71%), herring (41%), palm oil (39%), and pork (30%). Trans fatty acids (in hydrogenated oils) increase LDL-cholesterol (and lower high-density lipoprotein). Davi et al. (1997) showed that high blood cholesterol was associated with high levels of the Series 2 eicosanoids.

Other fatty acids lower or do not affect LDL. For instance, stearic acid makes up about 25% of the saturated fat in the diet and does not raise LDL-cholesterol. Higher levels of stearic acid are found in cocoa butter, pork, and beef. Linoleic acid (Group A fats) mildly lowers LDL-cholesterol and is found in many oils.

High-density lipoprotein (HDL)-cholesterol has a positive effect on cardiac health, and low levels are associated with CHD (Wilt et al. 1997). Exercise has a positive effect on HDL-cholesterol levels (Moore et al. 1983), and high-carbohydrate diets may lower HDL-cholesterol (Carranza-Madrigal et al. 1997). Bordia et al. (1997) demonstrated that in some patients, fenugreek significantly decreases blood lipids (total cholesterol and triglycerides) without affecting the HDL.

It is therefore important, when the patient's blood lipid levels are being assessed, that the total cholesterol and the LDL and HDL fractions be measured (along with fasting triglycerides).

High triglyceride levels are also positively correlated with CHD (Austin 1991). Alpha linolenic acid (ALA) (Group C fats) lowers triglycerides (Connor 1986), and carbohydrates raise triglycerides. In addition, the ratio of triglycerides to HDL is a strong predictor of myocardial infarction (Gaziano et al. 1997).

Given this important information, athletes should not have fears about consuming the proper amounts and quality of fat in their diet. An appropriate fat consumption can help improve endurance, performance, and overall health. Later in this chapter we will consider dietary fats and inflammation, and in the next chapter the relation between fats and supplementation.

PROTEIN

The protein needs of athletes are also an individual issue. Protein is a major component of cell structure, is vital for enzymes in all biochemical reactions, and helps regulate gene expression. Proteins may also be used for energy—perhaps up to 15% of an athlete's needs (Friedman and Lemon 1989). Many amino acids can be deaminated to form glucose when either blood glucose or glycogen levels are low. For example, as much as 90% of the daily requirement for leucine may be oxidized during 2 hr of moderate training.

Daily protein requirements for adults have been established by the World Health Organization at 0.75 g/kg body weight for Western diets (1985). Some countries have modified this recommendation: the United States to 0.8 g, Canada to 0.86 g, and Germany and Australia to 1.0 g (Linder 1991). These values correlate with levels consumed by average adults, who according to Guyton (1986) require a minimum of 30-55 g/day to maintain normal stores. However, many other experts call for major revisions to these recommendations (Young 1994), with some proposing much higher amounts for athletes, and imply that low intakes can have a detrimental effect on performance. Lemon (1996) states, "An increasing number of studies have appeared that indicate dietary protein needs are elevated in individuals who are regularly physically active. Together, these data suggest that the recommended daily allowance (RDA) for those who engage in regular endurance exercise should be about 1.2-1.4g protein/kg body mass/d (150%-175% of the current RDA) and 1.7-1.8g protein/kg body mass/d (212%-225% of the current RDA) for strength exercisers" (p. 169). Others have shown that daily protein intakes as high as 2 g/kg may still be inadequate in athletes training at 64% $\dot{V}O_2$max (Butterfield 1987). Also, endurance athletes may require higher protein intakes than bodybuilders (Tarnopolsky et al.

1988). Negative nitrogen balance may occur in young men who engage in resistance training while consuming dietary protein at the RDA (Tarnopolsky et al. 1992). The Canadian recommended nutrient intake for protein of 0.86 g/kg per day is insufficient for athletes (Phillips et al. 1993).

Greater gains in body mass occur during heavy resistance training in young men when 3.3 versus 1.3 g protein/kg per day is consumed (Fern et al. 1991). Low protein intake results in a loss of lean body mass and decreased power (Castaneda et al. 1995a). Women eating too little protein experience significant losses in lean tissue, poor immune response, and muscle dysfunction (Castaneda et al. 1995b).

Populations at greatest risk for consuming insufficient protein include any group that restricts energy intake (people on diets) or high-quality protein sources (vegetarians), as well as any group that has a requirement higher than normal due to another existing condition, such as individuals who are still growing. For endurance athletes, the increased oxidation of amino acids and higher mitochondrial protein content may result in needs higher than the RDA (Lemon 1996).

After meals that are low in or void of protein, levels of both essential and nonessential amino acids in plasma decrease continuously for up to 5 to 7 hr. In addition, muscle concentrations fall for up to 5 hr after the meal (Bergstrom et al. 1990).

Regarding these diverse opinions on protein requirements, Reeds and Beckett (1996) state, "Failure to resolve these difficulties stems in part from the word 'requirement,' which is used in different ways by different authors" (p. 67). Fortunately, by matching the protein needs of each patient rather than offering the same general recommendations for everyone, practitioners can avoid these academic conflicts.

There is much less evidence that daily protein intakes above 2 g/kg are beneficial (Lemon 1996), with the potential of negative effects. Excess protein, including that used for energy, is converted to fat and stored. Nutritional needs may also be increased in association with high protein intakes. Because vitamins B6, B12, and folic acid are involved in the metabolism of protein, increased protein intake may increase the requirements for these nutrients, which can be assessed by higher homocystine in the urine (Linder 1991). Increased water intake may be required in those with higher protein intakes, since excretion of higher nitrogen from the kidney may require more water. According to McArdle et al. (1991), excess protein may produce metabolic stress on liver and kidney function. The studies demonstrating these potential problems, however, have been done on patients with previously impaired kidney function. Jorda et al. (1988) showed that long-term feeding of very high protein to healthy animals had no adverse effects. The concerns regarding high protein intake and calcium loss may relate only to purified protein, or those individuals associated with atherosclerosis, and may not apply to most humans (Lemon 1996).

As discussed in the next chapter, the essential amino acid content of food is important. Foods containing the highest-quality protein contain a balance of essential amino acids. In this regard, the ideal protein food is egg, which is also among foods with the highest levels of digestibility; whey and beef are also among the highest-quality proteins. However, one can achieve an overall high-quality protein diet by consuming a proper balance of high- and so-called lower-quality protein foods. For example, a cereal and legume combination provides a high-quality protein meal. It is not necessary to create a high-quality protein combination at each meal but rather to do so in the course of the day or week. However, with these combinations of foods may come higher carbohydrate intakes.

Protein requirements may be influenced by digestion, absorption, and caloric intake. The first step in protein utilization is efficient digestion to the individual amino acids, which can then be followed by absorption. Kilocalorie intake has a significant influence on protein needs; low-kilocalorie diets may increase protein needs, and adequate kilocalories may reduce protein needs (Linder 1991).

An important relationship exists between dietary protein and reactions by the immune system (Barbeau 1997). Absorption of intact proteins may produce allergic or hypersensitivity reactions in some patients (Kaminogawa 1996). This response results in the production of immunoglobulin G, A, and E antibodies and can be measured in the serum of these individuals (Kolopp-Sarda et al. 1997). Common allergens include proteins from cow's milk, wheat gluten, and corn. Other important relationships between protein and immune function are discussed in the next chapter in connection with L-glutamine.

DIETARY FACTORS AFFECTING INFLAMMATION

A variety of natural food substances can either increase the inflammatory response or diminish it. Various dietary fats are converted to specific prostaglandins, leukotrienes, and thromboxanes, collectively called eicosanoids. In general, reduced essential fatty acid intakes increase the pro-inflammatory eicosanoids (Blond and Bezard 1991). An imbalance of dietary fatty acids can do the same.

Increasing Inflammatory Responses

The Series 2 eicosanoids have an inflammatory effect in the body, also creating associated edema and hyperalgesia (Portanova et al. 1996). These are produced from arachidonic acid, found in many foods, especially meats, shellfish, and dairy products. Balancing of Group A and Group C unsaturated fats to promote increased production of Series 1 and 3 eicosanoids exerts a strikingly protective effect on tissue inflammation and injury (Lefkowith et al. 1991). While traditionally viewed as unhealthy, the Series 2 eicosanoids have a beneficial function in stimulating immune activity, microbicidal activity, and recycling of damaged tissue (Bland 1997). However, an imbalance of these eicosanoids can result in dysfunction—specifically chronic inflammation, which is a common problem in athletes.

The Series 2 eicosanoids can also be increased from Group A fats through the action of delta-5-desaturase. This enzyme converts dihomo-gamma-linolenic acid to arachidonic acid, and is promoted by insulin.

The effect of trans fats, which are contained in large amounts in hydrogenated and partially hydrogenated oils such as margarine and many other foods as listed on ingredient labels, was discussed in chapter 6. These fats can cause significant eicosanoid imbalance; they should be considered as enhancers of the effects of the Group B fats, and they do not possess the functions of an essential fatty acid. In addition, they may exacerbate an essential fatty acid deficiency. Some of these fats, such as those found in fried foods, are formed from oils that have been heated to high temperatures (Chardigny et al. 1996). Most importantly, trans fats can inhibit the delta-6-desaturase and elongase enzymes; this restricts production of the anti-inflammatory Series 1 and 3 eicosanoids, resulting in a relatively higher level of Series 2 pro-inflammatory eicosanoids. The trans fats may also stimulate the delta-5-desaturase enzyme. (Although some trans fats occur in nature, they are very short chain fatty acids that are easily metabolized and that do not impair essential fatty acid function adversely as the processed long-chain trans fats do.)

Of great significance in sport is the increased production of the Series 2 eicosanoids as a natural result of any repetitive activity (Almekinders et al. 1993). Weight-bearing activity further increases the Series 2 eicosanoid level significantly (Thorsen et al. 1996) over levels obtained with non-weight-bearing workouts (i.e., swimming). Lower levels of Series 2 eicosanoids may be important for proper bone formation, but higher levels may cause bone loss (Desimone et al. 1993). Krieger (1997) demonstrated that calcium transport is also inhibited by these eicosanoids (specifically by prostaglandin E2). (Likewise, Claassen et al. [1995] showed that gamma-linolenic acid increases calcium absorption from the gastrointestinal tract and bone calcium, and reduces urinary calcium loss.)

Diminishing Inflammatory Effects

Sesamin, a lignan of sesame seed oil, inhibits the action of delta-5-desaturase and has anti-inflammatory effects (Chavali et al. 1997). This response, however, is most active in the conversion of dihomo-gamma-linolenic acid to arachidonic acid and for unknown reasons does not seem to affect the production of eicosapentaenoic acid (EPA) (Umeda-Sawada et al. 1995). Turmeric can also inhibit delta-5-desaturase (Shimizu et al. 1992). This spice may also inhibit the production of other inflammatory eicosanoids.

The use of sesame oil in the uncooked state is best, since heating sesame oil results in the production of sesamol, which is carcinogenic (Pariza 1996).

Sesamin also has some other interesting health benefits. It may increase vitamin E absorption (Kamal-Eldin et al. 1995) and enhance hepatic detoxication of chemicals as well as protect against oxidative stress (Chavali et al. 1997). Furthermore, it may reduce cholesterol synthesis, may repair liver alcohol damage, and has anti-cancer activity (Umeda-Sawada et al. 1995).

As described in chapter 6, the Series 2 eicosanoids encompass two important pathways. One results in the production of leukotrienes and requires the lipoxygenase enzyme. The other produces thromboxanes and the Series 2 prostaglandins, which in turn produce prostacyclin, countering the actions of the other Series 2 eicosanoids (Koester 1993). Prostacyclin may also promote cartilage repair. Figure 18.2 shows these relationships.

Certain foods in the diet may stimulate the production of prostacyclin, including ginger, garlic, and onions. These have been used in complementary sports medicine for many years. Ginger (*Zingiber officinale*) has been shown to have anti-inflammatory effects (Srivastava and Mustafa 1992), possibly through inhibition of Series 2 prostaglandins and/or stimulation of prostacycline. Bordia et al. (1997) demonstrated that a single dose of 10 g powdered ginger produced a significant reduction in platelet aggregation. Garlic (*Allium sativum*) and onion (*Allium cepa*) may significantly inhibit thromboxanes when eaten raw, with garlic being more potent in this effect (Bordia et al. 1996). Ali and Thomson (1995) also showed a significant reduction in thromboxanes, along with a 20% reduction in cholesterol, with the use of garlic.

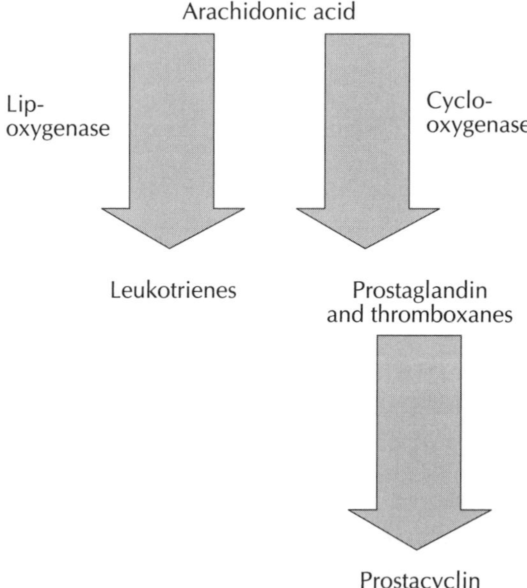

Figure 18.2 Conversion of Group B fats to their eicosanoids

Ginger also has anti-rhinoviral properties, making it a natural remedy without side effects for athletes with colds (Denyer et al. 1994). In addition, it contains a sulfur ester known as allicin, which has anti-microbial activity. Ginger has also been shown to have anti-emetic properties, improving the symptoms of nausea (Meyer et al. 1995; Sharma et al. 1997).

Group A and Group C unsaturated fats, described in chapter 6, increase the Series 1 and Series 3 eicosanoids, respectively, which have anti-inflammatory effects. Of particular importance are the Group C fats, which contain ALA. These fats are consumed with much less frequency, and their conversion is less effective with age.

Balancing Pro- and Anti-Inflammatory Effects

For obvious reasons, it is important for patients to balance their fats to establish a balance of pro- and anti-inflammatory hormones in the body. A combination of approximately equal amounts of Group A, B, and C fats has been recommended by the author (Maffetone 1997); this is a 2:1 ratio of unsaturated to saturated fat, frequently recommended. Simopoulos (1991) recommends a ratio of 1:1 for all omega-6 and omega-3 fats, noting that the ratio in diets of early humans was 1:1 but that the ratios of today's diets range from 10:1 to 25:1.

Three considerations are important for the dietary manipulation of pro- and anti-inflammatory eicosanoids in patients who require improved fatty acid and eicosanoid balance. Increased intake of Group A fats (high in linoleic acid) can reduce the incorporation of EPA into the cells (Mantzioris et al. 1995). This can shift the balance to higher Series 1 and reduced Series 3 eicosanoids. This may eventually increase the body's adipose tissue stores of linoleic acid and provide a continual source of this fat for metabolic activity. In some patients, however, levels of the Series 1 eicosanoids are reduced in the spring and fall (and may be associated with allergies).

In addition, increased arachidonic acid from animal fats can also reduce the levels of Series 1 and 3 eicosanoids. This may result in more pro-inflammatory and less anti-inflammatory activity. Also higher intakes of Group C fats can increase the conversion of Group C fats to Series 3 eicosanoids as well as reduce both delta-6- and delta-5-desaturase in conversion of Group A fats to Series 1 and 2 eicosanoids (Ulmann et al. 1994). This shifts the balance to higher Series 3 and reduced Series 1 (and 2) eicosanoids.

For a variety of reasons, either patients may not consume enough of the necessary fats, or their body may not properly convert the fats to the respective eicosanoids. For example, pyridoxine (vitamin B6) is necessary for the conversion of Group C fats to the Series 3 eicosanoids (Maranesi et al. 1993), with magnesium also being important. Unfortunately, the B6 and magnesium levels in foods have diminished (Welsh and Marston 1982). Low dietary protein may also have an adverse effect on essential fatty acids, increasing the requirement for these (Hill and Holman 1980), and may adversely affect the polyunsaturated-to-saturated fatty acid ratio (Bouziane et al. 1994). Siguel and Lerman (1996) showed that 25% of patients with chronic intestinal dysfunction had essential fatty acid deficiencies, indicating potential indigestion and malabsorption of other nutrients.

Recommending increases or decreases in specific foods to help balance the three groups of fats should be based partly on the patient's current diet as already described and partly on the need as determined during the assessment process. This includes the results of Group Ten of the Symptom Survey that includes common signs and symptoms of essential fatty acid needs, questions regarding aspirin's effect on the patient's symptoms, and any chronic or recurrent inflammation in the patient. Table 18.2 shows a fatty acid profile from a patient's dietary assessment.

Table 18.3 lists some common foods containing Group A, B, and C fats. Most foods contain all three types of fats; the listing here is based on the predominant fat contained in a food. For example, shrimp contains some EPA, but predominantly Group B fats; linseed (flax) oil contains Group A and C fats, but predominantly C (ALA).

Table 18.2 Contribution of Individual Fatty Acids in Your Diet (in grams)

Saturated fats		Monounsaturated fats		Polyunsaturated fats	
Butyric	0.33	Myristol	0.24	Linoleic (n-6)	8.67
Caproic	0.16	Palmitoleic	2.83	Linolenic (n-3)	1.00
Caprylic	0.13	Pentadecenoic	0.00	Moroctic	0.03
Capric	0.34	Heptadecenoic	21.31	Eicosatrienoic	0.00
Lauric	0.29	Oleic	25.32	Arachidonic (n-6)	0.55
Pentadecanoic	0.14	Gadoleic	0.51	EPA (n-3)	0.20
Myristic	1.63	Erucic	0.27	DPA	0.05
Palmitic	18.14	Nervonic	0.00	DHA	0.47
Margaric	0.29				
Stearic	6.38				
Arachidic	0.10				
Behenate	0.03				
Lignoceric	0.00				

Reprinted by permission of NutrAnalysis, Inc.

Table 18.3 Common Foods Containing Group A, B, and C Fats

Group A	Group B	Group C
Most vegetable seed oils (safflower, corn, peanut, etc.)	Meats, dairy, shellfish	Some oils (linseed, pumpkin seed); walnuts; beans; fish (salmon, mackerel, sardines); leafy vegetables

When essential fatty acid needs exist, the practitioner has several options and ideally should consider all of them. The first option is to balance the intake of dietary fats based on the assessment (or imbalance) of the patient's current diet. For example, if the patient is consuming twice as great an amount of Group B fats as of Group A and C fats, the recommendations might include decreasing foods high in Group B fats and increasing foods high in Group A and C fats. Or, if the ratio of A to C is 18:1, decreasing A fats and increasing C fats would be recommended.

The second approach is to remove the potential inhibitors of the enzymes required to form the Series 1 and 3 eicosanoids. These include trans fats, excess saturated fats, excess sugar and high-glycemic carbohydrates, low protein intake, and excess stress. In addition, excess intake of Group A or B fats can inhibit these conversions.

Other needs may include dietary and nutritional factors that increase the production of Series 1 and 3 eicosanoids. These may include dietary protein if the patient's levels are low. In addition, vitamins B6, C, low doses of E (discussed later), and the minerals magnesium and zinc may be useful; these are discussed in the next chapter.

Concentrated fatty acids in supplement form may also be valuable for patients with fatty acid imbalance. These may include linseed (flax) oil, fish oil, and black currant seed oil as discussed in the next chapter. Sesame seed oil, ginger, garlic, and onions are food sources that can improve eicosanoid balance.

Table 18.4 lists some common oils and their approximate Group A and C percentages. Table 18.5 lists some common foods and their approximate unsaturated and saturated percentages.

Table 18.4 Approximate Levels of Group A and C Fats in Common Foods

Food	% Group A	% Group C
Butter	2	1
Palm kernel oil	2	0
Pork fat	9	0.5
Chicken fat	22	1.5
Peanut oil	26	0
Olive oil (omega-9)	8	1
Margarine	25	1
Soybean oil	53	8
Soy	50	9
Canola oil	7	30
Walnut	5	50
Corn oil	39	1
Cottonseed	47	0.4
Palm oil	11	1
Wheat germ oil	42	1 (as EPA)
Sesame oil	42	0.4
Safflower oil	74	0.5
Linseed oil	14	58
Cod liver oil	2	20 (19% EPA)

Adapted from Linder MC (1991) and Erasuas U (1996).

Table 18.5 Some Common Foods and Their Approximate Unsaturated and Saturated Percentages

Oil	% Monounsaturated	% Polyunsaturated	% Saturated
Olive	77	9	14
Canola	62	32	6
Peanut	49	33	18
Corn	25	62	13
Soybean	24	61	15
Safflower	13	77	10
Palm	39	10	51
Coconut	6	2	92
Egg yolk	48.3	15.6	36.1
Beef	49.2	4.3	46.5
Cheese	30.1	3.1	66.8
Almonds	68.1	22.0	9.9
Cashews	61.6	17.7	20.7
Peanuts	50.6	31.6	17.7

When patients have a primary dietary problem, addressing these needs first makes other therapy generally much easier.

DIETARY FIBER AND OTHER DIETARY FACTORS

Certain components of the diet that are not digested by enzymes and have no clearly defined nutritional value are referred to as dietary fiber. These components include plant-wall material (cellulose, hemicellulose, pectin, and lignin) and other intracellular polysaccharides such as gums and mucilages (Gallaher and Schneeman 1996). Some of these substances are soluble in liquid (making the term "fiber" an inaccurate one), and others are not. The soluble-insoluble model of fiber has not been accepted by all, as some propose physiological and other chemical definitions of fiber.

Although dietary fibers are not digested by enzymes in the mouth, stomach, and small intestine, they are acted upon by bacterial fermentation in the colon. This results in energy and the production and absorption of some very important nutrients. The products include three short-chain fatty acids—butyrate, propionate, and acetate—that are metabolized by the colonic epithelium (butyrate), liver (propionate), and muscle (acetate). Bacteria also synthesize small amounts of the B vitamins and protein and significant amounts of vitamin K (Cummings and Macfarlane 1997). In humans, 5%-10% of the total energy of the body may come from colonic fermentation of fiber (Nordgaard and Mortensen 1995). This may be a significant factor for athletes.

Foods containing fiber include vegetables, fruits, grains, and legumes. According to Block et al. (1992), fibers from vegetables and fruits are associated with more health benefits than those from grains and legumes. Sigleo et al. (1984) showed that when high levels of fiber are consumed, small-intestine morphology may be significantly influenced. The villi in these individuals are much broader than in the typical Westerner, whose fiber intake is relatively low. This larger villus size can result in improved nutritional absorption. An important aspect of dietary fiber is its potential reduction of glycemic and insulinemic response following a meal (Hanai et al. 1997). The fiber must be present at the same meal in order for this effect to occur. These results may be due to delayed stomach emptying or to slower glucose absorption.

Other beneficial effects of fiber include a plasma cholesterol-lowering effect, improvement of colon function, and binding of bile acids (Gallaher and Schneeman 1996). In addition, Dudkin et al. (1997) demonstrated a protective role of fiber against the effects of radiation.

The fiber in some foods may have an undesirable effect. Lairon et al. (1985) showed that wheat contains an inhibitor of pancreatic lipase. Fiber in cereals may inhibit absorption of various minerals, including calcium, iron, zinc, and copper (Torre et al. 1991); the inhibition may be due to the effect of phytic acid in the fiber (especially prevalent in all grains). Magnesium may also be adversely affected by excess fiber (Drew et al. 1979). It may be best for those patients with increased mineral requirements to reduce their carbohydrate levels.

Many athletes do not meet the U.S. Department of Agriculture recommendation for the intake of dietary fiber, which is 11.5 g/1000 kcal of food in the diet. It is important to assess the patient's intake, as described earlier. The following menus are for two diets with two different amounts of fiber.

Daily Menu With 15 Grams of Fiber

- Breakfast: Vegetable omelet (made with two eggs and a serving each of spinach and tomato); two slices whole-grain toast; half a grapefruit
- Lunch: Mixed salad (leaf lettuce, carrots, sprouts, avocado, celery); tuna with healthy mayonnaise
- Dinner: small Caesar salad; small steak; asparagus

Daily Menu With 25 Grams of Fiber

- Breakfast: Vegetable omelet (made with three eggs and a large serving each of spinach and tomato); two slices whole-grain toast; whole grapefruit
- Snack: Apple
- Lunch: Mixed salad (leaf lettuce, carrots, sprouts, avocado, celery); tuna with healthy mayonnaise
- Dinner: Caesar salad, New York sirloin; asparagus and red peppers; brown rice

Caffeine can have a significant impact on certain patients. It is commonly used as an ergogenic aid, but often because of the presence of general fatigue. Patients who consume caffeine should be questioned about their energy levels and also about how decreasing or eliminating caffeine in their diet would affect their energy levels.

Caffeine is one of a group of compounds called methylxanthines and is found in coffee, tea, chocolate, colas, and a variety of over-the-counter drugs. Table 18.6 lists the amounts of caffeine in some of these items. Amounts can vary significantly according to such factors as individual brewing methods, source, and concentration.

Caffeine reaches a peak concentration in the body at about 1 hr after intake and has an influence on the nervous, muscular, and cardiovascular systems. Graham and Spriet (1995) reported that plasma saturation occurs between doses of 6 and 9 mg/kg; they showed also that endurance increased equally (by 22%) with the 3 and 6 mg/kg doses but that a 9 mg/kg dose resulted in no further improvement. In this study, the plasma epinephrine was not increased with 3 mg/kg of caffeine; epinephrine was greater at the 9 mg/kg dose, which also increased plasma glycerol and free fatty acids. The authors state, "Thus the highest dose had the greatest effect on epinephrine and blood-borne metabolites yet had the least effect on performance. The lowest dose had little or no effect on epinephrine and metabolites but did have an ergogenic effect" (p. 867). Note that epinephrine increases with caffeine intake. This could have adverse effects on an already stressed adrenal gland.

Table 18.6 Caffeine Levels in Some Beverages and Over-the-Counter Drugs

COFFEE (MG/CUP)	RANGE
Regular	85-240
Instant	60-100
Decaffeinated	3
TEA (MG/CUP)	**RANGE**
Regular	50-140
Iced	90
Instant	30
Herbal	0
OTHER	**RANGE**
Cola (mg/12 oz)	30-90
Chocolate drink	25-48
Chocolate candy	45-55
Drugs (standard dose mg/tablet)	15-280

Adapted from Linder 1991, Maffetone 1997, Wilmore and Costill 1994.

Jacobson et al. (1992) demonstrated that 7 mg/kg of caffeine helped some strength and power parameters, and Wiles et al. (1992) reported improved performance in 1500-m events. These improvements are most likely the result of increased utilization of fatty acids and sparing of glycogen.

The ergogenic effects of caffeine are present with urinary caffeine levels that are below the limit of 12 μg/ml allowed by the International Olympic Committee (Graham and Spriet 1995). In addition to the potential legal issue, caffeine may pose health risks that could ultimately adversely affect performance. The most significant is dehydration, as caffeine is a diuretic; these effects may be amplified in hot weather and at altitude. Calcium and magnesium loss may be increased in those who consume caffeine (Kynast-Gales and Massey 1994; Bergman et al. 1990), and caffeine may adversely affect bone metabolism (Massey et al. 1994). Immune function and the antioxidant system may also be negatively affected by caffeine intake (Rossowska and Nakamoto 1994; Sullivan et al. 1995).

The practitioner should be sure to note a patient's caffeine intake on the initial dietary analysis and should ask the patient during future visits about changes in caffeine habits. In patients with adrenal, immune, or other dysfunction (i.e., caffeine may cause gastrointestinal distress), reductions in or elimination of caffeine intake may be a consideration, with each patient requiring individual recommendations.

Alcohol (ethanol) is generally not used as an ergogenic aid, but athletes consume more alcohol than nonathletes (Rainey et al. 1996; Nattiv et al. 1997). Practitioners should be aware that diet surveys may not always indicate alcohol intake, especially in patients who are drinking under the legal age. Alcohol provides moderate amounts of energy (7 kcal/g). Moderate to large intakes may promote weight loss due to the substitution for carbohydrate, but this amount also inhibits fatty acid oxidation (Halstead 1996).

Recent studies show that mortality risk is greatest in those who abstain from alcohol and in those who consume more than two to three drinks per day, with the protective effect of moderate intake less in women (Klatsky et al. 1992; Doll et al. 1994; Gronbaek et al. 1995; Fuchs et al. 1995). Most of these data reflect coronary disease risk (Klatsky 1994). Alcohol in moderation may also have antioxidant effects (Moller et al. 1996). However, the risk of some cancers and liver stress may be elevated with moderate alcohol intake (Halstead 1996). Higher intakes increase the requirements for various nutrients including vitamin B1, folic acid, zinc, and niacin. As with all other recommendations, light to moderate alcohol consumption is a highly individual issue.

MENTAL AND EMOTIONAL ASPECTS OF DIET

The patient's mental and emotional state may be significantly influenced by the diet. This is also a very individual focus, but two common findings are related to fatty acid balance and carbohydrate content. Adams et al. (1996) showed that an imbalance of omega-6 and -3 fatty acids and of arachidonic acid and EPA was related to depression in patients. Christensen and Somers (1996) state the conclusions of their study: "Results revealed that depressed and nondepressed groups consume similar amounts of all nutrients except protein and carbohydrates. Nondepressed subjects consume more protein and depressed subjects consume more carbohydrates. The increase in carbohydrate consumption comes primarily from an increase in sucrose consumption" (p. 105).

Assessing patients' mental and emotional states in relation to all aspects of their lives is important, especially with regard to diet.

FINDING A MACRONUTRIENT BALANCE

Considering individual uniqueness, it seems clear that each patient's optimal balance must be determined individually rather than from general guidelines developed for a whole population. This is a three-step process:

- First, one considers any signs or symptoms observed and discussed during the consultation and examination.
- Next, a detailed assessment of the patient's current dietary habits is performed.
- Clinical decisions are made based on these and other factors (such as patient feedback, the type of activity the individual performs, and possibly results of the Two-Week test). These factors are described further on.

Uncovering a Dietary Imbalance

The first step in determining optimal dietary suggestions in a given patient is to relate the results of the consultation and examination. For example, if a patient's triglycerides are too high and he or she is frequently hungry and fatigued, the reason may be excess dietary carbohydrates. Or, if amenorrhea is present, fat content may be too low, as previously mentioned. Specific areas of the Symptom Survey may also indicate an imbalance of certain macronutrients. For example, the patient may have numerous complaints listed in Group Three and Group Nine (blood sugar and carbohydrate intolerance/insulin resistance, respectively), indicating potential excess carbohydrate intake. Group Ten includes symptoms that may be associated with increased essential fatty acid requirements and with too little dietary unsaturated fat.

As discussed earlier, the type of activity performed by the patient may have to do with the optimum recommendations. For example, endurance athletes who require very high levels of aerobic function, including runners, cyclists, triathletes, swimmers, and others whose training or competition lasts longer than about 10 min, may benefit from modifying their traditional high-carbohydrate/low-fat diet. Even football, basketball, baseball, and other team sport players require significant endurance even though they sometimes compete only for very brief periods with short bursts of activity. These athletes may be called upon numerous times during a longer event, and they generally have a long season and spend considerable time in training; all require a significant amount of endurance and aerobic function.

It is also important to consider the patient's preferences when helping to plan the diet. The beliefs of people who choose not to eat meat, for example, should be respected. Even diets that are strictly vegetarian can contain the proper balance of macro- and micronutrients, although significant discipline is required to maintain a proper diet.

Determining the Quality and Quantity of Macronutrients

The second step in finding the ideal balance of macronutrients is to assess the patient's current dietary habits from both a quality and a quantity standpoint. The procedure for gathering dietary information was discussed in chapter 7 as part of the patient history process. Once this information is collected, the patient's diet can be subjected to computer analysis (performing this task manually for each patient's diet record would take a great deal of time).

A variety of results can be obtained from a patient's diet record. Minimally, these should include total kilocalories; percentages of macronutrients; levels of specific vitamins and minerals, amino acids, and essential fatty acids; levels and ratio of omega-3 and -6 fats; percentages of monounsaturated, polyunsaturated, and saturated fat; amount of fiber.

A report given to patients that details their dietary makeup will greatly enhance their understanding of food quality and quantity and help them to make appropriate modifications. In addition, a reassessment of the diet in three to six months can be of value.

Making Dietary Decisions

Eating a number of smaller meals throughout the day—that is, four to eight rather than the traditional three or two (or sometimes one)—can be metabolically healthier (Jenkins 1997). However, this must not mean consuming more total kilocalories, unless that need exists. An increased number of meals is associated with significant reductions in postprandial insulin and glucose levels (i.e., a flatter curve) and with reduced body fat and obesity.

The Two-Week Test

An assessment tool called the Two-Week test has been developed and used by the author and other practitioners and patients for many years (Maffetone 1997); this test may also help determine the optimal carbohydrate intake for patients. The test is performed over a two-week period during which insulin levels remain relatively low because concentrated carbohydrate intake is significantly reduced. The test consists of four steps.

Step One: Before the test begins, the signs and symptoms that may indicate carbohydrate dietary excess are noted. These may include any of the following:

- Fatigue, insomnia, blood sugar-handling problems (frequent hunger and other indications from Group Three or Group Nine on the Symptom Survey)
- High fasting triglycerides (above 150-200 mg/dl [1.8 mmol/L]), high fasting insulin, abnormal blood sugar levels
- Orthostatic hypotension, high blood pressure
- Symptoms that occur immediately after meals: intestinal bloating, sleepiness, poor concentration, or feelings of depression

In addition, the patient's body weight should be measured, and the patient should be asked to perform the MAF test. Such measurements as vital capacity, oral pH, and others described earlier may also be valuable. These and any other signs or symptoms can be used to assess the success or failure of the Two-Week test.

Step Two: For a period of two weeks, the patient must avoid all concentrated carbohydrate (moderate and high GI) foods. These include

- bread, rolls, pasta, pancakes, cereal, muffins, rice cakes;
- all sweets, including all products that contain sugar (ketchup, honey, sports drinks, and prepared foods containing sweets as indicated on the labels);
- fruits and fruit juices;
- potatoes (all types), corn, rice, beans; and
- milk, half-and-half, yogurt.

Foods that may be eaten include

- whole eggs, cheeses, cream, meats (beef, turkey, chicken, lamb, etc.), fish, and shellfish (processed and prepackaged meats have added sugar and should be avoided);
- tomato and V8 juice;
- all vegetables (except potatoes and corn), cooked or raw, and tofu;
- nuts, seeds, nut butters; and
- oils, vinegar, mayonnaise, mustard (no hydrogenated oils).

The patient should be instructed as follows:

- Prepare for this test by shopping for the foods required so they are readily available.
- Avoid becoming hungry between meals. Unlimited smaller meals—snacks—of permitted foods may be necessary for some patients and are encouraged; patients who eat four to eight smaller meals are usually not hungry.
- Do not worry about the volume of food being consumed or about potential imbalances of macronutrients; they will be balanced in the next step.
- Be consistent; performing the test for less than two weeks may not provide a valid assessment. If the patient begins to have adverse reactions, the test should be ended.
- Consume enough vegetables (at least six servings per day) to maintain fiber intake and avoid constipation.
- Maintain a high volume of water intake.

Step Three: After the Two-Week test, the practitioner reevaluates the signs and symptoms addressed during the initial assessment.

- If there have been no changes (a negative test), or none that are significant, the patient may not be carbohydrate intolerant, and the previous level of carbohydrate intake may have been proper for the person's needs.
- If the patient shows improvement in signs or symptoms (a positive test), the carbohydrate intake may have previously been too high. In some cases, a dramatic improvement is evident, and some patients are more clearly carbohydrate intolerant.
- Some test results, such as cholesterol levels, commonly take more than two weeks to change. Triglyceride levels, however, can change significantly after two weeks.
- If the patient feels worse following the two weeks, the reason may be the drastic reduction in fiber and usually suggests that the person did not consume enough vegetable foods or became dehydrated. (On occasion, a fiber supplement may be useful, such as plain psyllium—a form that does not contain added sugar. This may be incorporated into the diet at any time.)
- If the Two-Week test is performed immediately following an examination, any results may be compared, especially muscle testing results.

Step Four: If the Two-Week test is positive, the next task is to determine how much concentrated carbohydrate the patient can tolerate without developing any of the signs or symptoms seen previously. This is accomplished as follows:

- The patient should begin adding small amounts of carbohydrates to the diet. This may include one or two pieces of 100% whole wheat toast with breakfast, or a small serving of brown rice with dinner. The patient should continue to avoid sugar, processed carbohydrates, and other high-glycemic foods.
- These added carbohydrates should not be eaten with consecutive meals.
- After each addition, the patient should watch for any of the symptoms that were present before taking the test. It is especially important to note symptoms that develop immediately after eating, such as intestinal bloating, sleepiness, poor concentration, or feelings of depression.
- The MAF test should also be performed and the results compared with earlier results.

After a period of another one to two weeks, the practitioner should reassess other significant tests, including body weight. Although this process is not designed specifically for weight loss, many patients lose weight as they go through these steps. Yang and Van Itallie (1976) showed that this eating profile for 10 days produced significant water loss, but 35% of the weight lost was from fat.

The goal of the patient is to become aware of whether, and when, their body has an adverse reaction to carbohydrate intake. By gradually adding more carbohydrates, patients will generally find a level of intake that does not adversely affect them. This level of carbohydrate intake may be significantly lower than the previous level. Most patients, with the help of the practitioner, can find an optimal level of carbohydrate intake.

After the level of carbohydrate intake has been established, the practitioner determines the levels of fats by looking at the results of the diet analysis and corrects the ratio as necessary. This often involves adding certain fats to the diet and removing others. Through this process, along with adjustments in carbohydrate intake, the amount of fat in the diet may be established. The same process is followed for protein. Typically, it may take several weeks to find an optimal balance of macronutrients.

Whatever the recommendations, both practitioner and patient should view this advice as one step in the process of finding optimal dietary balance. In a real sense, the dietary proposals can be viewed as a "trial" for the patient. After a period of time, the results can be analyzed and adjusted if necessary. Throughout this period, both practitioner and patient should ask several questions: Are there positive changes in the MAF test? In the laboratory evaluations? In responses to questions on the Symptom Survey or other forms? Is performance improved? Does the patient feel better?

Practitioners and members of their staff (or family) might consider following this process, including the Two-Week test if appropriate, for their own

Case History

Ralph's major complaint was fatigue, and he had back, hip, and knee pain that was helped by aspirin. His body fat content was 22% despite his training, which included running about 70 km (43 miles) and cycling 200 km (124 miles) per week. He was sleepy after meals and always hungry, and his Symptom Survey was full of other complaints in Groups Three, Nine, and Ten (blood sugar, fatty acids, and carbohydrate intolerance, respectively). There were a number of indicators for adrenal stress (decreased systolic blood pressure upon standing, insomnia, and other symptoms listed in Group Seven F). A long list of functional musculoskeletal problems was found, but Ralph's diet seemed to be a primary problem and was addressed first. His intake of carbohydrate, protein, and fat was 72%, 12%, and 16%, respectively. The ratio of omega-6 to omega-3 was approximately 30:1, and the lowest nutrients were B6 and magnesium. His MAF test for 5 km (3.1 miles) was 24:43. The first recommendations given to Ralph were to remove many of the Group A fats (beginning with those from the processed foods he was eating) and to add at least six servings of fresh leafy vegetables per day. He was given linseed oil, vitamin B6, sesame seed oil, and magnesium (Linum B6, Sesame Seed Oil, and Magnesium Lactate from Standard Process, Inc.) and was asked to begin the Two-Week test the next morning. Ralph returned in two weeks much improved; he had good energy and was much less hungry, and his previous day's MAF test had significantly improved to 22:51. Eighty percent of the musculoskeletal problems that had been evident two weeks earlier were not present, and lying-to-standing blood pressure changes were normal. Hands-on treatments were directed at correcting the remaining imbalances. Two weeks later, Ralph returned with a much better understanding of his level of carbohydrates. Two months later his diet was reevaluated, and it showed a macronutrient ratio of 38:25:37. His nutrient intake was balanced except for B6 and Group C fats, and he continued to take Linum B6. After several months, his body fat was reduced to 12%, and his MAF test continued to improve to under 20 min.

benefit as well as for a better understanding of patients' experiences.

CONCLUSION

Obtaining a balanced diet should be the focus of both the practitioner and the patient. This is accomplished first through a proper and extensive assessment of the patient's current diet for all of the key elements: macronutrient ratio, balance of Group A, B, and C fats, nutrient levels, and so on. Correcting dietary imbalance may result in increased athletic performance, improvement in body fat stores, lower injury rate, faster healing, and many other health and fitness benefits. A reassessment of the patient's diet on a regular basis may be optimal. All patients are unique, and their body requirements may change regularly. Learning to adjust to the body's needs is important, and the approach to doing so may best be considered as an ongoing process. The athlete's diet helps provide fuel during training and competition and throughout the recovery process as well. Repair of the normal training wear and tear, as well as maintenance of the various systems (such as hormonal, digestive, skeletal), also relies on nutrients from the diet.

Nutritional Supplement Therapy

If the diet does not supply the necessary nutrients for optimal health and fitness, nutritional supplements can help balance the patient's structural, chemical, and mental/emotional state. Sobal and Marquart (1994) surveyed studies of over 10,000 athletes at various levels of competition from 15 different sports and found that about half took nutritional supplements (more than the percentage for the general population). Elite athletes used supplements more than college or high school athletes. More women used supplements than men. It is critical to collect information on the patient's supplement intake, if any, during the initial assessment process and to update this information as necessary. An increased nutritional need may be due not only to a lack of dietary sources but also to a number of commonly encountered situations: decreased nutrient absorption by the gastrointestinal tract; increased nutrient excretion in sweat, urine, and feces; increased nutrient turnover; and biochemical adaptation to training. Human work performance is reduced with low levels of specific vitamins and minerals (van der Beek et al. 1988; Lukaski et al. 1996). It is the job of the complementary sports medicine practitioner to assess and treat these potential imbalances.

FUNCTIONAL NUTRITION

This chapter addresses nutrition from a functional standpoint, rather than from the perspective of disease and prevention of deficiency diseases, which are rare in industrialized countries. Specific nutrients may be required by a patient to improve physical, chemical, and mental/emotional function, even when blood tests are normal for these nutrients (Lukaski and Penland 1996). Many patients fall into the gap between overt deficiency and the levels of nutrient intake that allow optimal function. According to Lukaski and Penland, "One factor limiting efforts to determine human requirements for dietary intakes of mineral elements has been the unavailability of acceptable standards for evaluating the effects of marginal and mild deficiencies" (p. 2354). Certainly the same can be said for most, if not all, micronutrients.

While most studies in nutrition do not measure function, but rather disease or gross imbalances, some may still be of great value to the complementary sports medicine practitioner for understanding the abnormal mechanisms associated with these imbalances. Even more important is an understanding of the normal biochemical pathways, which can be applied clinically in our endeavor to balance the body's physical, chemical, and mental/emotional state.

Recommendations used in complementary sports medicine do not necessarily compare with the recommended daily allowances (RDAs), which are mostly disease based. For example, the RDA for vitamin C is 60 mg/day for adults. This dose is based on prevention of signs and symptoms of scurvy for at least four weeks if there is no vitamin C intake (Food and Nutrition Board 1989). In addition, Reeds and Beckett (1996) state that an RDA is designed explicitly to be applicable to populations rather than to individuals. However, the use of RDA values may have some benefit in that these can serve as a general guide when one is comparing patients' diets.

Unfortunately, the food intakes of some individuals do not even provide the RDA for some nutrients. This may be especially true in athletes who are restricting energy intake to achieve weight loss (Clarkson 1995) and in athletes involved in competition (Steen et al. 1995). In fact, weight loss by energy restriction reduces competitive ability (Rankin et al. 1996). In addition, substances that are not recognized as essential or that have no RDA may still be vital for human function. For example, boron has been shown to improve cognitive performance but has not been established as an important nutrient (Penland 1994).

NUTRITIONAL ASSESSMENT

As with all other therapies described in this text, the assessment process regarding supplement need is of primary importance. The dietary analysis described in the previous chapter gives both practitioner and patient an accurate history of many of the individual nutrients consumed in the diet. Further evaluations should complement the diet analysis. In addition, the oral nutrient challenge may be useful in helping the practitioner to determine which dietary supplements, if any, the patient may require.

Individual nutrients may be adversely affected by a number of factors that reduce their levels in food. For example, most vitamins are unstable to the heat of cooking, including vitamins A, C, thiamin (B1), riboflavin (B2), pyridoxine (B6), and E, as well as biotin, the carotenoids, folic acid, and pantothenic acid (B5). In addition, lysine and threonine are amino acids unstable to heat. Linder (1991) also reported the following:

- During cooking, sometimes significant amounts of nutrient may be destroyed or lost in liquids if these are not consumed. For example, half the riboflavin (vitamin B2) in beef, up to half of the vitamin C in broccoli, and up to 60% of the riboflavin in spinach may be lost from overcooking.
- Compared to fresh foods, foods lose nutrients in both freezing and canning. For example, niacin loss in frozen vegetables may be 26% and that in canning 51%.
- Foods stored for longer periods may lose nutrients. After 48 hr, lettuce may lose 30%-40% of its vitamin C content.
- Ripened foods generally have higher levels of nutrients. Tomatoes have more vitamin C and beta carotene when ripe compared to unripe; bananas have more vitamin C when ripe compared to medium ripe or overripe.
- Vitamin E is destroyed by commercial cooking, food processing, and deep-freezing (Mayes 1993c).

Like all other aspects of complementary sports medicine, addressing the nutritional status of each individual begins with assessment, as the first of several steps in balancing nutrition. Most of these assessments were described earlier (chapters 7, 8, 11, and 18). It is important to note again that blood tests may not always indicate nutritional needs, as low nutrient levels in the body may not always be reflected in these tests (Miyajima et al. 1989). The next step is application of a particular therapy, in this case providing a nutritional supplement. Finding the cause of the problem goes hand in hand with this step. For example, patients who have a need for iron may benefit from the proper type of iron supplement, but the cause of the low-iron state must also be found, if possible. In other words, providing supplementation is one part of the therapy, and addressing the cause (poor intake, poor absorption, blood loss, etc.) is the other. Finally, after a period of time when the supplementation has been stopped, a reassessment process must be performed to ensure that the whole problem has been corrected.

NUTRIENT ABSORPTION

Before discussion of specific nutrients in relation to carbohydrate, fat, and protein metabolism and other nutritional factors, the important issue of food digestion and nutrient absorption must be addressed. Even with optimal dietary intakes, if food is not first digested, and if the small intestine's absorptive mechanisms are not functional enough to obtain the diet's nutrients, nutritional imbalances can occur due to malabsorption. These problems could be identical to those associated with not eating enough of the necessary nutrients. In other words, nutritional imbalances may be due to not consuming enough nutrients, or not digesting them, or not absorbing them. (The utilization of nutrients after absorption is also important and is discussed throughout this chapter.) Two common causes of nutrient unavailability are dysfunction of the hydrochloric acid mechanism in the stomach, which is a key step in the digestive process, and dysfunction of the small-intestine villi (the structures that absorb nutrients) due to atrophy.

All these problems can cause a relatively minor (as compared to celiac disease) but clinically significant subclinical or functional malabsorption. An example is seen in specific conditions such as anemia, which has been termed subclinical celiac disease by Corazza et al. (1995). More often, however, this so-called malabsorption syndrome is accompanied by minor, transitory, and extraintestinal symptoms (Gasbarrini and Corazza 1993). Many patients who are not digesting efficiently do not have clear symptoms of gastrointestinal (GI) distress but more subtle indicators, such as excessive gas or stool odor. Many will not think to discuss these relatively minor intestinal problems especially when their main complaints, such as low back pain, are more distressing. Use of the symptom survey type of form and a complete history will enable the practitioner to uncover more of these significant problems.

Stress Effects

Among the potential causes of poor digestion and absorption of nutrients is any type of stress, which may result in altered production of hydrochloric acid. Stress can also lead to mucosal suppression in the small intestines, where most nutrients are absorbed (Bragg et al. 1991). Such suppression includes the absence of luminal substrates, decreased pancreatic and biliary secretions, and alterations in endocrine or paracrine activity that normally accompanies digestion and absorption. Malabsorption, most likely from diminished hydrochloric acid production, also increases with age (Ferraris 1997). Reduced hydrochloric acid may also be the result of caloric restriction (Higashide et al. 1997). In addition, GI blood flow is vital for digestion and especially absorption, and may be reduced in patients taking nonsteroidal anti-inflammatory drugs (Taha et al. 1993). Gastrointestinal blood flow is also shunted to skeletal muscles with the onset of activity—a reason to relax during and after meals.

Level of Hydrochloric Acid Production

Hydrochloric acid is a normal and vital part of the digestive process; without its action, nutrient availability may be greatly diminished. Malabsorption may be due to hypochlorhydria or achlorhydria—low levels or lack of gastric hydrochloric acid, respectively (Dickey et al. 1997). This results in diminished digestion not only in the stomach, but also in the small intestine, as the hydrochloric acid content of food (chyme) leaving the stomach is a significant stimulant for the production of pancreatic and other enzymes in the small intestine (Guyton 1986). Hypo- or achlorhydria may be considered if the fasting plasma gastrin is over 200 ng/L. The magnesium hydrogen breath test may also assess hypo- or achlorhydria (Humbert et al. 1994). Manual muscle testing may be most useful clinically in helping the practitioner assess and treat this problem, especially in its early functional state, and it is discussed later.

Hydrochloric acid dysfunction often results in diminished production, but in some cases an excess is produced (McColl 1997). This may be the result of autonomic (sympathetic-parasympathetic) imbalance. Recall the other indicators of autonomic dysfunction noted in previous chapters: signs and symptoms in Groups One and Two from the Symptom Survey, the heart rate of an overtrained athlete (too high with sympathetic stress and too low with parasympathetic stress), cold pressor test results (which could demonstrate a lack or excess of sympathetic response), and others.

Malabsorption of nutrients can be a direct result of diminished hydrochloric acid production. For example, hypo- or achlorhydria can have a significant effect on reducing the absorption of calcium and phosphate (Graziani et al. 1995), vitamin B12 (Saltzman et al. 1994), iron (Champagne 1989), and zinc and carbohydrate (Russell 1992).

Hypo- or achlorhydria may have other numerous adverse secondary effects not only in the stomach but throughout the GI tract, including bacterial overgrowth (Freston 1997), and is probably involved in gastric carcinogenesis (Brandi et al. 1996). Incidence of yeast and fungal infections (i.e., candida) is significantly higher in patients with hypo- or achlorhydria (Ramani et al. 1994; Ghoshal et al. 1994; Veselov and Ruchkin 1987). In addition, hypo- or achlorhydria is common in patients with rheumatoid arthritis (Henriksson et al. 1993; Svintsyts'kyi et al. 1994).

Supplementing the patient with hydrochloric acid tablets may improve the absorption of nutrients (Saltzman et al. 1994; Russell et al. 1994). The need for this supplementation may first be assessed from the history and examination. In chapter 11, the relationships between organs and muscles were described, and it was shown that the stomach is related to the pectoralis major clavicular (PMC). It is common to observe an inhibited PMC bilaterally when there is a need for hydrochloric acid. This muscle inhibition must be differentiated from the same inhibition indicating a possible mental/emotional stress; in some cases, though, the two problems occur together. In the case of PMC inhibition bilaterally, applying an oral chemical challenge using betaine hydrochloride, for example, may normalize muscle function. In this case, betaine hydrochloride is typically supplemented at a dose of 250-300 mg after each meal and approximately half that dose after a snack. (Betaine hydrochloride is the hydrochloride salt of betaine, which on hydrolysis yields hydrochloric acid.)

Taking antacids may be counterproductive for efficient digestion and absorption, especially when hypo- or achlorhydria already exists. It is important for patients to understand that "neutralizing" stomach acids cannot be achieved with any single acid-inhibitory drug or any combination of these drugs (Brunner et al. 1996). In mainstream medicine, a rationale for giving antacids is the fact that between feedings, the stomach normally does not produce any acidic secretion unless there is strong emotional stress that stimulates acid production (Guyton 1986).

Small-Intestine Efficiency and L-Glutamine

In addition to gastric function, small-intestine efficiency is required for optimal nutrient absorption. L-Glutamine is the primary metabolic fuel of the intestinal mucosa (Islam et al. 1997). This amino acid is important for intestinal function and especially nutritional absorption, specifically by improving the structure and function of the small-intestine villi—the sites of nutrient absorption (Buchman et al. 1995; Lacey and Wilmore 1990). During stress, including that from training and competition, the muscles synthesize and release L-glutamine, and the intestine takes up much of this amino acid. Supplementing L-glutamine may provide benefits for patients with diminished absorptive function (Maffetone 1990). The author has used doses of 500 mg to 1000 mg, two to four times daily between meals. In cases of primary functional malabsorption, oral nutrient testing with L-glutamine may normalize all muscle inhibition.

Foods high in glutamine include meats and fish, seeds and sprouted seeds, and cabbage. However, even if glutamine is prevalent in the diet, significant amounts can be lost in food as a result of cooking, as glutamine is heat labile. In addition, avoidance of food (skipping meals, fasting, etc.), which can inhibit intestinal function, may further reduce glutamine levels; an extreme example is a four-day fast, which can reduce glutamine levels by 50% (Shabert 1997).

L-Glutamine has been one of the most intensely studied nutrients in the field of nutrition in recent years (Ziegler et al. 1996). In addition to its use for intestinal stress and malabsorption, there are a number of other important aspects of L-glutamine to consider:

- Glutamine improves water, sodium, potassium, and chloride absorption (Islam et al. 1997) and may be useful during sport activity.
- Glutamine has a positive effect on the immune system of athletes (Newsholme 1994).

- L-Glutamine supplementation following exercise reduces infections (Castell et al. 1996).
- Plasma glutamine concentration is decreased in overtrained athletes and after long endurance training and racing (Parry-Billings et al. 1992).
- Low levels of glutamine may serve as a marker for overtraining (Rowbottom et al. 1996).
- Glutamine exerts protein anabolic effects (Ziegler et al. 1996).
- Glutamine improves nitrogen balance (van der Hulst et al. 1993).
- Glutamine has been shown to have marked anti-inflammatory activity and moderate analgesic activity (Jain and Khanna 1981), possibly because it inhibits nitric oxide synthesis (Meininger and Wu 1997).
- Kelso et al. (1989) demonstrated the anti-inflammatory effects of glutamine in skeletal muscle.
- In addition to affecting the small intestine, L-glutamine has positive effects on large-intestine function (Scheppach et al. 1994).

Practitioners can help patients improve their nutritional state by discussing not only what they eat, but how they consume meals and foods. Eating food in a stressful environment, such as during work, may be contraindicated for good nutrition because of potential intestinal dysfunction and the lack of optimal nutritional absorption. When eating patterns are evaluated, this problem is often observed. Listening to enjoyable music can be helpful in reducing stress levels (McKinney et al. 1997); music during the meal may be another approach patients can use to improve their digestion and absorption.

In the case of small-intestine dysfunction, the muscle relationships include the quadriceps and abdominals. In many instances of malabsorption, quadriceps and/or abdominal muscle inhibition is present. If these muscles are inhibited, it is important to evaluate the potential need for hydrochloric acid and/or L-glutamine using the oral challenge. Note that this muscle dysfunction can also alter body structure, affecting performance and increasing the risk of secondary mechanical injury.

In addition to supplementing with the nutrients mentioned (or others), it is important to correct other related problems associated with these muscles, that is, through Chapman's reflexes, acupuncture points, and emotion reflexes. Such correction may have a significant therapeutic effect not only on the muscle(s) but also on the GI system.

TYPES OF NUTRITIONAL SUPPLEMENTS

Many considerations come into play when one confronts the thousands of types of nutritional supplements available. These include the so-called natural and synthetic products, low and high dose, and various formulas. To simplify, think of nutritional supplements as consisting of just two basic types: food concentrates and products containing manufactured, or isolated, nutrients.

Food Concentrates and Phytochemicals

Food concentrates are produced from whole foods, concentrated and made available in tablet, capsule, powder, perle, or liquid form. Because they are made from foods, usually with the fiber and water removed, or are otherwise concentrated, these contain most or all the components found in the whole food. While science has discovered many of the important individual substances necessary for optimal nutrition, such as many of the common vitamins and minerals, it is very likely that a number of other important substances have not yet been discovered. Nonetheless, the undiscovered benefits are still available in food concentrates. Some of these substances are now referred to as phytochemicals or phytonutrients.

Food concentrates include products such as nutritional yeast, oil concentrates (from fish, linseed, black currant seed, sesame seed, etc.), herbs, animal concentrates (from organs and glands), and other products. It is important that these food supplements be processed without high heat, since many nutritional substances are heat labile and are changed or damaged when overheated.

Phytochemicals are technically thought of as "nonnutritive" substances in plants that possess health-protective benefits, although their therapeutic value is well recognized (Craig 1997). These phytochemicals are found in relatively high amounts in vegetables, nuts, and fruits and are made up of phenolic compounds, terpenoids, pigments, and other natural substances. They have been associated with protection from chronic disease such as heart disease, cancer, diabetes, and hypertension, along with other conditions. The foods and herbs with the highest health-protective activity include ginger, garlic, soybeans, licorice, citrus, green tea, cabbage, kale, Brussels sprouts, and other umbelliferous vegetables (carrots). Many in complementary sports medicine have used phytochemicals in their therapeutic approach for decades. Standard Process, Inc., the oldest nutritional supplement company in the United States, has been growing its own organic food and producing food concentrates containing phytonutrients since 1929.

Foods containing phytochemicals can no longer be viewed only from the standpoint of their nutrient content, including the traditional antioxidants; they should be seen as foods with important therapeutic properties (Messina and Messina 1996). Scientists have not isolated all the beneficial substances in phytonutrients. Among the benefits are their anti-inflammatory effect (Chan et al. 1995, 1997) and antioxidant-type qualities (Craig 1997). For example, cruciferous vegetables such as Brussels sprouts contain glucosinolates, which differ from antioxidants but function similarly, for example by reducing oxidative DNA damage (Verhagen et al. 1997). Nutritional supplements that contain phytonutrients may be of great value to the practitioner and patient in circumstances in which the patient is not consuming sufficient amounts of high-quality foods.

When taking supplements, since they are really foods or food derivatives, patients should be instructed to taste or chew them before swallowing. This provides the added stimulus observed in the oral nutrient challenge; the patient's body responds to the supplement upon tasting by improving muscle function. If the supplement is in a capsule, it can usually be opened or broken in the mouth; the same is true with a coated tablet. While the added benefit has not been researched, some practitioners have observed improved responses when patients taste their supplements before swallowing as compared to when they do not. The only products that should not be chewed are those containing betaine hydrochloride, discussed later, which may adversely affect tooth enamel.

Manufactured Nutritional Supplements

Manufactured or isolated nutritional products are the most common form of nutritional supplement on the market; these are also the source of nutrients used in fortification of processed foods. These products either are manufactured synthetically or are extracted from their food origins. Examples of these products are ascorbic acid (as vitamin C), vitamin B6, zinc, and almost all single or formula nutritional supplements in common use. These products are useful if a higher dose is required or if the patient is allergic to certain items contained in food concentrates, such as soy.

In the majority of cases, food concentrates provide relatively lower doses of individual nutrients than manufactured products do. For example, vitamin E in a food concentrate may contain 5 international units (IU) of all tocopherols in nature; but an isolated form may contain 400 IU of only alpha-tocopherol, one of eight tocopherols (vitamin E complex is discussed further on). Patients who require a particular supplement may benefit from either the food concentrate, the manufactured product, or occasionally both. This can be differentiated using an oral challenge or according to other preference on the part of both patient and practitioner. The use of whole-food concentrates is preferred if there is an option.

Toxic reactions to excess vitamin and mineral supplements sometimes occur (Snodgrass 1992), but are not common. These are usually the result of taking isolated or synthetic forms of nutrients, as described later, versus those naturally occurring in food concentrates of lower doses. Perhaps the most common excess is stored iron (as ferritin), which has been associated with an increased risk of heart disease (Salonen et al. 1992) and liver oxidative stress (Houglum et al. 1997).

A more common harmful effect of nutritional supplements is the false sense of balance the patient may derive; many patients think taking a once-a-day synthetic vitamin product, for example, may make up for the many imbalances in their diet. Patients must understand that in addition to the fact that most so-called "multiple" supplements are incomplete because they are manufactured from isolated or synthetic nutrients, there are many substances within foods that have not yet been discovered, or have been only recently discovered, that are not included in once-a-day supplements. Food concentrates in combination with a healthy diet, however, may provide all the substances normally found in food.

Glandular Preparations as Supplements

Although the use of animal glandular products remains popular with many nutrition-oriented practitioners, very little scientific research has been conducted showing positive or negative effects of these supplements on humans. While more studies are needed, the clinical benefits of these glandular supplements continue to be observed. These substances include products made from adrenal, pancreas, liver, thyroid, ovary, thymus, and other glands. Other products from animal organs are also processed and used. In the wild, these animal parts are the first to be eaten by most animals, with much of the muscle meat left to scavengers. Overall, organs and glands have much more nutritional value. For example, liver averages 2.8, 7.5, and 71 µg/g of thiamin, pyridoxine, and pantothenic acid, respectively; the same nutrients in muscle meat average 0.9, 3.3, and 4.7 µg/g, respectively (Linder 1991).

In mainstream medicine, the use of certain isolated substances from animals has proven effective for humans—for example, bovine and porcine insulin, estrogen, and other hormones. However, some practitioners have avoided the use of nonprescription nutritional animal supplements because of the lack of scientific evidence regarding their value. Recently, however, Song et al. (1998) demonstrated that powdered bovine prostate may contain biochemical constituents that exert positive metabolic effects in humans. Animal studies have shown that prostate concentrates from various animals may increase zinc absorption.

Thymus products are also used in complementary sports medicine. Thymus in association with immune function is especially important in athletes given the possible relationships to training stress discussed in chapters 5 and 23. Human thymus function gradually diminishes with age, resulting in the alteration of T-cell functions in the elderly. However, thymus function is still active in adults, and the loss of function can be reversed (Hirokawa et al. 1992). Thymomodulin, a calf thymus derivative (composed of several peptides), remains active when administered orally to humans (Kouttab et al. 1989). Thymomodulin has been used successfully for the treatment of food allergies (Genova and Guerra 1986) and respiratory infections (Fiocchi et al. 1986) and has been shown to regulate the maturation of human T cells (Cazzola et al. 1987).

Various types of preparations of a given gland are available and are used for various types of imbalances. Adrenal dysfunction, for example, may be treated with whole, desiccated adrenal gland or a glandular extract. Schmitt (1990) discusses three types of glandular preparations: aqueous tissue extracts, whole glandular concentrates, and so-called protomorphogens. In making these products, it is important for companies to avoid heating them above body temperature to prevent destruction of various nutrients, enzymes, and other substances contained in the gland while at the same time ensuring safety. The current use of each type in complementary sports medicine is briefly described in the following paragraphs. All these types of preparations are available without prescription except as noted. When muscle testing is used as an assessment tool, these preparations can have very different effects during an oral challenge.

Aqueous tissue extracts are available as two main types—those containing hormones and those that are hormone free. The extracts containing hormones are prescription items; these include thyroid, which contains thyroxine, and ovary, containing estrogen and progesterone. Their mode of action is clear; they are useful as a hormone replacement therapy, required by patients whose ability to produce their own hormones is greatly diminished.

More common is the use of nonprescription aqueous extracts that do not contain hormones. The reason for the beneficial actions is unknown. Common supplements in this category include thymus extracts, which may be successful in improving the immune system function. Others are ovary and prostate extracts.

Whole glandular extracts are dried, unprocessed products of individual glands, but do not contain hormones. They may be used by practitioners when increased gland function is desired but some may be contraindicated when a gland is overactive. For example, during certain stages of adrenal stress, certain hormones, such as cortisol and the catecholamines, are overproduced. In this situation, a whole adrenal concentrate may not be an appropriate choice. Rather, one of the other glandular preparations may be helpful. This supplement may function because of its content of raw materials needed by the organ or gland for balanced function, but this is speculation.

Protomorphogens are theoretically nucleoprotein extracts from the cells of specific organs and glands and are used when there is either excess or deficient function. They may have actions that are antigen-like, interacting with circulating antibodies to specific organs or glands that may interfere with their repair process. Like whole extracts, protomorphogens do not contain hormones.

The use of organ and glandular products may be considered if the patient has an inhibition of a muscle related to an organ or gland as discussed in chapter 11. For example, a sartorius muscle inhibition is sometimes associated with adrenal dysfunction, or a psoas muscle inhibition may be related to kidney dysfunction. In this case, an oral challenge using the appropriate organ or glandular supplement may be helpful to the practitioner in deciding which product, if any, may benefit the patient.

Case History

Sam played tennis four to five times per week for 2 to 3 hr each time and competed regularly. His job in advertising was very stressful, and he never ate a meal in a relaxed state. He had a variety of signs and symptoms including generalized muscle pain between workouts, and especially after competitions, and muscle cramping during play. He had bilateral shoulder pain, low back pain, fatigue, and difficulty falling asleep. Among the findings were an inhibition of the PMC bilateral, which normalized when Betaine Hydrochloride (Standard Process, Inc.) was used for oral challenge, and inhibition of all abdominal muscles, which normalized with an oral challenge of L-Glutamine Plus (Nutri-West). Calcium intake was relatively high, and Sam also took extra calcium supplements from a popular antacid. However, some of his complaints might have been associated with a need for calcium, as this mineral also was positive with an oral challenge; typically, muscle pain after workouts, muscle cramping, and difficulty falling asleep may be associated with a lack of calcium in the tissues. His shoulder pain might also have been associated with the bilateral PMC inhibition, and the low back pain with abdominal dysfunction. Sam was given Betaine Hydrochloride and L-Glutamine Plus. When he returned three weeks later, Sam reported that his muscle pains and cramping had completely resolved, falling asleep was about 75% improved, fatigue had improved by 50%, and his shoulder and low back had improved by about 90%. He was asked to continue his supplements for about two months, when he would return for another session. Sam was also instructed to sit quietly to eat each of his three meals, which was a very difficult change for him. Ultimately, Sam's signs and symptoms completely improved, as did his tennis game.

NUTRIENTS IMPORTANT FOR CARBOHYDRATE METABOLISM

Recall the obvious fact that the generation of adenosine triphosphate from glucose through various pathways is an important aspect of health and fitness. For this process to continue, a variety of nutrients are directly and indirectly essential. The most common ones are these:

- Thiamin (B1)
- Riboflavin (B2)
- Pyridoxine (B6)
- Cobalamin (B12)
- Niacin (B3)
- Biotin
- Pantothenic acid (B5)
- Choline
- Magnesium
- Manganese
- Iron
- Chromium

A low supply of any of these nutrients may adversely affect carbohydrate metabolism at various levels. For example, chromium deficiency may contribute to the prevalence of glucose intolerance in the American and Western European populations (Linder 1991).

Among the common nutrients related to carbohydrate metabolism and their high-quality food sources are the following:

- Vitamin B1—meats, fish, egg yolks, whole grains, brown rice
- Vitamin B2—meats, fish, egg yolks, cheese, yogurt, almonds
- Vitamin B6—meats, fish, brown rice, soybeans, whole grains
- Vitamin B12—beef, fish, egg yolks, cheese
- Niacin—meats, fish, nuts, seeds, brewer's yeast
- Biotin—egg yolks, liver, sardines, brown rice, legumes
- Pantothenic acid—meats, fish, egg yolks, soybeans, whole grains
- Choline—egg yolks, fish, organ meats, brewer's yeast, soybeans
- Magnesium—vegetables, seafood, nuts, seeds, whole grains
- Manganese—vegetables, egg yolks, legumes, nuts, whole grains
- Iron—meats, liver, fish, egg yolks
- Chromium—brewer's yeast, whole grains, grapes

One should note that fluoride has an inhibitory effect on carbohydrate metabolism, blocking the enolase enzyme in the glycolysis pathway (Mayes 1993a). The major source of this mineral for many individuals is fluoridated drinking water and toothpaste; tea and seafood contain relatively high levels. Oral contraceptives have a significant adverse effect on carbohydrate metabolism; those who take oral contraceptives have more than twice the risk of developing decreased glucose tolerance than nonusers have (Skouby et al. 1990).

NUTRIENTS IMPORTANT FOR ANTI-INFLAMMATORY ACTIVITY

The inflammatory and anti-inflammatory process was introduced in chapters 6 and 18 in connection with the conversion of dietary fats to eicosanoids. Also described were a number of nutrients important for the synthesis of the Series 1 and 3 eicosanoids, as well as approaches to manipulating these substances. Nutrients required for the delta-6-desaturase enzyme include vitamin B6, magnesium, and zinc; elongase requires vitamin B6, magnesium, and niacin.

As described in the previous chapter, sesamin, from sesame seed oil, can inhibit delta-5-desaturase, reducing the conversion of dihomo-gamma-linolenic acid to arachidonic acid and thus restricting the production of pro-inflammatory Series 2 eicosanoids. Eicosapentaenoic acid (EPA) also inhibits this enzyme. Unheated sesame seed oil in sealed perles may be best since this helps prevent the unsaturated fats from oxidizing.

Other nutrients are important for the action of cyclooxygenase, which helps convert dihomo-gamma-linolenic acid to the Series 1 eicosanoids and EPA to the Series 3 eicosanoids, including low-dose vitamin E (discussed later), vitamin C, niacin, vitamin B6, and magnesium.

If these nutrients are not available in sufficient amounts in the patient's diet, supplementation must be used. All the nutrients described here are available in supplement form without prescription. Figure 19.1 lists nutrients used by the body for the production of Series 1 and 3 eicosanoids, and figure 19.2 lists nutrients that inhibit delta-5-desaturase.

It is important to note that a low dose of vitamin E (i.e., natural and food sources; that is, less than 10 IU) is used in these reactions, as high doses (i.e., isolated and synthetic sources; above 200-400 IU) may inhibit the cyclooxygenase enzyme. Although vitamin E (the generic name for all tocopherols and tocotrienols) is labeled by the amount of alpha-tocopherol, there are at least eight different types of tocopherols in nature (Kamal-Eldin and Appelqvist 1996), in addition to those synthetically produced. Christen et al. (1997) showed that gamma-tocopherol (the most common form found in foods) was more effective than alpha-tocopherol (the most common isolated form in high-dose vitamin supplements) in antioxidant effects, and that large doses of alpha-tocopherol can displace gamma-tocopherol in plasma and other tissues. Wolf (1997) demonstrated that gamma-tocopherol was more effective in controlling oxidation of unsaturated fats.

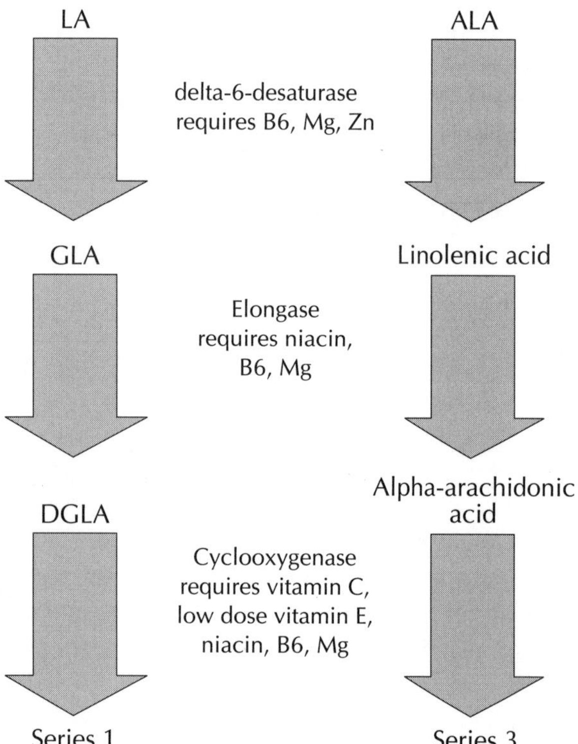

Figure 19.1 Nutrients important for the production of Series 1 and 3 eicosanoids: linoleic acid (LA), gamma-linolenic acid (GLA), dihomo-gamma-linolenic acid (DGLA), and Alpha linolenic acid (ALA)

Taking too much vitamin E may also lower thyroid hormone levels and slightly increase fasting triglyceride levels (Linder 1991). In high doses, vitamin E may become a pro-oxidant (Takahashi 1995). This is more often the case with alpha-tocopherol and less so with gamma-tocopherol (Kamal-Eldin and Appelqvist 1996). In addition, high doses of vitamin E have been shown to cause muscle weakness (Snodgrass 1992).

Vitamin E may be seen in nature as part of a "complex" (Schmitt 1990) that includes the tocopherols (providing antioxidant activity), the phospholipids (part of the cell-wall structure), steroid hormone precursors, and essential fatty acids. In foods, the amount of naturally occurring tocopherol is very small. For example, in a loaf of whole wheat bread (which contains a relatively high level of natural vitamin E), only 2-4 IU may be present.

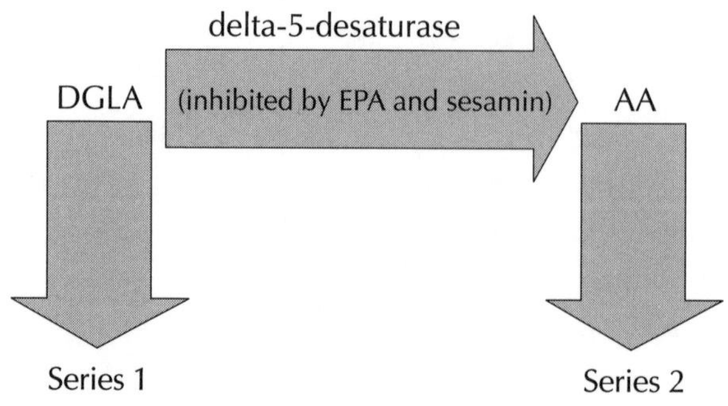

Figure 19.2 Inhibition of delta-5-desaturase

Each patient's need for vitamin E should be individually evaluated. Manual muscle testing may also help the practitioner determine the proper dose. It may be best to consume foods containing quality sources of natural vitamin E "complex," such as nuts, seeds, and vegetables. If a supplement is required, it is a good idea to use a natural source of low-dose vitamin E family, such as Cataplex E (Standard Process, Inc.), which contains 2.5 IU; if a high-dose vitamin E product is required for the short term, the patient should be carefully monitored.

Selenium is an important mineral associated with vitamin E function because it is an integral part of the antioxidant enzyme, glutathione peroxidase (van de Vijver et al. 1997). Supplementation of vitamin E may necessitate additional selenium.

Other supplements that may help in balancing the inflammatory and anti-inflammatory hormones include ginger and garlic. It may be best, and is relatively easy, to consume ginger in its raw state, but many patients are reluctant to eat raw garlic. Instead, they can use a supplement to avoid the odor associated with eating raw garlic as long as it has been processed without heating.

In some patients, an imbalance of eicosanoids may result from a lack of nutrients needed for enzyme activity. In other cases, the precursor fatty acid may be necessary (i.e., black currant seed oil for Series 1 and linseed oil or EPA for Series 3); sometimes a combination is required. Performing an oral challenge using these nutrients may be helpful in determining which nutrients to use for a given patient. Ginger, garlic, and onion can also be used in an oral nutrient challenge.

Many patients take fish oil as a source of EPA; but linseed oil, high in alpha-linolenic acid, is also very effective and predictable in increasing the body's levels of EPA, at levels comparable to those obtained with fish oil supplementation (Mantzioris et al. 1995).

Although not necessarily directly related to eicosanoid production, the nutrient choline may also have anti-inflammatory effects (Gaur et al. 1997) and is discussed later in this chapter.

Case History

Ellen had a number of physical and chemical injuries, including a chronic inflammatory condition. Previously she had had numerous hands-on treatment sessions with several professionals (including chiropractors, an osteopath, and a massage therapist), which would often provide temporary relief of her painful joints. Her dietary analysis showed that the ratio of Group A, B, and C fats was approximately 13:5:1. Oral challenge with aspirin resulted in temporary normalization of all 18 muscle inhibitions. Through an oral nutrient challenge, the nutrients listed in figure 19.1 were assessed. Three of these nutrients (fish oil, low-dose vitamin E, and zinc) normalized all muscles, whereas the others either had no effect or normalized some, but not all, of the inhibited muscles. In addition to the recommendations to reduce Group A and B fats, Ellen was given the three supplements that had been positive during the oral challenge. She was to take three capsules of EPA fish oil three times daily and one tablet each of Cataplex E and Zinc Liver Chelate (Standard Process, Inc.) three times daily. A number of structural problems that had been previously corrected (i.e., numerous spinal joint problems) were left untreated, while others not previously treated were corrected (including a cranial respiratory fault). Ellen returned in three weeks and stated that she was 70% improved; in another three weeks she was showing 95% improvement. She continued improving in both health and fitness without exacerbation.

AEROBIC SYSTEM NUTRITION

The so-called "red" aerobic muscle fibers derive their color from their high volume of blood vessels and especially the presence of myoglobin, a protein compound containing large amounts of iron. Myoglobin combines with oxygen released by the red blood cell, stores it, and transports it to the mitochondria. This is a necessary function that among other actions promotes the utilization of fats for energy. (Iron in hemoglobin is also important for delivery of oxygen.)

Unfortunately, use of iron has been heavily promoted in our society as a method of "increasing energy." There are many causes of fatigue, and regularly taking iron supplements may pose risks. The stored form of iron as ferritin in excess has been associated with an increased risk of heart disease (Salonen et al. 1992). It is important to assess the need for iron in the patient rather than just supplementing based on a symptom such as fatigue. This is best accomplished with a blood test that measures at least serum iron, hemoglobin and hematocrit, and ferritin (see chapter 8 regarding blood testing). Oral nutrient challenge may also be helpful to assess the potential need for iron, as blood levels may not always reflect all myoglobin or other needs. For example, non-anemic patients may demonstrate a need for iron despite not being anemic (Zhu and Haas 1997). This is sometimes referred to as "sports anemia" (Aruoma et al. 1988) and is another example of a functional nutritional need. As previously discussed, malabsorption of iron could be the cause of iron need. In patients without anemia who demonstrate a need for more iron, and in those whose blood tests continue to show low iron, it is important to rule out malabsorption and blood loss.

Biochemically, one of the most important aspects of the aerobic system is the mitochondria, the site of beta oxidation (and a major site of antioxidant activity). This organelle is traditionally described as the "powerhouse" of the cell, generating 80% of the adenosine triphosphate used for cellular activity from the Krebs cycle. In order to achieve optimal mitochondrial function, various nutritional factors are necessary. Mitochondrial dysfunction may be a reason for aerobic deficiency. Impaired oxidative metabolism, migraines, Parkinson's disease, multiple sclerosis, and other conditions may also be associated with mitochondrial dysfunction (Argov et al. 1997).

In general, many vitamins and minerals are necessary for mitochondrial function (van der Beek 1991). Included are those used in the Krebs cycle and nonessential amino acid synthesis and others previously discussed. Essentially, the macro- and micronutrients used by the aerobic muscle fibers and mitochondria are the same ones found in muscle foods—meat and fish. In addition to these nutrients, others may need to be supplemented in particular patients.

Carnitine is an amino acid that is necessary for the transportation of fat to the mitochondria for oxidation (beta oxidation) (Mayes 1993b). It is available in the diet (mostly from meat) and is also synthesized in the body from lysine and methionine, a process that requires iron and vitamin C (Linder 1991). Low dietary protein may result not only in a lower intake of carnitine, but also in lower amounts of raw materials (lysine and methionine) for its production; this may have adverse effects on mitochondrial oxidation of fats. The use of oral challenge in patients with suspected carnitine needs is especially important, since muscle carnitine levels can be extremely low while the serum carnitine concentration is normal (Miyajima et al. 1989). In these patients, L-carnitine supplementation may be helpful, but the cause of the problem must also be addressed through evaluation of diet (especially protein intake, iron, and vitamin C), digestion, and absorption.

LACTIC ACID AND NUTRITION

Lactic acid is continually produced in anaerobic muscle fibers, from small amounts in a resting state (1 mmol/kg) to much larger amounts during high-intensity anaerobic workouts (25 mmol/kg) (Wilmore and Costill 1994). Other tissues, including smooth muscle and tissues in the brain, skin, GI tract, and kidney, also produce lactic acid, as do the red blood cells (Mayes 1993a). Recall that pyruvic acid is produced during anaerobic glycolysis and when oxygen is greatly limited, pyruvic acid is converted to lactic acid.

Lactic acid decreases the pH of the muscle fiber, which reduces glycolytic enzyme function and may diminish calcium-binding capacity, in turn reducing muscle contraction. As discussed earlier, pain is not produced directly from lactic acid. Lactic acid is released into the blood and quickly buffered to sodium (or potassium) lactate. This lactate is not a "waste" product as many patients think, but is recycled (via the Cori cycle) in the liver to glucose and used for energy in the muscles and other tissues.

Most important is the fact that various nutrients are necessary for the proper metabolism of lactate and lactic acid. The most significant association is evident in the fact that thiamin (vitamin B1) deficiency significantly increases plasma lactate levels (Molina et al. 1994). Nakasaki et al. (1997) showed that therapeutic doses of thiamin were effective in significantly reducing high blood lactate levels; van der Beek et al. (1994) demonstrated that patients with low levels of thiamin, riboflavin (vitamin B2), and pyridoxine (vitamin B6) had elevated lactate levels (along with low aerobic power and oxygen consumption).

Good sources of thiamin include meats, nuts, seeds, vegetables, and whole grains (refining flour removes the thiamin, although some flour is enriched with thiamin). This vitamin is unstable in oxygen and moisture, with significant losses in cooking and freezing. Just as important are the potential natural anti-thiamin substances found in nature, referred to as thiaminase (Rindi 1996). This enzyme can destroy thiamin; it is found in red chicory, Brussels sprouts, and red cabbage and in small amounts in tea. It is also contained in clams, oysters, squid, and other mollusks (Alston and Abeles 1987), as well as in certain fish such as herring and smelt (Hirn and Pekkanen 1975). This enzyme is probably easily destroyed by heat. Individuals who may have high needs for thiamin should consider avoiding these foods in their uncooked state. Thiaminase may also be present in certain human intestinal bacteria that hydrolyze thiamin.

Supplementing with a large dose of thiamin may result in poor absorption (Rindi 1996). In addition to foods high in thiamin, it may be best to use a lower-dose product, such as a food extract, taken several times daily rather than in one morning dose.

A variety of studies have shown high lactate levels to be associated with depression, anxiety, phobias, and panic disorders, even in patients with no psychiatric history (Dager et al. 1989; Buller et al. 1989; Martinsen et al. 1989; Balon et al. 1989). This correlates with the fact that increased dietary carbohydrates increase lactate production while lower-carbohydrate diets reduce lactate production (Aitken and Thompson 1989).

AUTONOMIC BALANCE AND NUTRITION

Dysfunction in the autonomic nervous system is well documented in various conditions; it can be observed as early in life as in infancy (de Klerk et al. 1997) and is reduced with aging (Pfeifer et al. 1983).

Certain nutritional factors may be useful for the manipulation of autonomic function. For example, low phosphorus (which may result from increased calcium intake) may reduce sympathetic activity (Peuler et al. 1987). Low copper and ascorbic acid, however, can increase sympathetic function (Lukaski et al. 1988). Toth and Poehlman (1994) showed that vegetarians had increased sympathetic nervous system activity in comparison to nonvegetarians.

Supplements have been used for many years in complementary sports medicine to treat autonomic imbalance. Several nutrients have been shown to be most effective in this regard. To increase sympathetic and/or decrease parasympathetic activity, supplementation with phosphorus (i.e., phosphoric acid) is helpful. Capsaicin, the hot substance found in hot red peppers, may also increase sympathetic activity (Doucet and Tremblay 1997). To increase parasympathetic and/or decrease sympathetic activity, one can supplement with choline and potassium. Fasting may also reduce sympathetic activity, but only during the fasting state (Young and Landsberg 1997).

As a general guide, the Symptom Survey discussed in chapter 7 contains two groups of signs and symptoms that are sometimes evident in patients who have sympathetic and parasympathetic dysfunction: Group One and Group Two, respectively. Certain nutrients from the vitamin "B" family may also be associated with autonomic imbalance. The B complex, sometimes referred to as the "B" vitamins, is a group of water-soluble nutrients that include thiamin (B1), riboflavin (B2), niacin (B3) and niacinamide, pantothenic acid (B5), pyridoxine (B6), biotin, cobalamin (B12), and folic acid. There may be individual nutrients within a given single vitamin. For example, the phosphates of vitamin B6—pyridoxal phosphate (the major form), pyridoxine, and pyridoxamine phosphate—are the three main vitamins in the diet (Mayes 1993d).

Another subgrouping of the B complex, sometimes regarded as consisting of the "B" group (containing predominately thiamin, but also pantothenic acid, cobalamin, and others) and the "G" group (containing predominately riboflavin, but also niacin, folic acid, and others), is commonly used in complementary sports medicine as described by Schmitt (1990). In this case, thiamin and riboflavin are differentiated by their alcohol solubility and insolubility, respectively, but more importantly by their clinical actions on the nervous system. For example, thiamin may promote sympathetic activity, and riboflavin parasympathetic activity. As such, the "B" group may promote vasoconstriction, increase blood pressure, and elevate heart rate in patients who are in need of this nutrient. The "G" group may likewise promote vasodilation, lower blood pressure, and reduce heart rate in patients who need this nutrient.

Schmitt (1990) states, "The entire B complex is a valuable tool in many conditions, but the whole B complex will not be effective if the patient requires only one fraction or the other. Using separate sources of 'B,' 'G' and whole vitamin B complex gives the doctor three tools to work with instead of one" (p. 51). The separate subgroups are available from food sources as Cataplex B and Cataplex G (Standard Process, Inc.) and as isolated thiamin and riboflavin from many commercial companies.

Some clinical signs and symptoms are associated with the need for the "B" fraction of the vitamin B complex: "B" factors include carbohydrate intolerance, sleepiness after meals, and intolerance to noise; lack of vibration sense; frequent nocturnal urination; itchy skin; decreased breath-holding time; and frequent yawning or fatigue and/or decreased body temperature.

Some clinical signs and symptoms are associated with the need for the "G" fraction of the vitamin B complex: "G" factors include poor fat metabolism; ineffective digestion; anxiety and excessive worrying; restless/jumpy/shaky legs; jerkiness of whole body or limb upon falling asleep; cracking at corners of mouth; rash on skin from shaving; very thin upper lip; and/or burning or itchy eyes.

AMINO ACID SUPPLEMENTATION

Supplementing the diet with amino acids is very common in the sport community, but the research results have been mixed except for L-glutamine (discussed earlier). The lack of extensive positive research with other amino acids may indicate the importance of individualization. Practitioners should be very cautious about supplementing with individual amino acids because of the risk of worsening an amino acid imbalance unless careful assessments are made. This may be less of a problem with L-glutamine, which is utilized to a greater extent in the GI tract and is not completely absorbed. However, a number of studies are of interest:

- Supplementing the diet with 23 g of a complete protein source enhanced muscle mass gains compared to values in subjects who trained without the supplement (Meredith et al. 1992).
- Amino acid supplements can lower cortisol levels in swimmers (Kreider et al. 1993).
- Supplementing amino acids during endurance activities may improve negative protein balance and also supplies substrate fuel (Kreider et al. 1993).
- Male power athletes whose daily dietary protein levels were 1.26 g/kg had serum amino acid levels that were significantly lowered during intense training; leucine supplementation prevented the decrease in the serum leucine (Mero et al. 1997).
- Lehmann et al. (1993) demonstrated significant reductions in serum amino acids following an ultratriathlon.

Traditionally, amino acids are grouped as either "essential" (not made by the body; must be consumed in the diet) or "nonessential" (can be manufactured within the body). But all the amino acids are necessary for normal body function; these are listed further on. However, this terminology can be very misleading, for two important reasons. The production of so-called nonessential amino acids requires other nutritional substances, and lower levels of these other nutritional substances can result in lower levels of nonessential amino acids. Maintenance of normal levels of so-called essential amino acids is accomplished through absorption from the diet. Maintenance does not require further biochemical conversions that utilize other nutrients and enzymes when the amino acids are being used for protein synthesis, but does require numerous vitamins and minerals when the amino acids are being converted into other active compounds (i.e., norepinephrine and serotonin). For example, glutamine synthesis requires magnesium, serine production requires niacin, and glycine requires choline. In other cases, nonessential amino acids require essential amino acids for their production; cysteine (nonessential) is produced from methionine (essential) and serine (nonessential), and requires niacin.

In view of this, effective levels of nonessential amino acids may be more difficult to attain in comparison to essential amino acids when a typical Western diet is followed. Rodwell (1993) states, "It might be argued that the nutritionally nonessential amino acids are more important to the cell than the nutritionally essential ones, since organisms (e.g., humans) have evolved that lack the ability to manufacture the latter but not the former group" (p. 287).

It should also be noted that under certain conditions, the need for some nonessential amino acids may become much greater, or the rate of synthesis may be inadequate and these amino acids may be considered essential. For example, in situations of stress such as heavy training, glutamine requirements may be higher than normal so that glutamine may be considered "conditionally essential" (Lacey and Wilmore 1990). In children, histidine and arginine are essential, but they are considered nonessential in adults and are therefore viewed, overall, as "semiessential" (Rodwell 1993).

"Essential" amino acids are arginine, histidine, isoleucine, leucine, lysine, methionine, phenylalanine, threonine, tryptophan, and valine.

"Nonessential" amino acids include alanine, asparagine, aspartate, cysteine, glutamate, glutamine, glycine, proline, serine, and tyrosine.

If supplementation of amino acids is necessary, it can be done using individual amino acids (e.g., L-glutamine tablets) or whole-food concentrates containing all amino acids (i.e., complete protein concentrates). In some instances, a combination may be necessary. With oral nutrient testing, individual amino acids and whole-protein supplements can be used to help determine which may be best for the patient.

It should be emphasized that if a patient requires amino acids, the reason may be a dietary insufficiency. If such is the case, one should attempt to correct the imbalance. Although this may not show up on the dietary assessment, some patients do not effectively digest and absorb sufficient amino acids. Dietary protein must be acted upon by hydrochloric acid in the stomach, which activates the proteolytic enzymes of the stomach, pancreas, and small intestine. Stress, overtraining, or use of antacids, for example, may have an adverse effect on stomach hydrochloric acid as previously discussed.

CHOLINE AND "EXERCISE-INDUCED ASTHMA"

Choline is a major donor of methyl groups (i.e., for the production of methionine), a precursor for membrane synthesis, and a component of the neurotransmitter acetylcholine (Savendahl et al. 1997). Choline is found in foods (especially egg yolks and fish) and can be manufactured in the body from the amino acids serine and methionine, using vitamin B12 and folic acid (Linder 1991). Practitioners of complementary sports medicine have found that choline supplementation can provide great clinical benefits in patients with so-called exercise induced asthma (EIA). The use of choline for EIA has been shown to be effective by Gaur et al. (1997) and Gupta and Gaur (1997). This condition is also referred to as exercise-related or exercise-induced bronchial spasm or bronchoconstriction. Exercise-induced asthma, although not the most appropriate term, is the designation used in this text since it is the one most often encountered in the literature.

Exercise-induced asthma can be defined as a bronchial constriction and a decrease in some measure of air flow, with symptoms of wheezing, chest tightness, coughing, and difficulty in breathing, that is triggered by exercise (Weiler 1996). Up to 15% of athletes have this condition, but almost all people with asthma will have symptoms of EIA (Enright 1996). The assessment of EIA, as an exercise challenge, was discussed in chapter 8. Exercise-induced asthma is a common complaint, and the prevalence appears to be increasing worldwide (Anderson 1996).

Because medications such as cromolyn (an antihistamine) are often effectively used to treat EIA (Weiler 1996), it is not unusual that allergic reactions are sometimes a contributing factor. A number of studies have shown food reactions associated with EIA, especially to cheese (Tilles et al. 1995), celery (Kidd et al. 1983), and shrimp (McNeil and Strauss 1988). Reactions usually occur within a few minutes of exercise from foods ingested 2 to 3 hr before. Kidd et al. (1983) reported a case in which EIA was triggered after the ingestion of any food.

The author has used choline for patients with EIA in doses of 100-200 mg four times daily, and in severe cases 100-200 mg up to six to eight times per day or more. As previously mentioned, it is important for the patient to taste or chew the supplement before swallowing. Potential food hypersensitivity or allergies should be considered (see chapter 18). Vitamin C may also have a positive therapeutic effect in patients with EIA (Cohen et al. 1997).

ANTIOXIDANTS

It is now clear that anaerobic training and competition create increased oxidative stress (Packer 1997). This is attributable to the production of oxygen free radicals, which are also mediators of skeletal muscle damage and inflammation through the release of arachidonic acid (Dekkers et al. 1996). Free radicals may be related to postexercise muscle pain (Pyne 1994), can damage the sodium/potassium pump (Demopoulos 1983), and can promote disease processes (Mayes 1993d). Light and moderate training, however, can improve immune function by increasing the antioxidant enzymes (superoxide dismutase and catalase) (Hirokawa 1997).

Free radicals are atoms or molecules containing one or more unpaired electrons (Halliwell 1996). When a free radical reacts with other nonradical molecules, a new free radical is created with the potential for a devastating chain reaction. When this happens with the unsaturated fatty acids in cell membranes and lipoproteins, lipid peroxidation occurs. Recall from the previous chapter that this problem occurs in the low-densitylipoprotein-cholesterol—which is the reason it has the potential for damaging effects in blood vessel walls. Protein and DNA damage is also associated with free radical activity.

Free radical stress also can adversely affect collagen and joint function, promoting joint disease (Hawkins and Davies 1997), and may be associated with temporomandibular joint dysfunction (Milam et al. 1998).

In addition to the exercise itself, being outdoors can increase free radical stress from air pollution and non-ionizing radiation (ultraviolet and microwaves) (Moller et al. 1996). Copper and iron may also be involved in the production of hydroxyl radicals, which can have damaging effects as well (Berenshtein et al. 1997). It should be noted that vitamin C can be toxic if given to a patient with excess iron because of the potential oxidative stress posed by iron (Halliwell 1996). This may also occur from the oxidation of estrogen catechols by copper (Seacat et al. 1997).

Dietary antioxidants, and supplements, have a positive effect on "scavenging" these free radicals and may prevent much of the muscle damage associated with training and competition. The degree of free radical damage may be associated with training intensity—with exhaustive workouts and competition creating the most oxidative stress.

Antioxidant nutrients that have demonstrated benefits in reducing free radicals include vitamin E and selenium (Veera et al. 1992) and vitamin C (ascorbic acid) (Alessio et al. 1997). Vitamin C also helps to preserve alpha-tocopherol (May 1998). However, high doses of ascorbic acid may have a biphasic relationship between the concentration and the effect, suggesting that an excess may have opposite effects as compared to low doses, including the risk of kidney stones in some patients (Snodgrass 1992). In addition, intake of vitamin C above 250 mg results in significantly less absorption (Goldfarb 1992). It may therefore be best to take small doses of vitamin C several times per day.

Other nutritional substances contribute to antioxidant defense. Glutathione, for example, which has significant antioxidant activity, is a tripeptide consisting of cysteine, glutamic acid, and glycine and requires the mineral selenium for activation (Murray 1993). Carotenoids are also antioxidants, as are flavonoids (Cao et al. 1997), originally called vitamin P by Szenti-Gyorgy, who discovered them in 1936. These flavonoids, responsible for the colors in foods, are found in many vegetables, berries, citrus and other fruits, and red wine; they include phenols, rutin, hesperidin, quercetin, robinin, and others (Craig 1997). In addition, tumeric is a common spice that has significant antioxidant properties (Krishnaswamy 1996).

Dietary restriction as a way of slowing the aging process seems to be effective because of its ability to reduce oxidative stress (Yu 1996). However, dietary restriction must not be at the expense of adequate nutrition.

Oxidative stress can be assessed by direct measurement of free radicals and through measurement of lipid oxidation (Packer 1997); both are special tests. The so-called age pigments observed in some patients are usually end products of lipid peroxidation (Halliwell 1996). A clinical test using manual muscle testing for free radical stress has been used in applied kinesiology as originally proposed by Schmitt (1987a, 1987b). This test utilizes the olfactory challenge described in chapter 11. The substance used is hypochlorite, which is also one of the free radicals the body normally produces (available as regular commercial unscented bleach). If a patient quickly sniffs a mild bleach solution and a normal muscle becomes inhibited, a need for antioxidants may be indicated. (This muscle inhibition lasts only 10-15 sec.) When this test is positive, the practitioner can perform an oral nutrient test with individual antioxidants, or a complex of antioxidants, using another preexisting muscle inhibition during the challenge. If a positive test is found with specific antioxidants, these can be retested using the bleach olfactory challenge. The following shows how this test might work.

Assessment of Oxidative Stress

1. The patient is suspected of having a need for antioxidant supplementation.
2. The right pectoralis major sternal (PMS) is inhibited, and the right psoas is normal (any normal and inhibited muscle can be used).
3. The patient quickly sniffs a mild bleach (hypochlorite) solution that causes inhibition of the psoas muscle (and does not change the inhibited PMS). This inhibition lasts about 10-15 sec.
4. The practitioner performs an oral nutrient test for the following supplements, using the inhibited PMS muscle, with these results:
   - Vitamin C is negative.
   - The vitamin E/selenium combination is positive.
   - Beta carotene is negative.
   - A bioflavonoid complex is positive.
5. Both of the nutrients that were positive (vitamin E/selenium, bioflavonoids) are retested against bleach olfactory challenge as in step 3, with these results:
   - With vitamin E/selenium in the mouth, the patient quickly sniffs the bleach. This test does not cause inhibition of the psoas as in step 3.
   - The same procedure is followed using bioflavonoids, but this does not negate the inhibition.
6. The practitioner can presume that the vitamin E/selenium supplement may be effective as an antioxidant. The bioflavonoid may still be effective, since it produced normal muscle function during the challenge, but this may not be related to its antioxidant activity.

Some of the antioxidant nutrients, along with those that may assist antioxidants in their function, include alpha-tocopherol (vitamin E); vitamin C; carotenoids; cysteine, glutamic acid, and glycine; flavonoids (phenol, quercetin, hesperidin, rutin, robinin, and others); and selenium.

CONCLUSION

If and when an athlete does not consume a diet containing all the necessary nutrients, specific nutritional supplementation becomes an important therapy. The use of supplements begins with a complete assessment of the athlete's diet. Matching particular nutrients with the patient's specific need is the most effective approach. One should also remember that a nutritional oral challenge, using manual muscle testing, can help the practitioner decide which nutrients or food extracts to recommend for a specific patient. If a patient tastes a substance that his or her body will benefit from, the substance can normalize an inhibited muscle. Likewise, tasting a substance that is harmful may cause inhibition of a normal muscle.

20

Ergogenic and Therapeutic Nourishment

Ergogenic nourishment refers to the consumption of liquid or solid nutrients to assist in athletic performance. In a sense, a balanced dietary and nutritional state accomplishes this task to a great extent and should be a primary focus. Essentially, three types of ergogenic and therapeutic aids are available to athletes: water, various solutions (i.e., "sports" drinks), and solid food in the form of "energy" bars.

During prolonged activities, macronutrients may serve an added role, especially for long endurance workouts or competitions. Macronutrients are also important after a workout or a competition for replacement of glycogen stores. Perhaps more important is the fact that in some athletes, adrenal gland or sympathetic dysfunction may lead to sodium/potassium imbalances. It is not the intent of this chapter to prescribe specific drinks, solutions, or products for a given type of athlete, but rather to assist practitioners in helping athletes improve their fluid, electrolyte, and macronutrient balance before, during, and after workouts and competitions. It is important for the practitioner and athlete to work together in this endeavor.

WATER

One of the most important ergogenic aids is water, with sodium having importance for long endurance activities in hot environments. During activities lasting up to about 60-90 min, water may be the only additional ergogenic requirement. Water may be the most common nutritional "deficiency" in the athlete population and should therefore be considered the fourth macronutrient after carbohydrate, protein, and fats. Many people do not drink enough water, and others who perform very long workouts may have difficulty maintaining normal hydration despite drinking sufficient quantities. For athletes, the need to replace water is much greater than the need to replace any other nutritional substance.

A young man's body is typically 60% water, and may contain 42 kg (93 lb) of water; a young woman's body may contain slightly less at 50% of total weight. Approximately two-thirds of the water is intracellular (predominantly in muscle cells), and one-third is in extracellular compartments; a small amount is contained in the transcellular compartments (intestines, anterior chamber of the eye, and subarachnoid space), which may hold up to about 1 L of water (Luft 1996).

Approximately 60% of the body's need for water is supplied from liquids and 30% from foods. The other 10% is produced in the body from the cellular metabolism. Water loss at rest occurs from the kidneys (60%), through respiration (with equal amounts from skin and lungs, totaling 30%), through sweating (5%), and from the large intestine (5%). During activity, however, sweating increases significantly, accounting for 90% of the water lost (1-2 L/hr in prolonged training or competition).

Exercise Effects on Water Regulation

Thirst is activated by sodium and when the total-body water level is reduced. Even slight dehydration reduces plasma volume, triggering thirst. But thirst is sensed after dehydration is present. Once an athlete is dehydrated, it may take up to 48 hr to properly rehydrate using thirst as a guide (Wilmore and Costill 1994). If the amount of water lost becomes greater than the intake, the blood volume diminishes. With diminished blood volume, blood flow (and oxygen) to the muscles and organs is reduced, which raises the heart rate.

Endurance runners, for example, can reduce their pace by 2% for each percentage of body weight lost by dehydration (Wilmore and Costill 1994). Water losses of 6%-10% may occur in marathon events, even more in longer competitions. This translates to a runner's performing a 10-km race in 35 min under normal hydration but slowing to complete the same distance in almost 38 min when 4% dehydrated—a significant loss of performance. Many athletes who find a plateau or worsening in their Maximum Aerobic Function test are experiencing dehydration, which causes an elevated heart rate that forces them to slow the pace. The ability to expel heat is lost with dehydration since skin circulation is reduced, elevating the core temperature.

Team sports require players to perform multiple work bouts at near-maximal effort, with intervals of rest, over a period of time. Such activity patterns are associated with a significant loss of body water that could have a negative impact on temperature regulation and overall performance (Burke and Hawley 1997). Under certain conditions, such as playing in hot weather, the potential for heat stroke is higher; this sometimes fatal condition can be easily mistaken for head injury in contact sports (Savdie et al. 1991). Players have adequate opportunities to drink enough water to minimize or prevent dehydration. Studies across a number of sports show that fluid intakes of up to 1 L/hr can be achieved (Burke 1997). Therefore, consumption of this amount hourly—in small doses—may serve as a guide during competition in many sports.

In athletes with high aerobic function, water regulation is more efficient, including maintenance of body temperatures and lower sweat rates (Yoshida et al. 1995).

Proper Hydration

It is important for an athlete to drink water throughout the day, every day, and not wait until an upcoming event. Ingestion of large amounts of water at one time, however, can inhibit thirst and promote a diuretic response (Maughan et al. 1997). This may result, over time, in a lower net water volume. The best recommendation is to consume small amounts of water throughout the day, each day. In an average-weight athlete, the author suggests between 3 and 4 L/day as a minimum. In athletes who work out more than an hour or two each day, additional water may be required.

It is important to assess the need for water and to do so regularly. Studies have demonstrated that the traditional method of assessing for hydration status, by observing the color of the urine, is a good general guide. A definite yellow color can indicate dehydration, with a clear urine characterizing proper hydration (Armstrong et al. 1994). Urine color is also correlated with specific gravity and osmolality (both laboratory measures of hydration). This approach, however, does not preclude the use of laboratory evaluations that are more precise. Most importantly, patients can learn to assess their own urine color on a daily basis and increase water as necessary.

Practitioners can also use manual muscle testing and oral challenge with water to help determine the hydration status. In this case the outcome is either positive, indicating a need for more water, or negative, meaning that hydration may be adequate. This test may be useful during each session because dehydration is so common in athletes, and also because dehydration may develop at any time throughout the year. Note that when an athlete reaches a very early stage of dehydration, or "functional dehydration," all muscles will become inhibited. In this case, an oral challenge will temporarily normalize all muscles. (It is possible that this functional dehydration will not yet appear in a routine urinalysis.)

Recall from chapter 4 that fluoride inhibits the enolase enzyme in the glycolysis pathway. Athletes may wish to avoid fluoridated water and toothpaste and other unnatural sources that tend to be relatively high in fluoride.

ELECTROLYTES

Sodium and chloride are the dominant electrolytes in the extracellular fluid. Potassium is also present, but in much lesser quantity. The converse is true in the intracellular fluid, which contains high levels of potassium and very small amounts of sodium and chloride. Electrolyte regulation is controlled in part by sodium and chloride, which help regulate extracellular water, by hormonal mechanisms (especially through the adrenal hormone aldosterone), and by the sympathetic nervous system.

Dietary intake of sodium and its loss from the body help regulate both the thirst and the salt-appetite mechanism in the brain, with influence from angiotensin II from the kidney. To help maintain rehydration for some hours after water ingestion, as a precompetition solution, for example, drinks or foods should contain moderate levels of sodium, perhaps as much as 50-60 mmol/L (Maughan et al. 1997).

Sympathetic nervous system activity is important for regulating sodium and chloride, causing sodium retention through its action on the kidney (DiBona 1994). Reduced levels of sodium may also stimulate sympathetic activity. Sympathetic dysfunction, which is commonly associated with overtraining (see chapter 23), is potentially a significant source of electrolyte imbalance, as alluded to earlier.

Adrenal Hormone Effects on Sodium

The adrenal hormone aldosterone (along with angiotensin II activity) is important for electrolyte regulation, increasing sodium and chloride resorption from the kidney and potassium excretion (Guyton 1986). Reduction in levels of aldosterone, however, may occur in association with excess cortisol production (Parker et al. 1985) and is often seen in conditions of overtraining and other stress. This can result in excess sodium and chloride loss, increased potassium in extracellular fluid, and a diminished water volume in both extracellular fluid and the blood. In less severe cases, this functional problem can be treated conservatively by a complementary sports medicine practitioner. In extreme conditions, such as the total loss of adrenal activity (Addison's disease), without medical intervention, the result will be death.

Aldosterone also affects sweat gland function, much the same way as in the kidney; it causes resorption of some sodium and chloride and allows the loss of some potassium. This adrenal hormone also causes increased sodium absorption from the intestine. Nonetheless, most electrolytes lost in sweat are sodium and chloride (Wilmore and Costill 1994). Reduced aldosterone, as seen in some athletes under stress and overtraining, causes excess loss of sodium. With reduced aldosterone, diarrhea may result, causing significant losses of sodium and water.

It is hypothesized by the author that many conditions of so-called athlete's diarrhea are due to chronic adrenal dysfunction—a condition that may not be evident until the stress of competition. This is especially true in people competing in longer events. Diarrhea in athletes may also be related to excess parasympathetic stimulation (Wilmore and Costill 1994). This type of neurological stress exists in later stages of overtraining. The chronic loss of sodium during adrenal dysfunction has also long been considered the reason for salt craving by these patients (and is referred to on the Symptom Survey described in chapter 7). In addition, excess sodium in the urine may be due to adrenal dysfunction in the early stages; but in a chronic condition, or when excess aldosterone is present, very low urine sodium is observed. (Dietary fats also have an influence on sodium and chloride balance through activity of the eicosanoids.)

Hyponatremia

Hyponatremia (blood sodium concentration below 136 mmol/L) can occur during or after competitive events (Speedy et al. 1997) and can sometimes be observed at rest in a normal blood test in athletes showing no symptoms of hyponatremia. (Hyponatremia can exist in a symptomatic or asymptomatic state [Noakes 1992].) Early symptoms may include weakness or disorientation. In extreme cases, hyponatremia can result in such problems as rapid neurological deterioration, cardiovascular instability, and seizures (Surgenor and Uphold 1994).

Even during very early stages of hyponatremia, or in people with low normal sodium, practitioners may find a positive sodium oral challenge using manual muscle testing; muscle inhibition will normalize in an athlete who tastes a tablet of sodium chloride. Practitioners should consider regular evaluation of athletes using an oral challenge along with blood tests, especially during the competitive season. Low sodium levels may be due to restriction of sodium intake, adrenal dysfunction, or overtraining and can have adverse effects on performance and health.

The use of sodium during competition may also be important, especially in long endurance events, as hyponatremia can occur if too much water and too little sodium are consumed (Frizzell et al. 1986). Small amounts of sodium added to water speed gastric emptying and fluid absorption from the intestine (Lamb and Brodowicz 1986). The American College of Sports Medicine has taken the following position on sodium: "Inclusion of sodium (500-700 mg per liter) in the rehydration solution ingested during exercise lasting longer than 1 hour is recommended since it may be advantageous in enhancing palatability, promoting fluid retention, and possibly preventing hyponatremia in certain individuals who drink excessive quantities of fluid" (Convertino et al. 1996, p. I).

Athletes who test positive on the sodium challenge can use sodium tablets during endurance events. The well-hydrated athlete sucks on a salt tablet until losing the desire or taste for salt. Athletes may consume many salt tablets during long events. In one case, an athlete took more than 25 tablets, completing a 9-hr race in a personal best time and place and for the first time did not develop muscle cramps.

Even in early stages, patients with sodium loss often demonstrate orthostatic intolerance, sometimes on a functional level, as discussed in chapter 8. Regarding these patients, El-Sayed and Hainsworth (1996) state that "salt is suggested as a first line of treatment" (p. 134).

While large amounts of salt have been given to healthy individuals with no adverse effects (Luft 1996), some patients may be sodium sensitive. This problem may be detected in the initial assessment process, especially as hypertension (although not all people with hypertension are sodium sensitive); and care must be taken not to exceed the patient's limit of sodium.

Especially for endurance athletes, severe hyponatremia and dehydration are the only two potentially likely life-threatening medical emergencies (Sawka and Greenleaf 1992). These can be avoided if the practitioner helps to maintain the athlete in a state of optimal health and fitness—ensuring normal adrenal function, specifying a diet that best matches the person's needs, and educating the athlete on proper fluid and electrolyte intake during competition and long training workouts.

Potassium Requirements

In addition to sodium and chloride, some athletes may need added potassium. The same assessment procedures—measures of blood levels, dietary analysis, and oral challenge—can be used for potassium as for the others. As a general guide, with adrenal dysfunction (i.e., aldosterone), there is increased sodium loss and potassium retention (i.e., an excess potassium). Recall from chapter 17 that potassium is a potential nociceptor irritant and that excesses may be involved with the production of pain.

It is possible for excess adrenal function to produce excess aldosterone, as occurs during the initial stages of Selye's general adaptation syndrome (Selye 1976) and in early stages of overtraining states. This hyperadrenal state may also be associated with excess sympathetic stimulation that could potentially contribute to increased potassium loss.

In some situations, then, potassium may become depleted in athletes. It is important to evaluate each person individually and not rely on a general nutritional regimen.

Sodium and Potassium Balance

It is worth remembering that sodium and potassium have some "opposite" effects in the body. Thus, performing an oral challenge with these two substances will often produce opposing effects: either sodium will normalize an inhibited muscle (and potassium cause inhibition), or sodium will inhibit a muscle (and potassium normalize an inhibited muscle). The following is an example of this type of challenge.

Potassium/Sodium Oral Challenge

1. The patient has an inhibition of the pectoralis major clavicular (PMC) and a normal latissimus dorsi muscle.
2. The practitioner places a tablet of sodium chloride in the patient's mouth. As the patient tastes the tablet, the muscles are retested. One of three possible outcomes is likely:
   - The PMC normalizes and the latissimus dorsi remains normal.
   - The PMC remains inhibited and the latissimus dorsi becomes inhibited.
   - There is no change to either muscle.
3. If the test produces the first outcome (normalization of the PMC with the latissimus dorsi remaining normal), testing potassium may have the opposite effect: the PMC will be unchanged and the latissimus dorsi will become inhibited.
4. If the test produces the second outcome (the PMC remains inhibited and the latissimus dorsi becomes inhibited), testing potassium may result in the opposite effect: the PMC will normalize and the latissimus dorsi will be unchanged.
5. If the test results in the third outcome, the test is negative, and potentially neither sodium nor potassium may be required by the patient.
6. Much less common is the situation in which the patient's inhibited muscle normalizes to both sodium and potassium. This may indicate a need for both electrolytes.
7. If testing is positive, the practitioner might consider five avenues:
   - How can the diet be adjusted so that the patient obtains more of the nutrient that improved muscle function (i.e., added use of sea salt for sodium, more fresh fruits for potassium)? Note that sea salt and fruit each contain both electrolytes but that sodium is predominant in the former and potassium in the latter.
   - Is the athlete consuming too much of the nutrient that caused inhibition (i.e., too much fruit juice, or sodium salt)? Note that a good balance of sodium and potassium is usually obtained through consumption of a variety of vegetables.
   - It may be useful to supplement with sodium (added sea salt on food is preferred over salt tablets) or potassium tablets as indicated.
   - It may be appropriate to add more sodium or potassium to the athlete's electrolyte drink during and after long training or during competitions. In some cases, sodium or potassium tablets may be more convenient.
   - Is there some primary dysfunction, such as adrenal or autonomic imbalance, for example, that is causing excess sodium loss and increased potassium retention?
8. A follow-up reevaluation is important. Athletes tend to exhibit the same or very similar problems if there is a recurrence, so evaluation of potentially significant problems such as sodium/potassium imbalance should be ongoing.

"SPORTS" DRINKS

Many ready-made and powdered sports drinks are on the market—advertised and sold through a variety of tactics. They include many types of glucose or glucose polymer drinks, some with and some without various combinations of electrolytes and other nutrients. Unfortunately, many such drinks have very low or no sodium. No single drink matches the needs of everyone (except plain water). In most cases, these sports drinks are useful only during or immediately after longer training, or competition, and should not be used to supplement the normal diet or as a replacement for a meal. Most athletes can perform short workouts of an hour or less without needing anything except water (although the author has observed that those with very good aerobic function can train effectively much longer with water only). As previously discussed, consuming carbohydrates in drinks before workouts or competitions can have an adverse effect on performance.

It is important for the practitioner to determine which added nutrients, if any, an athlete requires during or immediately after activity. In long endurance events, such as a marathon, a long triathlon, or any ultramarathon event, most likely both carbohydrates and electrolytes will be required.

It is not difficult to customize a sports drink to match the patient's needs for carbohydrate and electrolytes. One does this by first testing individual ingredients such as sodium, potassium, and various carbohydrates with an oral challenge and then adding these ingredients to an existing product and testing the patient with the solution. Making a drink from basic ingredients (such as water, sugar, and sea salt) is another option and may be the first step in creating an ideal solution for an individual. In either case, there are three steps:

- The practitioner performs an oral challenge to observe whether the solution causes an inhibited muscle to normalize. This measures the potential therapeutic effect of the solution.
- The athlete should use the solution during several long workouts before using it during competition. This measures its potential ergogenic effect.
- The practitioner should retest the solution after a long workout, since the athlete is in a different physiological state under this condition. It may be that the need for additional electrolytes, for example, is observed only at this time.

Products made in gel form are also used by some athletes and are a modified version of a sports drink without the water. They are very concentrated, and sometimes other nutrients have been added. Like carbohydrate and electrolyte drinks, they are not replacements for water. Because they are not made up predominantly of water, the user may require more water intake.

The practitioner should test other potential needs of the athlete during and immediately after training. Other recommendations for fluids during and after activity can vary with each athlete. Some endurance athletes do not feel comfortable drinking during competition; some may swallow large amounts of air, causing potential gastrointestinal distress. The remedy is to have athletes "practice" drinking during training. In addition, many activities and competitions such as endurance events result in dehydration despite fluid intake, since it is almost impossible to balance water loss: the stomach is capable of emptying only about 800 ml (26 oz) of fluid per hour during vigorous workouts, while water loss may be as high as 2 L (68 oz) (McArdle et al. 1991). Nonetheless, some general suggestions to consider are the following:

- Drinking additional water, 400-600 ml (13-20 oz), approximately 20 min before training or competing in the heat may delay dehydration and rises in body temperature.
- Cool fluids, between 15 and 22 °C (59 and 72 °F), empty from the stomach more quickly than body-temperature fluids. Some athletes think this means they should drink very cold fluids, but this may stimulate stronger stomach contractions and thus create the potential for gastrointestinal discomfort.
- Some investigators have reported that stomach emptying increases for each 100 ml (3.3 oz) up to 600 ml (20 oz) volume (McArdle et al. 1991), although others have shown this not to be true (Duchman et al. 1997).
- High amounts of sugar (glucose, sucrose, or fructose) can reduce stomach emptying due to the high osmolality of sugar. A 10% glucose solution, for example, reduces gastric emptying by half.
- Older studies indicated that glucose polymers (maltodextrin) up to 7%-8% may not slow gastric emptying because of their low osmolality (McArdle et al. 1991); but others report the opposite effect (Murray et al. 1994) or no effect (Brouns et al. 1995), depending on how the research was carried out.
- The ingestion of glucose polymer drinks does not necessarily offer any advantage over ingestion of regular glucose solutions in terms of metabolic or water balance (Massicotte et al. 1989).

Case History

Jim's first year of college sports was plagued with fatigue and minor injuries of the knee, calf, and ankle, as well as numerous episodes of diarrhea—along with disappointing performances. His family doctor found no disease but found a low sodium blood level of 132 mmol/L. During my initial assessment, Jim described his regular intake of a popular sports drink, even during the day when he was not training or competing, and his water intake was negligible. His blood pressure changed from 126/82 lying to 110/78 standing, and there were numerous other abnormal findings. All Jim's muscles were inhibited, and upon oral challenge with water they all normalized. An oral challenge with potassium and water did not change any muscle inhibition. Sodium chloride also normalized all muscle inhibition. Because of time constraints, Jim had to be rescheduled for an appointment three days later. I recommended that during the interim, he drink 3 to 4 L of water per day in small doses, use liberal amounts of sea salt on his food, increase his vegetable intake, and avoid all sports drinks and fruit juice. When Jim returned, there were only a few inhibited muscles as all others normalized. Blood pressures were 124/80 lying and 126/82 standing. Jim stated that his energy level, injuries, and diarrhea were all about 75% improved. Within four weeks and two sessions his energy was 100%, there were no episodes of diarrhea, and his knee, calf, and ankles were asymptomatic. After two more sessions, Jim was tested following a hard workout. Sodium normalized two primary muscle inhibitions, and water tested negative. Through testing various sports drinks, we found one that did not cause muscle inhibition (many did) and added sodium (from sea salt) to this drink. Jim used his personal drink, along with water and other appropriate dietary and training changes, during his second college year with continued good energy, no injuries or diarrhea, and great performances.

- Small amounts of sodium may improve hydration, partly due to increased thirst. The amount necessary can vary among athletes, but approximately one-third of a teaspoon of sea salt per liter may be a general guide.
- Fructose may result in incomplete absorption and cause intestinal cramps or diarrhea (Ravich et al. 1983), or malabsorption of iron, magnesium, calcium, and zinc (Ivaturi and Kies 1992). In addition, fructose is converted much more slowly to blood glucose (Convertino et al. 1996).
- As discussed in chapter 19, L-glutamine improves water, sodium, potassium, and chloride absorption and may be useful during sports activity.
- The conflicts in the scientific literature probably indicate individual variations in athletes. Especially in the case of fluid replacement and electrolytes, each patient's need must be considered independently.

"ENERGY" BARS

There are dozens of so-called energy bars on the market. Unfortunately, most are in opposition to recommendations to eat foods in as unprocessed and as whole a state as possible. Most are made with very highly processed ingredients, often containing hydrogenated oils, high amounts of saturated fats, refined sugar (often disguised as maltodextrin or high-fructose corn syrup), or a combination of all of these; in addition, these bars are frequently low in fiber. Many are made predominantly of high-glycemic carbohydrates, with little or virtually no protein or good fats. More problematic is the fact that many athletes use these unbalanced products as meals; most bars do not qualify as a meal replacement since they are not made from real foods. Very few bars would meet the healthy criteria outlined in this text. Practitioners and athletes should consider recommending and using only products made from real food and avoid those containing high-glycemic and processed ingredients, especially those containing fats that interfere with the body's delicate eicosanoid balance.

Bars that are healthy may be useful for athletes in a number of situations:

- As a between-meal snack, especially for people who need to consume food every 2 to 3 hr
- As a healthy alternative to snacks or meals of "junk food"
- As an easily accessible food when other food is not available—for example, during work, school, or travel
- During long practice sessions or competitions
- After training or competition

Another important use for bars containing carbohydrates, protein, and fats is to help replace glycogen stores. At one time it was thought that only glucose drinks were effective for replacing glycogen stores after a workout or competition, but as previously discussed, a mixed meal can also be very effective. The convenience of a bar allows the athlete to immediately consume a healthy food, along with water, to accomplish this task.

CONCLUSION

While it is important to understand the current research, the athlete's needs are most important and may not always correlate with laboratory data. Through proper assessments and experience, athlete and practitioner can find the optimal fluid and solid nutritional regime. The final outcome is also determined through an oral challenge to observe whether a food or drink causes an inhibited muscle to normalize, giving a therapeutic effect; the athlete should use this substance(s) during long workouts, before using it during competition, to observe for a positive ergogenic effect. The practitioner should also perform an oral challenge using these substances again after a long workout to observe their therapeutic effects.

21

Practitioner's Role in Training and Competition

The practitioner plays a vital role in the athlete's training and competition. This is accomplished not necessarily by providing schedules but by ensuring that the athlete is in optimal structural, chemical, and mental/emotional balance. Maintaining this balance may become difficult as training and competition are added to the schedule; such difficulty provides clues to the practitioner and patient that additional therapies may be necessary to meet the added stress, or that the training and/or competitive routine are excessive given the individual's overall capability. On the basis of the evidence, the practitioner helps guide the athlete (sometimes with the help of a coach, trainer, or other professional) through the process of undergoing training and competition, making appropriate dietary and nutritional choices, and dealing with other factors discussed that are important before, during, and after workouts.

MAINTAINING PATIENT CARE

Traditional treatment programs are typically recommended for a specific injury or condition. Successful therapy may require a variety of treatments over a particular time period. Once the patient is symptom free, the patient and practitioner may end their relationship. If the problem recurs, the patient returns for therapy. This crisis-care approach is not usual in complementary sports medicine. Instead, the relationship becomes more holistic, with assessment and treatment of imbalances often far from the knee pain, for example. Most importantly, this process continues into the next phase when the patient increases training and contemplates competition.

Continual assessment and treatment during this period are important to successful training because the practitioner can help

- maintain the structural, chemical, and mental/emotional balance that was achieved with previous therapies;
- prevent a recurrence of the previous injury or condition;
- assess and correct subtle imbalances that result from more intense or longer training before they become more serious; and
- obtain additional information from the patient's body that may be useful in formulating training and competition schedules.

The body more easily develops imbalances, especially in previously injured areas, during stressful training periods. Many of these recurring imbalances are structural, occurring in the origin and insertion of muscles, musculotendinous junction, and muscle belly (Safran et al. 1989), and can be treated with GTO/spindle cell therapy as discussed in chapter 14. Chemical imbalances also are common. Newsholme (1994) demonstrated that high-intensity training suppresses the immune system, and Leaf et al. (1997) linked training with significant increases in lipid peroxidation (associated with free radicals) concomitant with intensity. Properly assessing the patient when these problems begin to develop leads to the discovery of imbalances in their earliest stages, when they are most easily corrected. This type of care can be provided every few weeks, though athletes such as boxers, football players, and hockey players may need more regular treatment during periods of intense training and competition. The athlete's mental/emotional state sometimes improves merely because maintenance of the athlete's optimal structural and chemical balance promotes a feeling of well-being and the knowledge that he or she is receiving optimal care.

Evaluation and treatment during this training phase also provide additional information that can be used to formulate the patient's training and competition schedules. For example, a runner who maintains a balanced state with a weekly average of 100 km (62 miles) may experience numerous structural imbalances when that distance is increased slightly. Restricting training to 100 km/week is necessary until the practitioner determines the reason the athlete is unable to handle increased training stress. The practitioner also can make adjustments to a patient's training schedule if the Maximum Aerobic Function (MAF) test begins to worsen, a possible indication of training that has been too intense. Hodgetts et al. (1991) showed that excessive high-intensity exercise diminishes the availability of fatty acid in muscle. This may impair aerobic function and be reflected in the MAF test.

A treatment administered immediately before an event may help create the most optimal state of balance during competition. Similarly, treatment that immediately follows competition may help correct imbalances caused by exertion, and will help restore the patient to optimal form so that training can resume normally. However, practitioners must be cautious about treating a patient for the first time when competition is within two or three days; the body may require several days to adapt to any significant changes in structure or chemistry and may not be capable of optimal functioning until then. If a new patient requires care but has an impending competition, it may be best to apply only the therapy absolutely necessary until after the event.

ACTIVE WARM-UP

A warm-up prepares the body for activity and is an integral part of every training session and competition. A good warm-up reduces the muscle soreness associated with the early stages of an exercise program and decreases the risk of injury (Wilmore and Costill 1994). Safran et al. (1988) showed with animal studies that greater stress is required to produce an injury in warmed-up muscles than in muscles that are not warmed. The warm-up may be the most important "therapeutic" aspect of exercise.

Eliminating a warm-up can result in an abnormal electrocardiogram, myocardial ischemia, and poor blood pressure response following exercise, even in healthy, fit individuals (McArdle et al. 1991). Cardiac patients need a proper warm-up to reduce the myocardial workload and oxygen (O_2) requirements and to provide adequate coronary blood flow before vigorous exercise.

An active warm-up is performed before any exercise or competition, aerobic or anaerobic. The heart rate is only slightly elevated at the onset of the warm-up and continues to increase until the maximum training heart rate is achieved at the end of the warm-up process. One of the significant benefits of an active warm-up is the elevation of body temperature, which serves a number of purposes (Shellock and Prentice 1985). The higher body temperature

- increases the dissociation of O_2 from hemoglobin and myoglobin,
- decreases the activation energy rates of metabolic chemical reactions,
- increases blood flow to working muscles,
- produces greater mechanical efficiency,
- increases the sensitivity of nerve receptors, and
- increases the speed of nervous impulses.

The warm-up also results in an increase in circulating fatty acids (useful for energy in aerobic muscle fibers) and vital capacity. Safran et al. (1988) showed a greater extensibility of collagenous tissue as well. This can also increase range of motion (ROM).

An active warm-up is not stretching, but instead consists of easy, whole-body activity that is similar to, or the same as, that which is to follow. A runner may warm up by jogging slowly or, in some cases, walking. Golfers also may walk—or jog if they are in good aerobic condition. An active warm-up will take at least 12 to 15 min or longer based on the duration of the total workout and how the athlete feels. Workouts lasting more than about 90 min require a longer warm-up. Athletes must develop the ability to sense when their body is prepared for more intense activity; most individuals experience this readiness as a looseness. Their gait becomes fluid, flexibility increases, and they feel warmer.

Isolated warm-up activities that consist of a modified version of the activity to come usually are performed after the active warm-up. For example, following a short walk, a golfer initially makes easy, short swings with the club and gradually increases the ROM, eventually making a normal stroke. After an active warm-up, a basketball player easily tosses and dribbles the ball and works up to passing and shooting it farther and harder.

A heart monitor can help the athlete greatly in the warm-up process by showing heart rate progression. Athletes can easily observe their heart rate and avoid a too rapid, or occasionally too leisurely, heart rate elevation. For example, an individual who begins warming up by jogging at a heart rate of 60 beats per minute (bpm) will see the heart rate gradually increase to 80, 100, and higher. After 15 min, the maximum aerobic heart rate is achieved and training intensity may be maintained (see figure 21.1).

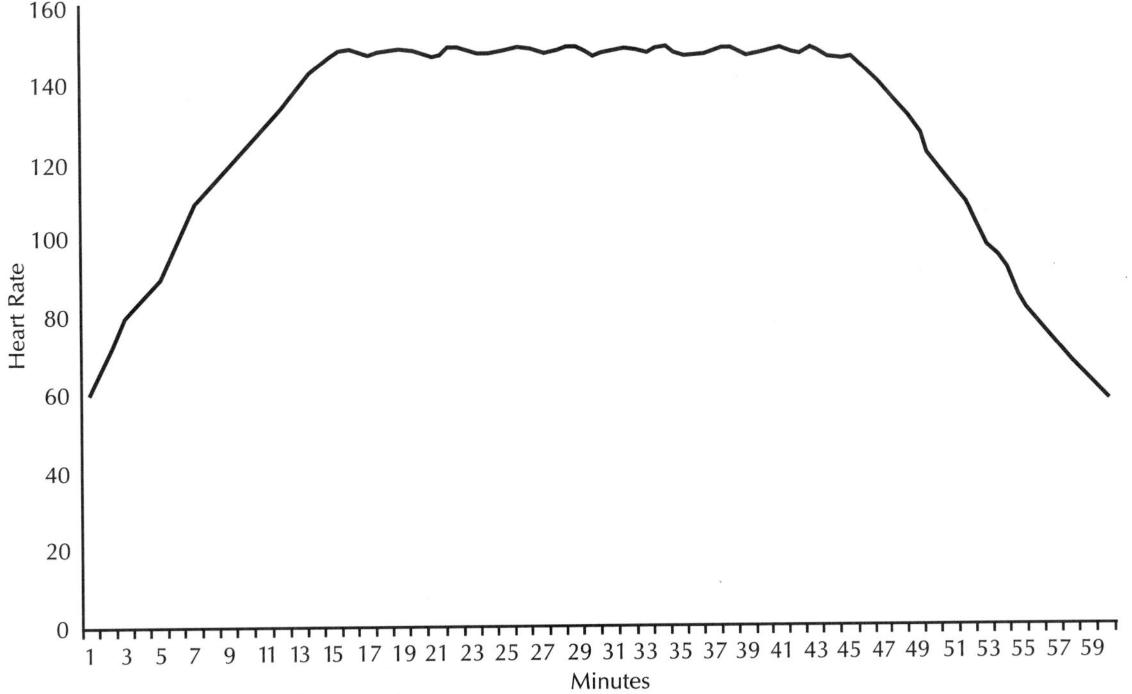

Figure 21.1 Heart rate changes during 15-min warm-up and 15-min recovery as part of a 60-min workout.

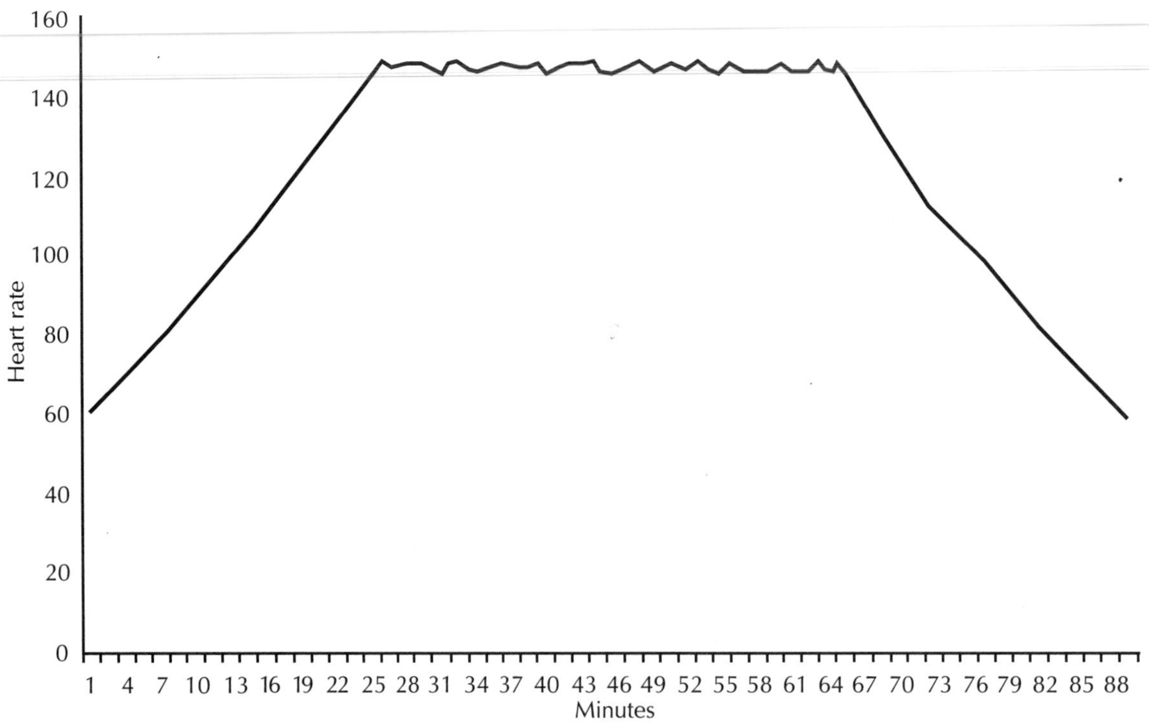

Figure 21.2 Heart rate changes during 25-min warm-up and 25-min recovery as part of a 90-min workout.

If a longer workout is planned, a warm-up of increased duration is recommended, as shown in figure 21.2.

An active warm-up, and especially an active recovery, can take a longer time in power and sprint athletes (who may have a higher population of anaerobic muscle fibers) because of a reduction in aerobic fibers that improve the circulatory response (Colliander et al. 1988).

ACTIVE RECOVERY

The process of active recovery, also referred to as cooling- or warming-down, is recommended after all training and most competition. Active recovery involves diminishing levels of activity while the heart rate is reduced. Passive recovery, or complete rest after the workout or competition, is a form of recovery that patients too often use. Passive recovery should be reserved for the situation in which one is completely exhausted following competition.

Case History

Patty is a distance runner with an aerobic training heart rate of 155 bpm. She begins her 90-min run with a resting heart rate of 58 bpm. A slow jog elevates that number to 70 bpm, and as she increases her speed, her heart rate matches the faster pace. After about 8 min, Patty's heart rate is 105 bpm, and after about 12 min it rises to 120 bpm. She begins to feel loose and her stride is comfortable. At 16 min, her heart rate is 140 bpm. It increases to about 150 bpm at 20 min, and she starts to feel good. Patty reaches her maximum training heart rate of 155 after about 24 min and maintains that rate 70 min into the run. She adjusts her pace over hills to keep her heart rate at 155. At 70 min, she begins to slow her pace and lower her heart rate. At 75 min, her heart rate is 135; it gradually decreases past 120 until she is under 100 bpm at 85 min. At the end of her run, Patty's heart rate is 85, and she walks for 5 min to bring it down to about 80 bpm. Patty feels that she could almost perform the same workout again without undue stress.

Compared to passive recovery, active recovery increases O_2 availability and circulation through the muscle fibers and rapidly removes blood lactate (Taoutaou et al. 1996; Yoshida et al. 1996). In intermittent sports such as football and basketball, active recovery from one bout of activity results in more anaerobic power output during the second bout (Ahmaidi et al. 1996); this phenomenon has also been shown in sprint cyclists (Bogdanis et al. 1996). Active recovery is highly dependent on the function of the aerobic muscle fibers (Colliander et al. 1988). It is important, therefore, to develop a good aerobic system, especially for power athletes.

The circulation response produced by active recovery increases the removal of lipid peroxidation by-products, which are produced in greater amounts with increasing intensity. An active recovery also helps prevent blood pooling in the extremities, particularly the legs, that can result in dizziness and fainting (Wilmore and Costill 1994).

Heart rate awareness can assist in active recovery, although it is not necessary, or usually possible, to reduce the heart rate to its pretraining level. As with the warm-up, a longer active-recovery period should be used to complete an extended workout. Note that the warm-up and recovery are considered part of the workout. For example, a 60-min workout includes a 15-min warm-up and 15 min of recovery. This leaves 30 min of training at the maximum aerobic heart rate level (or other intensities as planned).

ACTIVE WARM-UP AND RECOVERY IN COMPETITION

A warm-up is crucial before competition, and some athletes find that their warm-up lasts longer than their actual event. A 5-km race may last less than 15 min, for example, but a typical runner with a good aerobic system and competitive experience may take 45 min or longer to warm up. Shorter warm-ups that include walking may be used before events that are considerably longer, such as marathons or Ironman triathlons.

Athletes who compete in anaerobic events also may benefit from proper warm-ups and recovery periods. For example, a football player who is in and out of the game and a sprinter who must compete in several heats to qualify for the finals have similar needs: a good initial warm-up consisting of 20 to 30 min of increasingly intense activity that mimics the upcoming event. During the competitive period, competitions are followed by relatively brief active-recovery periods, and the cycle repeats itself until the game or event is over. Ideally, another period of active recovery should follow the last bout of activity.

As has been emphasized, a good warm-up is dependent on a highly developed aerobic system. If an athlete's heart rate soars to 180 bpm during an easy warm-up, the person clearly should not be performing that activity before a competition or training, as it may cause fatigue. This would usually indicate that the individual's aerobic system is not well developed.

STRETCHING

Stretching is a complex, controversial, and inconclusive issue. It is always individual. In the author's opinion, most endurance athletes do not need to stretch if they participate in a proper warm-up and active recovery, and only athletes who require a greater-than-normal ROM, such as dancers and track and field athletes, may need to stretch. In addition, the author has observed more injuries in athletes

Case History

John plays golf several times per week. He begins with 20 min of easy walking followed by 10 min at a faster pace. Then, with a four iron, he begins taking short, effortless practice swings and takes 10 min to work up to a full swing with a wood. John then hits balls on the practice range for another 10 to 15 min. If he doesn't feel his body is warm, he continues to practice on the driving range.

who stretch than in those who do not, as found also by Jacobs and Berson (1986).

Most athletes consider stretching and the resultant increase in ROM a form of injury prevention. However, sound epidemiologic evidence for the preventive effect of stretching is scarce and contradictory (Van Mechelen et al. 1993). Common injuries in sport occur in the muscles that respond to training stress and undergo a significant lengthening, possibly due to decreased muscle tone that results from postexercise fatigue (Skinner et al. 1986). This damage is significantly apparent around the knee joint, one of the most common injury sites (Van Mechlelen et al. 1993).

Range of motion measurements have no predictive value for injury (though previous injuries correlate with an increased risk for further damage) (Wiesler et al. 1996). Some studies demonstrate that increased flexibility produces more injuries (Jones et al. 1993, 1994). Goniometric (joint ROM) measurements show no significant differences between the injured and noninjured side of the body (Van Mechelen 1992).

Part of the controversy that surrounds stretching results from the difference between ballistic and static stretching, the two most common types of stretches (Shellock and Prentice 1985). Other types of stretching may exist, but they are variations of ballistic and static stretching.

Ballistic stretching involves repetitive, bouncing movements that use the body's momentum to repeatedly stretch a joint to, or beyond, ROM extremes. Though this may be the most harmful type of stretch, it is the most common—possibly because athletes often are in a hurry to begin their workouts. Ballistic stretching may activate the stretch reflex and increase tension and the risk for microtears in the muscle. Athletes who stretch ballistically will show a recurrent need for Golgi tendon organ/spindle cell therapy.

Static stretching involves very slowly stretching the muscle to a point of slight discomfort and then holding it for up to 30 sec. Each muscle group is sequentially stretched three to four times, and it is essential not to rush the routine. Static stretching may be either active or passive. Active static stretching contracts the antagonist muscle (i.e., to actively stretch the latissimus dorsi, the pectoralis muscles are flexed and adducted). Passive static stretching typically requires force by another person (or body part) to move a body segment to the end of, or beyond, its ROM. When performed properly, static stretching relaxes the muscle. However, note the substantial time commitment—one that many athletes do not make.

BUILDING AEROBIC FUNCTION

The muscular, circulatory, and energy aspects of the aerobic system, its dietary and nutritional components, and the importance of heart monitor assessments and the MAF test have been described throughout this text. Training is another vital aspect of aerobic function. The practitioner, athlete, coach, and other professionals must continually monitor for the structural, chemical, or mental/emotional aspects of overtraining—both single incidents and the culmination of many workouts—that may damage aerobic function.

Several factors help the athlete build a good aerobic system; the most important of these is finding the optimal maximum aerobic training heart rate. Measured with the MAF test, this is the heart rate at which training will continue to benefit the aerobic system without inducing health problems. Once the optimal training heart rate is found, the athlete must not train at levels that exceed this rate during the period of building aerobic function—a period of time referred to as the aerobic base. In fact, as noted previously, if exercise continues at a heart rate that is slightly above the maximum aerobic heart rate, the athlete may experience initial benefits, but complete development of the aerobic system may not occur.

Training at levels consistent with or lower than the optimal heart rate may sound easy, and athletes initially may complain about the slow pace, believing that an easy workout will not improve performance. However, aerobic function improves over time, and the pace will quicken while the person maintains the same heart rate. Similar changes have been noted in studies by Bell et al. (1991). Months later, the athlete may complain that the pace—at the same heart rate—is too fast.

Athletes confront other factors that may make it difficult to stay within their heart rate range, such as the social aspect of training. A patient's heart rate will rise too quickly if he or she runs or bikes up a hill too fast. When an athlete is training in a group, slowing down may cause social or psychological stress, and many athletes are unable to do it. This is why training alone in the early stages of building the aerobic system, or with others who are at similar fitness levels, is a good technique. Once the athlete's pace quickens, training with a group will not be a problem, as endurance and speed will have improved but now without elevating the heart rate to anaerobic levels.

It is important to use the MAF test to monitor the progress of the aerobic system. The test should show consistent progress with only an occasional plateau and never a regression. A worsening pace indicates a problem that must be identified immediately.

Endurance athletes who participate in a period of strict aerobic training that is void of any anaerobic workouts usually perform well in competition. In fact, the author has observed that more than 75% of runners who can compare regular distances and times experience personal bests in their first competitive performance after a period of strict aerobic training (having performed no anaerobic training).

The following case history was written by professional and world-class triathlete Mike Pigg and is excerpted from *Training for Endurance* (Maffetone 1996).

Case History

The training seemed slow at first at my designated heart rate of 155. There were times when I had to walk up hills during the run and zigzag on the bike just to stay in my aerobic range. In a little time, things started to change and I became stronger at the same heart rate—which became quite exciting. After five months of loyal training, I got my first big sign that the program was working.

Before going on the program, I would ride to my parents' summer place, which is 65 miles with three good climbs in it. My previous record was set with a good friend of mine. We had the total grudge match all the way to find who was "king of the bike." He would attack on the hills and I held a heart rate between 165 and 182 to establish a record of 3 hours and 15 minutes. When we arrived at the cabin, I would achieve a total "bonk." The best I could do for the rest of the day was eat, sleep, and eat, and even that was difficult. Three years later, after 5 months on the aerobic program, I attempted the same course again. This time solo and never went above 155 bpm, even on the long climbs. The results were interesting: I went 3:09 and felt good enough to go for a 10-mile run straight after. Slowly, I was becoming convinced that the theory was working.

By the first race of the season while following this plan, I was seeing good aerobic results in my workouts, but still had doubts about my competitiveness in a world-class field. You see, I still needed my "hammer sessions" to prove or build my confidence that I was ready to race at a professional level. The season opener was in Australia at Surfer's Paradise International Triathlon. My confidence was so blown that I didn't even want to get on the plane, but a swift kick from my wife, and I was off. The whole week prior to the race, I was fighting myself, saying that I wasn't going to do well because of a lack of anaerobic training. Finally, I told myself to shut up and go have a good time. To my surprise, I did have a good time, and I won. For some reason, the speed was there, and my endurance definitely was there. Plus a bonus, I was able to beat Mark Allen—the best in the world at the time—at his own game.

Football, basketball, and baseball players may find that the off-season is the best time to build the aerobic system and should begin training soon after the end of their regular season. Only after development of the aerobic system should anaerobic training and competition be added to a schedule as discussed in the next chapter.

AEROBIC INTERVALS

Aerobic intervals may be a useful addition to a training program when endurance athletes begin to progress to faster speeds at their maximum aerobic heart rate. As athletes progress, they can run, bike, or swim at faster speeds at the same heart rate, and eventually it may become physically more difficult to stay within the training heart rate range throughout the workout. The following routine is an example of an aerobic-interval workout, developed for a cyclist performing 2-hr workouts at a maximum aerobic heart rate of 145 bpm:

- Warm up for approximately 30 min.
- Ride at a heart rate of 145 bpm for 10 min (often a very fast pace).
- Reduce the heart rate to 120 to 130 bpm for 5 min.
- Perform the second and third steps four times.
- Cool down for 30 min.

This workout may be modified so that more or less time is spent in the second or the third step, depending on the athlete's comfort and fitness level. For example, some cyclists can maintain their maximum aerobic heart rate for 15 or 20 min; others can remain at that level for only 5 min. This workout may feel difficult, like an anaerobic ride; but recovery is generally quick, as with other aerobic workouts. Other sports such as running, biking, walking, and swimming can be performed similarly. In sports such as basketball, tennis, racquetball, and rowing, the same principles apply; practice sessions are done without exceeding the maximum aerobic heart rate, and in time, the same activity can be done with a much higher intensity and at the same heart rate. When competition begins, anaerobic intensities will be accomplished with less effort (i.e., at lower heart rates). In many cases, an athlete can eventually play a hard competitive match or game without becoming anaerobic.

WALKING AND AEROBIC FUNCTION

Walking is the simplest form of aerobic exercise. Ideal for beginners or for people undergoing rehabilitation or recovery from injury, walking can be used as part of the warm-up and active recovery for all types of training. It is also a useful way to extend workout times, particularly for individuals who are beginning to jog or run or for those on a weight-control program.

Walking may help relax some competitors before an event and aid in recovery afterward. A heart monitor is not necessary, as most patients' heart rates usually will not rise near or above their maximum aerobic heart rate during walking (though in some patients who are very unfit, an easy walk raises the heart rate too high, even on flat surfaces). Walking over hilly terrain, however, may easily elevate the heart rate.

Walkers can develop the aerobic system with regular workouts. However, before recommending a regular walking routine, practitioners should assess patients with a heart monitor to evaluate them during their routine on two or three separate occasions.

Some patients may consider carrying weights to increase the metabolic cost of the activity, but even small amounts of weight can distort natural posture and gait and may produce structural imbalance in susceptible patients. Carrying hand weights also may elevate the systolic blood pressure during activity (Sagiv et al. 1990; Graves et al. 1988). For these reasons, it may be more effective for walkers to begin jogging if and when they wish to perform more intense physical activity. At this point, the use of a heart monitor is essential to prevent aerobic workouts from becoming anaerobic.

Competitive walkers, including those who use a more normal walking gait and those who are Olympic walkers, can follow the same routines as described here.

BUILDING ANAEROBIC FUNCTION

Anaerobic training—that is, training above the aerobic maximum heart rate, and all weight training—should not be added to an athlete's training program until aerobic function is significantly improved. In fact, many endurance athletes find that training only aerobically is the best formula for success since most of their competitive energy (usually more than 95%) comes from the aerobic system (McArdle et al. 1991). With this strategy, they rely on competition to provide anaerobic stimulation. Also, one needs to consider that injuries most often occur in the anaerobic muscle fibers (Safran et al. 1988). Despite the fact that heart rate usually will not exceed the maximum aerobic training heart rate during strength training, lifting a weight is a short-duration activity that usually does not allow an athlete to reach the peak training heart rate zone.

Once anaerobic training is added to the athlete's program, aerobic system progress usually will plateau (sometimes after a brief improvement)—a change that is evident on the MAF test. This may occur in endurance athletes within three to four weeks of beginning anaerobic training; Lehmann et al. (1997) showed that an increased risk of overtraining may be expected after about three weeks of intensified anaerobic training. If the MAF test shows a decline in aerobic function, anaerobic exercise should be stopped. This may indicate that further anaerobic training is unnecessary or that there is some imbalance preventing the body from progressing further. In either case, it is important to avoid anaerobic workouts.

Anaerobic training often is associated with overtraining and the secondary structural, chemical, and mental/emotional imbalances that accompany it. Fry et al. (1991) showed that 77% of overtrained athletes participated in anaerobic sports. Increased cortisol is a primary marker of overtraining (Lehmann et al. 1997), and cortisol levels can normally increase significantly after anaerobic workouts such as weight training (Horne et al. 1997). Anaerobic training may be contraindicated for patients with adrenal dysfunction associated with high resting cortisol levels.

Though endurance athletes may often derive anaerobic benefits from competition or from very few anaerobic sessions, power athletes often require a more extensive anaerobic training period. Anaerobic training must be tailored to these individuals' needs. It is imperative that the training not adversely affect the athlete's health or aerobic function; the practitioner and athlete may use the MAF test and other assessments as a tool for monitoring and maintaining the training balance.

Aerobic function must be maintained during anaerobic training periods through participation in aerobic exercise between anaerobic sessions. Many strength athletes avoid aerobic training because they fear it will adversely affect their power development. This idea comes from older, short-term studies that demonstrated this potential problem (Dudley and Djamil 1985; Hickson 1980). However, these studies have not been reproduced, and newer, more

Case History

Ed was an Olympic weight lifter who had reached a performance plateau. He reluctantly ceased weight training and built his aerobic system by walking, jogging, and riding the stationary bike. His pace and overall health improved throughout the 4.5 months in which he exclusively trained his aerobic system. He then began weight training again, adding a warm-up and active-recovery period to his sessions, and continued to participate in five aerobic workouts per week. After three months, Ed could lift more weight during competition than he had in his last two years competing, and he achieved several personal records. He now schedules a four-month period every year in which he only trains aerobically, and his anaerobic training and performance have continued to improve.

effective studies addressing this issue have shown that strength develops regardless of a combination of aerobic and anaerobic training (McCarthy et al. 1995; Bell et al. 1991).

In fact, anaerobic benefits can increase with aerobic training, so power athletes should make every effort to maintain a balanced training program that includes anaerobic and aerobic components and warm-up and cool-down periods. It is possible for power to be reduced and recovery delayed with diminished aerobic fiber function (Colliander et al. 1988). Aerobic muscle fibers also remove circulating blood lactate, which can have a significant effect on power function (Simoneau et al. 1985).

MILD HYPERBARIC CHAMBERS

The portable mild hyperbaric chamber has become standard equipment for high-altitude expeditions during the decade since its development by University of Colorado professor R. Igor Gamow in the late 1980s (Taber 1990; King and Greenlee 1990). These devices have also been used successfully to eliminate excess carboxyhemoglobin (Jay et al. 1995), to treat acute altitude sickness in areas around ski resorts (Kasic 1991), to perform on-site management of injured scuba divers (Moon 1988), and in other conditions. It has also been shown that addition of hyperbaric conditions versus breathing only 100% O_2 at sea-level pressures has distinct therapeutic advantages (Yee and Brandon 1983).

The Gamow hyper bag has been used as a natural therapeutic and training aid for athletes. Wyndham et al. (1971) showed that miners' $\dot{V}O_2max$ uptake increased 11%-12% immediately after they rapidly descended from an altitude of 1763 m (5784 ft) to sea level. Even more significant were changes made above an altitude of 1600 m (5248 ft); $\dot{V}O_2max$ diminished approximately 11% for each 1000 m (3281 ft) increase in elevation (Wilmore and Costill 1994). Such data suggested that exposure to a high-pressure environment similar to that in a mild hyperbaric chamber could have therapeutic effects (see figures 21.3 and 21.4).

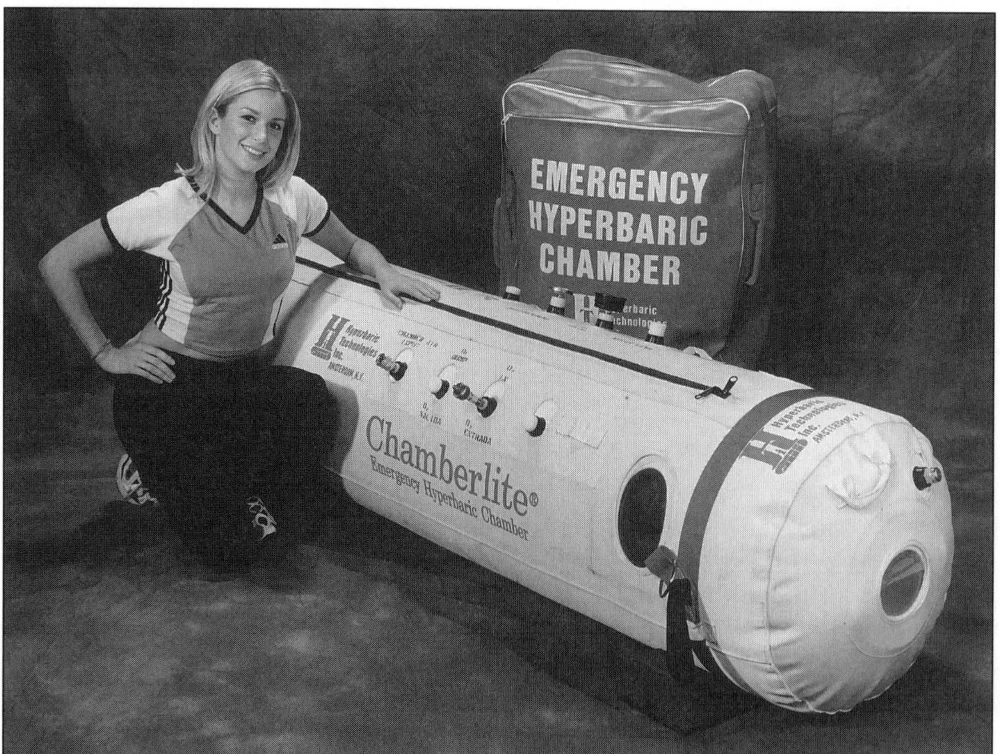

Figure 21.3 The Chamberlite bag is a medical device employing approximately 15 psi.
Reprinted by permission of Hyperbaric Technologies Incorporated.

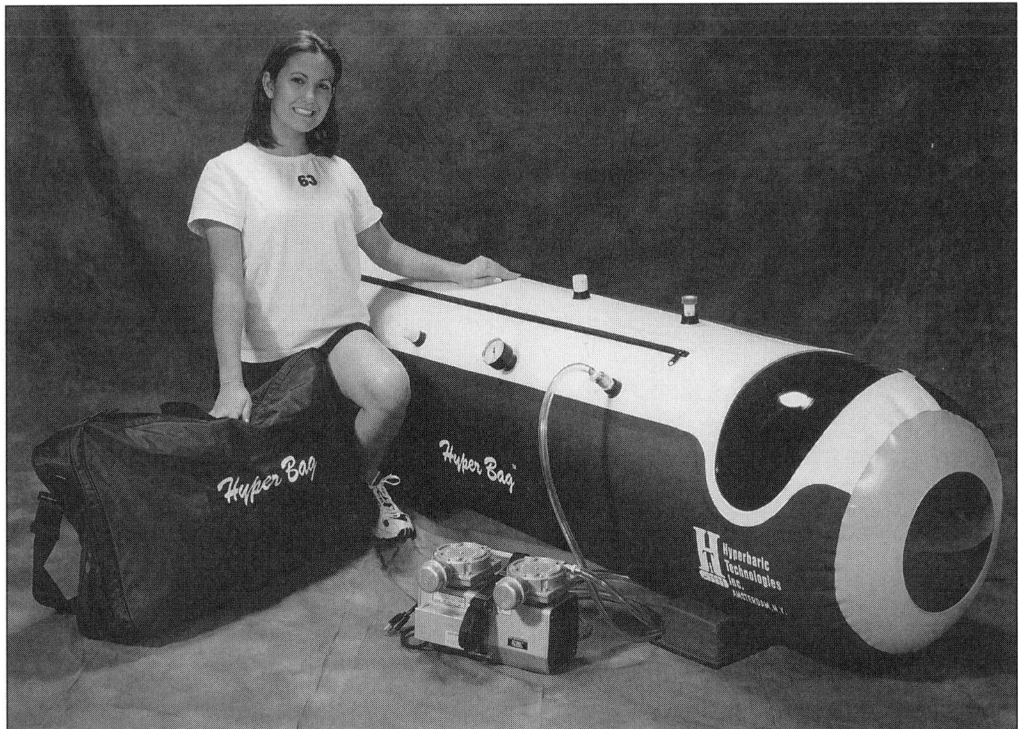

Figure 21.4 A Gamow hyper bag increases pressure to 3-4 psi.
Reprinted by permission of Hyperbaric Technologies Incorporated.

Although ambient air contains 20.9% O_2 at all altitudes, the reduced partial pressure of O_2 at higher altitudes (lower barometric pressure) causes reduced O_2 availability. Higher pressures, as already noted, increase O_2 uptake. The pressure inside a mild hyperbaric chamber increases anywhere from 3-4 pounds per square inch (psi) to about 15 psi, depending on the type of chamber used. Even a change of 3-4 psi, which mimics a descent from an altitude of over 1600 m (5248 ft) to sea level, can result in a significant change in O_2 uptake.

Exposure to a hyperbaric environment has significant therapeutic effects that are maintained after the exposure to that environment ceases. The most pronounced changes include improvement of abnormal muscle inhibition and facilitation as determined by manual muscle testing. The author has also observed that these changes may improve posture and gait, and even vital capacity (probably due to improved chest expansion).

The therapeutic process involves the athlete's resting in the chamber for approximately 45 min. This is typically done on a weekly basis. Use of the chamber is increased before and after important competitions or on longer or more intense training days. No negative effects have been noted.

CONCLUSION

The practitioner may play an active role in the patient's training and competition. Practitioners assist in maintaining patient care to preserve the balance achieved with previous treatment, to assess and correct developing imbalances in their earliest stages, and to continually obtain information from the patient's body that may be useful when formulating and revising training and competition schedules. Practitioners also can emphasize proper warm-up and cool-down sessions; help determine optimal aerobic and anaerobic training periods; determine the optimal aerobic training heart rate and chart the MAF test; and advise when competition should begin, end, or be modified, including planning the competitive schedule in some cases.

Training and Competition Schedules

For many athletes, the main goal of training is to develop the ability to compete successfully and without injury. To make both the training process and the competition effective, balanced training and competitive schedules are necessary and, like other aspects of treatment, should be developed based on the individual's needs. Even members of a competitive team must each have an individual program.

TRAINING SCHEDULES

Each training schedule should be developed on the basis of three components that will continually influence it: lifestyle, quality, and balance.

An athlete's training is heavily influenced by lifestyle, which includes everything he or she is committed to do throughout the day or week. Each of these commitments must be considered in the planning of an athlete's training schedule. For example, a cyclist also may be a father, husband, son, and entrepreneur and have a number of social obligations. A tennis player who is training for a local tournament may be a mother, wife, and executive. Professional athletes may have family obligations, along with other business responsibilities.

Ensuring the quality of the workout is another important aspect of the training schedule development process. Each workout should include a proper warm-up, exercise at the proper training heart rate, and active recovery. Some individuals ignore one or more of these components to save time, and the practitioner must delineate the importance of each. For example, if a tennis player and her partner have an 8 A.M. court time and she arrives at 7:50 A.M., she is likely to forego a warm-up and rush into play. Similarly, an executive who must catch the 7:18 A.M. train may rush his morning 5-km run if he wakes up late and there is not ample time for a proper warm-up and cool-down. Athletes who are tempted to shorten their warm-ups and cool-downs should be reminded that these two activities are integral parts of a complete and successful workout.

The third key to developing a beneficial training schedule is balance. Athletes must adhere to the training formula: Training = Workout + Recovery. If this formula is not followed, the result may be overtraining (too much exercise and/or too little recovery) or undertraining (an insufficient amount of exercise, i.e., three or fewer days per week). For patients with overtraining or undertraining aerobic deficiency, a minimum of three to four exercise sessions per week may be required to develop good aerobic function and achieve balanced fitness and health.

Ideally, an intuitive athlete may ultimately be able to train by instinct. However, this would require extreme discipline, including removing oneself physically and mentally from all potential negative external influences such as training partners, advertising, media, and the like.

TEAM TRAINING

Several factors come into play when one is devising training schedules for a team or other group of athletes. The most important is that each individual has to take a certain amount of responsibility for his or her own training. Each team member must be individually assessed, beginning with an aerobic evaluation that may be conducted by the coach, trainer, or others or by the individual athlete. The group may require a point-by-point explanation of the assessment process that enables the athletes to keep their own records (which should be maintained by the coach, trainer, and practitioner). Each athlete first performs a Maximum Aerobic Function (MAF) test. Athletes then are divided into groups of similar aerobic ability for training sessions. As improvements in aerobic function occur at varying intervals, some individuals may periodically need to change groups. This process is simplified if each team member uses a heart monitor and regularly performs the MAF test.

TRAINING DIARIES

Both the practitioner and athlete will benefit when the athlete maintains a training diary. Each becomes more familiar with the athlete's progress and unique needs, and the practitioner also may use the diary to assist in future evaluations of the treatment and training schedule. It is particularly important to refer to the athlete's goal in the diary. Athletes should record an entry for each workout, including the type (i.e., running, walking, biking, etc.) and duration of activity and heart rate measures. A separate chart should be maintained in the diary for all MAF test results. The athlete also should note subjective pre- and postexercise feelings and, if desired, other secondary measures, such as distance, pace, or speed.

Traditionally, a runner will record the distance and pace of the workout. However, it may be better to emphasize total time and heart rate, for two reasons:

- With measurement of only distance, total training volume will diminish over time as improved aerobic function increases speed, resulting in the completion of the same course in less time.
- When measuring only distance, some athletes feel pressured to complete a certain weekly mileage—or they compare themselves to other athletes, training partners, or younger versions of themselves. Heart rate is a more useful parameter than distance because it relates to the quality, rather than the quantity, of the activity.

COMPETITION SCHEDULES

Competitive athletes' schedules fall into two general types: those with a predetermined schedule of competitive events, such as ball players and track and field athletes, and those who choose to compete in a potentially unlimited number of events, including road running and, to a lesser extent, cycling and triathlons (therefore making their own schedules).

Athletes With a Predetermined Competition Schedule

Athletes in the first group have no choice regarding competition dates. If planned properly, however, the training schedule could provide athletes with a competitive advantage, making them less vulnerable to injury by allowing time to build the aerobic system, develop the anaerobic state, and recover from hard training in time for the onset of the competitive season.

An athlete whose competitive season runs from September through January, for example, begins aerobic training in February after a recovery period. The athlete should use a heart monitor during this aerobic training period to ensure high-quality workouts (which should feel relatively easy). It also is important to perform an initial MAF test so that progression or regression may be noted in the future. The athlete should be assessed and treated by a complementary sports medicine practitioner to correct any existing structural, chemical, and mental/emotional imbalances before they become significant conditions. The professional should also make recommendations for an optimal dietary and nutritional plan that enables the person to develop maximum aerobic function. This aerobic training period may last three to five months depending on anaerobic training needs.

It is important for the athlete to build the aerobic system for as long as possible before adding an anaerobic component to the training in May, June, or later. As anaerobic training is begun, the frequency of aerobic workouts is decreased. It is essential for the athlete to perform a warm-up and active recovery before and after all anaerobic sessions, and to be periodically reassessed and treated to correct any imbalances. This training schedule continues until just before competition begins in September.

During the one- to three-week period before competition, the athlete can reduce all training—referred to as "tapering"—to ensure effective recovery. This reduction may be as much as 50% or more. Walking may serve as a relaxation or meditation technique, and the athlete should use this time to contemplate the past and future seasons as positive, healthy experiences. If the proper schedule, treatments, and diet have been maintained, the athlete should enter the competitive season fit and healthy. Athletes must not be allowed to fear this taper period thinking they will lose fitness. Rather, they should understand that it will result in improved power, strength, and endurance as well as improvement in all other function.

Training volume and intensity are decreased during the competitive season, as the competition itself will help maintain and develop more anaerobic function. This is especially true on the day (or sometimes two days) before competition and the day (or two) after.

During the competitive season, all training sessions should begin with a 15-min (or longer depending on the individual's needs) easy warm-up and be followed by an active recovery. Activities such as walking and swimming are ideal after training, especially for power athletes. Regular assessment and treatment by a complementary sports medicine practitioner help correct functional imbalances that will occur, particularly in contact sports, even during training.

On competition days, athletes should follow their previously determined optimal meal plan and perform an athlete-specific warm-up prior to the event. If athletes have trained properly and have had appropriate preseason therapy, treatment on the day of the event will be necessary for only a very few, if any.

After the season, a period of one to three weeks of total recovery may be important for most athletes. This is a time when the discipline of training and competition is greatly diminished. The athlete may choose to not work out, or just to walk for an hour each day. It is a period of recovery and reflection.

One-Year Training Schedule for Predetermined Competition Season

1. Month 1: The athlete begins training after one to three weeks of total recovery immediately following the competitive season.
2. Months 2-5: Over the next few months, the athlete begins aerobic training using a heart monitor. At the end of this period, the athlete has significantly built and trained the aerobic system. At this time also, or sooner if required, the complementary sports medicine practitioner should conduct regular sessions with the athlete.
3. Month 5 or 6: After the aerobic system has been developed, the athlete begins work on the anaerobic system. This period could start slightly earlier or later, depending on the athlete. During this time, the number of aerobic workouts is reduced.
4. Month 8: By the eighth month of training, aerobic and anaerobic systems are well developed. With competition starting in three weeks (Month 9), the athlete should begin a recovery plan by significantly reducing all training.
5. Months 9-12: For the competitive season, the athlete must decrease all training. Warm-ups should be thorough and should take place immediately before an event. Athletes need to perform active recovery with activities such as walking or swimming.

Athlete-Designed Competition Schedule

Athletes who choose their competitions from the many available usually target specific major events throughout the season. For example, a runner's goal may be to compete in the New York City Marathon in November. Because this event is late in the season and because recovery from marathons takes longer than for shorter events, this race marks the end of the racing season. From among all the local competitions that are available almost weekly and are often no more than a short drive from home, this athlete must determine which events to attend during the competitive season leading up to the Marathon. Unfortunately, many athletes choose to compete in too many events, causing structural, chemical, and/or mental/emotional imbalances.

It is best to plan a balanced race schedule before the competitive season begins and not to deviate from it, even if training partners or others encourage participation in an additional event. The year probably will consist of two aerobic training periods and two competitive seasons.

The training schedule for this type of athlete, such as the one described earlier, may begin after the end of the previous competitive season, following a recovery period. The first of the year is often a good time to begin, as some athletes lose discipline during the holiday period from the end of November through the first of the year.

The athlete begins training the aerobic system; this is the first of two aerobic periods. He or she uses a heart monitor and continues to perform the MAF test. Total workout time is slowly increased in proportion to the duration of events in the first competitive period in April. For example, if the longest event is a 15-km running race that lasts about 1 hr, the longest training run need not exceed about 90 min or be performed more than once per week. Or, if the longest bike leg of a triathlete's event is expected to last 60 min, training rides should not be longer than 2 hr.

After a base period of aerobic training, three weeks of anaerobic training may be added if desired and if the MAF test has not regressed. It is preferable, however, to exclude anaerobic training for these endurance athletes and instead to use the three weeks for additional aerobic strengthening. If no anaerobic work is performed, one to three additional races usually can be added to the athlete's schedule—an option many endurance athletes prefer, especially after they have experienced this process.

Many endurance athletes incorporate anaerobic intervals into their programs. A runner, for example, may train on a track once, twice, or even three times during the week, performing fast short-distance (i.e., 400-m) runs at, near, and often faster than the pace at which they will be racing. The author's experience is that this approach produces a higher incidence of structural injury and chemical (aerobic/anaerobic) imbalance. According to McArdle et al. (1991), "Interval training may place a disproportionate stress on the fast-twitch muscle fibers; these are not the fibers predominantly recruited in endurance competition!" (p. 444).

Competition may last April through June, and during this time the athlete's total training volume is reduced by 50% to 70%. There should be at least one day off before the day of competition, and a day of very easy training should follow. A thorough warm-up and active recovery are recommended on the day of competition.

A second aerobic training period begins on July 1; the athlete's training volume slowly increases for two months. The second competitive season runs from September through November, and training volume again is reduced by 50% to 70%. This season ends with the marathon.

Year-Long Training Plan for an Athlete-Designed Competition Schedule

1. The fall competitive season is followed by one to three weeks of total recovery.
2. Development of the aerobic system begins on January 1.
3. The first competition season begins in mid-April; training volume is reduced by 50% to 70%.
4. The athlete returns to an aerobic training period by July 1 and slowly increases the training volume.
5. The second competition season begins in September; training volume is reduced by 50% to 70%.
6. The competitive season ends in November.
7. The practitioner regularly assesses and treats the athlete to address imbalances.

Case History

Marianne, though overtrained and seriously injured, was a world-class runner embarking on a spring season of road and track running. It was clear, even to her, that unless she made some significant training changes and received care, her career would soon end. Her first heart monitor test showed an 8:45 per mile—an extremely slow pace for such a high-caliber athlete. Marianne agreed to cancel her spring and summer season to build a good aerobic system so she could return in the fall in top form. With each month of aerobic training, her pace quickened and her structural, chemical, and mental/emotional imbalances gradually improved. By the end of September, her MAF test showed a 6:40-mile pace and she felt 99% improved. Marianne did not participate in any anaerobic training. She entered a 10-km race and won in 33 min, a personal best. She raced two more times, then continued her aerobic training through the winter. She began racing on a regular schedule the following spring with success and good health.

These examples of training and competitive schedules for these types of athletes are realistic for individuals who base their training and competitions on the calendar. Practitioners sometimes encounter overtrained athletes in the middle of their competitive season, or individuals whose beginning training point does not correlate with the calendars described here. These athletes must participate in an aerobic training period while other therapies are utilized. Successful treatments are difficult—almost impossible—to render without balancing aerobic and anaerobic function. Some athletes may need to sacrifice part (or sometimes all) of a season to remedy their imbalances—a loss they will not regret.

PREVENTING OVERTRAINING IN INDIVIDUAL ATHLETES

The most common problem athletes face when training for competition is overtraining, a condition that arises out of the widely held belief that "more is better." What many athletes do not realize, however, is that once the aerobic and anaerobic systems are strengthened, training volume and intensity can be diminished without loss of optimal functioning; this approach actually can improve function. More training does not result in more benefits, but in fact often produces an overtrained athlete. In most cases, during the one- to three-week period prior to competition, reducing an athlete's training level by 50% to 70% can provide additional benefits, a finding echoed by Lehmann et al. (1997). Research shows that maintaining high levels of training can quickly lead to poor performance and "staleness" in various sports (Costill et al. 1988; Fry et al. 1992; Snyder et al. 1995). Reducing training allows for a complete recovery, maintains fitness levels, and enables the practitioner to ensure that the athlete is structurally, chemically, and mentally/emotionally balanced before entering competition.

Balanced athletes reach a point in their training when everything seems right—the MAF test has improved, they are injury free, and performance is great. A well-balanced athlete will be able to sustain this level of fitness for long periods of time, ideally throughout the competitive season and with a continuation the following season, undergoing healthy recovery during each postseason. Unfortunately, many athletes reach a similarly high level of fitness, that is, performance, that is not matched by their health. They traditionally refer to this high level of fitness as a "peak"—a short period of improved performance. This is a misleading term, however, as it implies that optimal fitness is followed by an inevitable decline in function. These athletes who are at their "peak" are sometimes able to perform time trials with results that beat their competition efforts. This is not uncommon in overtrained individuals. The "peak" for a balanced athlete can last a long time, and can continue season after season.

Case History

Bob has a stressful career as a Wall Street trader, is a husband, a father of three young children, and an amateur triathlete. He races twice monthly from April through August and competes in an Ironman triathlon (an almost 10-hr swim, bike, run event) in the fall. Bob's workday begins at 8:30 A.M. He does not train on Monday, but from Tuesday through Thursday he swims for an hour at 6 A.M. and runs for an hour at 4:30 P.M. He takes an easy, hour-long bike ride on Fridays, which allows him to recover from his week and prepare for the weekend. Bob runs up to 90 min on Saturday mornings, less in the spring and early summer, and if he feels good and his schedule permits, he swims for an hour in the afternoon. He rides for 2 to 3 hr on Sunday mornings, increasing his duration in the late summer to prepare for the Ironman race. During race weeks, Bob does not train on Saturday if the event is on Sunday. Bob has not experienced any injuries, his energy is good, and he is able to perform at a high level—he is often ranked in the top five in his age group at major events.

CONCLUSION

Though most types of competition, especially events such as football and hockey games and boxing matches, can create significant structural, chemical, and mental/emotional stress, in most cases a balanced athlete should recover with no net loss of health or fitness; indeed, a gain should be the expected result. If this is not the case, and training or competition reduces the health or fitness of the athlete, a reevaluation of the whole athlete and his or her goals is in order. Remember that even if the athlete's ability matches the intensity of the workout or competition, imbalance is inevitable if he or she participates in too many training sessions, or especially too many competitions.

23

The Overtraining Syndrome

Though there is no standard definition of overtraining, it has been traditionally described as diminished performance that results from an increase in training volume and/or intensity (Fry and Kraemer 1997). As previously discussed, overtraining occurs when the Training = Workout + Recovery equation shows an imbalance resulting from excess number and/or intensity of workouts, lack of recovery, or both. This multifactorial problem is referred to as the overtraining syndrome and is associated with autonomic dysfunction (sympathetic and parasympathetic imbalance), hormonal imbalance (adrenal dysfunction in particular), and nutritional and dietary deficiencies.

ASSESSING THE OVERTRAINING SYNDROME

Assessment and treatment of the overtraining syndrome in its earliest stages are crucial to the prevention of further regression. The Maximum Aerobic Function (MAF) test is a useful tool for assessing overtraining as it begins to develop, and may provide the first objective sign. In order for this assessment to be effective, athletes at all levels must conduct the test every three to four weeks, and the practitioner (and coach or trainer, if applicable) should record the results.

A thorough, immediate assessment of the athlete is vital at the first sign of overtraining; it should cover all structural, chemical, and mental/emotional aspects of the patient, including posture and gait, diet and nutrition, training and competition schedules, and all lifestyle factors. One must differentiate between primary and secondary problems in order to determine the correct treatment.

To assist the practitioner and patient in understanding the full spectrum of overtraining, not just the more obvious late-stage conditions, this chapter characterizes overtraining in terms of three stages: functional overtraining, sympathetic overtraining, and parasympathetic overtraining.

FUNCTIONAL OVERTRAINING

A MAF test that demonstrates an abnormal plateau (or regression), as compared to the normal plateau, may be the first sign of overtraining; similar changes were observed by Hakkinen et al. (1985). This first stage is referred to as "functional overtraining." Interestingly, it is sometimes accompanied by a sudden and dramatic improvement in competitive performance that may convince the athlete—and others—that training is ideal. This temporary improvement may be due to an abnormally increased sympathetic function.

Another sign associated with functional overtraining is an imbalance between aerobic and anaerobic function indicated by muscle testing and/or by a comparison of maximum aerobic function and maximum anaerobic function. Recall that aerobic function can be measured with the MAF test and anaerobic function by competitive performance or time trial. An imbalance is evident, for example, if the runner performs the MAF test at 7 min/mile but races under 5 min/mile. It is not uncommon for talented athletes to compete at high levels but achieve proportionately slow scores on the MAF test, possibly because of excess sympathetic activity that often occurs during competition. This is an example of aerobic deficiency and anaerobic excess.

Other athletes, such as cyclists, are not as easy to assess because there are no definitive times to compare. A traditional time trial may be useful in this situation. Or, it may be best to compare training and racing performance within a group of cyclists. For example, if the 10th-slowest cyclist (riding at maximum aerobic function) performs as one of the best road racers among a group of 20 cyclists, diminished aerobic function relative to an excess of anaerobic function may be indicated. When one conducts this type of assessment, it is important to be sure that the other athletes in the group are not overtrained.

Functional overtraining probably is synonymous with overreaching, which has been shown to boost performance but often turns into overtraining (Stone et al. 1991). Decreased performance levels are not evident until middle and later stages of overtraining, for example during more obvious autonomic imbalance (Urhausen et al. 1997). Functional overtraining may also be associated with Selye's first "alarm-reaction" phase of the general adaptation syndrome (GAS) (Selye 1976).

FUNCTIONAL SIGNS AND SYMPTOMS

The overtraining syndrome typically results in poor performance and structural injury. In addition, secondary chemical injuries such as fatigue and infection, as well as altered mood states and reproductive function, are evident (Lehmann et al. 1997). Note that the diminished performance associated with overtraining does not occur only in competitive athletes; it is also seen in people performing everyday chores. The practitioner must also focus on factors unrelated to competition to assess the potential of overtraining.

In many cases, secondary structural injury results from primary chemical problems. In addition to relationships previously discussed between adrenal dysfunction and muscle inhibition, for example, immune dysfunction can also alter gait and increase the risk of structural problems (Weidner et al. 1997).

An athlete's lifestyle may also contribute to overtraining; this aspect of overtraining was recognized as early as 1923 (Parmenter 1923). To date, however, mainstream medicine has not produced a standard assessment or treatment process, perhaps because research on overtraining has yielded variable results, making the syndrome difficult to understand using that approach. For example, some studies demonstrate that performance reduction is associated with high cortisol levels whereas others do not show this relationship. It is evident that overtraining is a highly individual functional problem. It produces not just physical signs and symptoms, but "organ-related complaints which are without organic disease" (Urhausen et al. 1997, p. 253) and other functional imbalances, and it is best treated by a complementary sports medicine practitioner.

In addition to these symptoms of overtraining, other problems begin in the functional overtraining period and continue through all phases of overtraining. These functional symptoms often overlap with those that occur with the aerobic deficiency syndrome and adrenal dysfunction. Symptoms begin as subtle complaints and are revealed when the practitioner takes a thorough history and conducts a functional assessment. These complaints, which begin during functional overtraining and continue through the later stages of overtraining, include fatigue and an increase in body fat. An individual is fatigued in the morning, finding it difficult to "get out of bed"—or after meals, which may be a sign of carbohydrate intolerance. This may include a blood sugar-handling stress, which is indicated by fatigue between meals, constant hunger, and increased food cravings, especially for sweets. The athlete has an increase in body fat, despite increased training. There are recurrent nutritional problems that often are due to a secondary malabsorption of nutrients, and excess consumption of carbohydrates is coupled with low fat and protein intakes.

Among the functional signs and symptoms of overtraining are symptoms indicated on the Symptom Survey (Groups Three, Seven, Eight, and Nine) and structural injuries, especially those that recur. Adrenal dysfunction may inhibit the sartorius, tibialis posterior, and/or gracilis, increasing vulnerability to back, knee, ankle, and foot injuries. In addition, high cortisol levels generally occur in the early and middle stages of overtraining, and low cortisol levels are associated with late stages. Premenstrual syndrome and menopausal symptoms may be secondary complaints for women, and sexual dysfunction may be a symptom for both sexes. Mental and emotional stress, including mild or clinical depression and anxiety, is associated with overtraining also.

Other problems may include orthostatic hypotension (or its functional form), reduced body temperature, abnormal cold pressor test, low oral pH, low vital capacity, low dehydroepiandrosterone [DHEA(S)] levels, and other signs and symptoms of imbalance.

SYMPATHETIC OVERTRAINING

Overtraining, even during the functional overtraining stage, typically is associated with autonomic nervous system dysfunction (Kuipers and Keizer 1988). Excess sympathetic tone begins in the early stage and is dominant by the middle stage, and the late stage is associated with excess parasympathetic activity (Fry and Kraemer 1997).

Sympathetic overtraining begins during the later stages of the functional overtraining state and becomes increasingly dominant, causing increased sympathetic activity during the resting and training states. This is typically reflected in a high resting heart rate, restlessness, and hyperexcitability (Lehmann et al. 1997) and produces a regression of MAF test results. Sympathetic overtraining is more common in athletes who train with speed and power excess, those who train too often, those with contributing lifestyle stress, and most often those athletes who have a combination of these factors.

Dysfunction of the sympathoadrenergic system (the sympathetic nervous system and adrenal glands) is more dominant with sympathetic overtraining (Urhausen et al. 1997). This is why early detection and treatment of adrenal dysfunction are vital to the prevention of overtraining.

Hormonal changes play a major role in the full spectrum of overtraining. As sympathetic activity increases, cortisol (and catecholamine) output may rise to abnormal levels, further amplifying the normal elevation in cortisol that occurs prior to competition. The keen awareness and fine hand-to-eye coordination required in sports such as golf and racquetball are adversely affected by these hormone problems (McKay et al. 1997; Urhausen et al. 1997).

Generally, high cortisol levels have a catabolic effect on the system comparable to that produced by exhaustive, prolonged training. Regular cortisol measurement may be one of the best laboratory assessment tools; however, experience will allow practitioners to accurately predict the patient's cortisol levels on the basis of all other nonlaboratory assessment methods. High cortisol may also be associated with high insulin.

High insulin levels may be another sign of overtraining in some individuals. Moderate-intensity training usually suppresses insulin production during exercise, whereas maximal training intensities may increase the insulin response (Urhausen et al. 1997). The resulting insulin-mediated sympathetic response further stimulates the sympathetic nervous system. Generally, training improves insulin sensitivity. However, some non-obese individuals have a functional biochemical imbalance that is characterized by high insulin levels, much like those of obese individuals; Ruderman et al. (1981) refer to such people as "metabolically obese."

A good indicator of the anabolic/catabolic balance is the testosterone/cortisol ratio, with a reduction of 30% or more diagnostic for overtraining (Adlercreutz et al. 1986). Low testosterone levels, secondary to reduced DHEA(S), create significant problems for athletes because this hormone is important for muscle recovery and may help replace glycogen stores. Fortunately, depressed testosterone/cortisol levels are easily remedied with proper care.

PARASYMPATHETIC OVERTRAINING

The second stage of overtraining may be associated with Selye's "resistance phase" of GAS. This autonomic problem sometimes regresses to an excess parasympathetic overtraining condition (Stone et al. 1991).

Parasympathetic overtraining, accompanied by a relative lack of sympathetic tone, produces decreased resting heart rates, lowered cortisol and catecholamine levels, lack of desire to compete (and sometimes train), depression, and most notably exhaustion. It also is associated with reduced lactate response, making lactate assessment inaccurate. The MAF test has usually significantly regressed and plateaued at a poor level. This condition is associated with low resting heart rates (and low heart rate recovery from interval training or competition); some athletes misinterpret the low heart rate recovery and think that they are improving.

As discussed in chapter 20, a lack of sympathetic activity may result in increased sodium and chloride loss due to reduced aldosterone and may increase the athlete's vulnerability to functional or more traditional signs of hyponatremia. Parasympathetic overtraining may correspond to the "exhaustion" phase, the third phase in Selye's GAS.

AMENORRHEA IN ATHLETES

Menstrual dysfunction is frequently associated with overtraining, showing a positive correlation to high-intensity training (Arena et al. 1995). Overtrained female athletes often develop menstrual abnormalities including amenorrhea (the absence of menstrual bleeding), oligomenorrhea (a menstrual cycle between 35 and 90 days), and delayed menarche (Benson et al. 1996). This problem, like all others discussed in this text, is individual and multifactorial; no clear single cause-and-effect pattern has been found between amenorrhea and training, diet, nutrition, psychiatric factors, or other factors not reviewed here.

Amenorrhea may occur at a very early age. In a recent study of high-level athletes (Bale et al. 1996), only 20% of the gymnasts (average age 13.3 years) and 40% of the runners (average age 13.6 years) had started menstruating as compared with 95% of noncompetitive girls of similar ages.

The problems in many amenorrheic athletes may be considered a syndrome, comprising overtraining and disordered eating (especially reduced kilocalorie intake and excessively low fat intake), excessively low body weight and body fat (especially femoral fat stores: fat around the hips, buttocks, and thighs), and vegetarianism (Benson et al. 1996).

One of the most significant structural problems associated with amenorrhea is bone loss. Prolonged low estrogen and progesterone levels increase the risk of decreased bone density, stress fractures, muscle soreness, and physical fatigue (De Cree et al. 1995). Demineralization of bone is most common in the spine, wrist, and metatarsals. These imbalances can lead to structural problems in the skeleton later in life due to osteoporosis (Dueck et al. 1996). In addition, scoliosis is associated with amenorrhea in athletes (Arena et al. 1995). (It should be noted that men may also have reduced androgens, specifically testosterone, which adversely affects bone density, also causing bone loss [Wishart et al. 1995].)

Two significant chemical factors are associated with amenorrheic athletes: hormonal imbalance and nutritional deficiency. High cortisol levels are common in amenorrheic athletes (Ding et al. 1988). Elevated cortisol is associated with reduced DHEA(S), resulting in diminished androgen production, which adversely affects the menstrual cycle (Belanger et al. 1994). The reduced estrogen and progesterone profiles typical in amenorrheic athletes are very similar to those of postmenopausal women (Dueck et al. 1996).

In many cases, amenorrheic athletes consume an energy-deficient diet. Laughlin and Yen (1996) state, "Growing evidence suggests that menstrual disturbances in female athletes are related to the metabolic cost of high levels of energy expenditure without compensatory increases in dietary intake" (p. 4301). In some cases, however, amenorrheic athletes consume the same total kilocalories as those with normal menstrual cycles, but much less fat (up to 50% less) and protein, with higher carbohydrate intakes. Reduced fatty acid intakes can result in lower calcium absorption and lower bone calcium (Claassen et al. 1995). This is typically aggravated by low dietary calcium intake but may be associated with normal blood levels of calcium (Lukaski and Penland 1996).

Disordered eating itself is a complex mental/emotional issue, involving a full spectrum of problems from functional to pathological—from poor eating, dieting, and preoccupation with low fat to clinically diagnosed anorexia nervosa and bulimia. The endocrine equilibrium that regulates reproductive function can also be affected by other psychological factors; the stress associated with competition may be a significant variable as well (Arena et al. 1995).

In athletes without defined amenorrhea, other menstrual distress (so-called premenstrual syndrome) is nevertheless common and is also associated with increased consumption of carbohydrates (Johnson et al. 1995) and depression (O'Connor et al. 1989). The latter was mentioned earlier, as was the relation between reduced fatty acids and mental/emotional stress.

Amenorrhea is often thought of as having psychogenic origins, but it has been shown that nutritional and hormonal imbalance can be more of an etiological factor (Laughlin et al. 1998). The critical relationship between training and nutritional imbalance is best assessed and treated by practitioners of complementary sports medicine. According to Dueck et al. (1996), it is easy to see how non-pharmacological treatment can successfully reestablish normal hormonal profiles and menstrual activity in amenorrheic athletes.

ASSESSMENT OF OVERTRAINING

In addition to the MAF test, many of the tests described in earlier chapters may be used to assess the full spectrum of overtraining. These tests include the postural blood pressure test (to assess adrenal dysfunction), the cold pressor test and resting heart rate (to assess autonomic imbalance), and the oral pH and respiratory quotient, when available, to indicate substrate utilization (the process of diminishing fat and increasing glucose utilization begins in the functional overtraining state and is represented by a decrease in oral pH and a rise in respiratory quotient). In addition, one can compare more subtle current symptoms to the notes on the patient's Symptom Survey, especially for Groups One and Two, which relate to sympathetic and parasympathetic states, respectively.

Hormone tests that measure cortisol, testosterone, growth hormone, and catecholamines, as well as others that measure reduced neuromuscular excitability (Lehmann et al. 1997), may demonstrate overtraining. The functional overtraining state may not yet produce abnormal test results except for tests that measure function. One exception may relate to increased cortisol, which the author has found to be associated with poor MAF test results beginning with the lengthened plateau.

As mentioned earlier, one should always assess for the muscle imbalances associated with overtraining, such as inhibition of the sartorius, tibialis posterior, and gracilis. These imbalances often, but not always, result in poor functioning of the areas supported by the muscles: hip, low back, knee, calf, ankle, or foot.

An important tool for assessment of the functional overtraining and overtraining conditions that cannot be overemphasized is a good patient history. Practitioners often underscore the physical assessment and treatment process but fail to make

Case History

Dave monitored his MAF test every three weeks and noted improvements each time, with some brief plateaus. After about 18 months, five consecutive MAF tests showed a sustained plateau. During this same period, Dave competed and obtained sudden, exceptional results. Five weeks later, two competitions ended in his worst results in two years. Soon afterward, his left knee began to be painful; this was the first injury he had experienced and was the reason for his visit. His exam showed a lack of systolic pressure as he stood from a lying position; his left sartorius muscle was inhibited, and other indications of adrenal dysfunction were present. Dave was treated and scheduled for another session; his training schedule was not addressed. Three weeks later his systolic pressure fell 14 mmHg; his knee improved for a few days, but the pain returned. Dave now complained of insomnia, and his energy levels diminished; to maintain alertness, he began drinking several cups of coffee a day. His MAF test was now worse. He was treated, but training stress was not addressed. In three weeks he returned with a cold—the first he had had in a year—and stated that he had lost his desire to compete. After another week, still with a cold, he complained of severe pain in his right knee, and the left knee continued to be painful. His wife became concerned with his mood swings. Treatment relieved certain symptoms, but never for more than a week. Dave suffered for several weeks through the overtraining syndrome, with three more MAF tests that demonstrated regression in performance. Eventually, training was reduced by more than 70%, and with the combined effects of elimination of caffeine, strictness with diet, and work on lifestyle stress, Dave showed gradual improvement. His body ultimately became balanced and he continued progressing in training and competition with renewed success and enjoyment. Although only one case, Dave's situation illustrates the importance of the MAF test and the need for a multifactorial approach to assessment and treatment. It was early in his practice that the author saw Dave, and this case helped set the precedent for use of the MAF test and the heart monitor assessment.

proper use of conversation as an assessment tool. It is critical to be aware of the seemingly unimportant comments that the patient may make on any visit. The practitioner needs to ask questions that pertain to mood, energy levels, performance, and infections. The answers, combined with recent MAF test results and the functional tests, are crucial to discovering overtraining in its earliest stages.

Treatment of Overtraining

Therapy for overtraining includes restructuring the athlete's training schedule, modifying lifestyle factors including diet and nutrition, addressing stress, and rendering proper hands-on treatments. Although therapy should always be based on the assessment process, some specific avenues must be considered in athletes who are overtrained:

1. The athlete should decrease training time by 50% to 70%, or more if necessary.
2. The athlete should immediately cease all anaerobic training, including competition.
3. A helpful remedy for an overtrained athlete is walking. One should explain to a patient who is uncertain of its benefits that walking gently stimulates circulation and aerobic muscle fiber activity, is mentally beneficial (much like meditation), and can help redevelop the aerobic system—the first phase of retraining.
4. Retraining, that is, building the aerobic base, should last three to six months and does not include any anaerobic training or competition.
5. Adrenal and aerobic dysfunction is almost always associated with overtraining.
6. Some athletes require stimulation of emotional reflexes as described in chapter 11.

DIETARY AND NUTRITIONAL FACTORS

Individual dietary and nutritional factors are important considerations in overtrained athletes, but because each athlete is unique, no protocol exists. However, certain common factors that were discussed in chapters 18 and 19 are pertinent to overtraining.

Malabsorption is common in overtrained athletes. These athletes experience increased sympathetic stress that may result in mucosal suppression in the small intestines, where most nutrients are absorbed. Malabsorption can begin a series of secondary nutritional problems. Betaine hydrochloride may improve digestion and nutrient absorption in patients experiencing malabsorption.

Overtrained athletes often experience a decreased plasma glutamine concentration, especially after endurance training or competition. Glutamine supplementation may improve immune and small-intestine function and related muscle function.

Lifestyle also affects the patient's digestion. Eating while driving or working, for example, adversely influences digestion and nutrient absorption. The practitioner must assess lifestyle habits that may produce stress before, during, and after meals and must provide guidance in modifying the habits.

Caffeine consumption may be contraindicated for patients who have increased sympathetic stress. Reduction in or avoidance of stimulants such as coffee, tea, soda, and chocolate, as well as caffeine-containing over-the-counter and prescription drugs, may be necessary.

Overtraining may disrupt the normal balance of eicosanoids, through which the inflammatory/anti-inflammatory state is balanced. The practitioner should carefully evaluate the patient's dietary fat ratios and consider the potential need for omega-3 supplementation.

Zinc may help reduce the abnormally high levels of cortisol common to overtrained athletes (Brandao-Neto et al. 1990); however, timing is an important factor when one is supplementing with zinc. Cortisol should be measured throughout the day to determine abnormal peak levels; then the athlete should be directed to take zinc supplements 2 to 3 hr prior to cortisol peaks.

Reduction of high-glycemic foods and consumption of smaller, more frequent meals may help patients with abnormally high cortisol, especially those who have symptoms of depression. Moderating carbohydrate intake may also be helpful, as higher-carbohydrate diets may elevate cortisol levels (Tegelman et al. 1992). Inadequate caloric intake and eating disorders may also adversely affect hormone balance and decrease the metabolic clearance of cortisol (Urhausen et al. 1997).

The practitioner may discover a need for choline and potassium (the so-called alkaline-ash minerals) in overtrained athletes during the first two stages. Recurrent asthma symptoms may be an early indication of overtraining and usually respond well to choline supplementation. During parasympathetic overtraining, additional phosphorus may be necessary.

The combination of potential malabsorption, an athlete's general increased need for nutrients, and a poorly selected diet create the possibility of the need for virtually any nutrient.

RECOVERY FROM OVERTRAINING

Properly treated, athletes can sometimes recover rapidly from overtraining imbalances. This is especially true in the functional overtraining state. In many cases, modifying the training schedule, making appropriate nutritional and dietary adjustments, and applying hands-on therapy can result in an almost immediate improvement in function. This rapid progress will be demonstrated not only in the MAF test, but also in blood pressure changes, oral pH, and most other measures. Usually, these athletes either will not need to modify their competitive schedules or will need to make only minor adjustments in near-term competitions. For example, a patient who goes to a practitioner with an injury and is found to be in the functional overtraining stage can ordinarily be ready to compete in less than a month.

Athletes in the second, sympathetic-dominant stage of overtraining can also respond quickly to proper care. However, those who have upcoming competitions may be required to modify or cancel those early events to allow for a more complete recovery from overtraining. In this case, the structural problems typically respond quickly to proper therapy. However, building an acceptable aerobic base will take at least two and sometimes up to six months.

Those who are chronically overtrained and in the third parasympathetic stage are much more difficult to treat. They may need to cancel their next competitive season (as if they had a physical injury that prevented competing) and spend time building their aerobic system, reducing stress, improving their body chemistry through proper diet and nutrition, and learning about their body and its limits. These patients will require four to six months or more before resuming effective competition. In some cases, they may need a year or more.

This chapter provides insight into the characteristics of overtrained athletes and the assessment and therapy methods necessary for treatment. Table 23.1 is a review of the overtraining spectrum.

CONCLUSION

Because of the complex nature of an overtraining syndrome, it is difficult to formulate a specific treatment protocol. Individual variation dictates treatment. Remember that a longer plateau in MAF tests may be the first sign of overtraining—termed functional overtraining—and that both the practitioner and athlete should carefully evaluate this possibility. The practitioner should correct existing imbalances and modify the athlete's training schedule as indicated to prevent further regression and restore progress. The patient must comply with the modifications, or further deterioration into sympathetic overtraining and then parasympathetic overtraining is inevitable. Treatment for this chronic overtraining may last for months or even longer.

Table 23.1 Three Stages of Overtraining With Common Associated Factors

THREE STAGES OF OVERTRAINING			
	Functional	**Sympathetic**	**Parasympathetic**
Patient complaints	Typically structural: knee, ankle/foot, low back, etc.	Structural (similar to functional stage) and chemical (fatigue, hormonal, immune, etc.)	Structural, chemical, and mental (depression and anxiety)
MAF test	Plateau	Worsening	Plateaued at a very poor level
Common findings	Muscle inhibition and joint dysfunction. Lack of rise in systolic blood pressure on standing. High training volume and/or intensity. Increased performance.	Increased muscle inhibition; chronic joint dysfunction. Decreased systolic blood pressure on standing. Increased resting and training heart rate. Increased cortisol, insulin, and catecholamines. Decreased testosterone and DHEA(S). Performance plateaued or diminishing.	Worsening structural and chemical stress. Orthostatic hypotension. Decreased cortisol, DHEA(S), testosterone, and catecholamines. Decreased lactate response. Performance greatly diminished or not performing.
GAS	Alarm reaction	Resistance response	Exhaustion
Aerobic/Anaerobic	Beginnings of imbalance	Aerobic deficiency	Aerobic deficiency and anaerobic excess
Recovery	Immediate	Rapid, within 2-6 mo	Physical problems, 1-2 mo; other problems much longer, at least 4-6 mo, up to a year or more
Autonomics	Subtle imbalance	Increased sympathetic and decreased parasympathetic	Decreased sympathetic and increased parasympathetic

24

Training and Competitive Footwear

Athletes wear special training and competitive shoes to protect the plantar surface of the foot from the potentially damaging effects of stones, glass, and other objects and to protect the dorsum of the foot from the feet of other athletes. Most believe that athletic shoes also provide the extra support and stability necessary to prevent injury. Unfortunately, the opposite may be the case, as modern athletic footwear has been associated with frequent injury (Robbins and Waked 1998, 1997a, 1997b; Robbins et al. 1994). In fact, barefoot athletes generally are more resistant to injury than those who wear shoes. Some athletes also erroneously believe that advanced athletic footwear can improve athletic function.

FOOT FUNCTION

Ankle sprains may be the most common injuries in sport and may account for the greatest loss of playing time in comparison to any other injury. Foot and ankle imbalances, many of which are asymptomatic, also can cause a variety of secondary problems in the leg, knee, hip, pelvis, and spine and even in areas higher in the body. These foot and ankle imbalances may also result from wearing modern footwear.

Most importantly, practitioners can assess athletes who wear modern footwear—nearly all athletes—to determine which, if any, areas have become dysfunctional. These often include the tibialis and peroneal muscles, talus and calcaneal bones, and first metatarsals, although dysfunction in any area of the foot, ankle, leg, knee, pelvis, and spine is common. Dysfunction secondary to improper shoes begins asymptomatically. Correction of imbalances in this early stage can help prevent further dysfunction, symptomatic injury, and diminished performance.

During weight-bearing activity, sudden loading of the lower extremity normally produces a sharp rise of vertically transmitted force (impact). This normal stress induced by impact is the common denominator in injuries to the foot, ankle, leg, and knee. For example, the normal force on impact for an athlete during running is about two and one-half times the athlete's body weight applied statically (Robbins and Hanna 1987). Improper adaptation to this impact is associated with injuries such as plantar fascitis, shinsplints, stress fractures, metatarsalgia, osteoarthritis (including vertebral), and various knee injuries. Even sports such as cycling produce the same impact forces, but the rate of loading is lower. Robbins and Hanna (1987) state, "The high injury frequency in sports involving running and jumping has led many to conclude that the lower extremities, and particularly the foot to be of poor design, an unusually fragile structure unable to sustain the use associated with running without injury, thus requiring additional protective devices" (p. 148).

Thus the boom in so-called highly technological and very expensive athletic shoe manufacturing and marketing. The implied inability of the human frame to function effectively during natural activity is illogical. Robbins and Hanna (1987) also write, "The opinion that the lower extremities are inherently fragile goes against the authors' understanding of the concept of natural selection" (p. 149).

Wearing thick-soled, soft shoes causes the foot to hold a more rigid position and keeps it from adapting normally to the normal stress induced by sport activity (Robbins and Hanna 1987). This adversely affects muscle function. Basmajian and Bentzon (1954) were among the first to show this with electromyographic studies that demonstrated a lack of tonic activity of intrinsic muscles of the shod foot. Perhaps this is why there is a higher injury rate in North American runners compared to those in areas such as Europe, Asia, the West Indies, and Haiti, where barefoot and shod athletes coexist.

Jorgensen (1990) also showed that some heel counters caused a reduction in musculoskeletal transients and in the activity of the gastrocnemius, soleus, and quadriceps muscles at heel strike. A resulting 2.4% decrease in $\dot{V}O_2$max, a significant effect, is an example of how a seemingly minor structural change can significantly impact the whole system.

A primary reason for higher injury rates in shod athletes, therefore, is the lack of sensory feedback from the foot while the same level of shock absorption is present. The lack of sensory feedback—diminished kinesthetic sense of foot position—is the result of wearing modern athletic shoes. "Kinesthetic sense—and therefore position awareness—is derived almost entirely from muscle and tactile receptors" (Robbins et al. 1995, p. 242). This may be another mechanism by which muscular inhibition in the foot and leg can significantly contribute to structural imbalance and secondary injury. Kinesthetic awareness normally declines with age as a result of a loss of plantar tactile sensitivity, and may be a contributing factor to the frequency of falls that occur in later life. But young athletes wearing modern footwear show no kinesthetic awareness.

The fact that a shod foot does not significantly change shock absorption during activity is a significant aspect of increased injury in shod athletes (Robbins and Hanna 1987). Activity performed while barefoot normally produces proprioception from plantar sensation. The central nervous system relies on this information to adjust the body's posture and gait to provide compensation for the stress of the activity. Wearing a shoe prevents the transmission of this sensation. The load created by a barefoot athlete allows the foot to absorb shock naturally, a process that is not effective when shoes are worn.

ARCH FUNCTION

Arch support is a topic that often arises during discussions about shoes. Populations that live primarily barefoot have a high arch when the foot is unloaded that significantly flattens when the foot is loaded (Robbins and Hanna 1987). Unfortunately, many athletes confuse this normal response with "flat feet" or negatively refer to it as a "pronation problem." This normal response is similar in biped terrestrial primates that have foot structures similar to that of humans and are the only other species to possess Meissner corpuscles—a sensory nerve ending located at the dorsum of the foot, among other locations. The Meissner corpuscles discern spatial characteristics of touch sensation (Guyton 1986) and rapidly respond to the objects touched by the skin. According to Robbins and Hanna (1987), this plantar sensory feedback may induce intrinsic foot shock absorption related to the function of the medial arch. (Recall that the tibialis posterior is a primary muscle related to the structure and function of the medial arch.)

The arch response of individuals in shod populations is not the same, possibly because the arch support common to most athletic shoes blocks the sensation created by the Meissner corpuscles and interferes with the normal mechanisms of the medial arch on loading (i.e., flattening of the arch). Without these sensations, a higher amount of stress is placed on the foot, ankle, and other parts of the body.

TAPING AND OTHER JOINT SUPPORT

Ankle taping may help prevent injuries, but not through immobilization as once thought. Taping may prevent injuries by tractioning the skin of the foot and leg, providing cutaneous sensory cues of plantar surface position and better allowing the nervous system to adapt to movement (Robbins et al. 1995; Robbins and Waked 1998). Therefore, if taping is used as a therapy, it may be necessary to include the lower leg, ankle, and plantar areas. This process may be effective with the use of just two (sometimes three) strips of tape wrapped around the ankle and foot (anchored on the lower leg) rather than the many layers that are commonly applied.

Taping the ankles may help prevent injury by partially restoring impaired proprioception caused by modern athletic footwear. This may be the primary benefit provided by taping, since the support function is lost after as little as 20 min (Perlman et al. 1987). Robbins et al. (1995) showed that foot-position awareness was 107.5% worse in nontaped subjects with athletic footwear and 58.1% worse in those with the ankle taped, as compared to those who were barefoot.

Because the use of tape and other support devices reduces range of motion, such devices can also impair athletic performance. The effects can include reduced speed, agility, and vertical jumping, as well as reduced force production and total work (Robbins and Waked 1998). Moreover, the use of prophylactic devices in other joints may also increase the incidence of injury. For example, numerous studies clearly demonstrate that knee supports of various types increase the incidence of knee injury (Rovere et al. 1987; Grace et al. 1988; Teitz et al. 1987).

Rather than rely on taping, braces, expensive shoes, and other devices, practitioners are encouraged to determine the primary factor or factors that caused or are maintaining structural imbalances and correct them as discussed in earlier chapters. In many cases, the causes are found in areas apart from the secondary area of injury. In the author's experience, almost all functional imbalances in the foot may be corrected using the conservative measures described in this text (if correctly applied), including choosing the shoes that best match the athlete's needs—and without any additional foot or ankle support.

ORTHOTICS

Knowledge of most of the benefits of foot orthotics is empirical. This is not to discount the effectiveness of these devices, however. One potential problem with the use of orthotic devices is that the need for other therapies may be overlooked. People with past or current surgical needs, stroke or hemiparetic patients, or those who for various reasons will never have normal foot function are more difficult or even impossible to treat using only a conservative approach. In these patients, the orthotic may be more important in the rehabilitation process than the shoe (Hesse et al. 1996).

Neither shoe inserts (Clark et al. 1989) nor orthotics (Krivickas 1997), including those with shock-absorbing abilities (Gardner et al. 1988), have been shown to protect against the risks of injury. These devices may actually further reduce arch function and provide excessive cushioning, resulting in increased structural stress. Krivickas (1997) states, "Orthotics are often prescribed to improve lower extremity alignment. However, studies have not shown that orthotics have any effect on knee alignment and, while they can alter subtalar joint alignment, the clinical benefit of this remains unclear" (p. 132). In addition, electromyographic studies fail to show any significant differences in the average muscle activity of the tibialis anterior, peroneus longus, and gastrocnemius muscles (Tomaro and Burdett 1993) when orthotics are used. These and other factors lead most authors to believe that these devices do not prevent injuries (Thonnard et al. 1996; Robbins and Waked 1998).

OTHER ANKLE DYSFUNCTION

Ankle injuries are among the most common athletic injuries; Leanderson et al. (1993) showed that during a two-year period, 78% of basketball players experienced some type of ankle injury. Of these, 83% reported recurrent ankle problems. Many basketball players and other athletes wear "high-top" athletic shoes, thinking they provide additional ankle support. However, clinical trials have not demonstrated that high-top shoes are able to prevent ankle sprains (Barrett and Bilisko 1995). In addition, Brizuela et al. (1997) reported that high-top shoes produced lower eversion ranges but higher ranges of inversion on landing. Inversion sprains may be the most common form of ankle injury. These shoes also reduced the average jump height and increased the time needed to complete a running course in comparison to the corresponding values in participants who wore low-support shoes. Rovere et al. (1988) also showed that high-top athletic shoes were associated with increased rates of injury.

According to Robbins and Waked (1998), "The best solution for reducing ankle sprains in shod athletes is the use of more advanced footwear to retain maximal tactile sensitivity, thereby maintaining an awareness of foot position comparable to that of the barefoot state or perhaps even improving on it" (p. 63). In other words, injury is less common when athletes wear "low-tech" shoes that have flat soles with little-to-no cushioning or support systems as compared to the popular athletic shoes. The author's experience with athletes who wear these types of (very inexpensive) athletic footwear is that they are associated with a significant decrease in injury compared to the more common (expensive) shoes. Robbins et al. (1994) state that shoes with thin, hard soles provide superior foot and ankle stability.

Practitioners should consider a number of factors when discussing the issue of athletic footwear with patients. In many cases, the use of inexpensive, flat, nonsupportive athletic shoes may be healthier during training and competition and whenever shoes are worn. These are made by lesser-known companies. Most major shoe companies make some flat shoes with less support and cushioning that may be an improvement over their oversupported and cushioned models.

Athletes may benefit from spending more time being barefoot. This does not necessarily apply to training or competition unless the patient is used to this activity, but to idle time or other times when it is appropriate to remove one's shoes (i.e., at home or in some working conditions). Being barefoot will help the muscles, ligaments, and tendons adapt to the new position of the foot, since the athlete has often spent almost an entire lifetime in shoes with a higher heel. This is what some women experience who have worn high heels much of their life and decide (often because of low back or other problems) to switch to flatter shoes. This process can be started with the removal of the insert found in most shoes; this can reduce some cushioning and height and improve the fit of the shoe, as will be noted later.

Those athletes sponsored by shoe companies should consider switching to more appropriate footwear, but if none is available, athletes can ask the shoe company to make them a special shoe appropriate for their foot and sport. Peer pressure may be a significant factor when athletes choose which shoes they will wear; this is especially true in younger athletes. For example, a high school basketball player may be reluctant to wear low-top shoes when everyone else wears high-tops.

When imbalances in the foot and ankle develop, improving muscle and joint dysfunction most often provides sufficient natural support to allow healing of the injury, even if those problems are far from the foot and ankle dysfunction. If further foot and ankle support is required, taping for a short period of time (no more than five days) may be an effective adjunct. Most importantly, proper overall assessment and therapy of the athlete and his or her lifestyle can help in correcting foot, ankle, and other problems associated with normal training and competition. In patients with more serious foot and ankle problems, such as people requiring surgery, a complementary approach can be taken; in some cases, carefully improving foot and ankle function before surgery, and in most cases after, can significantly improve recovery time, restoration of function, and return to activity as well as preventing risk of additional injury.

Manual muscle testing also may be used to assess shoe compatibility. While the patient is barefoot and in a neutral weight-bearing position, the pectoralis major clavicular (PMC) or another convenient muscle is tested. After the patient puts on both shoes, the PMC muscle is retested. If muscle inhibition is produced with the shoes on as compared to off, the shoe may not be compatible—perhaps because of fit or an improperly matched support system. (If the PMC and other muscles are inhibited with the patient barefoot, the muscles should be retested with the patient in a non-weight-bearing state, such as lying, to rule out potential weight-bearing faults—perhaps an ankle joint dysfunction or certain pelvic or spinal joint problems previously discussed.)

PROPER FIT

Poorly fitting shoes are potentially another source of significant structural stress. Asymptomatic imbalances created by improper athletic shoe fit can cause significant problems that are difficult to assess and that often result in imbalances higher in the body structure. Chapter 16 addressed the effects of improperly fitted athletic shoes on the first metatarsal joint and other areas. A survey of over 100 runners conducted by the author (Maffetone 1996) showed that 52% trained or raced in shoes that were too small. The practitioner must evaluate all of the athlete's shoes, including those worn while not training, to determine whether they fit properly. Athletic shoes should be evaluated throughout the year for wear patterns (observe the manufacturer's insert for abnormal wear patterns) and pressure or tears in the front of the shoe (those that come from the first toenail indicate that a shoe is too short).

How to Buy Athletic Shoes

1. Always measure both feet while standing on a hard floor. Most adults do not measure their feet when buying new shoes, even though their size may have changed. Consequently, people often wear the wrong-size shoe for years, even decades. The practitioner may have patients measure their shoe size two to three times during a day to note size fluctuations. (Significant fluctuations must be differentiated from serious health problems, such as significant swelling or pathological changes.) The largest measurement should be used as a general guide when one is buying shoes. However, there are no standards. Manufacturers vary their sizes.
2. Allow time for a proper fitting. Find a hard surface to walk on (carpet can make shoes feel more comfortable), and go outside if necessary. Try on the size you normally wear. Even if it feels good, try the next half-size larger. Continue to try half-size-larger shoes until the shoe obviously is too large; then go back to the previous half-size. This one is usually the best fit. Remember to try on shoes with varying widths as necessary.
3. It may be best for an individual to wear shoes of two different sizes if the variance between the person's feet is more than a half-size. If the variance is less than one half-size, fit the larger foot.
4. Some female athletes find that men's shoes fit better than women's both for training and for competition. However, the shoe must fit properly. Some women's feet do not fit men's shoes, and some stores do not carry men's shoes in sizes small enough to fit women.
5. Be prepared to shop at more than one store. Most outlets carry only some of the many shoes on the market. Mail-order shoe outlets may be less expensive, but it is often necessary to return shoes until the correct size is found.
6. Once you find the shoe that fits properly, buy several pairs. Shoes are manufactured based on style, color, and other trends that are used to market them, so shoes frequently come and go. When buying multiple pairs of a shoe, try on each pair, as size may vary slightly.

CONCLUSION

There are hundreds of athletic training shoes on the market, and the practitioner must be able to educate patients about the misinformation propagated by the media and by advertisements for these products. This is especially relevant to cost, as most athletes think the best, most protective shoes are more expensive. Contrary to this belief, however, studies show that in comparison to the cheapest shoes, the more expensive running shoes are actually associated with more than twice the injuries (Robbins and Waked 1997a).

Clearly, improperly fitting shoes increase an athlete's risk for injury. Even when fit is good, the modern athletic shoe, with medial arch support and a relatively thick, soft sole, can increase the risk of injury. In fact, shock-absorbing and impact-cushioning materials used in popular athletic shoes are not engineered to fit the human foot and account for a 123% greater injury frequency in comparison to plain, less expensive shoes (Robbins and Waked 1997b). Materials that increase the height of the shoe's sole (Robbins et al. 1994), as well as rigid or semi-rigid construction that interferes with normal foot and ankle movement (Robbins and Waked 1998), also increase an athlete's risk of injury.

Carbohydrate Intolerance in Athletes

In this text, the inability of the body to properly metabolize dietary carbohydrates is referred to as carbohydrate intolerance (CI). From its earliest, most subtle dysfunctional state, through insulin resistance and hyperinsulinemia, to late stages of disease, CI is best seen as one condition rather than as separate entities, the way it is currently viewed. The term *carbohydrate intolerance* is used because patients can relate to it better than to the many other names. Also, the term incorporates the word *carbohydrate*, a key focus in assessment and therapy, with the excess consumption of dietary carbohydrates, or high-glycemic foods, potentially causing or worsening the problem.

A variety of terms have been used to refer to the various degrees of CI throughout its full spectrum. Reaven (1988) uses the term Syndrome X to describe middle and late stages of CI, which include insulin resistance, hyperinsulinemia, heart disease, hypertension, hyperlipoproteinemia, stroke, breast cancer, polycystic ovary, and diabetes. Although CI occurs in all types of people, it is more prevalent in blacks across all age groups (Svec et al. 1992). Certain types of individuals, possibly for a variety of reasons, (such as genetics, stress, phospholipid makeup), may be more susceptible than others to CI (Daly et al. 1997). Following are some of the terms used to denote CI from its early functional stage to late disease stage:

- Hypoglycemia
- Hyperinsulinemia
- Insulin resistance
- Metabolically obese, normal weight (person)
- Carbohydrate-lipid metabolism disturbance
- Type IV hyperlipoproteinemia
- Non-insulin-dependent diabetes and other Syndrome X conditions

Insulin resistance, a main feature of CI beginning in the first stage, is a metabolic state in which insulin in physiologic concentrations fails to produce a normal response (Simopoulos 1994). Specifically, glucose is not as efficiently carried across the cell membrane into the muscle fiber (and other cells) by insulin because of a fault in the cell's receptors. The exact mechanism of this problem is not completely understood, although Borkman et al. (1993) first showed that the condition is associated with low levels of Group C fats in muscle cell membranes. This leads to a resistance in the action of insulin, which is usually accompanied by an increase in insulin production (Nestler 1994).

Carbohydrate intolerance is relatively common in the population, with exact numbers varying depending on definitions and opinions of its incidence and on when the condition can first be assessed. In some patients, normal glucose tolerance tests are obtained in the presence of excess insulin, indicating insulin resistance (Zimmet et al. 1992). In other cases, normal insulin levels exist in the presence of slightly impaired glucose tolerance (Swinburn et al. 1995). Bassett et al. (1990) demonstrated the existence of a category of patients who are "otherwise normal" but have carbohydrate dysfunction as indicated, sometimes transiently, by a distinct pre-beta band on lipoprotein electrophoresis (these are very low density lipoproteins). These authors considered this a transitional state between normal and abnormal. The existence of a pre-beta lipoprotein may also be considered diagnostic of type IV hyperlipoproteinemia (Berkow 1992). These are the early stages of CI.

Patients with CI are at great risk for developing diseases in later years (Hughes et al. 1994). For example, patients with CI have an estimated 10-fold greater risk for developing NIDDM. Some of these patients who become diabetic have had clearly measurable hyperinsulinemia for up to 20 years before the onset of diabetes (Zimmet et al. 1992). It is difficult to estimate how many dysfunctional but disease-free years there have been before the onset of the early overt manifestations.

The exact relationships and progression of CI with regard to insulin, insulin resistance, glucose dysfunction, and other factors described here can vary with the individual biochemistry of the patient, and there are no clear patterns applicable to all patients with CI. For example, some studies have shown that insulin resistance is accompanied by low levels of dehydroepiandrosterone sulfate [DHEA(S)] (Block, Clemons, and Sperling 1987), while others found an association with high DHEA(S) (Lindgren et al. 1990). It is vital that the practitioner avoid following the predetermined approaches that are sometimes available for assessment, therapy, or work with lifestyle factors.

Complementary sports medicine practitioners frequently see patients who are carbohydrate intolerant. Many people in their "middle ages" who decide to begin an exercise program may seek professional guidance. Some people begin this process on their own and become injured. Some patients require rehabilitation (i.e., cardiac or other rehabilitation) and seek advice from a holistic professional.

Parents who are insulin resistant or have Syndrome X conditions (especially heart disease, hypertension, hyperlipidemia, or diabetes) may seek early care for their active adolescent children (or those who require an exercise program) from a holistic practitioner to complement their regular checkups.

Athletes who are older and becoming more carbohydrate intolerant are looking for answers to the onset of related signs and symptoms. Treatment of the patient with CI in its earliest stages can help prevent the secondary structural, chemical, and mental/emotional problems, improve performance, prevent disease in later years, and significantly improve the quality of life. High insulin levels may be associated with overtraining. Moderate-intensity training usually suppresses insulin production during exercise, whereas maximal training intensities may increase the insulin response (Urhausen et al. 1997).

Laboratory assessment procedures to determine the presence of CI may reveal normal ranges in the earliest stage and demonstrate abnormalities only in the middle and especially the later stage. At the earliest onset, with the lack of laboratory information the practitioner must rely on other signs and symptoms described in this chapter. Traditionally, the insulin-glucose clamp and the intravenous glucose tolerance test are commonly used, but these require a hospital or similar setting and are not practical for most clinicians. The best and most practical clinical laboratory test is the fasting ratio of serum insulin to glucose. This test may begin to show abnormalities in the middle stage of CI. Low thyroid hormone is also associated with CI (Muller and Seitz 1984). (Note that the symptoms of CI, like others described in this text, may also be attributable to other factors.)

Three stages of CI are described here: an early functional stage, the transitional stage from functional CI to a subclinical condition with the onset of reversible disease conditions, and the more classical disease state. The latter is recognized in mainstream medicine and is predominantly irreversible, although treatment can improve some factors and slow the progress of others. Conservative care in the first two stages is usually the only necessary treatment, but if the problem is untreated and progresses to the third stage, medical intervention complemented by conservative care is most appropriate.

STAGE 1 CARBOHYDRATE INTOLERANCE

Stage 1, the earliest functional condition of CI, has very subtle signs and symptoms. It may be observed in young patients, sometimes in adolescents, but its onset may not manifest until later in life. Only a careful history and dialogue, with the patient's collaboration, will make assessment possible during this stage.

The patient's birth weight may predict CI (Phillips and Barker 1997). Elevated sympathetic nervous system activity in utero is one mechanism linking low birth weight to insulin resistance later in life. Studies on this topic showed that adults with birth weights of 2.5 kg (5.5 lb) or less were at higher risk for CI than those who weighed 3.3 kg (7.5 lb) or more, independent of current body mass index and waist-to-hip ratio, and also independent of potential confounding variables including smoking, alcohol consumption, and social class. Van Reempts et al. (1997) demonstrated that infants who had experienced chronic intrauterine stress (i.e., maternal stress) exhibited higher sympathetic tone and decreased ability to counter stressful situations after birth. This may also result in more vulnerability to CI.

Family history of NIDDM also predisposes a person to CI. For example, first-degree relatives of NIDDM patients have an approximately 40% lifetime risk of developing insulin resistance and diabetes (Perseghin et al. 1997). However, most of these patients begin to show CI as adolescents (Lindgren et al. 1990). Unfortunately, some patients (and their parents) may not be sure of a history of insulin resistance. A history of any Syndrome X condition (heart disease, stroke, hypertension, hyperlipidemia, breast cancer, etc.) might also be a significant factor that predisposes one to CI.

The signs and symptoms of Stage 1 CI can be very elusive, especially in their earliest forms; some patients have only one or two complaints, although some have many more. Among these are so-called blood sugar-handling stress, which may cause increased hunger between meals; feelings of faintness, weakness, or shakiness if meals are delayed or skipped; increased cravings for sweets (and sometimes caffeine); and other symptoms noted on the symptom survey type of form. Many of these symptoms may be attributable to an increased sympathetic response to a drop in blood sugar (Tepperman and Tepperman 1987).

A very common symptom of CI is postprandial gastrointestinal (GI) "bloating," sleepiness, and inability to concentrate. Changes in mood following meals or consumption of sweets may also be common, especially in children; in adults, the same problem may cause feelings of depression. The early stages of CI are often associated with blood sugar swings, sometimes within the normal limits but with rapid changes. In comparison, the second stage of CI may show abnormal low-glycemic states, and the third stage sometimes high-glycemic states.

Increases in growth hormone (GH) are accompanied by insulin resistance (Lindgren et al. 1990). High levels of GH also occur during puberty. This may be a compounding factor that increases CI in adolescence. Other factors may be high-glycemic food intake (i.e., sweets), emotional stress, and others to be outlined later. Exercise also increases GH, with exercise intensity being directly related to production (Fry and Kraemer 1997). The highest levels of GH are seen following high-intensity resistance training. This may be one association between CI and overtraining.

In the early stages of CI, mental and emotional symptoms are evidenced in some patients by depression due to hypoglycemia, hypodopaminergia, and hyposerotonergia (Holden 1995). Holden states, "The fundamental problem does not lie with the neurotransmitter per se, but rather with uncontrolled fluctuations of brain glycaemic levels acting in conjunction with insulin resistance" (p. 379). (In Stage 3, hyperglycemia is much more common, since by this stage, insulin resistance is significant and the patient is often more clearly diabetic.) In addition, the cumulative stress of so-called life changes is associated with the development of CI and insulin resistance (Ravaja et al. 1996). Temperament, as described by Ravaja and Keltikangas-Jarvinen (1995), in children 6-15 years is also associated with the development of CI; in this study hyperactivity, aggression, and anger were related to the development of CI. Also, high insulin levels have been correlated with attention deficit disorder (ADD), violence, and early alcohol abuse (Virkkunen 1986).

Fatigue is a very common complaint in the early stages of CI. More importantly, patients—especially those in their late 30s and 40s—state that their health and/or fitness has "suddenly" declined from previous years. Patients who are more sensitive and aware of body function will voice this earlier than others. However, this comment is often ignored by many doctors who consider these problems part of the aging process. As described later in this chapter, aging is usually associated with CI, but only due to existing imbalances.

Despite these difficulties in assessment, CI is still a problem to consider in all patients. Measurement of fasting insulin levels may sometimes be a useful assessment tool in this stage (Laakso 1993), and may indicate borderline or above-average levels (although in some CI patients, fasting insulin levels appear normal and only postprandial levels are slightly elevated). In a study of 65 young girls, average age 15 years, Schiavon et al. (1996) reported that "the insulin concentrations in the study patients were remarkably higher than the values reported in the medical literature" (p. 335). According to Bergstrom et al. (1996), "Features typical of the insulin resistance syndrome are already present in adolescents" (p. 908). The adolescents with a high serum insulin had a higher attained height and weight during infancy and childhood. In addition, correlations of insulin levels predictive of hypertension (a common factor in Stage 3) have been shown in children as young as 3 years (Taittonen et al. 1996); insulin levels predictive of hyperlipidemia have also been found in children and adolescents ages 6-24 years (Raitakari et al. 1995).

In this stage, however, many patients with CI are, by mainstream medical standards, "otherwise normal" (Nestler 1994). However, by the standards defined in this text, a patient with CI may have structural, chemical, and mental/emotional dysfunction. Ruderman et al. (1981) first termed these individuals "metabolically-obese" because their weight is normal but their metabolism is similar to that of people who are obese, as seen particularly in larger fat cells and biliary (cholesterol) stones. Those with calcium renal stones or a history of such problems may also be carbohydrate intolerant (Schwille et al. 1997). Early stages may also reveal high calcium in the urine. Other laboratory measurements may be of value in the first stage and often are by the second stage. Typically, the high-density lipoprotein (HDL)-cholesterol fraction is lowered and fasting triglycerides are higher (Katzel et al. 1994). Fasting triglyceride levels above 150 mg/dl may be among the first laboratory signs of CI. Serum uric acid levels are also elevated in patients with CI (Facchini et al. 1991), and these patients may have a history of gout.

Carbohydrate intolerance is sometimes associated with sleep deprivation and may explain the reduced time to exhaustion in athletes with sleeping difficulty (VanHelder and Radomski 1989). This is especially a concern for competitors involved in international travel across time zones during the competitive season.

Unfortunately, as glucose uptake is diminished with higher insulin levels and insulin resistance, adipose tissue uptake is increased (Rohner-Jeanrenaud 1995). As a result, some patients with CI may complain of increased body fat, especially in the abdomen. Measurement of the waist-to-hip ratio (described in chapter 8) may reveal a borderline or high ratio, or, when previous measurements are available, an increasing ratio. The waist-to-hip ratio is a measure of body fat distribution and reflects all-cause mortality including that from cardiovascular and noncardiovascular diseases

(Duncan et al. 1995). It specifically correlates with CI (Sparrow et al. 1986). The waist-to-hip ratio is obtained by taking two measurements: the circumference of the patient's waist at the umbilicus and the hip circumference (Nestler 1994). A ratio greater than 0.9 in men and 0.8 in women indicates the android body type (sometimes referred to as android obesity—but many of these patients are relatively lean, especially in Stage 1 and often in Stage 2) and is associated with CI. The android body type is larger on top and is sometimes referred to as "apple shaped" in contrast to the gynecoid body type, which has a lower waist-to-hip ratio and is referred to as "pear shaped."

The onset of autonomic nervous system imbalance probably occurs in Stage 1. In general, CI is associated with an increased sympathetic function and decreased parasympathetic tone (Moan et al. 1996; Verwaerde et al. 1997). One study indicated that this may be observed in adolescents (13-18 years) who show increased sympathetic activity associated with increased insulin, subscapular skinfold, and resting heart rate; the authors stated that sympathetic overactivity may be associated with the onset of insulin resistance (Keltikangas-Jarvinen et al. 1996). While insulin itself can increase sympathetic activity, the increased sympathetic stress also antagonizes insulin-mediated glucose uptake in the skeletal muscles (Lembo et al. 1996). The sympathetic increase in the early and mid stages may decline in Stage 3 as discussed later—a pattern similar to that found in overtraining.

In addition, diminished parasympathetic activity during Stages 1 and 2 may contribute to CI. Xie and Lautt (1996) speculate that parasympathetic regulation of a liver-generated factor controls insulin effectiveness in skeletal muscle and that dysfunction of this mechanism may be involved with insulin resistance.

It should also be noted that muscle sympathetic activity at rest is lowest in healthy young individuals and highest in elderly and insulin-resistant subjects (Fagius et al. 1996). However, in response to carbohydrate intake, muscle sympathetic activity is normally significantly increased in healthy individuals but weak in those with insulin resistance.

Carbohydrate intolerance can produce not only altered glucose uptake in the muscle, but also muscle dysfunction, altered energy production, and increased risk of injury. As a result, physical symptoms are also common in Stage 1. General skeletal muscle weakness may precede and predict the development of insulin resistance (Lazarus et al. 1997). This can be measured by handgrip dynamometry. Muscle inhibition related to adrenal and other dysfunction is also evident. As a result, it is often the secondary complaints that bring the patient to seek professional help. For example, knee or low back pain secondary to adrenal stress is common. These imbalances may be very subtle but in Stage 1 are the start of a vicious cycle that may continue and intensify throughout all three stages of CI.

Patients with insulin-induced sympathetic activity also have higher heart rates (Facchini et al. 1996). This may be reflected in training quality and is associated with the functional overtraining stage described in chapter 23. As a result, during Stage 1 the Maximum Aerobic Function (MAF) test often shows a plateau or a considerable decrease in progress. Performance may also plateau, although as with the functional overtraining state, there may be a very temporary and significant elevation in performance ability due to the increased sympathetic activity contributing to increased muscle power. Patients are usually in an early stage of adrenal dysfunction (cortisol output is usually high in response to low blood sugar episodes) and often have aerobic deficiency (sometimes due to excess anaerobic training). Exercise assessment findings may indicate exercise hypertension while resting blood pressure is normal as described in chapter 8.

In some patients, CI can prevent not only the progression of aerobic benefits, but also other advantages normally incurred through exercise. This is most true for the expected improvements in lipid profiles, for example (Hughes et al. 1994). Some patients complain that despite proper exercise, other benefits do not materialize, including improved energy, weight loss, and improved mental/emotional state.

Certain drugs may contribute to CI. Diuretics, beta blockers, sympathomimetics, and corticosteroids are among the more commonly prescribed drugs that

Case History

Harvey had chronic knee pain that disallowed the additional training required to pursue his goal of running a marathon. His shorter-distance performances had also plateaued, but otherwise Harvey had no complaints. Assessment indicated adrenal dysfunction with an associated inhibition of the sartorius muscle, and treatment followed. However, there was little or no response after two sessions. On the third session, Harvey casually mentioned getting sleepy after meals, an observation he had neglected to note on his forms. Also, he recalled a family history of diabetes. He was asked to perform the Two-Week test, and the results were significantly more energy (Harvey stated that he had been unaware his energy was so poor), feeling good after meals, and a sudden and rapid loss of his knee pain 10 days into the test. These results were something of a surprise in a 31-year-old, very lean, relatively healthy patient. Dietary adjustments were made as necessary. Within the next three months, Harvey's MAF test improved dramatically, and a few months later he completed a marathon in about 3 hr.

may increase the risk of CI (Chan et al. 1996). In addition, sex hormones, especially oral contraceptives, can significantly increase insulin resistance (Skouby et al. 1990). It is crucial to obtain all information about prescription (and other) drugs initially and during follow-up visits as appropriate.

In this early stage of CI, practitioners do not have the luxury of research scientists who can measure autonomic response to various stress, insulin resistance via the insulin-glucose clamp, and other complex, expensive, and more invasive assessments. Rather, a good history cannot be overemphasized and must be relied upon to provide the practitioner with this information. In many cases, however, even elaborate laboratory measurements cannot take the place of an effective assessment. Especially important may be the use of the Two-Week test described in chapter 18.

STAGE 2 CARBOHYDRATE INTOLERANCE

In Stage 2 of CI there are clearer functional imbalances, and the condition is more easily assessed. Patients may have more numerous well-defined complaints attributable to blood sugar-handling stress, adrenal dysfunction, aerobic deficiency, autonomic imbalance, and other problems, including the many potential secondary problems associated with these imbalances. As these patients progress through Stage 2, they often develop elevated insulin levels, body fat stores, blood pressure and blood fats (especially triglycerides), and clear insulin resistance.

The insulin resistance in this stage may be associated with extensions of sleeping problems from Stage 1, with sleep apnea (sleep-disordered breathing) being common in these patients (Stoohs et al. 1996). This condition is traditionally assessed through nocturnal monitoring using a sleep apnea recorder.

The chronic excessive sympathetic stimulation of the skeletal muscles in Stage 2 can lead to two problems: it can increase insulin resistance and can produce a greater proportion of fast-twitch fibers, which are insulin resistant (Palatini and Julius 1997). This latter problem can worsen the aerobic deficiency common in the sympathetic phase of overtraining syndrome, and possibly contribute to excess lactate levels.

Abnormal production of sex hormones is associated with CI (Corbould et al. 1998); menstrual irregularities and infertility are sometimes noted in this stage and are more obvious in later stages

Case History

Julia complained of chronic low back pain and excess body fat despite more than 12 hr of training per week. She had previously maintained a diary of MAF test results, which had plateaued at about 8 min/mile. She ate a high-carbohydrate diet and had numerous symptoms of adrenal dysfunction and blood sugar-handling stress. She performed the Two-Week test with significant improvements in symptoms. One week later, her MAF test was almost a full minute faster. Julia continued to improve; she experienced losses in body fat and gains in sport performance. Two months later she became pregnant (she had not previously disclosed that she and her husband had tried unsuccessfully to conceive for several years).

(Hollmann et al. 1997; Schiavon et al. 1996). The so-called polycystic ovary syndrome is strongly associated with CI (Franks et al. 1996). The author has clinically observed, in women who have been unable to conceive, a relatively high rate of pregnancy soon after the Two-Week test process described in chapter 18. Velazquez et al. (1994) also showed that improvement in insulin resistance resulted in improvement in reproductive function. As a result, appropriate cautions should be given to CI patients of child-bearing age who are performing the Two-Week test or otherwise improving their carbohydrate function.

As increased sympathetic activity and CI evolve, resting and training heart rates increase further than in Stage 1. This may be related to the sympathetic overtraining described in chapter 23 and is associated with a diminishing MAF test and usually performance.

Cognitive impairment may be evident in this stage of CI and is highly prevalent among elderly persons, even in patients who are not diabetic (Kalmijn et al. 1995). This condition may sometimes be evident even in patients who are in their 50s and 60s. It is often associated with a history of elevated cortisol.

STAGE 3 CARBOHYDRATE INTOLERANCE

In this stage, a clear disease condition is more common, with regression to hyperinsulinemia, hypertension, hyperlipidemia, and more serious problems associated with Syndrome X, including heart disease and stroke. Overt type 2 diabetes mellitus may occur in this stage as a result of previous maximal insulin secretion that drastically and suddenly declines due to pancreatic beta-cell decompensation (Zimmet et al. 1992).

Sympathetic tone may rapidly decrease in Stage 3, as portrayed in later stages of hypertension (Julius and Nesbitt 1996). A classic sign in patients in Stage 3 is that the thermic effect of food is also greatly diminished along with sympathetic function (de Jonge and Bray 1997). This parallels the patterns seen in the later stages of overtraining in which parasympathetic activity dominates. Diminished thermic effect of food is also associated with hypothyroid states (Iossa et al. 1996) and is linked to significant increases in body fat, or obesity—often a secondary sign of the third stage of CI (Seidell et al. 1992).

Mental and emotional conditions may be more extreme in this stage of CI. Holden (1995) states that “mania and positive schizophrenia represent a continuum of liability associated with hyperglycemia, hyperdopaminergia, and hyperserotonergia” (p. 379). This is in contrast to the type of mental and emotional stress characteristic of the earlier stages. Holden’s contention is that “mental illness, in its many guises, is a general manifestation of a diabetic brain state which has been termed ‘cerebral diabetes’ ” (p. 379). This later stage of CI is often associated with excess blood lactate secondary to aerobic deficiency and anaerobic excess, which were discussed earlier with regard to their

Case History

Theresa was a 78-year-old woman with hypertension, high blood total cholesterol and triglycerides, and very low HDL-cholesterol. She complained about numerous musculoskeletal problems throughout her spine that rendered her unable to function in everyday life (unable to drive, shop, etc.), and her body fat content was very high. Treatment was rendered accordingly, with an emphasis on reductions in carbohydrates and increases in fats and proteins. Theresa was given a walking program of 20 min/day, which was gradually increased to 45 min over the next year. During this time, her body fat was reduced, blood fats returned to normal levels, and blood pressure normalized. Theresa began playing golf (a former passion) and within six months was regularly playing nine holes without a cart (walking).

link to depression, anxiety, phobias, and panic disorders, even in patients with no psychiatric history (see chapter 19).

TREATMENT OF CARBOHYDRATE INTOLERANCE

In one sense, treatment of a patient with CI involves the same process as with any other patient: a proper assessment, with appropriate treatment and lifestyle considerations. Some specific aspects of treatment should be mentioned, however, as they are directly related to CI in all stages.

Diet therapy may be the most significant therapy for CI patients. Dietary considerations should always begin with a computerized assessment of the patient's current diet as described in chapter 18. The three most important elements for diet therapy to address are the carbohydrate content of the diet, food frequency, and the balance of fats.

One of the most important aspects of the treatment plan for patients with CI is finding the ideal ratio of macronutrients, especially the proper level of carbohydrate intake, for each patient. It has long been known that reducing dietary carbohydrates reduces insulin levels in CI patients (Grey and Kipnis 1971), and this approach has been very useful in complementary sports medicine. More recently, Coulston et al. (1993) showed that a high-carbohydrate diet increases insulin production even in relatively healthy men and women. High-carbohydrate, low-fat diets can also worsen CI (Reaven 1997). Walker et al. (1996) reported that a high-carbohydrate, low-fat diet increased the waist-to-hip ratio in CI patients. It is especially important to reduce or eliminate added sugars and sugar-containing foods and drinks as well as other high-glycemic items. (The only exception is for athletes during long workouts or competitions, as tolerated.)

The excess insulin that accompanies CI and high-carbohydrate diets has been implicated in a number of disease states (Reaven 1997). In addition, diets lower in carbohydrate than the traditional "athlete's" diet may improve athletic performance (Muoio et al. 1994; Lambert et al. 1994; Griffiths et al. 1994; Pendergast et al. 1996). These topics were discussed in chapter 18 with emphasis on the Two-Week test and glycemic index. It should be emphasized again that there are no special diets or formulas that can be applied to every CI patient—that instead one must find each person's optimal balance of macronutrients.

The other primary dietary recommendation for patients with CI concerns food frequency, which may be as important as what foods are eaten. For example, the high-insulin peak after a meal can be moderated by eating a number of smaller meals rather than the traditional three (or less) consumed during the day (Jenkins 1997). One can achieve a greater than 50% decrease in postprandial insulin production by spreading meals of equal kilocalories over the day, that is, by having six smaller meals rather than two or three large ones. This regime stabilizes postprandial blood glucose and fatty acid levels and improves the economy of glucose clearance. Total cholesterol reduction and increased HDL-cholesterol also result from increased meal frequency (McGrath and Gibney 1994).

It is important, however, that increasing the number of meals not translate into increased total kilocalorie intake. This means that the "main" meals must be smaller (unless the patient's kilocalorie intake is already too low) than the in-between meals (sometimes referred to as snacks). In some patients, six small "meals" daily can significantly improve CI (Bertelsen et al. 1993). Eating a larger number of smaller meals may also have a positive effect on body-weight status (Drummond et al. 1996). It is important for the practitioner to work closely with patients to help determine the meal strategies that best match their particular needs. In some patients, a whole-food, low-glycemic "energy" bar (see chapter 20) is a suitable small meal and helps make this process more practical, especially with products containing adequate fiber.

It is preferable to refer to the smaller meals consumed between the three traditional ones as "meals" rather than "snacks," as many patients equate snacks with unhealthy foods. The meals referred to here include smaller versions of a larger main meal, or some healthy combination of real-food carbohydrates, proteins, fats, and fiber appropriate for the patient.

Adequate levels of dietary fiber are essential for patients with CI and can reduce insulin resistance (Stoll 1997). This effect appears to be the result of a reduced rate of glucose absorption that is achieved by spreading the nutrient absorption over time. If the patient's current level of fiber intake is not satisfactory, appropriate dietary recommendations are in order, as discussed in chapter 18.

The balance of dietary fats is the third priority for patients with CI. Dietary fats and related supplements were discussed in detail in chapters 18 and 19, respectively. Most important regarding CI and dietary fat balance are the following points:

- Increased Group A fats (omega-6 fatty acids) can worsen CI (Storlien et al. 1997).
- Increased Group B fats (saturated) can worsen CI (Parker et al. 1993).
- Palm oils and lard in the diet are associated with higher insulin levels and can worsen CI (palm oils can produce fasting hyperinsulinemia) (Ikemoto et al. 1996).
- Increased Group C fats (omega-3) can improve CI (Huang et al. 1997).
- Increased monounsaturated fats can improve CI (Storlien et al. 1997).

Pan et al. (1995) showed that delta-5-desaturase is associated with insulin resistance. Recall that this enzyme is primarily involved in conversion of dihomo-gamma-linolenic acid (from Group A fats) to arachidonic acid (a Group B fat). Chapters 18 and 19 outlined the benefits of sesame seed oil in inhibiting delta-5-desaturase activity without interfering with the production of eicosapentaenoic acid from Group C fats.

Consequently, CI patients must reduce common food oils (corn, safflower, peanut, etc.) and avoid all palm oils. Reduction in dietary saturated fats is necessary when levels of Group B fats are too high. Increases in linseed and fish oils and extra virgin olive oil (high in monounsaturated oil) are typical recommendations following assessment of the patient's diet. Avoidance of a low-fat diet is important in CI patients (Berkow 1992), as discussed in chapter 18.

Other nutritional factors that may improve CI include the following:

- Antioxidants: CI is associated with enhanced lipid peroxidation secondary to greater free radical formation, and results in so-called premature aging (Preuss 1997). Antioxidants (including alpha-lipoic acid) may also help prevent neurological dysfunction in people with diabetes and improve autonomic imbalance (Ziegler and Gries 1997).

- Chromium and vanadium: The minerals chromium and vanadium may improve insulin sensitivity (Preuss 1997). While chromium requirements may be higher during exercise, loss of chromium through the urine is also greater (Rubin et al. 1998).
- Magnesium: Low levels of magnesium are associated with CI (Rosolova et al. 1997).
- Zinc: A deficiency in zinc is associated with CI and may be improved with zinc supplementation (Song et al. 1998).
- Biotin: Increased biotin intake can improve glucose dysfunction associated with CI (Zhang et al. 1996). Raw egg whites, sometimes consumed by athletes, contain the glycoprotein avidin, which can bind biotin in the GI tract and prevent its absorption (Mei et al. 1994).
- Choline: Insulin resistance may be reversed by choline (Xie and Lautt 1996).

Ensuring that the diet contains adequate amounts of the nutrients listed is the first step in balancing the nutritional needs of the CI patient. If this is not possible with diet, or if patients require more of these nutrients, supplementation may be necessary.

Finally, alcohol may have an adverse effect on CI. Duncan et al. (1995) demonstrated that wine drinkers had lower waist-to-hip ratios than people who did not drink wine and consumed mostly beer. Alcohol was discussed in some detail in chapter 18.

TRAINING

As described here and in other chapters, improving aerobic function is vital for good health and fitness; this is especially true for the patient with CI. There is increasing evidence that CI is associated with diminished aerobic muscle fibers and increases in anaerobic fibers (Kriketos et al. 1996; Storlien et al. 1996). These conditions are related to the aerobic deficiency and anaerobic excess described in chapter 12. Patients with CI must develop as much aerobic function as possible to increase the percentage of aerobic muscle fibers. A cautious approach should be taken if anaerobic training is added to the schedule.

The traditional view that aging itself increases CI and insulin resistance is not universally accepted because of the exercise factor. Davy et al. (1996) showed that age-related increases in total body fat accompany decreases in lean tissue mass (muscle) and that these increases may be a result of the reduced physical activity typical of aging rather than the inevitable consequence of the aging process. Cononie et al. (1994) reported that older patients (60-80 years) with CI began to show positive effects on their carbohydrate metabolism after only seven days of exercise. When exercise training has been part of a regular healthy lifestyle, there appears to be little or no change in insulin action with age (Broughton and Taylor 1991). Specifically, masters athletes in their 60s who have maintained regular training do not manifest CI, and they have lower waist-to-hip ratios compared to age- and body fat-matched controls (Pratley et al. 1995). However, Rogers et al. (1990) showed that these types of athletes had a deterioration in glucose tolerance after only 10 days of inactivity, and in some cases the impairment was significant.

Carbohydrate intolerance is often associated with adrenal and aerobic dysfunction and may even be related to overtraining; all these links have been discussed in previous chapters. Thus each patient is assessed and treated accordingly. Carbohydrate intolerance itself, however, is often a primary problem, with numerous secondary signs and symptoms that possibly include adrenal and aerobic dysfunction. These imbalances may, for example, cause further dysfunction such as knee pain, which typically brings the patient to seek professional care. Table 25.1 lists the common factors associated with the three stages of CI.

TYPE 1 DIABETES

A less common form of diabetes mellitus is type 1, formerly called insulin-dependent, juvenile-onset, or Type I diabetes ("Report of the Expert Committee on the Diagnosis and Classification of Diabetes Mellitus" 1997). Approximately 10% of those classified as diabetic have type 1 diabetes (Granner 1993). Like the non-insulin-dependent type 2 diabetes, this condition is a disorder of carbohydrate metabolism.

Table 25.1 Some Common Factors Associated With Different Stages of Carbohydrate Intolerance

	Stage 1	Stage 2	Stage 3
Signs	Very subtle; blood sugar-handling stress; postprandial GI "bloating," sleepiness, or ↓concentration; fatigue; sleep irregularities; temperament problems in adolescence; ADD; hormonal imbalance (esp. menstrual); "sudden decline in health or fitness"	Extension of Stage 1 but more obvious and more advanced; polycystic ovary; infertility; cognitive impairment (middle aged and elderly); ↑mental/emotional stress	Onset of more clearly defined disease: i.e. Syndrome X; mental and emotional "illness"
Assessment	History (↓birth weight, ↑stress, family, renal or biliary stones, ↑uric acid/gout); possibly fasting insulin/glucose, ↓HDL, ↑triglycerides; ↑body fat/waist-to-hip ratio; general muscle weakness; muscle inhibition; early adrenal and thyroid dysfunction	Extension of Stage 1; insulin/glucose and blood fats frequently abnormal; blood pressure borderline or mild hypertension	Traditional medical tests to diagnose disease states
Training	Functional overtraining; MAF progress slowed or plateaued; ↑resting/training heart rate; onset of aerobic deficiency	Sympathetic overtraining problems; MAF regressing; ↑resting/training heart rate; aerobic deficiency	Parasympathetic overtraining; ↓ or no exercise; aerobic deficiency and anaerobic excess
Autonomics	↑Sympathetic/↓parasympathetic	↑Sympathetic/↓parasympathetic	↓Sympathetic/↑parasympathetic
Treatment	Conservative care	Usually conservative care only	Traditional medical care complemented by conservative care

Unlike NIDDM, type 1 diabetes usually has an onset under the age of 30 years, is not associated with significant overweight or obesity, and is accompanied by hyperglycemia—often with ketoacidosis, the increase of ketones that acidifies the blood (Berkow 1992). It is an autoimmune disorder in which 80% or more of the insulin-secreting beta cells of the pancreas are destroyed (Jimenez 1997). Common signs and symptoms may include fatigue, excessive hunger, extreme thirst, frequent urination, weight loss, and visual changes.

The care of athletes with type 1 diabetes is usually complementary in nature. A specialist plays a major role in the patient's care especially as it relates to the requirements for insulin. Thus an in-depth review on type 1 diabetes is beyond the scope of this text. Those interested in additional information should consult the references cited here and other texts that specifically address this issue (including Campaigne and Lampman 1994). It should be noted, however, that the complementary sports medicine practitioner may have more contact with the type 1 diabetic athlete than the specialist does, as the assessment and treatment applications described in this text are applicable to them.

The numerous benefits of exercise for patients with type 1 diabetes include an increase in insulin sensitivity and a reduction of blood glucose levels (Fahey et al. 1996). In addition, those patients who exercise regularly may develop fewer and less severe diabetes-related complications (Moy et al. 1993). However, common potential complications in these athletes include exercise-induced hypoglycemia, or hyperglycemia and postexercise hypoglycemia due to increased insulin sensitivity (Fahey et al. 1996). Anaerobic activities may be most stressful in this regard. Signs and symptoms of hypoglycemia include rapid heart rate, sweating, shakiness, headache, dizziness, and tingling in the face, tongue, and lips.

To prevent exercise-induced hypoglycemia, patients must be reminded of the need to always use a heart rate monitor in conjunction with the 180-formula in order to remain aerobic. A number of other factors are important during exercise. Guidelines for the athlete with type 1 diabetes include the following (Jimenez 1997):

- Avoid exercise during the peak of insulin action.
- Adjust carbohydrate intake as necessary before exercise.
- Adjust insulin dose before exercise (less may be required).
- Assess blood sugar before and after exercise (and during, if possible).
- Have access to 10-15 g of fast-acting carbohydrate (e.g., 120 ml [4 oz] of fruit juice) during exercise in the event of hypoglycemia.
- Wear medical identification.

In the event hyperglycemia occurs, it is usually associated with blurry vision, sleepiness, increased thirst and urination, and headache.

Diabetics may have altered posture and gait because of sensory deficits in the feet (Simmons et al. 1997). Some athletes, especially beginners, must take care to avoid activities that may increase the risk of injury resulting from an altered gait in actions, such as walking or running—especially on a treadmill, ski machine, stair-stepper, or similar apparatus. The area most frequently injured in diabetic athletes is the foot; the most common injury is fracture of the fifth metatarsal (Wolf 1998). In these cases, use of the stationary bike, swimming, or another non-weight-bearing activity may be more appropriate.

Dietary choices for the person with type 1 diabetes, as for any other athlete, are highly individual. It is recommended that the complementary sports medicine practitioner consult with both the medical specialist and the patient to arrive at an optimal approach.

CONCLUSION

A clinical model of CI as one condition, beginning with its earliest imbalances through the late disease stage, is useful. This description is presented not as an academic exercise but as a way of assisting practitioners in their assessment and treatment of CI in its earliest stage. As Nestler (1994) states, "In the near future, the standard of care may be to screen patients for the presence of subtle or sub-clinical insulin resistance" (p. 61). This process is currently employed in complementary sports medicine. More importantly, it should be recognized that CI is not uncommon in athletes who are regularly training and who may not show classic signs and symptoms of insulin resistance or hyperinsulinemia, but are structurally, chemically, and mentally/emotionally imbalanced as a result of dysfunction of carbohydrate metabolism.

26

Weight and Fat Control

In complementary sports medicine, patients with body fat imbalance—those referred to as overweight or overfat, or those classified as obese—are approached using the same assessment, treatment, and lifestyle methods as with any other patient; any dysfunction in their structural, chemical, and mental/emotional state is improved and normal function restored. When this is accomplished, body fat is usually reduced. This method is far superior to the traditional "weight-loss" programs used by great numbers of people. In most cases of imbalance, excess stored body fat is the problem; fewer patients present with too little body fat.

Patients usually consider excess body "weight" and body "fat" as synonymous. The issue, however, is body fat, as the patient's weight is influenced more by the body's water content than by fat. In addition, the obsession with "less is best" regarding body fat is seen in many athletes, including noncompetitors. While athletic performance is influenced by and dependent on the proportion and total amount of fat-free mass and fat mass, imbalances caused by forced reduction of body fat can produce serious problems.

EXCESS FAT

Clearly, above-normal levels of body fat are harmful to health, especially in later adult life (Wannamethee and Shaper 1990). Unfortunately, over a quarter of the adult population in the United States is overfat, and the number is increasing. Body fat levels above 25% in men and 35% in women may be considered obesity, although other estimates are used (McArdle et al. 1991). Childhood obesity has also increased 20% during the last decade and is now prevalent in about 25% of children in the United States (Bar-Or et al. 1998). Because of individual variations (i.e., physical and chemical body makeup), no "normal" body fat levels should be established; the concept of a "desirable" level is preferable. These optimal levels of body fat are approximately 15% for men and 25% for women (McArdle et al. 1991).

Complementary sports medicine practitioners are as capable as any other professional of treating most patients with imbalances causing excess fat, if not more so. In many ways, these patients are metabolically similar to athletes with aerobic deficiency, macro- and micronutrient imbalance, carbohydrate intolerance, and adrenal dysfunction. Therefore the recommendations for a patient whose goal is to lose fat are no different than for anyone else; the patient is treated and not the condition. A proper and extensive assessment is made and is followed by the appropriate treatment, along with the necessary lifestyle recommendations regarding eating and exercise.

It is important to avoid using the word "diet" with patients who may have been following many weight-loss diets that resulted in failure. True success in body fat balance occurs when one reduces stored fat to healthier levels without lowering lean body mass or inducing dehydration, and when this balance is maintained year after year. The majority of weight-loss programs may succeed in reducing the number of kilograms or pounds, but this does not always reflect a relative body fat loss. More importantly, the lost weight often returns, frequently with additional body fat gains. This is an example of the unhealthy aspects of "dieting."

It is also important for the practitioner to view the patient as a person with imbalances and not as a "weight-control patient" or an "overweight or obese patient." It is even more important to encourage patients to view themselves the same way. Moreover, it is best to refer to these patients as athletes. These seemingly minor details may provide great mental and emotional benefits to the patient. The patient should also gain an understanding of the body's metabolic function; this can be accomplished after the initial assessment. Incorrect ideas about kilocalories and dietary fat, and other common misconceptions promoted by the "diet" industry, may have unhealthy consequences.

Although women have lower sedentary metabolic rates than men (Ferraro et al. 1992), the approach to patient care should not be gender oriented. Metabolic rate is determined mostly by body fat content in all ages and both sexes (Molnar and Schutz 1997). In addition, the traditional idea that weight control is easily accomplished by reducing kilocalories is oversimplified, as metabolic state—that is, how these kilocalories are utilized, carbohydrate tolerance, nutritional status, and other issues—is highly significant. More importantly, large amounts of weight loss, as seen in many fast weight-loss diets, are often short-term, in part because metabolic rate remains low for long periods in these patients (Elliot et al. 1989).

Perhaps the most important mental/emotional factor is getting a commitment from the patient. Will the person make his or her program a lifestyle change and therefore a priority? Unfortunately, many patients are looking for just another diet program to follow in hopes of finding the one that works

Case History

Frank was told by his company doctor to lose 25 lb, but was left to do so on his own. After following several diet programs, with some short-term success, Frank now weighed more than when he had started. His body fat content was measured at 28%, and the forms he completed indicated a variety of other problems including fatigue, borderline hypertension and blood fats, and a family history of diabetes. Frank's first two appointments had to be changed because of his work schedule, and he arrived late for his rescheduled appointment. Much of the conversation during the initial consultation centered around his commitment to the program. This made Frank uncomfortable, and he appeared taken aback by the idea of commitment. He stated that he often could not find time to exercise, usually could not eat lunch because of his business, and ate most meals in restaurants and "on the run." He was asked to think about making this endeavor not just another program but a priority in his life—one that would require him to make time for exercise and meals and to consume healthy foods, and that otherwise it would not be worth pursuing. Frank was told to call for his next appointment after he considered these "requirements." Unfortunately for Frank, he never made another appointment.

for them, and to many the idea of a lifelong healthy lifestyle may be foreign. Without an understanding of the holistic approach including all associated factors, some patients may not be ready for a real commitment. It is important for the practitioner to assess this issue during the initial consultation and not accept patients who are unwilling or unable to make their program a priority.

Without cooperation from the patient, including an honest relationship between patient and professional, both will expend unnecessary time, energy, and money with no truly successful outcome. Moreover, these patients may be taking up places in the schedule that could best be used by a more dedicated patient.

ASSESSMENT OF BODY FAT

It is best to use body fat content as a primary assessment tool, with scale weight as a secondary measurement, if used at all. As described in chapters 8 and 25, the waist-to-hip ratio may be the best single measurement reflecting metabolic function, especially with reference to carbohydrate intolerance (CI), a common cause of increased stored fat. It is important to emphasize to the patient that measurements of body fat should not be taken daily or even weekly, since fat loss takes place over a longer period of time. Frequent measurements may produce or maintain preoccupation, as is often the case with patients who are on a diet and weigh themselves once or twice a day.

The devices and formulas ordinarily used to measure body fat are very general and are neither precise nor comparable to one another. For example, a study of bioelectrical impedance using 12 common formulas showed that the formulas that performed well in one group gave poor results in another, and vice versa (Pichard et al. 1997). Skinfold thickness, measured by calipers and using various formulas, may also produce varying fat content results. For example, two identical skinfold thicknesses may have significantly different concentrations of fat cells, and these external measurements of subcutaneous fat do not take into account internal adipose tissue content (Clarys et al. 1987). In comparing methods using calipers to underwater weighing for body density, Stout et al. (1995) found an error of 4.9% body fat—too large for accurate estimates. Even the use of more complex assessments, such as dual-energy X-ray absorptiometry, does not yield precise measurements of body fat (Kohrt 1998). Although computerized analysis of magnetic resonance images is more accurate, this also results in some variability (Elbers et al. 1997); in any case, these tests are much less practical.

In all, most methods underestimate body fat content (Fogelholm et al. 1997). The use of any device to obtain body fat content should be considered only a general measure, and the patient must understand that small changes are not relevant and may be due to error. In an office setting, a slight improvement in accuracy may be obtained if the same device is used in all evaluations, and by the same person (i.e., staff member, practitioner, etc.).

The respiratory quotient (RQ), however, is very accurate for assessing the patient's metabolic changes throughout the treatment program (Valtuena et al. 1997). Although this test does not relate to body fat content, as described in chapter 8, it determines the percentage of energy derived from fat and glucose. As metabolism improves, RQ generally diminishes. Patients with a lower RQ utilize more fat, which may protect against increased fat storage (Seidell et al. 1992). Likewise, the oxidation of fats for energy is lower in those with high body fat (Ranneries et al. 1998). This is reflected in a higher RQ not only in overfat patients, but also in those at higher risk of future substantial body fat gains—making high RQ a predictor of future fat gains (Seidell et al. 1992). It should be noted, however, that some obese patients have low RQs, which may be a compensation to prevent further fat gain (Ravussin and Swinburn 1993). As such, RQ should be only one of many assessment tools.

COMPETITIVE ATHLETES AND WEIGHT LOSS

Restricting kilocalories as a means of losing body weight can result in diminished athletic performance (Rankin et al. 1996). Athletes who restrict energy intake to promote weight loss can also decrease bone density (Talbott et al. 1998). The problem in some sports, especially in wrestling and ballet, is the increased mental/emotional pressure to attain low body weights. As a consequence of this pressure, these athletes, at all ages, implement many unhealthy habits, including food restriction, dehydration (fluid restriction), bulimic behaviors, and others. The Wisconsin minimum weight program as described by Oppliger et al. (1998) restricts weight loss in wrestlers by incorporating a minimal weight limit (determined from percent body fat) with a nutrition education program. This type of program may serve as a healthy guide for those in sport.

Clearly, in comparison to inactive people, many athletes are more preoccupied with thoughts of eating and body weight, feel they have more difficulty controlling their body weight, abuse laxatives more often for weight control, and more often report disordered eating. In a recent study, Abraham (1996) found that two-thirds of ballet dancers were using at least one method of weight control.

A variety of over-the-counter weight-loss products are used by athletes, laxatives and diuretics being the most common. In a study by Martin et al. (1998), an average of 29% of female athletes from several sports reported using weight-reducing products; percentages in some sports, including volleyball (71%), were very high. While most of these products do not reduce body fat, they can cause dehydration and potassium deficiency.

DIET AND NUTRITION

Dietary assessment should be made initially, to provide a view of the patient's style of eating along with his or her levels of nutrients. It is especially important to note meal frequency, water intake, and a possible major focus on low-fat food items. One also notes any healthy items the patient prefers to eat, in addition to those the person does not enjoy. It is important to emphasize the healthy foods that appeal to the patient and to avoid recommending those that do not. For example, if the patient likes avocados but avoids them thinking they are "fattening," avocados may be an excellent addition to a healthy eating plan; discussion of such choices offers an opportunity to explain the benefits of dietary fat. Or, if the patient does not like tofu, the practitioner should not recommend it as a protein option. A healthy eating plan can usually be structured for any patient around that individual's likes and dislikes. Often, patients need encouragement to try foods and combinations they have never tasted, such as spaghetti squash, Brussels sprouts, vegetables with breakfast, and fresh ginger in salad dressing.

Among the most common problems associated with increased body fat is CI. Patients eating a high-carbohydrate, low-fat diet usually utilize less fat for energy and rely more on glucose (i.e., have a high RQ). This correlates with studies by McNeill et al. (1988) and Aitken and Thompson (1989), who found that increased dietary carbohydrates raise RQ whereas a lower-carbohydrate, higher-fat diet lowers RQ, indicating more use of fats for energy. In addition, high-carbohydrate, low-fat diets may worsen CI (Reaven 1997). This may be a consequence of the insulin-lowering benefits of lower-carbohydrate diets compared to other weight-loss diets (Golay et al. 1996). Despite these and other clear indications that argue against low-fat, high-carbohydrate diets, these regimes are still used for weight control by many professionals (Carmichael et al. 1998). Unfortunately, the low-fat philosophy leads many patients to consume larger amounts of prepared low-fat foods, which are often made from high amounts of sugars, elevating glycemic index (Rolls and Miller 1997). This practice can further worsen CI.

It may therefore be important for many patients to begin the process of reducing body fat with a Two-Week test or other method of finding the optimal level of carbohydrate intake. In addition, controlling the postprandial insulin peak and potential extreme glucose fluctuations is very important for two reasons. This strategy will help control any regression in CI and prevent additional storage of fat (from dietary carbohydrate), and it can control hunger, cravings, and binge eating. Recall from chapter 25 that food frequency is an important element in the dietary habits of patients with CI. Spreading out the full day's food intake into many smaller meals rather than one, two, or three large ones can help produce a significantly flatter postprandial curve and control insulin and glucose peaks. Eating many smaller meals can also have a positive effect on body-weight control (Drummond et al. 1996). Many diet programs restrict meals and substitute high-carbohydrate drinks or other snacks, which are often a major metabolic stress for CI patients. It is important to emphasize that patients need to eat real food and real-food products throughout the day rather than rely on convenience items that are usually unhealthy, especially in relation to the content of fats (i.e., excess Group A and B fats, trans fats), often contributing to CI.

Other nutritional factors are often neglected in the pursuit of weight and fat loss. As discussed in chapter 18, fiber improves carbohydrate metabolism by decreasing the glycemic index of a meal. A general guide for the amount of fiber intake is at least 11.5 g for each 1000 kcal of food. Water is another important item, especially if protein intake is increased—which is often the case when total carbohydrate is lowered. Another concern is total nutrient intake. In their desire to restrict food, many people also restrict nutrient intake. This makes the initial and follow-up computerized dietary assessments very important. Patients must be made aware of the importance of the many nutrients necessary for balanced metabolism of carbohydrates, proteins, and fats as discussed in previous chapters.

It should also be noted that the pungent principle of hot red peppers, capsaicin, may have a positive effect in those patients with excess body fat, since it increases energy expenditure (Doucet and Tremblay 1997). This may be associated with increased sympathetic function, which is diminished in some patients with excess body fat.

TRAINING

Complementary sports medicine practitioners often have patients who are noncompetitive athletes. Many are individuals who must lose body weight and fat to get healthy and fit. The approach in these individuals regarding training needs is no different than for other patients.

For the majority of patients with excess body fat, the primary training focus is developing a good aerobic system, as many have excess anaerobic function and aerobic deficiency. Kriketos et al. (1996) found that individuals with high body fat had increased proportions of anaerobic and decreased aerobic muscle fibers. The process of developing aerobic function should include regularly performing the Maximum Aerobic Function (MAF) test, which will help measure progress and warn of impending plateau or regression of aerobic function. It is important to note that improvements in the MAF test usually precede body fat loss. The same factors are applied to these patients regarding the use of the MAF test as for any other athlete.

Case History

Michele's weight and body fat had increased over the previous three years. Numerous diet programs did not work, but aerobic dance may have helped prevent further gains. Michele's recurring neck pain was becoming more constant, perhaps exacerbated by job stress, and fatigue was more of a regular problem. All blood and urine tests were normal. Michele's diet analysis revealed a significant imbalance between Group A and C fats, and a diet that was approximately 70% carbohydrate, 15% protein, and 15% fat. Her heart rate during aerobic dance class often reached 160—much higher than the aerobic maximum rate of 135 as determined by the 180-formula. Initial treatment consisted of balancing the dietary macronutrients by eliminating all high-glycemic carbohydrates and restricting Group A fats, adding supplements of linseed oil and vitamin B6 (Linum B6; Standard Process, Inc.) and magnesium (Magnesium Lactate; Standard Process, Inc.), and using a heart monitor to ensure that a 135 heart rate was not exceeded during exercise. On Michele's second session one month later, her scale weight had decreased by about 4 kg (9 lb), her energy was 80% improved, and her neck pain was 50% improved; there were then additional improvements each month. After about a year, Michele's body fat had decreased by more than 10%, and all other problems were nearly 100% improved. A dietary reevaluation revealed that the ratio of macronutrients that made Michele feel the best and also reduced body fat was approximately one-third each of carbohydrate, protein, and fat.

Case History

Jan was, by her estimation, about 20 lb overweight, and her body fat content of approximately 30% had been increasing each year. It was clear from the first consultation that the scale was an obsession, as Jan weighed herself three to four times per day. If her weight increased slightly (even by 1 lb), she would drink more coffee and reduce her food intake. But whatever her approach, scale weight and body fat continued to increase each year. She agreed to stop using the scale and to measure her waist-to-hip ratio on the first day of each month only. Jan resigned herself to finding an appropriate lifestyle that would improve not just her body weight and fat, but her health and fitness too. Over the next 10 months, Jan lost almost 3 in. from her waist and 1 in. from her hips. In addition to the obvious loss of body fat, her waist-to-hip ratio diminished. After many of her friends commented positively about her weight loss and asked how much weight she had lost, Jan finally stepped on the scale; she had "only lost 7 pounds" and was distressed. It took some time to explain again the relationship between the body fat content, reflected in the waist-to-hip ratio, and body weight made up mostly of water and muscle. Reducing body fat with diet and exercise—and increasing lean body mass with exercise—could easily produce this outcome.

Some patients who use exercise exclusively as a way of reducing body fat and improving energy and aerobic function may be unsuccessful. Lamarche et al. (1992) reported that of 31 obese women, 20 lost substantial body fat, but 11 actually gained body fat, after six months of only aerobic training (they all showed similar improvements in $\dot{V}O_2$max). Unless the whole person is considered, including needs such as diet and nutrition, success may not be optimal.

Overtraining is often seen in patients with too little body fat; excess exercise is common in both competitive and noncompetitive athletes who are focused on reducing body fat. Because of the high stress levels of patients with too little body fat, as for those with excess fat, adrenal dysfunction is common.

Fortunately, for the majority of patients, high body fat is reduced through balancing of structural, chemical, and mental/emotional aspects. There are no special requirements regarding diet, nutrition, or exercise other than addressing the individual's needs. Rather, applying some of the basic assessment, treatment, and lifestyle methods described in this text is often highly effective.

It is important to continually assure patients that even though they are eating what seem to them excess amounts of food, especially dietary fat, the strategy will not have negative effects.

CONCLUSION

The scenarios presented in this chapter serve only as examples of the types of problems observed in patients with excess body fat. Although these situations are very common, any type of structural, chemical, or mental/emotional imbalance can adversely affect the body's metabolism, impacting fat content, as can genetics. Rarely is there only one problem; this is almost always a multifactorial issue.

27

The Athlete's Triad of Dysfunction

The most common primary problem confronting the complementary sports medicine practitioner is the triad of aerobic deficiency, adrenal dysfunction, and overtraining. These imbalances share many structural, chemical, and mental/emotional signs and symptoms, including their stages of progression as discussed in previous chapters. This chapter looks at these three problems as one primary entity and provides a clinical overview of the approach to patient care.

SECONDARY STRUCTURAL PROBLEMS

In most cases, a thorough history will indicate this triad of dysfunction, with numerous complaints that are caused by a lack of aerobic function, adrenal distress, and training imbalance. The most common secondary structural problems include ankle, knee, hip, and back pain, although any joint dysfunction—spinal, pelvic, or extravertebral—may be troublesome, especially in view of the fact that the aerobic muscle fibers provide the physical support for the joint. In some cases, an acute injury brings an athlete to the practitioner's office for help, and the conclusion is that preexisting but asymptomatic imbalances predisposed the athlete to injury.

In the majority of these cases in which secondary complaints provoked the athlete to seek help, relief can be very rapid, and care directed at the secondary site of injury (e.g., a knee joint) is unnecessary. For example, a patient with chronic knee pain due to adrenal dysfunction may have swelling and localized pain in the knee joint. Traditional remedies may include ice, nonsteroidal anti-inflammatory drugs, and other therapy directed at the symptom, but often without permanent recovery. But if primary problems are improved, a rapid increase in knee function, including a rapid healing, will occur—often with no need for therapy on the knee itself.

Case History

Barry's knee pain was chronic, preventing him from performing his normal training volume and intensity, as well as from competing. The onset of pain had occurred over a period of about six weeks. The lateral knee was slightly swollen and warm; the pain worsened with activity and improved slightly during rest. In the course of the history, it became obvious that Barry was in the middle stages of overtraining; his training heart rates were all above aerobic levels and his resting rate was elevated. He also had numerous adrenal stress symptoms including sleeping difficulties, dizziness upon standing, and fatigue. His body fat content had recently increased. Just before the onset of knee pain, he had had two competitive events that were dramatic improvements over all preceding ones. In the past, numerous therapies directed at the knee had sometimes provided short-term relief. Specifically, a variety of specialists had applied their therapy, including chiropractors (who balanced the spine and pelvis), a podiatrist (who used orthotics), and an orthopedist (who recommended ice, rest, and nonsteroidal anti-inflammatory drugs). Barry's training shoes, including the ones worn when not training, were too small, and he was immediately given advice on buying the proper shoe. Inhibition of the tibialis posterior and sartorius responded to the stimulation of adrenal reflexes (acupuncture and Chapman's). On the basis of dietary analysis, carbohydrates were reduced and fats balanced. Within 3 days, Barry's knee was 90% improved. After 10 days, appropriate heart monitor training was increased significantly without knee pain, which was now 100% improved. Higher volumes were added without reoccurrence of muscular imbalances or pain. After 2.5 months, competition was initiated and then continued without reoccurrence of previous problems.

In addition to structural problems, fatigue may be the chemical symptom most common in the triad of dysfunction, since it is also the most common complaint in each condition separately. Although structural complaints are most typical in the earliest stage, chemical problems may be ultimately more significant than mechanical ones. In addition to fatigue, increases in body fat, hormonal imbalances, and blood sugar-handling stress are often evident. In some cases, athletes are almost unaware of their low mental or physical energy level unless asked about it. This can be measured using the Maximum Aerobic Function (MAF) test and first recognized as an aerobic dysfunction. The low energy level is another manifestation of fatigue. Most important is the understanding that the fatigue and other chemical problems are secondary symptoms.

Mental or emotional symptoms are also typical in the middle and especially the late stages of the triad. Feelings of depression are most common, and anxiety is associated with the athlete's frustration in not understanding the injury or poor performance dilemma.

It is important to recognize that stress is a key factor contributing to the triad of dysfunction. When stress affects the body, the adrenal glands compensate, or attempt to do so. Depending on their success, the patient may recover from the stress or may continue to regress. As previously discussed, Selye's general adaptation syndrome (GAS) parallels these problems, and is often associated with the triad of athletic dysfunction.

Secondary symptoms are often the only ones patients can relate to, and patients may become very focused on these details. Some are much more sensitive about their body and overtly aware of all their signs and symptoms. These patients might be described as obsessive, and although some may indeed be, most are just very aware of their body and

Case History

Jay was a new member of a top motor sport team. However, as he worked his way to higher levels in the sport, the stress associated with his intense desires produced a triad of dysfunction. He lifted weights and ran almost daily, at a very high heart rate, to a point of overtraining. The added travel stress was high, and the resulting adrenal dysfunction was obvious during assessment. Aerobic muscle testing, along with the obvious history of training imbalance, indicated aerobic deficiency and anaerobic excess. Jay favored making whatever changes were necessary to reduce his structural, chemical, and mental/emotional stress and balance his body. However, he was very concerned about the word "stress" and asked that this word not be used in front of other team members and especially the media. Jay felt that the word was not understood, or accepted, and that many in sport considered stress a sign of mental/emotional weakness.

are trying to make sense out of a seemingly complex situation. Practitioners can use this awareness to their own advantage in making an assessment, as all these secondary problems can have meaning and can help one to piece together the primary clinical picture. However, it is important also to educate the patient about the real value of these signs and symptoms and about the fact that most of the primary problems are usually asymptomatic. Otherwise such individuals may continue to be branded as obsessive or complaining patients. When they understand the meaning of various signs and symptoms, they focus less on their secondary problems and direct their attention to the same goals as the practitioner.

Many athletes, however, are more comfortable complaining about their secondary structural problems. In many sport environments, especially for team sports, complaining about structural problems is tolerated and almost accepted as "part of the game." However, chemical or mental/emotional stresses are often considered a sign of weakness and are discussed less frequently, usually in confidence.

Which particular dysfunction in the triad starts this process? It depends on the patient and his or her lifestyle. In many situations, it will be difficult or impossible to know which precise mechanism had developed at the onset of the patient's problems. Here are three case history summaries that portray different scenarios:

- Case History 1: James had an imbalanced training schedule (overtraining) that ultimately resulted in an imbalance of aerobic and anaerobic function (aerobic deficiency). The increased adrenal activity maintained compensation, but ultimately this level of adrenal function could not be continued (adrenal dysfunction).
- Case History 2: Pat's dietary and nutritional habits, combined with job stress, led to adrenal dysfunction. Recommendations to lift weights to reduce stress may have led to aerobic deficiency. The addition of endurance training to existing stress resulted in overtraining.
- Case History 3: Sally embarked on an exercise program for the first time, combining aerobic dance with weights. Unfortunately, the workouts were all anaerobic, and she became aerobically deficient. She became exhausted within a few months (adrenal dysfunction) but, being very disciplined, persisted. Her training equation quickly became imbalanced (overtraining).

It is not necessary that a precise name be attached to the patient's condition. For example, whether Sally developed aerobic deficiency first or whether the problem was actually an overtraining condition is not important. There are many overlapping imbalances within the triad and in most other patient profiles. Most importantly, it is not the condition that is treated, but rather the patient, and it is the structural, chemical, and mental/emotional imbalances that are assessed.

STAGES OF THE TRIAD

It can help practitioners in understanding a patient's various states of imbalances to view the triad of dysfunction as three stages, each blending with the one after and/or before. These are general guidelines and are not intended to define the precise pattern of dysfunction, as the structural, chemical, and mental/emotional aspects of patients can vary considerably.

Over a period of time—typically months to years—some athletes go through various stages of dysfunction that are predictable. During these stages, referred to simply as stages 1, 2, and 3, different types of aerobic, adrenal, and training dysfunction can be observed that follow a logical pattern of decline. While some athletes never enter this state of dysfunction, most at some time find themselves in the first or second stage, and some advance into the third stage. These stages may pertain to any patient—the professional athlete, the amateur who also has a full-time job, the weekend warrior, and even the beginning exerciser. As will be seen, these stages correlate with those of aerobic, adrenal, and training dysfunction.

Triad Stage 1

Stage 1 is the onset of the triad, in which one, two, or all three factors—aerobic, adrenal, and training stress—begin to have adverse effects on the patient. As with any other imbalance, the very early states are most difficult for the practitioner to assess. The treatment of patients in these early stages is fortunately relatively easy once the proper assessment is made. In addition, there is an excellent prognosis; the patient can not only return to normal function, but most often experiences improved function resulting in better performances.

The first stage is often associated with Selye's first stage of GAS, the alarm reaction. The patient's system has been structurally, chemically, and/or mentally stressed. The adrenal glands begin producing more of certain hormones, such as cortisol, at certain times of the day and evening to help adapt to the stresses placed upon them. These stresses may be cumulative: job stress, plus training stress, plus nutritional stress, and so on. If adrenal compensation is not effective, continual stress may result in further increases in cortisol followed by diminished dehydroepiandrosterone sulfate (DHEA[S]). Associated with increased adrenal activity is a heightened sympathetic nervous system.

Assessment of the patient may reveal some functional adrenal problems, notably the lack of increase in systolic blood pressure upon standing. Complaints of structural problems begin to occur in this stage, often due to inhibition of the muscles related to adrenal function: tibialis posterior, sartorius, and gracilis. The areas most vulnerable are the ankle, knee, hip, and low back, with the beginning of an inflammatory process in the joints involved. This pattern of structural stress can continue through all stages, becoming more chronic, with the chemical inflammatory stress amplifying as well.

This period often correlates with an increase in training volume and/or intensity, as the patient has adapted to lower levels of training stress and is capable of more. The patient's performance has often improved just before or during this stage. In some cases, a dramatic but short-lived increase in performance is noted, leading the patient to believe his or her program is working very well. This is probably attributable to the increased sympathetic activity, which can temporarily improve muscle power. However, the MAF test begins to plateau in this stage, and may be the first real sign of aerobic imbalance. This may correlate with a positive aerobic/anaerobic challenge indicating aerobic deficiency. Also associated with this stage in some patients is the first stage of carbohydrate intolerance (CI). If the adrenal response is not sufficient to compensate for the stress, or if training stress or imbalance continues, the patient can enter the next stage.

Triad Stage 2

Stage 2 is a state in which many patients seek help from a health care practitioner. The patient has chronic structural problems (an extension of those in stage 1) associated with more obvious inflammation and compounded by chemical symptoms, notably fatigue, increased body fat, hormonal imbalance, and immune dysfunction; patients get sick more often. Those who are disciplined can usually completely recover from the problems encountered in this stage, but only if they take the time (up to four months or more) to develop the aerobic system with training, along with other necessary changes. Like people treated effectively in stage 1, these patients can not only recover, but also ultimately improve their performances significantly.

The second stage may be associated with the resistance response of GAS. The structural, chemical, and/or mental/emotional stress has increased, but increased adrenal hormone is not sufficient to compensate for all stress, so the adrenal glands enlarge (hypertrophy) to compensate for the ongoing stress. Cortisol is elevated much of the time, along with insulin in some patients, and the increased sympathetic activity is reflected in increased catecholamine levels. This correlates with the second stage of overtraining, the sympathetic type. Parasympathetic activity may be lowered, as are some hormones including DHEA(S) and testosterone. As a result, menstrual irregularities are common. Adrenal indications may worsen: the systolic blood pressure often decreases upon standing, and the structural problems are more chronic and debilitating in this stage.

The patient's performance has often plateaued or diminished during this stage, and although it is difficult to do so, many patients try to maintain high levels of training. They usually show elevated resting and training heart rates. As a result, the MAF test is worse, a clear sign of aerobic deficiency—which correlates with a positive aerobic/anaerobic challenge that demonstrates the same. Some patients are in the first stage or may have advanced to the second stage of CI.

Many patients remain in a chronic state of dysfunction and continue in this stage indefinitely. Others add to these stresses by training harder or longer, reducing their fat intake, increasing carbohydrates, or maintaining other faulty habits and continue to regress and enter the third stage.

Triad Stage 3

Stage 3 is a much more serious condition, one in which complete recovery may not be possible. Some of the patient's chronic structural problems (a continuation of problems from stage 1) may have reached a degenerative state. The chemical problems, including late second-stage and third-stage CI, are more serious. Depression, anxiety, or other emotional problems are common. The prognosis is fair to good, with the necessary longer-term care and patient discipline; but it is not uncommon for these patients to never be as athletic again as before.

The third stage may be associated with the exhaustion stage of GAS. The adrenal glands can no longer compensate for much stress and are in a state of depletion. Levels of cortisol, DHEA(S), testosterone, and the catecholamines are diminished, as is sympathetic activity. There is a relative increased parasympathetic function, which correlates with the third stage of overtraining. The patient often has orthostatic hypotension.

The patient's performance is usually very poor, but more often the person has withdrawn from competition. Training at this stage is usually diminished owing to structural, chemical, or mental/emotional restraints. It is not uncommon to find these patients no longer working out and to hear them referring to themselves as "former athletes." Because of the autonomic shift, they usually have a diminished resting heart rate. The MAF test has regressed to a very poor plateau, and the aerobic/anaerobic challenge demonstrates both an aerobic deficiency and anaerobic excess. Although resting lactate levels may be higher than normal, the lactate response to exercise is diminished. Some patients are in the second stage or may have advanced to the third stage of CI, possibly due to the increase in anaerobic fibers and the decline of aerobic ones. Unfortunately, many patients remain in this chronic state with continual reductions in their quality of life.

Table 27.1 outlines some of the factors associated with the three stages of the triad of athletic dysfunction.

Table 27.1 Some Noteworthy Factors Associated With the Triad of Athletic Dysfunction

	Stage 1	Stage 2	Stage 3
Adrenal	"Alarm" reaction; No ↑ systolic blood pressure on standing; ↑cortisol, ↓DHEA(S). ↑sympathetic; inhibition of tibialis posterior, sartorius, gracilis	"Resistance" response; ↓systolic blood pressure on standing; ↑cortisol, insulin, catecholamines; ↓DHEA(S), testosterone; ↑sympathetic/↓parasympathetic activity; inhibition of tibialis posterior, sartorius, gracilis	"Exhaustion" stage; orthostatic hypotension; ↓Cortisol, testosterone, DHEA(S), catecholamines; ↓sympathetic/↑parasympathetic; inhibition of tibialis posterior, sartorius, gracilis
Aerobic	MAF plateau; possible aerobic deficiency noted	MAF decreased; aerobic deficiency	Aerobic deficiency and anaerobic excess; MAF to very poor level
Training	Functional overtraining ("overreaching"); lactate normal; ↑training volume and/or intensity	Sympathetic overtraining; lactate normal; ↑resting and training heart rate	Parasympathetic overtraining; ↓lactate response; ↓training and ↓resting heart rate
Other symptoms	Stage 1 CI; beginnings of structural problems; dramatic ↑ in performance (temporary)	Chronic structural problems; chemical problems: fatigue, ↑ body fat, hormonal imbalance; Stage 1-2 CI; performance plateau or ↓; menstrual problems	Chronic structural and chemical problems; mental stress; Stage 2-3 CI; performance ↓↓ or none
Prognosis	Complete and immediate	Complete; 2-4 mo minimally	Fair–good with longer-term care

CONCLUSION

When the triad of athletic dysfunction presents itself, it is usually a condition with a variety of secondary structural, chemical, and mental/emotional signs and symptoms; many of these are very subtle, especially in the first stage. Avoiding the potential pitfalls of treating these end-result problems is crucial for a successful clinical outcome. In many cases, athletes who develop these secondary symptoms seek help from practitioners because of these problems rather than for their cause, which often remains less obvious.

28

Physical, Chemical, and Mental/Emotional Injuries: A Retrospect

As a clinician, it is important to consider the scientific relationships involved in human function. More important, however, is the process of obtaining an optimal outcome in a patient presenting with pain, dysfunction, and imbalance. This chapter highlights the 10 most common clinical impairments seen in clinical practice and presents case histories that portray these relationships. Specifically, the most common structural, chemical, and mental/emotional injuries are outlined, and the condition of pain is addressed as a separate entity. Contrary to popular opinion, the presence of pain is not required in order for a patient to be considered injured; many imbalances and types of dysfunction can exist without pain, especially problems in their earliest stages. These problems have been discussed throughout this text in their clinical and scientific context.

The majority of patients in a typical complementary sports medicine practice can be treated successfully using the therapies described in this text. This chapter can serve as a review and future reference source, as the individual assessment and therapeutic aspects of complementary sports medicine may sometimes be quite numerous and complex. Table 28.1 lists the injuries most frequently encountered by the complementary sports medicine professional. These injuries often do not occur as single entities; rather, two, three, or more overlap and occur together. Also note that most of these injuries are secondary problems even though they may be the chief manifestations in the presenting complaints.

Table 28.1 Common Structural, Chemical, and Mental/Emotional Injuries and Their Treatment (Frequent Causes Noted in Parentheses)

Structural	
ASSESSMENT	TREATMENT
1. Localized muscle inhibition (trauma)	Origin & insertion therapy
2. Specific muscle inhibition (secondary to organ/gland, joint complex dysfunction [JCD], acupuncture, or nutrition/diet imbalance)	Treat primary cause
3. Joint complex dysfunction: cranium, pelvis, extravertebral, spine, cranium (muscle imbalance, TMJ problems)	If primary: gentle or non-force manipulation, lifestyle factors (shoes, bruxism); if secondary: address primary needs such as muscle imbalance
Chemical	
ASSESSMENT	TREATMENT
4. Inflammation (over- or undertraining, eicosanoid imbalance due to diet and lifestyle factors)	Balance fats: ↑ and ↓ specific fats as needed; supply necessary nutrients; modify lifestyle factors
5. Fatigue (structural, chemical, and mental causes)	Assess and treat cause(s)
6. Triad of athletic dysfunction	Assess and treat causes
Mental	
ASSESSMENT	TREATMENT
7. Misinformed athlete (social trends, media, advertisements)	Education
8. Feelings of depression and blood sugar-type mental or emotional stress symptoms (adrenal and autonomic dysfunction, neurotransmitter imbalance)	Improve adrenal dysfunction; balance diet (especially carbohydrates and omega-3 fats)
9. Depression and anxiety (overtraining, CI, aerobic deficiency, ↑lactate)	Treat cause; possible need to treat emotional reflexes

STRUCTURAL INJURIES

Perhaps the most common structural injury encountered by practitioners is muscle inhibition due to localized micro- or macrotrauma, often making it a primary problem. This is frequently the result of acute trauma, such as a collision between two athletes in a team event, a fall from a bike or during a cross-country run, or a strain or sprain occurring during anaerobic training or competition. More often, however, this problem results from more chronic activities, such as those performed by the athlete during the overtraining process and is an accumulation of localized stress. In many cases, poor aerobic muscle fiber development, a problem associated with aerobic deficiency states, may be a major contributing factor.

Muscle "tightness" (overfacilitation or sometimes spasm) may follow inhibition. This secondary tension is usually symptomatic. However, the primary muscle inhibition is usually asymptomatic, especially in its early stages, although the joint(s) it supports will often be dysfunctional and symptomatic.

The specific site of injury is often at the origin and/or insertion of the muscle, that is, the musculotendinous junction. Successful correction of this problem usually results in immediate improvement in muscle function, including improved range of motion and significant reduction or elimination of pain. A rapid reduction in associated factors, including swelling, follows over the subsequent 24-48 hr.

Assessment is made by taking the history and by manually testing the muscle(s) in question. Therapy-localizing the origin and/or insertion helps the practitioner establish the precise location of therapy.

Correction of this type of muscle inhibition is accomplished with manual pressure at the origin and/or insertion of the muscle, using a technique referred to as Golgi tendon organ (GTO)/spindle cell therapy. Muscle inhibition is treated by pushing the muscle away from its attachment and releasing it (allowing a rebound effect). This produces facilitation. It is important to be precise in the location of the therapy, to ensure that all muscle fibers are stimulated. The muscle is retested to verify that it has normalized. The patient is asked to perform some activity immediately after the procedure, and the muscle is then retested. A return of muscle inhibition means that additional therapy is needed. In some cases, patients are asked to perform a brief bout of their normal training or competition activity (i.e., swinging a golf club, throwing a ball, running) so that the effectiveness of therapy can be evaluated. In most cases, applying the proper therapy will allow the patient to resume almost immediately a significant amount of training or competition without further damage.

SECONDARY MUSCLE INHIBITION

Another common pattern of muscle inhibition occurs secondary to other, primary dysfunction, including organ or gland dysfunction (i.e., adrenal, thyroid, gastrointestinal), joint dysfunction (i.e., ankle or spinal, including cranial), acupuncture meridian imbalance, or dietary or nutritional imbalance. This type of muscle inhibition must be differentiated from the muscle problems described earlier, and can also result in further secondary muscle tightness and joint dysfunction.

The treatment of this problem is not localized but rather is directed to the causes. This means treatment of Chapman's reflexes associated with the organs or glands, correction of the specific joint dysfunction, balancing of the acupuncture meridians through stimulation of certain points, or dietary and nutritional modifications through diet recommendations and the use of supplements. For example, shoulder pain due to a teres minor muscle inhibition may require stimulation of Chapman's reflexes for the thyroid and stimulation of acupuncture points on the TH meridian.

JOINT COMPLEX DYSFUNCTION

Another very common structural problem is joint complex dysfunction (JCD). Primary joint problems are usually the result of trauma, similar to the trauma causing localized muscle inhibition. Secondary JCD, the most common type, is usually the result of muscle inhibition such that the muscle does not support a joint or allow it to move in its normal range. These problems may not be observed on static X-ray examination since they are of a functional type, although later stages may demonstrate degeneration, a displaced vertebra, or other pathology. Joint complex dysfunction can occur in any joint and may produce pain and dysfunction, limiting ranges of motion and potentially and ultimately causing other secondary problems (muscle imbalance, inflammation, joint degeneration, etc.). In the very early stages, this problem may not produce pain but instead causes other dysfunction such as diminished range of motion or loss of maximum muscle function. This early JCD, if not corrected by the body or with the help of a practitioner, typically worsens—producing more dysfunction, including pain.

Joint complex dysfunction commonly occurs in the pelvis (sacroiliac), extravertebral joints (talus or first metatarsal), spine, wrist, or temporomandibular joint (TMJ). The most important therapeutic consideration is whether this joint problem is primary or, as is often the case, secondary. If it is secondary, the primary problems must be addressed therapeutically. With successful therapy, the secondary structural problem is usually self-correcting. However, as discussed further on, concurrent inflammation usually accompanies JCD, and this may not self-correct and may require further chemical intervention.

Primary JCD most often occurs in the foot and ankle, taking the form of a talus bone dysfunction, for example. This type of problem may be treated with gentle manipulation or non-force technique as discussed in earlier chapters. Associated primary lifestyle stresses are often contributing factors and include the type of shoes worn by the patient; shoes may be oversupported, may fit improperly, or both. "Weaning" the patient into a flatter, more healthy shoe may take time, as the leg and foot muscles must adapt to the changes.

CRANIAL DYSFUNCTION

Another common type of primary JCD is cranial dysfunction, usually associated with phases of respiration as described in previous chapters. Most frequently seen is the inspiration-assisted cranial fault, which is also the easiest to assess and correct. This problem typically causes numerous secondary muscle inhibitions; it may be associated with local pain or be a contributing factor to other pain syndromes, including JCD in the spine. With use of a secondary muscle inhibition as a tool, patients are asked to inhale and hold their breath; normalization of the inhibited muscle as a result is a positive sign for this common fault. There may be other versions of respiratory faults, and some cranial faults are not associated with the breathing mechanism (i.e., the sagittal suture fault).

Cranial dysfunction may be a long-standing problem, possibly caused by stress during birth or by trauma to the head or neck at any time in life. Occasionally, muscle imbalance may be causal or contributory, especially inhibition of the sternocleidomastoid, upper trapezius, or neck extensors, or tightness of the temporalis. Temporomandibular joint imbalance, due to oral health problems such as a missing tooth or bruxism, may also contribute to cranial dysfunction or may be a primary problem in itself.

INFLAMMATION

One of the most common, and damaging, chemical injuries in sport is inflammation. This term, however, should be preceded by the word "excess," as the inflammatory process is part of the normal recovery from training and competition. Allowing the body to balance the inflammatory process may be the ideal approach rather than the use of nonsteroidal anti-inflammatory drugs (NSAIDs), which inhibit both inflammatory and anti-inflammatory eicosanoids. Excess inflammation occurs when eicosanoid balance is not maintained because of imbalances of Group A, B, or C fats; or because of an insufficiency of nutrients necessary to convert the Group A and C fats to the anti-inflammatory eicosanoids (i.e., Series 1 and 3); or because of increased inhibitory products or lifestyle factors that inhibit the production of Series 1 and 3 eicosanoids (i.e., trans fats, excess insulin, stress, etc.). In most patients, a combination of these factors contributes to excess inflammation and the resultant conditions.

Various names are attached to conditions associated with, and often caused by, excess inflammation—the "itis" problems. These include Achilles tendinitis, plantar fascitis, and arthritis, among others. Unfortunately, it is common in mainstream medicine to treat these conditions locally rather than to consider the cause of the excess inflammatory process (or other recurring structural imbalances that produce inflammation). In many cases, patients use aspirin or other NSAIDs to reduce the inflammation and/or the associated pain. If these drugs are successful in their actions, this effect should inform the complementary sports medicine practitioner that the patient's fats may not be balanced and that the patient is a good candidate for dietary/nutritional therapy.

Apart from patients who are training regularly, those who are inactive and unfit may have inflammation as a result of the "deconditioning syndrome." This is sometimes observed, for example, in the spinal joints. Eicosanoid imbalance is also evident in most of these patients.

Although the acute phase may last up to 72 hr, the body may require many months to completely recover from an inflammatory process, even one that is not dramatic. For example, a chronic low back problem that includes an inflammatory process may take up to a year to fully recovery chemically. The signs and symptoms, however, can often be significantly improved within hours or days, with function restored quickly. Subsequently, dietary and nutritional balance must be maintained, not only to ensure complete recovery, but also to prevent the chemical injury from recurring.

FATIGUE

Another very common chemical injury is fatigue. It is an end-result symptom of potentially many imbalances on a structural, chemical, and mental/emotional level. Physically, poor diaphragm muscle function may contribute and may be related to cranial respiratory dysfunction. Chemical causes are the most common. While traditional conditions, such as anemia, are often mentioned but never diagnosed, functional problems are most often the cause—carbohydrate intolerance (CI), aerobic deficiency, and overtraining (the triad of athletic dysfunction) being the most prevalent of these causes. Mental or emotional stress may cause adrenal dysfunction, producing fatigue. In addition, imbalances in neurotransmitters could result in a mental fatigue, as noted in connection with mental injuries later in this chapter.

The symptom of fatigue itself may become a stress, leading to a vicious cycle. Thus adrenal dysfunction is often associated with this problem, especially chronic fatigue. Patients' overall quality of life is often affected by fatigue, which impacts their structural, chemical, and mental/emotional capacities—potentially leading to problems with work, family, or social life, and not just in sport.

Fatigue is usually associated with a high respiratory quotient—a diminished ability to generate energy from fatty acids, thus a greater reliance on glucose. This is reflected in less effective training and competition performances and assessed by a worsening Maximum Aerobic Function (MAF) test. In addition, many patients with fatigue have increased body fat content.

Perhaps this chemical injury, fatigue, impels more patients to seek self-remedies than any other, especially when medical tests fail to find the cause. Remedies include "diets," low calorie or low fat, both often resulting in more fatigue in many patients. Self-prescribing nutrients is also common, with iron being a popular supplement. This can be dangerous in many patients, especially men, because of the potential of excess iron storage (as ferritin) and its relationship to heart disease and oxygen free radicals. Perhaps the most common "remedy" for fatigue is caffeine—patients drink more coffee, tea, and cola in an attempt to "get more energy." This puts further stress on an already dysfunctional adrenal gland and can worsen the problem.

Other dietary factors may also be a cause of fatigue; a common one is functional malabsorption. This is sometimes associated with hypo- or achlorhydria, causing secondary malabsorption of various nutrients. Autonomic imbalance may contribute to this problem. Dehydration is another dietary factor common in patients who are fatigued.

TRIAD OF ATHLETIC DYSFUNCTION

A third chemical injury, perhaps the most common syndrome in sport, encompasses aerobic deficiency, adrenal dysfunction, and overtraining, as discussed in chapter 27 as the triad of athletic dysfunction. In its early stages, this condition is treated easily and is completely reversible. Proper care should not only restore normal function in the patient's athletic ability; but when the body's structural, chemical, and mental/emotional states are well balanced, performance can reach its highest level. In the third stage of this triad, however, the chemical problems are difficult to treat, and longer-term care is necessary to restore health; often fitness never returns to very high levels. In some cases, quality of life is greatly diminished and the disease process is well defined.

MENTAL AND EMOTIONAL INJURIES

Although not usually thought of as injuries, problems may develop in patients with mental and emotional stress, including anxiety and depression, due to confusion and misunderstandings about their body. This type of injury is not uncommon. The 46-year-old physically injured masters athlete who is told that she is too old for competition, the young professional athlete—now considering retirement—who is unable to find relief from debilitating knee pain, and the overtrained athlete who no longer knows where to turn for help are examples of people in whom these frustrations can lead to mental/emotional injury. Many of these injuries are secondary but nonetheless significant, and pose a major problem for many patients.

The most common cause of this type of problem is a misunderstanding or indoctrination regarding normal body function. This can originate from sport tradition in the form of social trends, especially the "no pain, no gain" philosophy. Regular comments by sports announcers suggesting that an athlete is "tough" because he always "plays hurt" stay in the minds of many patients and, most unfortunately, children just being introduced to sport. Advertising campaigns that promote products through unhealthy commentary, quite evident in the athletic shoe market as already described, are another good example. Many companies spend billions of dollars to advertise their products seductively, and successfully, leaving the athlete miseducated—and eventually confused and stressed.

It is the job of the practitioner to educate the patient regarding balanced health and fitness (recall that the word "doctor" means teacher). This includes the realities of foot function and shoes, diet/nutrition and energy, and training and performance, to name three major issues patients may not properly understand. Practitioners who have an effective and well-trained (i.e., educated) staff can teach patients a great deal. Making reliable information available to patients can be crucial in the education process; in addition to one-on-one education, such information can take the form of notes on particular topics, copies of articles and books, and lectures by staff or practitioner.

A similar mental and emotional stress occurs in athletes with chronic structural and chemical dysfunction who have unsuccessfully consulted many types of practitioners, taken many drugs and nutritional supplements, followed many diets, and read many books, but are no better off—and frequently worse off—than when they started. This stress compounds any existing stresses, especially those associated with overtraining, CI, or adrenal dysfunction.

SECONDARY MENTAL AND EMOTIONAL PROBLEMS

Other common mental and emotional stresses are those secondary to blood sugar-handling problems triggered by excess sympathetic nervous system activity and adrenal dysfunction. These are listed on the symptom survey or other forms completed by patients and are discussed during the initial history taking. They include irritability before meals or if eating is delayed, moodiness with intake of too many sweets, feelings of depression between meals or immediately after consumption of particular foods, and anxiety. Thyroid dysfunction may cause similar symptoms, including reduced initiative. So-called premenstrual syndrome (PMS) may be associated with these mental/emotional injuries, developing during certain phases of the menstrual cycle.

Some symptoms evolve as a result of neurotransmitter imbalance, especially between serotonin and norepinephrine. This may result from consumption of a diet too high in carbohydrates or from changes in blood sugar balance in the brain. Whatever the cause, this type of imbalance is relatively easy to assess according to the basic procedures discussed throughout this text.

More advanced depression or anxiety may exist secondary to conditions such as overtraining and CI. High lactate levels also can produce psychiatric symptoms. These mental and emotional injuries can be evident in patients with no psychiatric history.

PAIN AS AN INJURY

As a separate entity, pain evokes structural, chemical, and mental/emotional responses and is reviewed separately here. In addition to its protective and recuperative role, preventing the athlete from undergoing additional training or competitive stress, pain can be viewed as an injury in the same way as the other nine impairments. Pain and the use of pain control techniques in complementary sports medicine were discussed in chapter 17.

The primary and most obvious task with a patient in pain is to rule out more serious problems that may require emergency care or referral to a specialist. Having done so, the practitioner assesses and treats the cause of the pain. There is no special treatment for pain as such other than to correct existing imbalances. In many cases, correction improves or eliminates most of the pain. However, in some cases, acupuncture therapy may reduce or eliminate pain that continues after the use of appropriate therapy. For example, sometimes pain is due to inflammation and other damage in a tendon, ligament, muscle, or joint. Correcting the soft tissue and joint dysfunction may reduce the pain, but some pain may continue. Use of acupuncture methods may eliminate the remaining pain.

In another case, if the patient has a painful fibula fracture, for example, and is also under the care of an orthopedist, the complementary use of acupuncture pain control can be very helpful. Such therapy may be especially beneficial in obviating the need for aspirin or other NSAIDs, which can slow or delay the healing process.

CLINICAL NOTES

Following are five case histories exemplifying situations that typically confront the complementary sports medicine practitioner. Note especially the on-the-field care in the first case, and the difference between the main complaint of the patient ("injury") and the primary findings in the other four cases.

The first case demonstrates the importance and potential effectiveness of acute or on-the-field care that may be necessary during an event (e.g., basketball, baseball, football), between events (e.g., track and field), or at other times, such as during an Olympics or a long stage race. In some cases a practitioner who travels with a team or individual athlete can transform a hotel room or recreational vehicle into an office setting.

Case History 1

Gary was in the final round of basketball for his school when he "pulled" his right hamstring and was in pain. He was unable to run with a normal gait or without pain, and also risked further injury if he played the next game that afternoon. Gary's right hamstring muscles were tested in the locker room and found to be inhibited; the testing was also very painful. Inhalation normalized the muscle and allowed a normal test with little pain. Therapy localization to the origin of the lateral hamstring (biceps femoris) and to the insertion of its short head were the only positive areas. The cranial fault was corrected and GTO therapy applied. The muscles then tested normal. Gary was asked to lightly run in place, which he could accomplish with an 80% reduction in pain. The hamstrings test continued to be normal. Gary was asked to mimic his actions during play (especially quick movements). Within about 30 sec, the pain returned. The hamstrings were tested and found to be inhibited again. Respiration no longer affected the muscle. Therapy localization to the insertion of the medial hamstrings was positive and corrected with GTO therapy. This allowed Gary to move quickly in a normal gait with about an 80% reduction in pain. An hour later, the hamstring muscles continued to be normal, and no cranial fault was present. However, a pectoralis major clavicular (PMC) tested standing was inhibited but was normal in the non-weight-bearing condition. This was due to a calcaneal imbalance in the right foot, which was corrected with light manipulation. After this therapy, the weight-bearing PMC test was normal. Gary was able to play the whole game with no additional pain or further injury.

Case History 2

Andrea, age 36, presented with chronic bilateral knee pain. Previous X-rays had been negative. Her main concern was the knee pain, although a longtime goal was running a marathon. During the history, Andrea admitted to symptoms of exercise-induced asthma (EIA) that she had experienced since her teens but had not listed on her initial forms. Daily medication improved the symptoms. She also noted adverse reactions to dairy products, a worsening of symptoms during stress, and gradual weight gain over the past five years. The history and examination revealed signs and symptoms of adrenal dysfunction. Andrea had insomnia, difficulty with night vision, and symptoms of blood sugar dysfunction including constant hunger, moodiness, and feelings of depression if she missed meals. She was often light-headed upon standing quickly. Among the primary examination findings were orthostatic hypotension, a very low vital capacity and breath-holding time, below-normal oral temperature at 36.2 °C (97.2 °F), and inhibition of both the sartorius and the right tibialis posterior muscles. Dietary assessment revealed a high-carbohydrate, low-fat, and low-protein diet that included low-fat milk with cereal each morning. Andrea also consumed a popular sports drink before each workout. Her fat ratio showed very high Group A and B fats. Numerous secondary structural problems were noted (not described beyond this point), including a pelvic Category II fault, several spinal joint problems, and a talus bone dysfunction. A separate session was scheduled to explain the meanings of these problems, relate them to Andrea's signs and symptoms, provide clear recommendations about future sessions and expectations, and ensure that Andrea understood her role and was willing to cooperate. After agreeing, Andrea was scheduled for another session.

At her next treatment session Andrea was given dietary recommendations, with explanations, that included avoiding all dairy products, increasing Group C fats and reducing Group A and B fats, increasing proteins, and avoiding all sugar and sugar-containing food (including her sports drink). Correction of both sartorius and tibialis posterior muscle inhibition was achieved by stimulating Chapman's reflexes, and there was a positive oral challenge for choline (one tablet to be chewed every 3 hr for the first five days, then four times daily). After Andrea ran in place for 2 min, the right tibialis posterior muscle inhibition returned. This was corrected using GTO/spindle cell therapy. A recommendation for flatter running shoes was given.

Training recommendations included using a heart monitor and not exceeding a heart rate of 140, avoiding all anaerobic training (including weights) and racing, and performing a MAF test. Andrea was scheduled for her next session in three weeks. It should be noted that this session totaled about 60 min.

At the next session, Andrea stated that her left knee was 90% improved and the right 50%; EIA symptoms were 50% improved. Systolic blood pressure difference from lying to standing was about the same at 110 mmHg. Vital capacity and breath-holding were normal, and temperature remained the same. Dietary and training compliance seemed good. Her MAF test was 9:50 per mile.

Several key factors were assessed and treated. The right sartorius was inhibited (the left was normal) and required stimulation of the right acupuncture point CX 9. The tibialis posterior muscles were normal. Running on a treadmill for 30 min caused the right sartorius inhibition to recur, which normalized only with zinc (one tablet, four times a day; Zinc Liver Chelate, Standard Process, Inc.) Andrea was scheduled for another session in five weeks. At her next session, Andrea stated that her EIA was 95% resolved and that her knee pain had improved 100% during the previous three weeks.

She claimed a reduction of body weight of 7 lb. Her MAF test was 9:05 per mile. Systolic pressure increased 6 mmHg upon standing, vital capacity and breath-holding remained normal, and temperature was 36.6 °C (98.0 °F). Muscle function was normal. Andrea decided on her own to discontinue her asthma medication.

Andrea continued to progress with an occasional brief but minor feeling of right knee pain and/or EIA symptoms during times of work stress (usually resulting from out-of-town travel). After about 10 months, Andrea's MAF test was 8:40 per mile. It was agreed that regular sessions about every two months would help maintain body balance. During these sessions, relatively minor imbalances were assessed and corrected, and about once each year her diet was reevaluated. Andrea's training was gradually increased and competition added, and about 18 months after the first session she successfully ran her first marathon.

Case History 3

Jack presented with chronic fatigue and three years of diminishing performances. He had always believed that performance was directly related to age, but two older training partners who had improved their performances had made the referral. Jack's fasting triglyceride level was 324 mg/dl. His fatigue significantly worsened after meals, especially after lunch, when he had to rest for about an hour before resuming work. Despite cycling about 15 hr/week, maintaining a consistent weight, and avoiding high-fat foods, Jack stated that his body fat had increased from about 12% to over 20% in the past five or six years. Jack's mother was diabetic. Examinations revealed many imbalances that appeared secondary to CI. After these issues were discussed and the possibility of CI was outlined, Jack agreed to perform the Two-Week test and was scheduled for his next session three weeks later. In addition, he would use a heart monitor during all his workout sessions and avoid all anaerobic training. Despite his understanding of what was required, during the subsequent three-week period Jack had to ask a staff member on several occasions to help him organize his eating plan and answer other questions, especially regarding fears of worsening his triglycerides.

During his next session, Jack noted a dramatic improvement in energy. The majority of imbalances seen in the previous session's assessments were not evident. Of the remaining problems, PMC bilateral, quadriceps, and abdominal inhibition were primary. Some were corrected by stimulating Chapman's reflexes and appropriate acupuncture points (for the quadriceps and abdominals); the PMC inhibition responded only to an oral challenge using betaine hydrochloride, which was given (two tablets after each meal, Betaine Hydrochloride, Standard Process, Inc.). Other dietary suggestions were discussed, especially the importance of balancing fats, eating meals without stress, and avoiding "hidden" sugars in foods. Jack was scheduled for a fasting blood test the following morning. Several days later Jack was informed that his triglyceride level was 185 mg/dl.

Jack's performances ultimately improved dramatically, surpassing his peak achievements of a decade before. His next triglyceride test showed a level of 140 mg/dl, which remained. Jack continued sessions about every six to eight weeks. During these, minor imbalances were found and corrected. After a couple of years, Jack stated that performing the Two-Week test about every six or eight months helped keep him "on track" regarding his diet, especially in early January after the holiday stress.

Case History 4

Barbara was most concerned about her weight gain. She was unable to exercise because of a chronic Achilles tendon problem that worsened during any physical activity. Her premenstrual stress was high, and her menstrual periods were profuse. Her goals were just to get healthy and fit; she was not interested in competition like her husband, who had referred her. She was persuaded not to use scale weight but rather waist measurement as a gauge of fat loss. Important findings on her initial assessment were a very low oral temperature of 35.7 °C (96.4 °F) and postural hypotension. Dietary assessment revealed a ratio of omega-6 and omega-3 fats that was approximately 30:1. Positive oral nutrient challenges for linseed oil, calcium, and iron were obtained, and supplements were recommended (Linum B6, three capsules three times daily; Calcium Lactate, two tablets three times daily; Ferrofood, one capsule with breakfast—all Standard Process, Inc.). Dietary recommendations included reducing Group A and Group B and increasing Group C fats. Barbara had inhibition of numerous muscles related to the hormonal system—primarily the tibialis posterior, teres minor, and gluteus medius. Correction of the tibialis posterior, which entailed correction of a cranial respiratory fault and manipulation of the talus bone, allowed Barbara to walk on a treadmill without Achilles pain. However, she was unable to walk even at a slow, easy pace without her heart rate exceeding 145—her maximum aerobic training rate. It was recommended that she walk 20 min five to six days per week at a slower pace using a heart monitor. She was asked to perform a MAF test immediately and another one just before her next session in four weeks.

At her next session, Barbara stated that her Achilles had been symptom free for the past two weeks. Her temperature was the same, but systolic blood pressure had increased 4 mmHg upon standing. Other assessments revealed a nutritional need for niacin and vitamin B6 (through an oral challenge using a recurrent inhibited teres minor muscle); one tablet twice daily was recommended (Niacinamide B6; Standard Process, Inc.). Barbara had just used up all her previous supplements, which were not replaced. Her first MAF test had been about 7:10 per quarter mile and the second about 6:30. Her waist measurement was about .5 in. less than before. She was scheduled for another session in six weeks.

At this session, Barbara stated that her past two menstrual periods were much improved, with about a 50% improvement in PMS symptoms. Her last two MAF tests had been 6:05 and 5:28 per quarter mile. Her Achilles was asymptomatic. Her tibialis posterior, teres minor, and gluteus medius muscles were normal. Her waist measurement was reduced a total of about 1 in.

Barbara continued to show steady improvements. She lost an amount of body fat that was acceptable to her, the Achilles problem never returned, and the menstrual problems were about 85% improved after six months. Barbara chose not to continue further sessions because of insurance denial of coverage. Fourteen months later she returned as a patient, stating that during the previous two months her PMS had worsened and that her Achilles, over the past month, had been aching after her walks. Evaluation of her diet showed imbalances similar to those found initially, with similar physical findings. She was treated, and she returned in six weeks feeling much improved. Two months later she felt better, and subsequently continued her care about every two months despite not having insurance coverage.

Case History 5

Walter had chronic thoracic, lumbar, and sacroiliac pain that prevented him from continuing his training and competition, which he had ended two years previously. In addition, he was chronically fatigued, was gaining weight, was depressed, and sought almost continual professional care of various types with limited success. On the basis of the history, Walter appeared to be in the later stages of the triad of athletic dysfunction. There were numerous signs and symptoms of adrenal stress, aerobic deficiency, and overtraining, as well as many secondary structural problems and indications for nutritional needs. His initial examination yielded four primary findings. First, he was dehydrated, and it was recommended that he drink at least 3 L of water throughout the day—more if his urine remained yellow. Second, he had an inhibited PMC bilateral, which responded to betaine hydrochloride (two tablets with each meal and one with each small meal or snack; Betaine Hydrochloride, Standard Process, Inc.). Third, his abdominal muscles were bilaterally inhibited; these responded to L-glutamine (500 mg in the morning and 500 mg in the evening on an empty stomach with water, L-Glutamine Plus; Nutri-West). These last two nutrients normalized all other inhibited muscles. The fourth finding was a primary cranial-sacral respiratory fault causing inhibition of both hamstring groups. Correction of these muscles also required treatment of other factors: the PMC muscles were secondary to a cranial-sacral fault, and the quadriceps and abdominal muscles were secondary to Chapman's reflexes. Walter was also given a variety of dietary recommendations including eating every 2 hr, avoiding all high-glycemic foods, and lowering his carbohydrate intake. It was recommended that he not attempt any workouts at that time. He was rescheduled for another session in one week.

At his second session, Walter's back pain was about 40% improved, and his energy was slightly improved (25%). He also claimed a 50% improvement in his mental/emotional state. Assessment revealed a recurrent inhibition of the abdominal muscles bilaterally. These were normalized by correction of a sagittal suture fault, which immediately and significantly improved his back pain. Numerous other structural and chemical problems were corrected. The importance of water and the dietary advice were further emphasized. At this time, it was recommended that Walter begin walking slowly for 20-30 min each day. This was initially a difficult concept in view of the high level of training and competition that Walter was used to. However, he eventually agreed that it was the best starting point. He would return in two weeks.

At his next session, Walter was feeling much improved; back pain was 90% improved, energy was 75% improved, and his mental/emotional state remained 50% improved. He had walked 30 min each day since his previous visit and was eager to train more. He had a reoccurrence of the PMC bilateral. Betaine hydrochloride did not affect the muscle inhibition, but the emotional stress points did; these were treated for about a minute, normalizing the PMC muscles. Walter was asked to think about his past training and competitions, and this caused the PMC muscle to become inhibited again. It was determined that ST 1 required treatment, and this point was tapped for about 1 min. The mental/emotional challenge no longer caused muscle inhibition. Walter was told to continue his walking and his adherence to other recommendations and was rescheduled for three weeks later.

On his next visit, Walter admitted having gone to the gym three days earlier to lift light weights for 30 min. He stated that he was feeling better than he had in a number of years (improvements in his back, energy, and mental/emotional state were over 90%). His back pain had returned that evening and continued. A recurrence of the cranial-sacral fault and sagittal suture was corrected, with complete alleviation of back pain. The importance of maintaining a balanced program was reemphasized. Numerous other problems were found and corrected, and Walter was rescheduled for four weeks later, but would receive a phone call after two weeks to check on his program.

Walter slowly but consistently improved, experiencing total recovery from back pain, fatigue, and mental/emotional stress. There were occasionally some minor recurrences of one, two, or all three symptoms during times of stress. Although he never attained the same level of fitness as before, his health progressed dramatically. He continued care about every month. Eventually, Walter began coaching in his spare time, working with young athletes and hoping to help them understand balanced sport philosophy.

Table 28.2 lists the results of the five patients' primary and secondary problems, the treatments found to be effective, the results, and the total time for maximum resolution including the number of visits.

Table 28.2 Five Case History Summaries

	Secondary problems (complaints)	**Primary problems**	**Therapy**	**Results**	**Time/Number of sessions**
Case 1—Gary	Acute hamstring "pull"	Structural imbalance	Cranial; origin and insertion therapy; calcaneal manipulation	Function restored 100%	3 hr/1 session
Case 2—Andrea	Chronic bilateral knee pain; exercise-induced asthma	Adrenal dysfunction	Physical treatment; choline, zinc; dietary modification; avoid anaerobic work for 4-5 mo	Knee: 100% resolution; asthma: 95% resolution	4 wk/3 sessions
Case 3—Jack	Chronic fatigue; high triglycerides; poor competitive performances	Carbohydrate intolerance	Dietary modification; avoid anaerobic work for 3-4 mo	All: 100% resolution	3 wk/2 sessions
Case 4—Barbara	Achilles tendon pain; weight gain; premenstrual stress	Aerobic deficiency; hormonal imbalance	Linseed oil, B6; increase dietary fats; walking program	Achilles: 100%; acceptable weight loss; PMS: 85% resolved	Achilles: 2 wk/1 session; weight/PMS: 6 mo/4 sessions
Case 5—Walter	Chronic low back pain; failing performances; chronic exhaustion	Triad of dysfunction	Physical treatment; several nutritional supplements; significant dietary change; avoid all anaerobic work for 6 mo	Low back, fatigue, and mental stress: 100% resolution	8-10 sessions; continued care as necessary

CONCLUSION

Obviously not all patients respond as well as those just described. However, these case histories are representative of those seen in a complementary sports medicine practice. There are always some patients whose problems are not compatible with the type of care complementary sports medicine offers and who are therefore not accepted. These individuals may be only seeking to eliminate their symptoms of knee pain, fatigue, or diminished performance and not willing to participate in the process. Others are too firmly entrenched in their workout ethics, eating habits, or social relationships within sport to break away from these "addictions." Clearly, some of these patients are willing to sacrifice their health for an attempt at more fitness.

Rather than expend time and energy on patients unwilling to care for themselves, practitioners are encouraged to put great effort into helping those who do wish to understand their body and to make appropriate changes for the optimal balance of health and fitness with long-lasting performance improvements. They will reap the great benefits that complementary sports medicine offers.

References

CHAPTER 1

Burkitt DP, Walker A, Painter N (1974). Dietary fiber and disease. *JAMA* 229:1068-1074.

Harman WW (1991). *A re-examination of the metaphysical foundations of modern science: Causality issues in contemporary science.* Research report. Sausalito, CA: Institute of Noetic Sciences.

Leadbetter JD, Leadbetter WB (1986). The philosophy of sports medicine care: An historical review. *Maryland Medical Journal,* 45(8):618-631.

McGee H (1984). *On food and cooking,* p. 550. New York: Collier Books.

Selye H (1976). *The stress of life.* New York: McGraw-Hill.

Siffert RS, Kaufman JJ (1996). Acoustic assessment of fracture healing. Capabilities and limitations of "a lost art." *Am. J. Orthop.* 25(9): 614-618.

Snook G (1984). The history of sports medicine. *Am. J. Sports Med.* 12(4): 252-254.

Walther DS (1988). *Applied kinesiology synopsis,* p. 12. Pueblo, CO: Systems DC.

CHAPTER 2

Costill DL, Maglischo E, Richardson A (1991). *Handbook of sports medicine: Swimming.* London: Blackwell.

Coyle EF, Coggan AR, Hopper MK, Walters TJ (1988). Determinants of endurance in well-trained cyclists. *J. Appl. Physiol.* 64(6): 2622-2630.

Fries J, Crapo L (1981). *Vitality and aging: Implications of the rectangular curve.* San Francisco: Freeman.

McArdle WD, Katch FI, Katch VL (1991). *Exercise physiology.* 3d ed., p. 756. Philadelphia: Lea & Febiger.

Wilmore JH, Costill DL (1994). *Physiology of sport and exercise,* pp. 303-304. Champaign, IL: Human Kinetics.

CHAPTER 3

Bernstein JH, Shuval JT (1997). Nonconventional medicine in Israel: Consultation patterns of the Israeli population and attitudes of primary care physicians. *Soc. Sci. Med.* 44(9): 1341-1348.

Carlston M, Stuart MR, Jonas W (1997). Alternative medicine instruction in medical schools and family practice residency programs. *Fam. Med.* 29(8): 559-562.

Cashman SJ (1988). Nomenclatures of anatomical distortions of the spine: A comparison. *J. Manip. Physiol. Ther.* 11(1): 31-35.

Christie VM (1991). A dialogue between practitioners of alternative (traditional) medicine and modern (western) medicine in Norway. *Soc. Sci. Med.* 32(5): 549-552.

Crossman J (1997). Psychological rehabilitation from sports injuries. *Sports Med.* 23(5): 333-339.

DeJarnette B (1979). *Sacro occipital technique.* Nebraska City, NE: Privately published.

Dorland's illustrated medical dictionary (1994). 28th ed., p. 1596. Philadelphia: Saunders.

Eisenberg DM, Kessler RC, Foster C, Norlock FE (1993). Unconventional medicine in the United States. Prevalence, costs, and patterns of use. *N. Engl. J. Med.* 328(4): 246-252.

Field T, Ironson G, Scafidi F, Narocki T, Goncalves A, Pickens J, Fox M, Schanberg S, Kuhn C (1996). Massage therapy reduces anxiety and enhances EEG pattern of alertness and math patterns. *Int. J. Neurosci.* 86: 197-205.

Geddes N, Henry JK (1997). Nursing and alternative medicine. Legal and practice issues. *J. Holistic Nurs.* 15(3): 271-281.

Hampf G (1993). A biopsychological approach to temporomandibular joint pain and other chronic facial pain. Part II: Broadening of spectrum of treatments. *Proc. Finn. Dent. Soc.* 89(1-2): 15-28.

Himmel W, Schulte M, Kochen MM (1993). Complementary medicine: Are patients' expectations being met by their general practitioners? *Br. J. Gen. Pract.* 43(371): 232-235.

Ironson G, Field T, Scafidi F, Hashimoto M, Kumar M, Kumar A, Price A, Goncalves A, Burman I, Tetenman C, Tatarca R, Fletcher M (1996). Massage therapy is associated with enhancement of the immune system's cytotoxic capacity. *Int. J. Neurosci.* 84: 205-217.

Janda V (1996). Evaluation of muscular imbalance. In *Rehabilitation of the spine,* ed. C Liebenson, p. 12. Baltimore: Williams & Wilkins.

Kronenberg F, Mallory B, Downey J (1994). Rehabilitation medicine and alternative therapies: New words, old practices. *Arch. Phys. Med. Rehabil.* 75(8): 928-929.

Laemmel K (1996). Interview in medicine. *Schweiz. Rundsch. Med. Prax.* 85(27-28): 863-869.

Leisman G, Ferentz A, Zenhausern R, Tefera T, Zemcov A (1995). Electromyographic effects of fatigue and task repetition on the validity of strong and weak muscle estimates in applied kinesiology muscle testing procedures. *Percept. Mot. Skills* 80: 963-977.

Lewit K (1991). *Manipulative therapy in rehabilitation of the locomotor system.* 2d ed., p. 81. Oxford, England: Butterworth-Heinemann.

Newsholme EA (1996). Breaking Olympic records: Improved understanding of psychology and nutrition will mean no end to record breaking. *Br. Med. J.* 313(1): 246.

Seaman DR (1997). Joint complex dysfunction, a novel term to replace subluxation/subluxation complex: Etiological and treatment considerations. *J. Manip. Physiol. Ther.* 20(9): 634-644.

Smith LL, Keating MN, Holbert D, Spratt DJ, McCammon MR, Smith SS, Israel RG (1994). The effects of athletic massage on delayed onset muscle soreness, creatine kinase, and neutrophil count: A preliminary report. *J. Orthop. Sports Phys. Ther.* 19(2): 93-99.

Travell J, Rinzler SH (1952). Myofascial genesis of pain in the neck and shoulder girdle. *Postgrad. Med.* 11: 425.

Verhoef MJ, Sutherland LR (1995). Alternative medicine and general practitioners. Opinions and behaviour. *Can. Fam. Physician* 41: 1005-1011.

Walther DS (1988). *Applied kinesiology synopsis,* p. 12. Pueblo, CO: Systems DC.

CHAPTER 4

Abernathy P, Thayer R, Taylor A (1990). Acute and chronic responses of skeletal muscles to endurance and sprint exercises. *Sports Med.* 10(6): 365-389.

Bonde-Petersen F, Robertson CH Jr (1981). Blood flow in "red" and "white" calf muscles in cats during isometric and isotonic exercise. *Acta Physiol. Scand.* 112(3): 243-251.

Borensztajn J (1979). Lipoprotein lipase and hypertriglyceridemias. *Artery* 5: 346-353.

Colliander EB, Dudley GA, Tesch PA (1988). Skeletal muscle fiber type composition and performance during repeated bouts of maximal, concentric contractions. *Eur. J. Appl. Physiol.* 58: 81-86.

Foster C, Costill DL, Fink WJ (1979). Effects of preexercise feedings on endurance performance. *Med. Sci. Sports* 11(1): 1-5.

Fox EL (1979). *Sports physiology.* Philadelphia: Saunders.

Gollnick PK (1985). Metabolism of substrates: Energy substrate metabolism during exercise and as modified by training. *Fed. Proc.* 44: 353-357.

Haggmark T, Eriksson E, Jansson E (1986). Muscle fiber type changes in human skeletal muscle after injuries and immobilization. *Orthopedics* 9: 181-185.

Hughes VA, Fiatarone MA, Ferrara CM, McNamara JR, Charnley JM, Evans WJ (1994). Lipoprotein response to exercise training and a low-fat diet in older subjects with glucose intolerance. *Am. J. Clin. Nutr.* 59: 820-826.

Hurley BF, Nemeth PM, Martin WH, Hagberg JM, Dalsky GP, Holloszy JO (1986). Muscle triglyceride utilization during exercise: Effect of training. *J. Appl. Physiol.* 60: 562-567.

Karlsson J, Nordesio L, Saltin B (1974). Muscle glycogen utilization during exercise and physical training. *Acta Physiol. Scand.* 90: 210-217.

Lambert EV, Speechly DP, Dennis SC, Noakes TD (1994). Enhanced endurance in trained cyclists during moderate intensity exercise following 2 weeks adaptation to a high fat diet. *Eur. J. Appl. Physiol.* 69: 287-293.

Mayes PA (1993). Metabolism of unsaturated fatty acids & eicosanoids. In *Harper's biochemistry,* 23d ed., eds. RK Murray, DK Granner, PA Mayes, VW Rodwell, pp. 164-171. Norwalk, CT: Appleton & Lange.

McArdle WD, Katch FI, Katch VL (1991). *Exercise physiology.* 3d ed., pp. 125-131. Philadelphia: Lea & Febiger.

Mountcastle VB, ed. (1974). *Medical physiology.* Vol. I. 13th ed., p. 620. St. Louis: Mosby.

Muoio DM, Leddy JJ, Horvath PJ, Awad AB, Pendergast DR (1994). Effect of dietary fat on metabolic adjustments to maximal $\dot{V}O_2$ and endurance in runners. *Med. Sci. Sports Exerc.* 26(1): 81-88.

Newsholme E (1977). The regulation of intracellular and extracellular fuel supply during sustained exercise. *Ann. NY Acad. Sci.* 301: 81-87.

Simoneau JA, Lortie G, Boulay MR, Marcotte M, Thibault MC, Bouchard C (1985). Human skeletal muscle fiber type alteration with high-intensity intermittent training. *Eur. J. Appl. Physiol.* 54: 250-253.

Utriainen T, Holmang A, Bjorntorp P, Makimattila S, Sovijarvi A, Lindholm H, Yki-Jarvinen H (1996). Physical fitness, muscle morphology, and insulin-stimulated limb blood flow in normal subjects. *Am. J. Physiol.* 270 (5 Part 1): E905-E911.

Vukovich MD, Costill DL, Hickey MS, Trappe SW, Cole KJ, Fink WJ (1993). Effect of fat emulsion infusion and fat feeding on muscle glycogen utilization during cycle exercise. *J. Appl. Physiol.* 75(4): 1513-1518.

CHAPTER 5

DeAndrade JR, Grant C, Dixon ASJ (1965). Joint distention and reflex muscle inhibition in the knee. *J. Bone Joint Surg.* 47: 313. Abstract.

Fisher NM, White SC, Yack HJ, Smolinski RJ, Pendergast DR (1997). Muscle function and gait in patients with knee osteoarthritis before and after muscle rehabilitation. *Disabil. and Rehabil.* 19(2): 47-55.

Guyton AC (1986). *Textbook of medical physiology,* pp. 612-613. Philadelphia: Saunders.

Ibid. pp. 686-697.

Janda V (1986). Some aspects of extracranial causes of facial pain. *J. Prosthet. Dent.* 56: 484.

Jull G, Janda V (1987). Muscles and motor control in low back pain. In *Physical therapy for the low back: Clinics in physical therapy,* eds. LT Twomey, JR Taylor. New York: Churchill Livingstone.

Kendall FP, McCreary EK, Provance PG (1993). *Muscles, testing and function.* 4th ed. Baltimore: Williams & Wilkins.

Lehmann MJ, Lormes W, Opitz-Gress A, Steinacher JM, Netzer N, Foster C, Gastmann U (1997). Training and overtraining: An overview and experimental results in endurance sports. *J. Sports Med. Phys. Fitness* 37: 7-17.

Liebenson C (1996). Rehabilitation of the spine. In *Integrating rehabilitation into chiropractic practice,* ed. C Liebenson. Baltimore: Williams & Wilkins.

McColl KE (1997). Helicobacter pylori and acid secretion: Where are we now? *Eur. J. Gastroenterol. Hepatol.* 9(4): 333-335.

Sahrmann S (1987). Posture and muscle imbalance: Faulty lumbar pelvic alignments. *Phys. Ther.* 67: 1840.

Selye H (1976). *The stress of life.* New York: McGraw-Hill.

Spencer JD, Hayes KC, Alexander IJ (1984). Knee joint effusion and quadriceps reflex inhibition in man. *Arch. Phys. Med. Rehabil.* 65: 171.

Tepperman J, Tepperman H (1987). *Metabolic and endocrine physiology,* pp. 249-296. Chicago: Year Book Medical.

Walther DS (1988). *Applied kinesiology synopsis,* p. 12. Pueblo, CO: Systems DC.

CHAPTER 6

Almekinders LC, Banes AJ, Ballenger CA (1993). Effects of repetitive motion on human fibroblasts. *Med. Sci. Sports Exerc.* 25(5): 603-607.

Amadio P Jr, Cummings DM, Amadio P (1993). Nonsteroidal anti-inflammatory drugs. Tailoring therapy to achieve results and avoid toxicity. *Postgrad. Med.* 93(4): 73-76.

Barron JL, Noakes TD, Levy W, Smith C, Miller RP (1985). Hypothalamic dysfunction in overtrained athletes. *J. Clin. Endocrinol. Metab.* 60(4): 803-806.

Bassett DR, Block WD, Dean EN, White AA (1990). Recognition of borderline carbohydrate-lipid metabolism disturbance: An incipient form of Type IV hyperlipoproteinemia? *J. Cardio. Pharm.* 15(5): 8-17.

Belanger A, Candas B, Dupont A, Cusan L, Diamond P, Gomez JL, Labrie F (1994). Changes in serum concentrations of conjugated and unconjugated steroids in 40- to 80-year-old men. *J. Clin. Endocrinol. Metab.* 79(4): 1086-1090.

Berkow MD (1992). *The Merck manual of diagnosis and therapy,* pp. 434-437. Rahway, NJ: Merck & Co., Inc.

Bernton E, Hoover D, Galloway R, Popp K (1995). Adaptation to chronic stress in military trainees. *Ann. NY Acad. Sci.* 774: 217-231.

Bezard J, Blond JP, Bernard A, Clouet P (1994). The metabolism and availability of essential fatty acids in animal and human tissues. *Reprod. Nutr. Dev.* 34(6): 539-568.

Bland, JS (1997). Insulin, endocrine function, and age-related dysfunctions. Fourth International Symposium on Functional Medicine, May 15-17, Aspen, CO.

Blond JP, Bezard J (1991). Delta 5-desaturation of dihomogammalinolenic acid (20:3(n-6)) into arachidonic acid (20:4(n-6)) by rat liver microsomes and incorporation of fatty acids in microsome phospholipids. *Biochem. Biophys. Acta* 1084(3): 255-260. Abstract.

Blond JP, Henchiri C, Bezard J (1989). Delta 6 and delta 5 desaturase activities in liver from obese Zucker rats at different ages. *Lipids* 24(5): 389-395.

Bordoni A, Biagi PL, Turchetto E, Hrelia S (1988). Aging influence on delta-6-desaturase activity and fatty acid composition of rat liver microsomes. *Biochem. Int.* 17(6): 1001-1009.

Bouziane M, Prost J, Belleville J (1994). Dietary protein deficiency affects n-3 and n-6 polyunsaturated fatty acids hepatic storage and very low density lipoprotein transport in rats on different diets. *Lipids* 29(4): 265-272.

Bove AA (1984). Increased conjugated dopamine in plasma after exercise training. *J. Lab. Clin. Med.* 104: 77.

Broughton DL, Taylor R (1991). Review: Deterioration of glucose tolerance with age: The role of insulin resistance. *Age and Ageing* 20: 221-225.

Buster JE, Casson PR, Straughn AB (1992). Postmenopausal steroid replacement with micronized dehydroepiandrosterone: Preliminary oral bioavailability and dose proportionality studies. *Am. J. Obstet. Gynecol.* 166(4): 1163-1170.

Chavali SR, Zhong WW, Utsunomiya T, Forse RA (1997). Decreased production of interleukin-1-beta, prostaglandin-E2 and thromboxane-B2, and elevated levels of interleukin-6 and -10 are associated with increased survival during endotoxic shock in mice consuming diets enriched with sesame seed oil supplemented with Quil-A saponin. *Int. Arch. Allergy Immunol.* 114(2): 153-160.

Claassen N, Coetzer H, Steinmann CM, Kruger MC (1995). The effect of different n-6/n-3 essential fatty acid ratios on calcium balance and bone in rats. *Prostaglandins Leukot. Essent. Fatty Acids* 53(1): 13-19.

Cordova A, Alvarez-Mon M (1995). Behaviour of zinc in physical exercise: A special reference to immunity and fatigue. *Neurosci. Biobehav. Rev.* 519(3): 439-445.

Coulston AM, Liu GC, Reaven GM (1993). Plasma glucose, insulin and lipid responses to high-carbohydrate low-fat diets in normal humans. *Metabolism* 32: 52-56.

Craig BW, Everhart J, Brown R (1989). The influence of high-resistance training on glucose tolerance in young and elderly subjects. *Mech. Aging Dev.* 49(2): 147-157.

Dajani EZ, Wilson DE, Agrawal NM (1991). Prostaglandins: An overview of the worldwide clinical experience. *J. Assoc. Acad. Minor Phys.* 2(1): 23.

De Cree C, Lewin R, Barros A (1995). Hypoestrogenemia and rhabdomyelysis (myoglobinuria) in the female judoist: A new worrying phenomenon? *J. Clin. Endocrinol. Metab.* 80(12): 3639-3646.

Dekkers JC, van Doornen LJ, Kemper HC (1996). The role of antioxidant vitamins and enzymes in the prevention of exercise-induced muscle damage. *Sports Med.* 21(3): 213-238.

Desimone DP, Green VS, Hannon KS, Turner RT, Bell NH (1993). Prostaglandin E2 administered by subcutaneous pellets causes local inflammation and systemic bone loss: A model for inflammation-induced bone disease. *J. Bone Miner. Res.* 8(5): 625-634.

Despret S, Dinh L, Clement M, Bourre JM (1992). Alteration of delta-6 desaturase by vitamin E in rat brain and liver. *Neurosci. Lett.* 145(1): 19-22.

Dillard CJ, Litov RE, Savin WM, Dumelin EE, Tappel AL (1978). Effects of exercise, vitamin E and ozone on pulmonary function and lipid peroxidation. *J. Appl. Physiol.* 45: 927-932.

Ding JH, Sheckter CB, Drinkwater BL, Soules MR, Bremner WJ (1988). High serum cortisol levels in exercise-associated amenorrhea. *Ann. Intern. Med.* 108(4): 530-534.

Di Pietro S, Suraci C (1990). Metabolic abnormalities in first-degree relatives of type 2 diabetics. *Boll. Soc. It. Biol. Sper.* 7: 631-638.

Eder K, Kirchgessner M (1996). Zinc deficiency and the desaturation of linoleic acid in rats force-fed fat-free diets. *Biol. Trace Elem. Res.* 54(2): 173-183.

Funk CD (1993). Molecular biology in the eicosanoid field. *Prog. Nucleic Acid Res. Mol. Biol.* 45: 67-98.

Gardiner NS, Duncan JR (1988). Enhanced prostaglandin synthesis as a mechanism for inhibition of melanoma cell growth by ascorbic acid. *Prostaglandins Leukot. Essent. Fatty Acids* 34(2): 119-126.

Ghiselli A, D'Amicis A, Giacosa A (1997). The antioxidant potential of the Mediterranean diet. *Eur. J. Cancer Prev.* 6(1): S15-S19.

Granner DK (1993). Hormones of the pancreas and gastrointestinal tract. In *Harper's biochemistry*, eds. RK Murray, DK Granner, PA Mayes, VW Rodwell. 23rd edition, pp. 562-563. East Norwalk, CT: Appleton & Lange.

Gray JB, Martinovic AM (1994). Eicosanoids and essential fatty acid modulation in chronic disease and the chronic fatigue syndrome. *Med. Hypotheses* 45(2): 219.

Groop L, Forsblom C, Lehtovirta M (1997). Characterization of the prediabetic state. *Am. J. Hypertens.* 10 (9 Part 2): 172S-180S.

Hakkinen K, Pakarinen A, Alen M, Kauhanen H, Komi PV (1988). Neuromuscular and hormonal adaptations in athletes to strength training in two years. *J. Appl. Physiol.* 65(6): 2406-2412.

Hoogeveen AR, Zonderland ML (1996). Relationships between testosterone, cortisol and performance in professional cyclists. *Int. J. Sports Med.* 17(6): 423-428.

Hughes VA, Fiatarone MA, Ferrara CM, McNamara JR, Charnley JM, Evans WJ (1994). Lipoprotein response to exercise training and a low-fat diet in older subjects with glucose intolerance. *Am. J. Clin. Nutr.* 59: 820-826.

Innis SM (1996). Essential dietary lipids. In *Present knowledge in nutrition,* 7th ed., eds. EE Ziegler, LJ Filer. Washington, DC: International Life Sciences Institute.

Jenkins RR, Friedland R, Howard H (1984). The relationship of oxygen uptake to superoxide dismutase and catalase activity in human muscle. *Int. J. Sports Med.* 95: 11-14.

Johnson MM, Swan DD, Surette ME, Stegner J, Chilton T, Fonteh AN, Chilton FH (1997). Dietary supplementation with gamma-linolenic acid alters fatty acid content and eicosanoid production in healthy humans. *J. Nutr.* 127(8): 1435-1444.

Kasper S, Rogers SL, Yancey AL, Schulz PM, Skwerer RG, Rosenthal NE (1988). Phototherapy in subsyndromal seasonal affective disorder (S-SAD) and "diagnosed" controls. *Pharmacopyschiatry* 21(6): 42809

Keizer H, Janssen GM, Menheere P, Kranenburg G (1989). Changes in basal plasma testosterone, cortisol and dehydroepiandrosterone sulfate in previously untrained males and females preparing for a marathon. *Int. J. Sports Med.* 10(3): S139-S145.

Kirwan JP, Costill DL, Flynn MG, Mitchess JB, Fink WJ, Neufer PD, Houmard JA (1988). Physiological response to successive days of intense training in competitive swimmers. *Med. Sci. Sports Exerc.* 20: 255-259.

Koester MC (1993). An overview of the physiology and pharmacology of aspirin and nonsteroidal anti-inflammatory drugs. *J. Athl. Training* 28(3): 252-260.

Konig D, Berg A, Weinstock C, Keul J, Northoff H (1997). Essential fatty acids, immune function, and exercise. *Exerc. Immunol. Rev.* 3: 1-31.

Krieger NS (1997). Parathyroid hormone, prostaglandin E2, and 1,25-dihydroxyvitamin D3 decrease the level of Na+-Ca2+ exchange protein in osteoblastic cells. *Calcif. Tissue Int.* 60(5): 473-478.

Laaksonen DE, Atalay M, Niskanen L, Uusitupa M, Hanninen O, Sen CK (1996). Increased resting and exercise-induced oxidative stress in young IDDM men. *Diabetes Care* 319(6): 569-574.

Lawler JM, Cline CC, Hu Z, Coast JR (1997). Effect of oxidative stress and acidosis on diaphragm contractile function. *Am. J. Physiol.* 273(2 Pt 2): R630-636.

Lemann J, Piering WF, Lennon EJ (1969). Possible role of carbohydrate-induced calciuria in calcium oxalate kidney-stone formation. *N. Engl. J. Med.* 280: 232.

Lopez Jimenez JA, Bordoni A, Hrelia S, Rossi CA, Turchetto E, Zamora Navarro S, Biagi PL (1993). Evidence for a detectable delta-6-desaturase activity in rat heart microsomes: Aging influence on enzyme activity. *Biochem. Biophys. Res. Commun.* 192(3): 1037-1041.

Maffetone P (1996). *Training for endurance.* Stamford, NY: David Barmore Productions.

Maffetone P (1997). *In fitness and in health.* 3d ed. Stamford, NY: David Barmore Productions.

Mahfouz MM, Kummerow FA (1989). Effect of magnesium deficiency on delta 6 desaturase activity and fatty acid composition of rat liver microsomes. *Lipids* 24(8): 727-732.

Maniongui C, Blond JP, Ulmann L, Durand G, Poisson JP, Bezard J (1993). Age-related changes in delta 6 and delta 5 desaturase activities in rat liver microsomes. *Lipids* 28(4): 291-297.

Mantzioris E, James MJ, Gibson RA, Cleland LG (1995). Differences exist in the relationships between dietary linoleic and alpha-linolenic acids and their respective long-chain metabolites. *Am. J. Clin. Nutr.* 61: 320-324.

Maranesi M, Barzanti V, Coccheri S, Marchetti M, Tolomelli B (1993). Interaction between vitamin B6 deficiency and low EFA dietary intake on kidney phospholipids and PGE2 in the rat. *Prostaglandins Leukot. Essent. Fatty Acids* 49(1): 531-536.

Marra CA, de Alaniz MJ (1989). Influence of testosterone administration on the biosynthesis of unsaturated fatty acids in male and female rats. *Lipids* 24(12): 1014-1019.

Mayes PA (1993). Metabolism of unsaturated fatty acids & eicosanoids. In *Harper's biochemistry,* 23d ed., eds. RK Murray, DK Granner, PA Mayes, VW Rodwell, pp. 232-240. Norwalk, CT: Appleton & Lange.

McArdle WD, Katch FI, Katch VL (1991). *Exercise physiology.* 3d ed., p. 727. Philadelphia: Lea & Febiger.

Medeiros LC, Liu YW, Park S, Chang PH, Smith AM (1995). Insulin, but not estrogen, correlated with indexes of desaturase function in obese women. *Horm. Metab. Res.* 27(5): 235-238.

Mills DE, Huang YS, Narce M, Poisson JP (1994). Psychosocial stress, catecholamines, and essential fatty acid metabolism in rats. *Proc. Soc. Exp. Biol. Med.* 205(1): 56-61.

Mills PC, Smith NC, Casas I, Harris P, Harris RC, Marlin DJ (1996). Effects of exercise intensity and environmental stress on indices of oxidative stress and iron homeostatis during exercise in the horse. *Eur J. Appl. Physiol.* 74(1-2): 60-66.

Moller P, Wallin H, Knudsen LE (1996). Oxidative stress associated with exercise, psychological stress and life-style factors. *Chem. Biol. Interact.* 102(1): 17-36.

Nestler JE (1994). Assessment of insulin resistance. *Scientific American*, Science and Medicine. September/October: 58-67.

Nestler JE, Jakubowicz DJ (1996). Decreases in ovarian cytochrome P450c17a activity and serum free testosterone after reduction of insulin secretion in polycystic ovary syndrome. *N. Engl. J. Med.* 335: 617-623.

Nestler JE, Strauss JF (1991). Insulin as an effector of human ovarian and adrenal steroid metabolism. *Endocrinol. Metab. Clin. North Am.* 20(4): 807-823.

Newsholme E (1994). Biochemical mechanisms to explain immunosuppression in well-trained and overtrained athletes. *Int. J. Sports Med.* 3: S142-147.

Nieman DC (1997a). Exercise immunology: Practical applications. *Int. J. Sports Med.* 18(1): S91-S100.

Nieman DC (1997b). Immune response to heavy exertion. *J. Appl. Physiol.* 82(5): 1385-1394.

Orentreich N, Brind JL, Rizer RL, Vogelman JH (1984). Age changes and sex differences in serum dehydroepiandrosterone sulfate concentrations throughout adulthood. *J. Clin. Endocrinol. Metab.* 59(3): 551-555.

Packer L (1997). Oxidants, antioxidant nutrients and the athlete. *J. Sports Sci.* 15(3): 353-363.

Parker LN, Levin ER, Lifrak ET (1985). Evidence for adrenocortical adaptation to severe illness. *J. Clin. Endocrinol. Metab.* 60: 947-952.

Pedersen BK, Rohde T, Zacho M (1996). Immunity in athletes. *J. Sports Med. Phys. Fitness* 36(4): 236-245.

Poisson JP, Huang YS, Mills DE, de Antueno RJ, Redden PR, Lin X, Narce M, Horrobin DF (1993). Effect of salt-loading and spontaneous hypertension on in vitro metabolism of [1-14C]linoleic and [2-14C]dihomo-gamma-linolenic acids. *Biochem. Med. Metab. Biol.* 49(1): 57-66.

Pulkkinen MO, Maenpaa J (1983). Decrease in serum testosterone concentration during treatment with tetracycline. *Acta Endocrinol.* (Copenhagen) 103(2): 269-272.

Reaven GM (1988). Role of insulin resistance in human disease. *Diabetes* 37: 1595-1607.

Reaven GM (1995). Pathophysiology of insulin resistance in human disease. *Physiol. Rev.* 75: 473-486.

Reaven GM (1997). Do high carbohydrate diets prevent the development or attenuate the manifestations (or both) of syndrome X? A viewpoint strongly against. *Curr. Opin. Lipidol.* 8(1): 23-27.

Roberts AC, McClure RD, Weiner RI, Brooks GA (1993). Overtraining affects male reproductive status. *Fertil. Steril.* 60(4): 686-692.

Rogers MA, King DS, Hagberg JM, Ehsani AA, Holloszy JO (1990). Effect of 10 days of physical inactivity on glucose tolerance in master athletes. *J. Appl. Physiol.* 68(5): 1833-1837.

Rosen LW, Smokler C, Carrier D, Shafer CL, McKeag DB (1996). Seasonal mood disturbances in collegiate hockey players. *J. Athl. Training* 31(3): 225-228.

Rosenthal NE, Sack DA, Gillin JC, Lewy AJ, Goodwin FK, Davenport Y, Mueller PS, Newsome DA, Wehr TA (1984). Seasonal affective disorder. A description of the syndrome and preliminary findings with light therapy. *Arch. Gen. Psychiatry* 41(1): 72-80.

Rudin DO (1982). The dominant diseases of modernized societies as omega-3 essential fatty acid deficiency syndrome: Substrate pellagra. *Med. Hypotheses* 8: 17-47.

Seals DR, Hagberg JM, Allen WK, Hurley BF, Dalsky GP, Ehsani AA, Holloszy JO (1984). Glucose tolerance in young and older athletes and sedentary men. *J. Appl. Physiol.* 56(6): 1521-1525.

Sen CK (1995). Oxidants and antioxidants in exercise. *J. Appl. Physiol.* 79(3): 675-686.

Shepard RJ, Shek PN (1996). Impact of physical activity and sport on the immune system. *Rev. Environ. Health* 11(3): 133-147.

Simopoulos AP (1994). Is insulin resistance influenced by dietary linoleic acid and trans fatty acids? *Free Radical Biology & Medicne.* 17 (4):367-372.

Simopoulos AP (1997). Omega-6/omega-3 fatty acid ratio and trans fatty acids in non-insulin-dependent diabetes mellitus. *Ann. NY Acad. Sci.* 827: 327-338.

Song MK, Rosenthal MJ, Naliboff BD, Phanumas L, Kang KW (1998). Effects of bovine prostate powder on zinc, glucose, and insulin metabolism in old patients with non-insulin-dependent diabetes mellitus. *Metabolism* 47(1): 39-43.

Stallknecht B, Kjaer M, Mikines KJ, Maroun L, Ploug T, Ohkuwa T, Vinten J, Galbo H (1990). Diminished epinephrine response to hypoglycemia despite enlarged adrenal medulla in trained rats. *Am. J. Physiol.* 259 (5 Part 2): R998-R1003.

Storlien LH, Kriketos AD, Calvert GD, Baur LA, Jenkins AB (1997). Fatty acids, triglycerides and syndromes of insulin resistance. *Prostaglandins Leukot. Essent. Fatty Acids* 57(4-5): 379-385.

Swinburn BA, Gianchandani R, Saad MF, Lillioja S (1995). In vivo beta-cell function at the transition to early non-insulin-dependent diabetes mellitus. *Metabolism* 44(6): 757-764.

Tiidus PM, Pushkarenko J, Houston ME (1996). Lack of antioxidant adaptation to short-term aerobic training in human muscle. *Am. J. Physiol.* 271(4 Part 2): R832-R836.

Ulmann L, Blond JP, Maniongui C, Poisson JP, Durand G, Bezard J, Pascal G (1991). Effects of age and dietary essential fatty acids on desaturase activities and on fatty acid composition of liver microsomal phospholipids of adult rats. *Lipids* 26(2): 127-133.

Umeda-Sawada R, Takahashi N, Igarashi O (1995). Interaction of sesamin and eicosapentaenoic acid against delta 5 desaturation and n-6/n-3 ratio of essential fatty acids in rat. *Biosci. Biotechnol. Biochem.* 59(12): 2268-2273.

Urhausen A, Gabriel H, Kindermann W (1997). Blood hormones as markers of training stress and overtraining. *Sports Med.* 20(4): 251-276.

Ves-Losada A, Peluffo RO (1993). Effect of L-triiodothyronine on liver microsomal delta 6 and delta 5 desaturase activity of male rats. *Mol. Cell Biochem.* 121(2): 149-153.

Wasserman DH, O'Doherty RM, Zinker BA (1995). Role of the endocrine pancreas in control of fuel metabolism by the liver during exercise. *Int. J. Obes. Relat. Metab. Disord.* 19(4): S22-30.

Weidner TG, Gehlsen G, Schurr T, Dwyer GB (1997). Effects of viral upper respiratory illness on running gait. *J. Athl. Training* 32(4): 309-314.

Wilmore JH, Costill DL (1994). *Physiology of sport and exercise,* pp. 136-137. Champaign, IL: Human Kinetics.

Yu BP (1996). Aging and oxidative stress: Modulation by dietary restriction. *Free Radic. Biol. Med.* 21(5): 651-658.

Zimmet PZ, Collins VR, Dowse GK, Knight LT (1992). Hyperinsulinaemia in youth is a predictor of Type 2 (non-insulin-dependent) diabetes mellitus. *Diabetologia* 35: 534-541.

CHAPTER 7

Baron S, Hales T, Hurrell J (1996). Evaluation of symptom surveys for occupational musculoskeletal disorders. *Am. J. Ind. Med.* 29(6): 609-617.

Bingham SA, Cassidy A, Cole TJ, Welch A, Runswick SA, Black AE, Thurnham D, Bates C, Khaw KT, Key TJ, et al. (1995). Validation of weighed records and other methods of dietary assessment using the 24 h urine nitrogen technique and other biological markers. *Br. J. Nutr.* 73(4): 531-550.

De Castro JM (1994). Methodology, correlational analysis, and interpretation of diet diary records of the food and fluid intake of free-living humans. *Appetite* 23(2): 179-192.

Fowler PB (1997). Evidence-based diagnosis. *J. Eval. Clin. Pract.* 3(2): 153-159.

Franzblau A, Salerno DF, Armstrong TJ, Werner RA (1997). Test-retest reliability of an upper-extremity discomfort questionnaire in an industrial population. *Scand. J. Work Environ. Health* 23(4): 299-307.

Laemmel K (1996). Interview in medicine. *Schweiz. Rundsch. Med. Prax.* 85(27-28): 863-869.

Laubli T, Thomas C, Hinnen U, Hunting W, Zeier H, Mion H (1991). Assessment of musculoskeletal disorders using a questionnaire (German). *Soz. Praventivmed.* 36(1): 25-33.

Terezhalmy GT, Schiff T (1986). The historical profile. *Dent. Clin. North Am.* 30(3): 357-368.

Winkler P (1979). The importance of history-taking in the diagnosis of inflammatory-rheumatic disease: A prospective study of 100 patients. *Dtsch. Med. Wochenschr.* 104(37): 1301-1306.

CHAPTER 8

Alpher VS, Nelson RB 3d, Blanton RL (1986). Effects of cognitive and psychomotor tasks on breath-holding span. *J. Appl. Physiol.* 61(3): 1149-1152.

Anderson LC, Garrett JR, Johnson DA, Kauffman DL, Keller PJ, Thulin A (1984). Influence of circulating catecholamines on protein secretion into rat parotid saliva during parasympathetic stimulation. *J. Physiol.* (London) 352: 163-171.

Asztely A, Tobin G, Ekstrom J (1996). The role of circulating catecholamines in the depletion of parotid acinar granules in conscious rats in the cold. *Exp. Physiol.* 81(1): 107-117.

Barnes B (1942). Basal temperature versus basal metabolism. *JAMA* 119: 163.

Barnes B, Barnes C (1972). *Heart attack rareness in thyroid-treated patients.* Springfield, IL: Charles C Thomas.

Barron JL, Noakes TD, Levy W, Smith C, Millar RP (1985). Hypothalamic dysfunction in overtrained athletes. *J. Clin. Endocrinol. Metab.* 60(4): 803-806.

Bartlett D Jr (1977). Effects of Valsalva and Mueller maneuvers on breath-holding time. *J. Appl. Physiol.* 42(5): 717-721.

Benfante R, Reed D, Brody J (1985). Biological and social predictors of health in an aging cohort. *J. Chronic Dis.* 38(5): 385-395.

Berkow MD (1992). *The Merck manual of diagnosis and therapy,* pp. 434-437. Rahway, NJ: Merck & Co., Inc.

Brandon JE, Loftin JM, Curry J Jr (1991). Role of fitness in mediating stress: A correlational exploration of stress reactivity. *Percept. Mot. Skills* 73(3 Part 2): 1171-1180.

Bunch TW (1980). Blood test abnormalities in runners. *Mayo Clin. Proc.* 55(2): 113-117.

Burchfiel CM, Enright PL, Sharp DS, Chyou PH, Rodriguez BL, Curb JD (1997). Factors associated with variations in pulmonary function among elderly Japanese-American men. *Chest* 112(1): 87-97.

Burrows B, Cline MG, Knudson RJ, Taussig LM, Lebowitz MD (1983). A descriptive analysis of the growth and decline of the FVC and FEV1. *Chest* 83(5): 717-724.

Chen Y, Horne SL, Dosman JA (1993). Body weight and weight gain related to pulmonary function decline in adults: A six year follow up study. *Thorax* 48(4): 375-380.

Chorot P, Sandin B, Fernandez-Trespalacios JL (1992). Pavlovian conditioning of phobic fear: Effects on skin and salivary pH. *Int. J. Psychosom.* 39(1-4): 56-61. Abstract.

Chyou PH, White LR, Yano K, Sharp DS, Burchfiel CM, Chen R, Rodrigues BL, Curb JD (1996). Pulmonary function measures as predictors and correlates of cognitive function in later life. *Am. J. Epidemiol.* 143(8): 750-756.

Convertino VA (1993). Endurance exercise training: Conditions of enhanced hemodynamic responses and tolerance to LBNP. *Med. Sci. Sports Exerc.* 25(6): 705-712.

De Cree C, Lewin R, Barros A (1995). Hypoestrogenemia and rhabdomyelysis (myoglobinuria) in the female judoist: A new worrying phenomenon? *J. Clin. Endocrinol. Metab.* 80(12): 3639-3646.

De Lorenzo F, Hargreaves J, Kakkar VV (1997). Pathogenesis and management of delayed orthostatic hypotension in patients with chronic fatigue syndrome. *Clin. Auton. Res.* 7(4): 185-190.

Dickson DN, Wilkinson RL, Noakes TD (1982). Effects of ultra-marathon training and racing on hematologic parameters and serum ferritin levels in well-trained athletes. *Int. J. Sports Med.* 3(2): 111-117.

Ding JH, Sheckter CB, Drinkwater BL, Soules MR, Bremner WJ (1988). High serum cortisol levels in exercise-associated amenorrhea. *Ann. Intern. Med.* 108(4): 530-534.

Douglas PD (1989). Effect of a season of competition and training on hematological status of women field hockey and soccer players. *J. Sports Med. Phys. Fitness* 29(2): 179-183.

Duncan BB, Chambless LE, Schmidt MI, Folsom AR, Szklo M, Crouse JR III, Carpenter MA (1995). Association of the waist-to-hip ratio is different with wine than with beer or hard liquor consumption. *Am. J. Epidemiol.* 142: 1034-1038.

Fasano ML, Sand T, Brubakk AO, Kruszewski P, Bordini C, Sjuaastad O (1996). Reproducibility of the cold pressor test: Studies in normal subjects. *Clin. Auton. Res.* 6(5): 249-253.

Feiner JR, Bickler PE, Severinghaus JW (1995). Hypoxic ventilatory response predicts the extent of maximal breath-holds in man. *Respir. Physiol.* 100(3): 213-222.

Foldes J, Istvanfy M, Halmagyi M, Varadi A, Gara A, Partos O (1987). Hypothyroidism and the heart. Examination of left ventricular function in subclinical hypothyroidism. *Acta Med. Hung.* 44(4): 337-347.

Gay SB, Sistrom CL, Holder CA, Suratt PM (1994). Breath-holding capability of adults. Implications for spiral computed tomography, fast-acquisition magnetic resonance imaging, and angiography. *Invest. Radiol.* 29(9): 848-851.

Gottlieb DJ, Sparrow D, O'Connor GT, Weiss ST (1996). Skin test reactivity to common aeroallergens and decline of lung function. The Normative Aging Study. *Am. J. Respir. Crit. Care Med.* 153(2): 561-566.

Guyton AC (1986). *Textbook of medical physiology,* p. 849. Philadelphia: Saunders.

Hagberg JM, Yerg JE, Seals DR (1988). Pulmonary function in young and older athletes and untrained men. *J. Appl. Physiol.* 65(1): 101-105.

Hajek P (1989). Breath holding and success in stopping smoking: What does breath holding measure? *Int. J. Addict.* 24(7): 633-639.

Hawkins H (1947). *Applied nutrition,* pp. 29-46. Palmyra, WI: Lee Foundation.

Hendrix TR (1974). The absorptive function of the alimentary canal. In *Medical physiology,* ed. VB Mountcastle, p. 1155. St. Louis: Mosby.

Herkenhoff F, Limia EG, Mill JG (1994). Arterial pressure reactivity to experimental stress tests in normotensive humans with arterial pressure hyperreactivity during submaximal exercise. *Braz. J. Med. Biol. Res.* 27(6): 1425-1430.

Hitsuda Y (1994). Non-respiratory factors and pulmonary function tests. *Rinsho. Byori.* 42(4): 407-412.

Hubinger L, Mackinnon LT, Lepre F (1995). Lipoprotein(a) [Lp(a)] levels in middle-aged male runners and sedentary controls. *Med. Sci. Sports Exerc.* 27(4): 490-496.

Irving RA, Noakes TD, Rodgers AL, Swartz L (1986). Crystalluria in marathon runners. *Urol. Res.* 14(6): 289-294.

Jacob G, Robertson D, Mosqueda-Garcia R, Ertl AC, Robertson RM, Biaggioni I (1997). Hypovolemia in syncope and orthostatic intolerance role of the renin-angiotensin system. *Am. J. Med.* 103(2): 128-133.

Jones DA, Rollman GB, Brooke RI (1997). The cortisol response to psychological stress in temporomandibular dysfunction. *Pain* 72(1-2): 171-182.

Jorgensen U (1990). Body load in heel-strike running: The effect of a firm heel counter. *Am. J. Sports Med.* 18(2): 177-181.

Keizer H, Janssen GM, Menheere P, Kranenburg G (1989). Changes in basal plasma testosterone, cortisol, and dehydroepiandrosterone sulfate in previously untrained males and females preparing for a marathon. *Int. J. Sports Med.* 10(Suppl. 3): S139-S145.

Kesavachandran C, Shashidhar S (1997). Respiratory function during warm-up exercise in athletes. *Indian J. Physiol. Pharmacol.* 41(2): 159-163.

Kolopp-Sarda MN, Moneret-Vautrin DA, Gobert B, Kanny G, Brodschii M, Bene MC, Faure GC (1997). Specific humoral immune responses in 12 cases of food sensitization to sesame seed. *Clin. Exp. Allergy* 27(11): 1285-1291.

Lange P, Groth S, Mortensen J, Appleyard M, Nyboe J, Schnohr P, Jensen G (1990). Diabetes mellitus and ventilatory capacity: A five year follow-up study. *Eur. Respir. J.* 3(3): 288-292.

Leaf DA, Allen D (1998). Respiratory exchange ratio slope: A new concept in the determination of physical fitness and exercise training. *Ann. Sports Med.* 3(4): 210-214.

Levine BD (1993). Regulation of central blood volume and cardiac filling in endurance athletes: The Frank-Starling mechanism as a determinant of orthostatic tolerance. *Med. Sci. Sports Exerc.* 25(6): 727-732.

Luft D, Lay A, Benda N, Kort C, Hofmann V, Hardin H, Renn W (1996). Pain intensity and blood pressure reactions during a cold pressor test in IDDM patients. *Diabetes Care* 19(7): 722-725.

Lukaski HC, Penland JG (1996). Functional changes appropriate for determining mineral element requirements. *J. Nutr.* 126: 2354S-2364S.

Madanmohan D, Thombre DP, Balakumar B, Nambinarayanan TK, Thakur S, Krishnamurthy N, Chandrabose A (1992). Effect of yoga training on reaction time, respiratory endurance and muscle strength. *Indian J. Physiol. Pharmacol.* 3(4): 229-233.

Maffetone P (1996). *Training for endurance,* pp. 151-153. Stamford, NY: David Barmore Productions.

Maffetone P (1997). *In fitness and in health.* 3d ed., p. 257. Stamford, NY: David Barmore Productions.

Malmberg LP, Hedman J, Sovijarvi AR (1993). Accuracy and repeatability of a pocket turbine spirometer: Comparison with a rolling seal flow-volume spirometer. *Clin. Physiol.* 13(1): 89-98.

Mayes PA (1993). Digestion & absorption. In *Harper's biochemistry,* 23d ed., eds. RK Murray, DK Granner, PA Mayes, VW Rodwell, pp. 609-614. Norwalk, CT: Appleton & Lange.

McArdle WD, Katch FI, Katch VL (1991). *Exercise physiology.* 3d ed., p. 727. Philadelphia: Lea & Febiger.

Ibid. p. 557.

Ibid. p. 273.

Ibid. p. 153.

McCarthy JP, Bamman MM, Yelle JM, Le Blanc AD, Rowe RM, Greenisen MC, Lee SM, Spector ER, Fortney SM (1997). Resistance exercise training and the orthostatic response. *Eur. J. Appl. Physiol.* 76(1): 32-40.

Mishra N, Mahajan KK (1996). Cardiovascular response to orthostatic stress following cold challenge in diabetics. *J. Indian Med. Assoc.* 94(1): 3-5.

Miyajima H, Sakamoto M, Takahashi Y, Mizoguchi K, Nishimura Y (1989). Muscle carnitine deficiency associated with myalgia and rhabdomyolysis following exercise. *Rinsho. Shinkeigaku* 29(1): 93-97.

Muller MJ, Seitz HJ (1984). Thyroid hormone action on intermediary metabolism. Part I: Respiration, thermogenesis and carbohydrate metabolism. *Klin. Wochenschr.* 62(1): 11-18.

Mundal R, Kjeldsen SE, Sandvik L, Erikssen G, Thaulow E, Erikssen J (1994). Exercise blood pressure predicts cardiovascular mortality in middle-aged men. *Hypertension* 24(1): 56-62.

Murphy PJ, Campbell SS (1997). Nighttime drop in body temperature: A physiological trigger for sleep onset? *Sleep* 20(7): 505-511.

Murphy PJ, Myers BL, Badia P (1996). Nonsteroidal anti-inflammatory drugs alter body temperature and suppress melatonin in humans. *Physiol. Behav.* 59(1): 133-139.

Nazar K, Kaciuba-Uscilko H, Ziemba W, Krysztofiak H, Wojcik-Ziolkowska E, Niewiadomski W, Chwalbinska-Moneta J, Bicz B, Stupnicka E, Okinczyc A (1997). Physiological characteristics and hormonal profile of young normotensive men with exaggerated blood pressure response to exercise. *Clin. Physiol.* 17(1): 1-18.

Nestler JE (1994). Assessment of insulin resistance. *Scientific American,* Science & Medicine, September/October, 58-67.

Ng AV, Callister R, Johnson DG, Seals DR (1994). Endurance exercise training is associated with elevated basal sympathetic nerve activity in healthy older humans. *J. Appl. Physiol.* 77(3): 1366-1374.

Northover B, O'Malley BP, Rosenthal FD (1983). Alterations in systolic time intervals in primary hypothyroidism as a consequence of warming. *J. Clin. Endocrinol. Metab.* 56(1): 185-188.

O'Connor PJ, Morgan WP, Raglin JS, Barksdale CM, Kalin NH (1989). Mood state and salivary cortisol levels following overtraining in female swimmers. *Psychoneuroendocrinology* 14(4): 303-310.

O'Malley BP, Davies TJ, Rosenthal FD (1980). TSH responses to temperature in primary hypothyroidism. *Clin. Endocrinol.* (Oxford) 13(1): 87-94.

Orlando P, Perdelli F, Gallelli G, Reggiani E, Cristina ML, Oberto C (1994). Increased blood lead levels in runners training in urban areas. *Arch. Environ. Health* 49(3): 200-203.

Perez-Padilla R, Cervantes D, Chapela R, Selman M (1989). Rating of breathlessness at rest during acute asthma: Correlation with spirometry and usefulness of breath-holding time. *Rev. Invest. Clin.* 41(3): 209-213.

Peters JR, Walker RF, Riad-Fahmy D, Hall R (1982). Salivary cortisol assays for assessing pituitary-adrenal reserve. *Clin. Endocrinol.* (Oxford) 17(6): 583-592.

Polinsky RJ, Kopin IJ, Ebert MH, Weise V (1980). The adrenal medullary response to hypoglycemia in patients with orthostatic hypotension. *J. Clin. Endocrinol. Metab.* 51(6): 1401-1406.

Puvi-Rajasingham S, Mathias CJ (1996). Effect of meal size on post-prandial blood pressure and on postural hypotension in primary autonomic failure. *Clin. Auton. Res.* 6(2): 111-114.

Rashed HM, Leventhal G, Madu EC, Reddy R, Cardoso S (1997). Reproducibility of exercise-induced modulation of cardiovascular responses to cold stress. *Clin. Auton. Res.* 7(2): 93-96.

Raven PB, Pawelczyk JA (1993). Chronic endurance exercise training: A condition of inadequate blood pressure regulation and reduced tolerance to LBNP. *Med. Sci. Sports Exerc.* 25(6): 713-721.

Rebuck DA, Hanania NA, D'Urzo AD, Chapman KR (1996). The accuracy of a handheld portable spirometer. *Chest* 109(1): 152-157.

Rijcken B, Schouten JP, Weiss ST, Speizer FE, van der Lende R (1988). The relationship between airway responsiveness to histamine and pulmonary function level in a random population sample. *Am. Rev. Respir. Dis.* 137(4): 826-832.

Saito I, Ito K, Saruta T (1983). Hypothyroidism as a cause of hypertension. *Hypertension* 5(1): 112-115.

Sakai K, Maguchi M, Kohara K, Nishida W, Wakamiya R, Hara-Nakamura N, Mukai M, Yokoyama A, Hiwada K (1996). A case of idiopathic orthostatic hypotension manifesting sick sinus syndrome due to sympathetic nervous dysfunction. *Nippon Ronen. Igakkai Zasshi.* 33(2): 105-109.

Saltin B, Hermansen L (1966). Esophageal, rectal and muscle temperature during exercise. *J. Appl. Physiol.* 21: 1757.

Sanderson JE, Woo KS, Chung HK, Chan WM, Tse KK, White HD (1997). Endothelium-dependent dilation of the coronary arteries in syndrome X: Effects of the cold pressor test. *Cardiology* 88(5): 414-417.

Schoene RB, Giboney K, Schimmel C, Hagen J, Robinson J, Schoene RB, Sato W, Sullivan KN (1997). Spirometry and airway reactivity in elite track and field athletes. *Clin. J. Sport Med.* 7(4): 257-261.

Seals DR (1990). Sympathetic activation during the cold pressor test: Influence of stimulus area. *Clin. Physiol.* 10(2): 123-129.

Sehnert KW, Croft AC (1996). Basal metabolic temperature vs. laboratory assessment in "posttraumatic hypothyroidism." *J. Manipulative Physiol. Ther.* 19(1): 6-12.

Shadick NA, Sparrow D, O'Connor GT, DeMolles D, Weiss ST (1996). Relationship of serum IgE concentration to level and rate of decline of pulmonary function. The Normative Aging Study. *Thorax* 51(8): 787-792.

Shimizu M, Kitazumi H, Kawabe T, Niitsuma K, Kawaguchi T, Nishiyama K, Kajita M, Noro C, Tsuyusaki T, Kikawada R (1992). Comparison of treadmill exercise, handgrip, and cold-pressor tests: With particular reference to the effects on hemodynamics, respiratory gas exchange, and sympathetic nervous activity. *J. Cardiol.* 22(2-3): 557-568.

Sparrow D, Glynn RJ, Cohen M, Weiss ST (1984). The relationship of the peripheral leukocyte count and cigarette smoking to pulmonary function among adult men. *Chest* 86(3): 383-386.

Sparrow D, O'Connor GT, Rosner B, De Molles D, Weiss ST (1993). A longitudinal study of plasma cortisol concentration and pulmonary function decline in men. The Normative Aging Study. *Am. Rev. Respir. Dis.* 147(6 Part 1): 1345-1348.

Sparrow D, Silbert JE, Weiss ST (1982). The relationship of pulmonary function to copper concentrations in drinking water. *Am. Rev. Respir. Dis.* 126(2): 312-315.

Sparrow D, Weiss ST, Vokonas PS, Cupples LA, Ekerdt DJ, Colton T (1988). Forced vital capacity and the risk of hypertension. The Normative Aging Study. *Am. J. Epidemiol.* 127(4): 734-741.

Stanley NN, Cunningham EL, Altose MD, Kelsen SG, Levinson RS, Cherniack NS (1975). Evaluation of breath holding in hypercapnia as a simple clinical test of respiratory chemosensitivity. *Thorax* 30(3): 337-343.

Staubli M, Roessler B, Kochli HP, Peheim E, Straub PW (1985). Creatine kinase and creatine kinase MB in endurance runners and in patients with myocardial infarction. *Eur. J. Appl. Physiol.* 54(1): 40-45.

Taskar V, Clayton N, Atkins M, Shaheen Z, Stone P, Woodcock A (1995). Breath-holding time in normal subjects, snorers, and sleep apnea patients. *Chest* 107(4): 959-962.

Telford RD, Cunningham RB (1991). Sex, sport, and body-size dependency of hematology in highly trained athletes. *Med. Sci. Sports Exerc.* 23(7): 788-794.

Urhausen A, Gabriel H, Kindermann W (1997). Blood hormones as markers of training stress and overtraining. *Sports Med.* 20(4): 251-276.

Vacek L (1997). Incidence of exercise-induced asthma in high school population in British Columbia. *Allergy Asthma Proc.* 18(2): 89-91.

Vana S, Foldes J, Nemec J, Zamrazil V, Bednar J, Zimak J (1990). Subclinical hypothyroidism. *Vnitr. Lek.* (Czech) 36(6): 566-572.

Van Antwerpen VL, Theron AJ, Richards GA, Van Der Merwe CA, Van der Walt R, Anderson R (1995). Relationship between the plasma levels of beta-carotene and lung functions in cigarette smokers. *Int. J. Nutr. Res.* 65(4): 231-235.

van den Berg A, Smit AJ (1997). Bedside autonomic function testing in patients with vasovagal syncope. Pacing. *Clin. Electrophysiol.* 20(8 Part 2): 2039-2042.

Walther DS (1988). *Applied kinesiology synopsis,* p. 477. Pueblo, CO: Systems DC.

Ibid. pp. 470-479.

Weiler JM (1996). Exercise-induced asthma: A practical guide to definitions, diagnosis, prevalence, and treatment. *Allergy Asthma Proc.* 17(6): 315-325.

Weiss ST, Segal MR, Sparrow D, Wager C (1995). Relation of FEV1 and peripheral blood leukocyte count to total mortality. The Normative Aging Study. *Am. J. Epidemiol.* 142(5): 493-498.

Wilmore JH, Costill DL (1994). *Physiology of sport and exercise,* pp. 104-106. Champaign, IL: Human Kinetics.

Yang TM, Chang MS (1990). The mechanism of symptomatic postural hypotension in the elderly. *Chung Hua I Hsueh Tsa Chih* (Taipei) 46(3): 147-155.

CHAPTER 9

Guskiewicz KM, Riemann BL, Perrin DH, Nashner LM (1997). Alternative approaches to the assessment of mild head injury in athletes. *Med. Sci. Sports Exerc.* 29(7 Suppl.): S213-221.

Guyton AC (1986). *Textbook of medical physiology,* pp. 615-616. Philadelphia: Saunders.

Hsieh CY, Phillips RB (1990). Reliability of manual muscle testing with a computerized dynamometer. *J. Manip. Physiol. Ther.* 13(2): 72-82.

Jeong BY (1991). Respiration effect on standing balance. *Arch. Phys. Med. Rehabil.* 72(9): 642-645.

Kendall FP, McCreary EK, Provance PG (1993). *Muscles, testing and function.* 4th ed., pp. 4-5. Baltimore: Williams & Wilkins.

Ibid. p. 7.

Lattanzio PJ, Petrella RJ, Sproule JR, Fowler PJ (1997). Effects of fatigue on knee proprioception. *Clin. J. Sport Med.* 7(1): 22-27.

Lawson A, Calderon L (1997). Interexaminer reliability of applied kinesiology manual muscle testing. *Percept. Mot. Skills* 84: 539-546.

Leisman G, Ferentz A, Zenhausern R, Tefera T, Zemcov A (1995). Electromyographic effects of fatigue and task repetition on the validity of strong and weak muscle estimates in applied kinesiology muscle testing procedures. *Percept. Mot. Skills* 80: 963-977.

Leisman G, Shambaugh P, Ferentz A (1989). Somatosensory evoked potential changes during muscle testing. *Int. J. Neurosci.* 45: 143-151.

Lepers R, Bigard AX, Diard JP, Gouteyron JF, Guezennec CY (1997). Posture control after prolonged exercise. *Eur. J. Appl. Physiol.* 76(1): 55-61.

Li X, Hamdy R, Sandborn W, Chi D, Dyer A (1996). Long-term effects of antidepressants on balance, equilibrium, and postural reflexes. *Psychiatry Rev.* 63(2-3): 191-196.

Liebenson C (1992). Pathogenesis of chronic back pain. *J. Manip. Physiol. Ther.* 15: 299-308.

Marino M, Nicholas JA, Gleim GW, Rosenthal P, Nicholas SJ (1982). The efficacy of manual assessment of muscle strength using a new device. *Am. J. Sports Med.* 10(6): 360-364.

Meigal AY, Lupandin YV, Hanninen O (1996). Head and body positions affect thermoregulatory tonus in deltoid muscles. *J. Appl. Physiol.* 80(4): 1397-1400.

Nakamura T, Meguro K, Yamazaki H, Okuzumi H, Tanaka A, Horikawa A, Yamaguchi K, Katsuyama N, Nakano M, Arai H, Sasaki H (1997). Postural and gait disturbance correlated with decreased frontal cerebral blood flow in Alzheimer disease. *Alzheimer Dis. Assoc. Disord.* 11(3): 132-139.

Nicholas JA, Sapega A, Kraus H, Webb JN (1978). Factors influencing manual muscle tests in physical therapy. *J. Bone Joint Surg.* 60(2): 186-190.

Perot C, Meldener R, Goubel F (1991). Objective measurement of proprioceptive technique consequences on muscular maximal voluntary contraction during manual muscle testing. *Agressologie* (French) 32(10): 471-474.

Petrella RJ, Lattanzio PJ, Nelson MG (1997). Effect of age and activity on knee joint proprioception. *Am. J. Phys. Med. Rehabil.* 76(3): 235-241.

Robbins S, Waked E, McClaran J (1995). Proprioception and stability: Foot position awareness as a function of age and footwear. *Age and Ageing* 24(1): 67-72.

Sakellari V, Bronstein AM, Corna S, Hammon CA, Jones S, Wolsley CJ (1997). The effects of hyperventilation on postural control mechanisms. *Brain* 120 (Part 9): 1659-1673.

Saxton JM, Clarkson PM, James R, Miles M, Westerfer M, Clark S, Donnelly AE (1995). Neuromuscular dysfunction following eccentric exercise. *Med. Sci. Sports Exerc.* 27(8): 1185-1193.

Schmitt WH Jr (1996). Three variations of manual muscle testing. *Proceedings of the International College of Applied Kinesiology—U.S.A.* Vol. 1, p. 63. Shawnee Mission, KS.

Seaman DR (1997). Joint complex dysfunction, a novel term to replace subluxation/subluxation complex: Etiological and treatment considerations. *J. Manip. Physiol. Ther.* 20(9): 634-644.

Shupert CL, Horak FB (1996). Effects of vestibular loss on head stabilization in response to head and body perturbations. *J. Vestib. Res.* 6(6): 423-437.

Simmons R, Richardson C, Pozos R (1997). Postural stability of diabetic patients with and without cutaneous sensory deficit in the foot. *Diabetes Res. Clin. Pract.* 36(3): 153-160.

Wadsworth CT, Krishnan R, Sear M, Harrold J, Nielsen DH (1987). Intrarater reliability of manual muscle testing and hand-held dynametric muscle testing. *Phys. Ther.* 67(9): 1342-1347.

Walther DS (1988). *Applied kinesiology synopsis*, p. 277. Pueblo, CO: Systems DC.

Weidner TG, Gehlsen G, Schurr T, Dwyer GB (1997). Effects of viral upper respiratory illness on running gait. *J. Athl. Training* 32(4): 309-314.

CHAPTER 10

Gray's anatomy. The anatomical basic of medicine and surgery. (1995). 38th edition. New York: Churchill Livingston.

Hall SJ. (1995). *Basic Biomechanics*, pp. 182-184. St. Louis: Mosby.

Kendall FP, McCreary EK, Provance PG (1993). *Muscles, testing and function.* 4th ed., pp. 288-289. Baltimore: Williams & Wilkins.

Richardson AB, Jobe FW, Collins HR (1980). The shoulder in competitive swimming. *Am. J. Sports Med.* 8: 159-161.

Walther DS (1988). *Applied kinesiology synopsis,* p. 324. Pueblo, CO: Systems DC.

CHAPTER 11

Armentia A (1997). Usefulness of specific bronchial challenge in monitoring immunotherapy in occupational asthma. *J. Investig. Allergol. Clin. Immunol.* 7(5): 325-326.

Baumgarten CR, O'Connor A, Dokic D, Schultz KD, Kunkel G (1997). Substance P is generated in vivo following nasal challenge of allergic individuals with bradykinin. *Clin. Exp. Allergy* 27(11): 1322-1327.

Bell IR, Schwartz GE, Bootzin RR, Wyatt JK (1997). Time-dependent sensitization of heart rate and blood pressure over multiple laboratory sessions in elderly individuals with chemical odor intolerance. *Arch. Environ. Health* 52(1): 6-17.

Biasioli S, Schiavon R, Petrosino L, Cavallini L, Zambello A, De Fanti E, Giavarina A (1997). Free radicals and oxidative stress challenge dialysis patients: Effects of two different membranes. *SAIO J.* 43(5): M766-772.

Callahan RJ (1985). *How executives overcome the fear of public speaking and other phobias.* Wilmington, DE: Enterprise.

Deschaumes-Molinaro C, Dittmar A, Vernet-Maury E (1991). Relationship between mental imagery and sporting performance. *Behav. Brain Res.* 45(1): 29-36.

Deschaumes-Molinaro C, Dittmar A, Vernet-Maury E (1992). Autonomic nervous system response patterns correlate with mental imagery. *Physiol. Behav.* 51(5): 1021-1027.

Dorland's illustrated medical dictionary (1994). 28th ed. Philadelphia: Saunders.

Elmquist JK, Scammell TE, Saper CB (1997). Mechanisms of CNS response to systemic immune challenge: The febrile response. *Trends Neurosci.* 20(12): 565-570.

Freeman R, Komaroff AL (1997). Does the chronic fatigue syndrome involve the autonomic nervous system? *Am. J. Med.* 102(4): 357-364.

Guyton AC (1986). *Textbook of medical physiology,* p. 747. Philadelphia: Saunders.

Hall H, Papas A, Tosi M, Olness K (1996). Directional changes in neutrophil adherence following passive resting versus active imagery. *Int. J. Neuosci.* 85(3-4): 185-194.

Hourihane JOB, Kilburn SA, Nordlee JA, Hefle SL, Taylor SL, Warner JO (1997). An evaluation of the sensitivity of subjects with peanut allergy to very low doses of peanut protein: A randomized, double-blind, placebo-controlled food challenge study. *J. Allergy Clin. Immunol.* 100(5): 596-600.

Lawson A, Calderon L (1997). Interexaminer reliability of applied kinesiology manual muscle testing. *Perceptual and Motor Skills* 84: 539-546.

Leisman G, Fernetz A, Zenhausern R, Tefera T, Zemcov A (1995). Electromyographic effects of fatigue and task repetition on the validity of estimates of strong and weak muscles in applied kinesiology muscle testing procedure. *Perceptual and Motor Skills* 80:963-977.

Leisman G, Shambaugh P, Ferentz A (1989). Somatosensory evoked potential changes during muscle testing. *Inter. J. Neuroscience* 45:143-151.

Lombardi E, Morgan WJ, Wright AL, Stein RT, Holberg CJ, Martinez FD (1997). Cold air challenge at age 6 and subsequent incidence of asthma. A longitudinal study. *Am. J. Respir. Crit. Care Med.* 156(6): 1863-1869.

Lukaski HC, Hall CB, Siders WA (1991). Altered metabolic response to iron-deficient women during graded, maximal exercise. *Eur. J. Appl. Physiol.* 63: 140-145.

Mattes RD (1997). Physiologic responses to sensory stimulation by food: Nutritional implications. *J. Am. Diet. Assoc.* 97: 406-410, 413.

Motyka T, Yanuck S (1998). Expanding the neurological examination using functional neurologic assessment part 1: Methodological consideration. *Intern J. Neuroscience.*

Newsholme EA (1994). Biochemical mechanisms to explain immunosuppression in well-trained and overtrained athletes. *Int. J. Sports Med.* 15: 142-147.

Parry-Billings M, Blomstrand E, McAndrew N, Newsholme EA (1990). A communicational link between skeletal muscle, brain, and cells of the immune system. *Int. J. Sports Med.* 11(Suppl. 2): S122-S128.

Pavlov IP (1910). The centrifugal (efferent) nerves to the gastric glands and the pancreas. In *The work of the digestive glands,* trans. WH Thompson, pp. 48-59. Philadelphia: Griffin.

Perot C, Meldener R, Goubel F (1991). Objective measurement of proprioceptive technique consequences on muscular maximal voluntary contraction during manual muscle testing. *Agressologie* (French) 32(10): 471-474. Abstract.

Pichichero ME, Pichichero DM (1998). Diagnosis of penicillin, amoxicillin, and cephalosporin allergy: Reliability of examination assessed by skin testing and oral challenge. *J. Pediatr.* 132(1): 137-143.

Ruegg RG, Gilmore J, Ekstrom RD, Corrigan M, Knight B, Tancer M, Leatherman ME, Carson SW, Golden RN (1997). Clomipramine challenge responses covary with Tridimensional Personality Questionnaire scores in healthy subjects. *Biol. Psychiatry* 42(12): 1123-1129.

Schmitt WH Jr. (1997). Is it sympathetic or parasympathetic? *Proceedings of the International College of Applied Kinesiology - U.S.A.* Vol. 1, pp. 131-140. Shawnee Mission, KS.

Schmitt WH, Yanuck S (1998). Expanding the neurological examination using functional neurologic assessment part 2: Methodological consideration. *Intern J. Neuroscience.*

Schwaiblmair M, Beinert T, Vogelmeier C, Fruhmann G (1997). Cardiopulmonary exercise testing following hay exposure challenge in farmer's lung. *Eur. Respir. J.* 10(10): 2360-2365.

Shlik J, Aluoja A, Vasar V, Vasar E, Podar T, Bradwejn J (1997). Effects of citalopram treatment on behavioural, cardiovascular and neuroendocrine response to cholecystokinin tetrapeptide challenge in patients with panic disorder. *J. Psychiatry Neurosci.* 22(5): 332-340.

Szabo A (1993). The combined effects of orthostatic and mental stress on heart rate, T-wave amplitude, and pulse transit time. *Eur. J. Appl. Physiol.* 67(6): 540-544.

Vacek L (1997). Incidence of exercise-induced asthma in high school population in British Columbia. *Allergy Asthma Proc.* 18(2): 89-91.

Wada L, King JC (1986). Effect of low zinc intakes on basal metabolic rate, thyroid hormones and protein utilization in adult men. *J. Nutr.* 116: 1045-1053.

Warner L, McNeill ME (1988). Mental imagery and its potential for physical therapy. *Phys. Ther.* 68(4): 516-521.

Weidner TG, Gehlsen G, Schurr T, Dwyer GB (1997). Effects of viral upper respiratory illness on running gait. *J. Athl. Training* 32(4): 309-314.

CHAPTER 12

Colliander EB, Dudley GA, Tesch PA (1988). Skeletal muscle fiber type composition and performance during repeated bouts of maximal, concentric contractions. *Eur. J. Appl. Physiol.* 58: 81-86.

Hodgetts V, Coppack SW, Frayn KN, Hockadag DR (1991). Factors controlling fat mobilization from human subcutaneous adipose tissue during exercise. *J. Appl. Physiol.* 71: 445-451.

Lukaski HC, Hall CB, Siders WA (1991). Altered metabolic response to iron-deficient women during graded, maximal exercise. *Eur. J. Appl. Physiol.* 63: 140-145.

Maffetone P (1996). A hypothesis for the clinical evaluation of aerobic and anaerobic function. *Sports Chiro. Rehab.* 10(2): 74-77.

Maffetone P (1997). *In fitness and in health.* 3d ed. Stamford, NY: David Barmore Productions.

Sisto SA, LaManca J, Cordero DL, Bergen MT, Ellis SP, Drastal S, Boda WL, Tapp WN, Natelson BH (1996). Metabolic and cardiovascular effects of a progressive exercise test in patients with chronic fatigue syndrome. *Am. J. Med.* 100(6): 634-640.

CHAPTER 13

Bell JM, Bassey EJ (1996). Postexercise heart rates and pulse palpation as a means of determining exercising intensity in an aerobic dance class. *Br. J. Sports Med.* 30(1): 48-52.

Bird SR, Hay S (1987). Pre-exercise food and heart rate during submaximal exercise. *Br. J. Sports Med.* 21(1): 27-28.

Boone T, Frentz KL, Boyd NR (1985). Carotid palpation at two exercise intensities. *Med. Sci. Sports Exerc.* 17(6): 705-709.

Boulay MR, Simoneau JA, Lortie G, Bouchard C (1997). Monitoring high-intensity endurance exercise with heart rate and thresholds. *Med. Sci. Sports Exerc.* 29(1): 125-132.

Cavanagh PR, Kram R (1985). Mechanical and muscular factors affecting the efficiency of human movement. *Med. Sci. Sports Exerc.* 17: 326-331.

Cordero DL, Sisto SA, Tapp WN, LaManca JJ, Pareja JG, Natelson BH (1996). Decreased vagal power during treadmill walking in patients with chronic fatigue syndrome. *Clin. Auton. Res.* 6(6): 329-333.

Dorland's illustrated medical dictionary (1994). 28th ed. Philadelphia: Saunders.

Fry AC, Kraemer WJ (1997). Resistance exercise overtraining and overreaching. *Sports Med.* 23(2): 106-129.

Gaesser GA, Wilson LA (1988). Effects of continuous and interval training on the parameters of the power-endurance time relationship for high-intensity exercise. *Int. J. Sports Med.* 9: 417-421.

Goldberg L, Elliot DL, Kuehl KS (1988). Assessment of exercise intensity formulas by use of ventilatory threshold. *Chest* 94(1): 95-98.

Guyton AC (1986). *Textbook of medical physiology,* pp. 237-240. Philadelphia: Saunders.

Heinert LD (1988). Effect of stride length variation on oxygen uptake during level and positive grade treadmill running. *Res. Q. Exerc. Sport* 59: 127-132.

Karvonen MJ, Kentala E, Mustala O (1957). The effects of training heart rate: A longitudinal study. *Annales Medicinae Experimentalis et Biologiae Fenniae* (French) 35: 307-315.

Karvonen J, Vuorimaa T (1988). Heart rate and exercise intensity during sports activities. Practical application. *Sports Med.* 5(5): 303-311.

Keast D, Cameron K, Morton AR (1988). Exercise and the immune response. *Sports Med.* 5: 248-267.

Kuipers H, Keizer HA (1988). Overtraining in elite athletes: Review and directions for the future. *Sports Med.* 6: 79-92.

Leaf DA, Allen D (1988). Respiratory exchange ratio slope: A new concept in the determination of physical fitness and exercise training. *Ann. Sports Med.* 3(4): 210-214.

Lee JY, Jensen BE, Oberman A, Fletcher GF, Fletcher BJ, Raczynski JM (1996). Adherence in the training levels comparison trial. *Med. Sci. Sports Exerc.* 28(1): 47-52.

Lehmann MJ, Lormes W, Opitz-Gress A, Steinacher JM, Netzer N, Foster C, Gastmann U (1997). Training and overtraining: An overview and experimental results in endurance sports. *J. Sports Med. Phys. Fitness* 37: 7-17.

Maffetone P (1996). *Training for endurance*, p. 62. Stamford, NY: David Barmore Productions.

McArdle WD, Katch FI, Katch VL (1991). *Exercise physiology.* 3d ed., pp. 169-172. Philadelphia: Lea & Febiger.

Ibid. p. 296.

Ibid. p. 705.

Miller WC, Wallace JP, Eggert KE (1993). Predicting max HR and the HR-VO2 relationship for exercise prescription in obesity. *Med. Sci. Sports Exerc.* 25(9): 1077-1081.

Moore AD Jr, Lee SM, Greenisen MC, Bishop P (1997). Validity of a heart rate monitor during work in the laboratory and on the Space Shuttle. *Am. Ind. Hyg. Assoc. J.* 58(4): 299-301.

Newsholme EA (1994). Biochemical mechanisms to explain immunosuppression in well-trained and overtrained athletes. *Int. J. Sports Med.* 15: S142-S147.

Oldridge NB, Haskell WL, Single P (1981). Carotid palpation, coronary heart disease and exercise rehabilitation. *Med. Sci. Sports Exerc.* 13(1): 6-8.

Ring C, Brener J (1996). Influence of beliefs about heart rate and actual heart rate on heartbeat counting. *Psychophysiology* 33(5): 541-546.

Sandvik L, Erikssen J, Ellestad M, Erikssen G, Thaulow E, Mundal R, Rodahl K (1995). Heart rate increase and maximal heart rate during exercise as predictors of cardiovascular mortality: A 16-year follow-up study of 1960 healthy men. *Coron. Artery Dis.* 6(8): 667-679.

Seaward BL, Sleamaker RH, McAuliffe T, Clapp JF 3d (1990). The precision and accuracy of a portable heart rate monitor. *Biomed. Instrum. Technol.* 24(1): 37-41.

Stone MH, Keith RE, Kearney JT (1991). Overtraining: A review of the signs, symptoms and possible causes. *J. Appl. Sports Sci. Res.* 5(1): 35-50.

Weidner TG, Gehlsen G, Schurr T, Dwyer GB (1997). Effects of viral upper respiratory illness on running gait. *J. Athl. Training* 532(4): 309-314.

Whaley MH, Kaminsky LA, Dwyer GB, Getchell LH, Norton JA (1992). Predictors of over- and underachievement of age-predicted maximal heart rate. *Med. Sci. Sports Exerc.* 24(10): 1173-1179.

Wilmore JH, Costill DL (1994). *Physiology of sport and exercise,* p. 177. Champaign, IL: Human Kinetics.

Ibid. p. 304.

CHAPTER 14

Aragao W (1991). Aragao's function regulator, the stomatognathic system and postural changes in children. *J. Clin. Pediatr. Dent.* 15(4): 226-231.

Borg-Stein J, Stein J (1996). Trigger points and tender points: One and the same? Does injection treatment help? *Rheum. Dis. Clin. North Am.* 22(2): 305-322.

de Wijer A, Steenks MH, de Leeuw JR, Bosman F, Helders PJ (1996). Symptoms of the cervical spine in temporomandibular and cervical spine disorders. *J. Oral Rehabil.* 23(11): 742-750.

Gerwin RD (1994). Neurobiology of the myofascial trigger point. *Baillieres Clin. Rheumatol.* 8(4): 747-762.

Gerwin RD (1997). Myofascial pain syndromes in the upper extremity. *J. Hand Ther.* 10(2): 130-136.

Goodheart GJ Jr (1976). *Applied kinesiology workshop procedure manual.* 12th ed. Gross Point, MI: Privately published.

Hong CZ (1996). Pathophysiology of myofascial trigger point. *J. Formos. Med. Assoc.* 95(2): 93-104.

Ishii H (1990). A study on the relationships between imbalance of stomatognathic function and asymmetry of craniofacial morphology, and the center of gravity of the upright posture. *Osaka Daigaku Shigaku Zasshi* 35(2): 517-556.

Johnson LR, Westrum LE (1980). Brain stem degeneration patterns following tooth extractions: Visualization of dental and periodontal afferents. *Brain Res.* 194(2): 489-493.

Lee-Knight CT, Harrison EL, Price CJ (1992). Dental injuries at the 1989 Canada games: An epidemiological study. *J. Can. Dent. Assoc.* 58(10): 810-815.

Safran MR, Garrett WE, Seaber AV, Glisson RR, Ribbeck BM (1988). The role of warmup in muscular injury prevention. *Am. J. Sports Med.* 16(2): 123-129.

Safran MR, Seaber AV, Garrett WE Jr (1989). Warm-up and muscular injury prevention. An update. *Sports Med.* 8(4): 239-249.

Salonen MA, Raustia AM, Huggare J (1993). Head and cervical spine postures in complete denture wearers. *Cranio.* 11(1): 30-33.

Travell JG, Simons DG (1983). *Myofascial pain and dysfunction: The trigger point manual.* Baltimore: Williams & Wilkins.

Wabeke KB, Spruijt RJ (1993). Dental factors associated with temporomandibular joint sounds. *J. Prosthet. Dent.* 69(4): 401-405.

Walther, D (1983). *Applied kinesiology, volume II: Head, neck, and jaw pain and dysfunction: The stomatognathic system.* Pueblo, CO: Systems DC.

Walther, D (1988). *Applied kinesiology synopsis,* pp. 385-386. Pueblo, CO: Systems DC.

Ibid. pp. 146-158.

Westling L (1992). Temporomandibular joint dysfunction and systemic joint laxity. *Swed. Dent. J. Suppl.* 81: 1-79.

Westrum LE, Canfield RC (1977). Electron microscopy of degenerating axons and terminals in spinal trigeminal nucleus after tooth pulp extirpations. *Am. J. Anat.* 149(4): 591-596.

Westrum LE, Canfield RC, O'Connor TA (1980). Projections from dental structures to the brain stem trigeminal complex as shown by transganglionic transport of horseradish peroxidase. *Neurosci. Lett.* 20(1): 31-36.

Westrum LE, Johnson LR, Canfield RC (1984). Ultrastructure of transganglionic degeneration in brain stem trigeminal nuclei during normal primary tooth exfoliation and permanent tooth eruption in the cat. *J. Comp. Neurol.* 230(2): 198-206.

CHAPTER 15

DeJarnette MB (1981). *Sacro occipital technique.* Nebraska City, NE: Privately published.

Upledger J (1987). *Cranialsacral therapy II: Beyond the dura.* Chicago: Eastland Press.

Upledger J, Vredevoogd J (1983). *Cranialsacral therapy.* Chicago: Eastland Press.

Walther, D (1988). *Applied kinesiology synopsis,* p. 365. Pueblo, CO: Systems DC.

CHAPTER 16

Maffetone P (1996). *Training for endurance.* Stamford, NY: David Barmore Productions.

Walther, D (1988). *Applied kinesiology synopsis,* p. 425. Pueblo, CO: Systems DC.

CHAPTER 17

Amadio P Jr, Cummings DM, Amadio P (1993). Nonsteroidal anti-inflammatory drugs. Tailoring therapy to achieve results and avoid toxicity. *Postgrad. Med.* 93(4): 73-76.

Bentley S (1996). Exercise-induced muscle cramp. Proposed mechanisms and management. *Sports Med.* 21(6): 409-420.

Brandt KD (1987). Nonsteroidal antiinflammatory drugs and articular cartilage. *J. Rheumatol.* 14: 132-133.

Cleak MJ, Eston RG (1992). Muscle soreness, swelling, stiffness and strength loss after intense eccentric exercise. *Br. J. Sports Med.* 26(4): 267-272.

Clyman B (1986). Role of non-steroidal anti-inflammatory drugs in sports medicine. *Sports Med.* 3: 342-346.

Dajani EZ, Wilson DE, Agrawal NM (1991). Prostaglandins: An overview of the worldwide clinical experience. *J. Assoc. Acad. Minor Phys.* 2(1): 23.

David MJ, Vignon E, Peschard MJ, Broquet P, Louisot P, Richard M (1992). Effect of non-steroidal anti-inflammatory drugs (NSAIDS) on glycosyltransferase activity from human osteoarthritic cartilage. *Br. J. Rheumatol.* 31(Suppl. 1): 13-17.

Dieppe P, Cushnaghan J, Jasani MK, McCrae F, Watt I (1993). A two-year placebo-controlled trial of non-steroidal anti-inflammatory therapy in osteoarthritis of the knee joint. *Br. J. Rheumatol.* 32: 595-600.

Goodheart (1977). *Applied kinesiology workshop procedure manual*, 13th edition. (Privately published.)

Guyton AC (1986). *Textbook of medical physiology,* pp. 592-605. Philadelphia: Saunders.

Hertel J (1997). The role of nonsteroidal anti-inflammatory drugs in the treatment of acute soft tissue injuries. *J. Athl. Training* 32 (2): 350-358.

Hugenberg ST, Brandt KD, Cole CA (1993). Effect of sodium salicylate, aspirin, and ibuprofen on enzymes required by the chondrocyte for synthesis of chondroitin sulfate. *J. Rheumatol.* 20(12): 2128-2133.

Khan MI (1997). Fracture healing: Role of NSAIDs. *Am. J. Orthop.* 26(6): 413.

Koester MC (1993). An overview of the physiology and pharmacology of aspirin and nonsteroidal anti-inflammatory drugs. *J. Athl. Training* 28(3): 252-259.

Kuipers H (1994). Exercise-induced muscle damage. *Int. J. Sports Med.* 15(3): 132-135.

McArdle WD, Katch FI, Katch VL (1991). *Exercise physiology.* 3d ed., p. 486. Philadelphia: Lea & Febiger.

Miles MP, Clarkson PM (1994). Exercise-induced muscle pain, soreness, and cramps. *J. Sports Med. Phys. Fitness* 34(3): 203-216.

Murphy PJ, Badia P, Myers BL, Boecker MR, Wright KP Jr (1994). Nonsteroidal anti-inflammatory drugs affect normal sleep patterns in humans. *Physiol. Behav.* 55(6): 1063-1066.

Murphy PJ, Myers BL, Badia P (1996). Nonsteroidal anti-inflammatory drugs alter body temperature and suppress melatonin in humans. *Physiol. Behav.* 59(1): 133-139.

Portanova JP, Zhang Y, Anderson GD, Hauser SD, Masferrer JL, Seibert K, Gregory SA, Isakson PC (1996). Selective neutralization of prostaglandin E2 blocks inflammation, hyperalgesia, and interleukin 6 production in vivo. *J. Exp. Med.* 184(3): 883-891.

Pyne DB (1994). Exercise-induced muscle damage and inflammation: A review. *Aust. J. Sci. Med. Sport* 26(3-4): 49-58.

Safran MR, Garrett WE, Seabar AV, Glisson RR, Ribbeck, BM (1988). The role of warmup in muscular injury prevention. *Am. J. Clin. Nutr.* 32 (9): 123-129.

Schmitt WH Jr (1988). *The functional neurology of pain and pain control.* Original paper presentation, International College of Applied Kinesiology, Summer Meeting 1988, Shawnee Mission, KS.

Schmitt WH Jr (1989). *Nociceptor stimulation blocking technique.* Original paper presentation, International College of Applied Kinesiology, Winter Meeting 1989, Shawnee Mission, KS.

Smith LL, Brunetz MH, Chenier TC, McCammon MR, Houmard JA, Franklin ME, Israel RG (1993). The effects of static and ballistic stretching on delayed onset muscle soreness and creatine kinase. *Res. Q. Exerc. Sport* 64(1): 103-107.

Smith RL, Kajiyama G, Lane NE (1995). Nonsteroidal antiinflammatory drugs: Effects on normal and interleukin 1 treated human articular chondrocyte metabolism in vitro. *J. Rheumatol.* 22(6): 1130-1137.

Standard Process, Inc. 1200 West Royal Lee Drive, Palmyra, WI 53516. 800-848-5061.

Swaak AJ (1997). Anti-inflammatory medication after muscle injury. A treatment resulting in short-term improvement but subsequent loss of muscle function. *J. Bone Joint Surg. Am.* 79(8):1270-1271.

Taha AS, Angerson W, Nakshabendi I, Beekman H, Morran C, Sturrock RD, Russell RI (1993). Gastric and duodenal mucosal blood flow in patients receiving non-steroidal anti-inflammatory drugs—influence of age, smoking, ulceration and Helicobacter pylori. *Aliment. Pharmacol. Ther.* 7(1): 41-45.

Wright V (1995). Historical overview of non-steroidal anti-inflammatory drugs. *Br. J. Rheumatol.* 34(Suppl. 1): 2-4.

CHAPTER 18

Adams P, Lawson S, Sanigorski A, Sinclair A (1996). Arachidonic acid to eicosapentaenoic acid ratio in blood correlates positively with clinical symptoms of depression. *Lipids* 31 Suppl: S157-S161.

Ali M, Thomson M (1995). Consumption of a garlic clove a day could be beneficial in preventing thrombosis. *Prostaglandins Leukot. Essent. Fatty Acids* 53(3): 211-218.

Almekinders LC, Banes AJ, Ballenger CA (1993). Effects of repetitive motion on human fibroblasts. *Med. Sci. Sports Exerc.* 25(5): 603-607.

Arena B, Maffulli N, Maffulli F, Morleo MA (1995). Reproductive hormones and menstrual changes with exercise in female athletes. *Sports Med.* 19(4): 278-287.

Austin MA (1991). Plasma triglyceride and coronary heart disease. *Arterioscler. Thromb.* 11: 2-14.

Barbeau WE (1997). Interactions between dietary proteins and the human system: Implications for oral tolerance and food-related diseases. *Adv. Exp. Med. Biol.* 415: 183-193.

Benson JE, Engelbert-Fenton KA, Eisenman PA (1996). Nutritional aspects of amenorrhea in the female athlete triad. *Int. J. Sport Nutr.* 6(2): 134-145.

Bergman EA, Massey LK, Wise KJ, Sherrard DJ (1990). Effects of dietary caffeine on renal handling of minerals in adult women. *Life Sci.* 47(6): 557-564.

Bergstrom J, Furst P, Vinnars E (1990). Effect of a test meal, without and with protein, on muscle and plasma free amino acids. *Clin. Sci.* (Colch.) 79(4): 31-337.

Bernardis LL, Bellinger LL (1996). The lateral hypothalamic area revisited: Ingestive behavior. *Neurosci. Biobehav. Rev.* 20(2): 189-287.

Bird SR, Hay S (1987). Pre-exercise food and heart rate during submaximal exercise. *Br. J. Sports Med.* 21(1): 27-28.

Bjorntorp, P (1991). Importance of fat as a support nutrient for energy: Metabolism of athletes. *J. Sports. Sci.* 9: 71-76.

Bland, JS (1997). *Functional modulation of immune and inflammatory process.* Fourth International Symposium on Functional Medicine, May 15-17, Aspen, CO.

Block G, Patterson B, Subar A (1992). Fruit, vegetables and cancer prevention: A review of the epidemiological evidence. *Nutr. Cancer* 18: 1-19.

Blond JP, Bezard J (1991). Delta 5-desaturation of dihomogammalinolenic acid (20:3[n-6]) into arachidonic acid (20:4[n-6]) by rat liver microsomes and incorporation of fatty acids in microsome phospholipids. *Biochem. Biophys. Acta* 1084(3): 255-260.

Bordia A, Verma SK, Srivastava KC (1997). Effect of ginger (Zingiber officinale Rosc.) and fenugreek (Trigonella foenumgraecum L.) on blood lipids, blood sugar and platelet aggregation in patients with coronary artery disease. *Prostaglandins Leukot. Essent. Fatty Acids* 56(5): 379-384.

Bordia T, Mohammed N, Thomson M, Ali M (1996). An evaluation of garlic and onion as antithrombotic agents. *Prostaglandins Leukot. Essent. Fatty Acids* 54(3): 183-186.

Borensztajn J (1979). Lipoprotein lipase and hypertriglyceridemias. *Artery* 5: 346-353.

Bosch AN, Dennis SC, Noakes TD (1993). Influence of carbohydrate loading on fuel substrate turnover and oxidation during prolonged exercise. *J. Appl. Physiol.* 74: 1921-1927.

Bosch AN, Dennis SC, Noakes TD (1994). Influence of carbohydrate ingestion on fuel substrate turnover and oxidation during prolonged exercise. *J. Appl. Physiol.* 76: 2364-2372.

Bouziane M, Prost J, Belleville J (1994). Dietary protein deficiency affects n-3 and n-6 polyunsaturated fatty acids hepatic storage and very low density lipoprotein transport in rats on different diets. *Lipids* 29(4): 265-272.

Broadhurst CL (1997). Balanced intakes of natural triglycerides for optimum nutrition: An evolutionary and phytochemical perspective. *Med. Hypotheses* 49(3): 247-261.

Butterfield GE (1987). Whole-body protein utilization in humans. *Med. Sci. Sports Exerc.* 19(5): 157-165.

Carranza-Madrigal J, Herrera-Abarca JE, Alvizouri-Munoz M, Alvarado-Jimenez MR, Chavez-Carbajal F (1997). Effects of a vegetarian diet vs. a vegetarian diet enriched with avocado in hypercholesterolemic patients. *Arch. Med. Res.* 28(4): 537-541.

Castaneda C, Charnley JM, Evans WJ, Crim MC (1995a). Elderly women accommodate to a low-protein diet with losses of body cell mass, muscle function, and immune response. *Am. J. Clin. Nutr.* 62(1): 30-39.

Castaneda C, Dolnikowski GG, Dallal GE, Evans WJ, Crim MC (1995b). Protein turnover and energy metabolism of elderly women fed a low-protein diet. *Am. J. Clin. Nutr.* 62(1): 40-48.

Chardigny JM, Sebedio JL, Grandgirard A, Martine L, Berdeaux O, Vatele JM (1996). Identification of novel trans isomers of 20:5n-3 in liver lipids of rats fed a heated oil. *Lipids* 31(2): 165-168.

Chavali SR, Zhong WW, Utsunomiya T, Forse RA (1997). Decreased production of interleukin-1-beta, prostaglandin-E2 and thromboxane-B2, and elevated levels of interleukin-6 and -10 are associated with increased survival during endotoxic shock in mice consuming diets enriched with sesame seed oil supplemented with Quil-A saponin. *Int. Arch. Allergy Immunol.* 114(2): 153-160.

Christensen L, Somers S (1996). Comparison of nutrient intake among depressed and nondepressed individuals. *Int. J. Eat. Disord.* 20(1): 105-109.

Claassen N, Coetzer H, Steinmann ML, Kruger MC (1995). The effect of different n-6/n-3 essential fatty acid ratios on calcium balance and bone in rats. *Prostaglandins Leukot. Essent. Fatty Acids* 53: 13-19.

Connor WE (1986). Hypolipidemic effects of dietary omega-3 fatty acids in normal and hyperlipidemic humans: Effectiveness and mechanisms. In *Health effects of polyunsaturated fatty acids in seafoods,* eds. AP Simopoulos, RR Kifer, RE Martin, pp. 173-210. Orlando, FL: Academic Press.

Cook NE, Rogers QR, Morris JG (1996). Acid-base balance affects dietary choice in cats. *Appetite* 26(2): 175-192.

Coulston AM, Liu GC, Reaven GM (1993). Plasma glucose, insulin and lipid responses to high-carbohydrate low-fat diets in normal humans. *Metabolism* 32: 52-56.

Craig WJ (1997). Phytochemicals: Guardians of our health. *J. Am. Diet. Assoc.* 10(2): S199-S204.

Cummings JH, Macfarlane GT (1997). Role of intestinal bacteria in nutrient metabolism. *J. Parenter. Enteral. Nutr.* 21(6): 357-365.

Davi G, Alessandrini P, Mezzetti A, Minotti G, Bucciarelli T, Costantini F, Cipollone F, Bon GB, Ciabattoni G, Patrono C (1997). In vivo formation of 8-Epi-prostaglandin F2 alpha is increased in hypercholesterolemia. *Arterioscler. Thromb. Vasc. Biol.* 17(11): 3230-3235.

Davis, CM (1928). Self selection of diet by newly weaned infants. *Am. J. Diseases Childr.* 36 (4): 651-679.

Denyer CV, Jackson P, Loakes DM, Ellis MR, Young DA (1994). Isolation of antirhinoviral sesquiterpenes from ginger (Zingiber officinale). *J. Nat. Prod.* 57(5): 658-662.

Desimone DP, Greene VS, Hannon KS, Turner RT, Bell NH (1993). Prostaglandin E2 administered by subcutaneous pellets causes local inflammation and systemic bone loss: A model for inflammation-induced bone disease. *J. Bone Miner. Res.* 8(5): 625-634.

Deuster PA, Kyle SB, Moser PB, Vigersky RA, Singh A, Schoomaker EB (1986). Nutritional intakes and status of highly trained amenorrheic and eumenorrheic women runners. *Fertil. Steril.* 46: 636-643.

Diaz MN, Frei B, Vita JA, Keaney JF Jr (1997). Antioxidants and atherosclerotic heart disease. *N. Engl. J. Med.* 337(6): 408-416.

Doll R, Peto R, Hall E, Wheatley K, Gray R (1994). Mortality in relation to consumption of alcohol: 13 years' observations on male British doctors. *Br. Med. J.* 309: 911-918.

Dreon DM, Fernstrom HA, Williams PT, Krauss RM (1997). LDL subclass patterns and lipoprotein response to a low-fat, high-carbohydrate diet in women. *Arterioscler. Thromb. Vasc. Biol.* 17(4): 707-714.

Drew LM, Kies C, Fox HM (1979). Effects of dietary fiber on copper, zinc, and magnesium utilization by adolescent boys. *Am. J. Clin. Nutr.* 32(9): 1893-1897.

Dudkin MS, Shchelkunov LF, Denisiuk NA, Korzun VP, Saglo VI (1997). Dietary fibers as radiation protectors. *Vopr. Pitan.* 2: 12-14.

Erasuas, U (1996). *Fats and Oils,* p. 231. Vancouver: Alive Books.

Expert Panel on Detection, Evaluation, and Treatment of High Blood Cholesterol in Adults (1994). The second report of the National Cholesterol Education Program (NCEP) expert panel on detection, evaluation, and treatment of high blood cholesterol in adults. *Circulation* 89: 1239-1445.

Fern EB, Bielinski RN, Schutz Y (1991). Effects of exaggerated amino acid and protein supply in man. *Experientia* 47: 168-172.

Foster C, Costill DL, Fink WJ (1979). Effects of preexercise feedings on endurance performance. *Med. Sci. Sports* 11(1); 1-5.

Foster-Powell K, Miller JB (1995). International tables of glycemic index. *Am. J. Clin. Nutr.* 62: 871S-893S.

Friedman JE, Lemon PWR (1989). Effect of chronic endurance exercise on retention of dietary protein. *Int. J. Sports Med.* 10(2): 118-123.

Fromentin G, Nicolaidis S (1996). Rebalancing essential amino acids intake by self-selection in the rat. *Br. J. Nutr.* 75(5): 669-682.

Fuchs CS, Stampfer MJ, Colditz GA (1995). Alcohol consumption and mortality in women. *N. Engl. J. Med.* 332: 1245-1250.

Gallaher DD, Schneeman BO (1996). Dietary fiber. In *Present knowledge in nutrition,* eds. EE Ziegler, LJ Filer Jr, p. 87. Washington, DC: International Life Sciences Institute.

Gaziano JM, Hennekens CH, O'Donnell CJ, Breslow JL, Buring JE (1997). Fasting triglycerides, high-density lipoprotein, and risk of myocardial infarction. *Circulation* 96(8): 2520-2525.

Golay A, Eigenheer C, Morel Y, Kujawski P, Lehmann T, de Tonnac N (1996). Weight-loss with low or high carbohydrate diet? *Int. J. Obes. Relat. Metab. Disord.* 20(12): 1067-1072.

Graham TE, Spriet LL (1995). Metabolic, catecholamine, and exercise performance responses to various doses of caffeine. *J. Appl. Physiol.* 78(3): 867-874.

Grandjean AC (1997). Diets of elite athletes: Has the discipline of sports nutrition made an impact? *J. Nutr.* 127(5 Suppl.): 874S-877S.

Granner DK (1993). Hormones of the pancreas & gastrointestinal tract. In *Harper's biochemistry,* eds. RK Murray, DK Granner, PA Mayes, VW Rodwell, pp. 563-564. Norwalk, CT: Appleton & Lange.

Griffiths AJ, Humphreys SM, Clark ML, Frayn KN (1994). Forearm substrate utilization during exercise after a meal containing both fat and carbohydrate. *Clin. Sci.* 86: 169-175.

Gronbaek M, Deis A, Sorensen TI, Becker U, Schnohr P, Jensen G (1995). Mortality associated with moderate intakes of wine, beer, or spirits. *Br. Med. J.* 310: 1165-1169.

Grundy SM (1996). Dietary Fat. In *Present knowledge in nutrition,* eds. EE Ziegler, LJ Filer Jr, pp. 44-57. Washington, DC: International Life Sciences Institute.

Grynberg A, Demaison L (1996). Fatty acid oxidation in the heart. *J. Cardio. Pharm.* 28(1): S11-S17.

Guyton AC (1986). *Textbook of medical physiology,* p. 862. Philadelphia: Saunders.

Halstead CH (1996). Alcohol: Medical and nutritional effects. In *Present knowledge in nutrition,* eds. EE Ziegler, LJ Filer Jr, pp. 547-556. Washington, DC: International Life Sciences Institute.

Hanai H, Ikuma M, Sato Y, Iida T, Hosoda Y, Matsushita I, Nogaki A, Yamada M, Kaneko E (1997). Long-term effects of water-soluble corn bran hemicellulose on glucose tolerance in obese and non-obese patients: Improved insulin sensitivity and glucose metabolism in obese subjects. *Biosci. Biotechnol. Biochem.* 61(8): 1358-1361.

Harper AE, Peters JC (1989). Protein intake, brain amino acid and serotonin concentrations and protein self-selection. *J. Nutr.* 119: 677-689.

Hawley JA, Palmer GS, Noakes TD (1997). Effects of 3 days of carbohydrate supplementation on muscle glycogen content and utilisation during a 1-h cycling performance. *Eur. J. Appl. Physiol.* 75(5): 407-412.

Heinrichs SC, Koob GF (1992). Corticotropin-releasing factor modulates dietary preference in nutritionally and physically stressed rats. *Psychopharmacology* (Berlin) 109(1-2): 177-184.

Hill EG, Holman RT (1980). Effect of dietary protein level upon essential fatty acids (EFA) deficiency. *J. Nutr.* 10(5): 1057-1060.

Holder MD, DiBattista D (1994). Effects of time-restricted access to protein and of oral-sensory cues on protein selection. *Physiol. Behav.* 55(4): 659-664.

Holt S, Brand J, Soveny C, Hansky J (1992). Relationship of satiety to postprandial glycaemic, insulin and cholecystokinin responses. *Appetite* 18: 129-141.

Jacobs I, Lithell H, Karlsson J (1982). Dietary effects on glycogen and lipoprotein lipase activity in skeletal muscle in man. *Acta Physiol. Scand.* 115: 85-90.

Jacobson BH, Weber MD, Claypool L, Hunt LE (1992). Effect of caffeine on maximal strength and power in elite male athletes. *Br. J. Sports Med.* 26(4): 276-280.

Jenkins DJA (1997). Carbohydrate tolerance and food frequency. *Br. J. Nutr.* 77(Suppl. 1): S71-S81.

Jeppesen J, Schaaf P, Jones C, Zhou MY, Chen YD, Reaven GM (1997). Effects of low-fat, high-carbohydrate diets on risk factors for ischemic heart disease in postmenopausal women. *Am. J. Clin. Nutr.* 65(4): 1027-1033.

Joannic JL, Auboiron S, Raison J, Basdevant A, Bornet F (1997). How the degree of unsaturation of dietary fatty acids influences the glucose and insulin responses to different carbohydrates in mixed meals. *Am. J. Clin. Nutr.* 65: 1427-1433.

Jorda A, Zaragoza R, Portoles M, Baguena-Cervellera R, Renau-Piqueras J (1988). Long-term high-protein diet induces biochemical and ultrastructural changes in rat liver mitochondria. *Arch. Biochem. Biophys.* 265(2): 241-248.

Kamal-Eldin A, Pettersson D, Appelqvist LA (1995). Sesamin (a compound from sesame oil) increases tocopherol levels in rats fed ad libitum. *Lipids* 30(6): 499-505.

Kaminogawa S (1996). Food allergy, oral tolerance and immunomodulation—their molecular and cellular mechanisms. *Biosci. Biotechnol. Biochem.* 60(11): 1749-1756.

Klatsky AL (1994). Epidemiology of coronary heart disease—influence of alcohol. *Alcohol Clin. Exp. Res.* 18: 88-96.

Klatsky AL, Armstrong MA, Friedman GD (1992). Alcohol and mortality. *Ann. Intern. Med.* 117: 646-654.

Koester MC (1993). An overview of the physiology and pharmacology of aspirin and nonsteroidal anti-inflammatory drugs. *J. Athl. Training* 28(3): 252-259.

Kolopp-Sarda MN, Moneret-Vautrin DA, Gobert B, Kanny G, Brodschii M, Bene MC, Faure GC (1997). Specific humoral immune responses in 12 cases of food sensitization to sesame seed. *Clin. Exp. Allergy* 27(11): 1285-1291.

Krieger NS (1997). Parathyroid hormone, prostaglandin E2, and 1,25-dihydroxyvitamin D3 decrease the level of Na+-Ca2+ exchange protein in osteoblastic cells. *Calcif. Tissue Int.* 60(5): 473-478.

Kynast-Gales SA, Massey LK (1994). Effect of caffeine on circadian excretion of urinary calcium and magnesium. *J. Am. Coll. Nutr.* 13(5): 467-472.

Lairon D, Lafont H, Vigne JL (1985). Effects of dietary fibers and cholestyramine on the activity of pancreatic lipase in vitro. *Am. J. Clin. Nutr.* 42: 629-638.

Lambert EV, Speechly DP, Dennis SC, Noakes TD (1994). Enhanced endurance in trained cyclists during moderate intensity exercise following 2 weeks adaptation to a high fat diet. *Eur. J. Appl. Physiol.* 69: 287-293.

Larue-Achagiotis C, Martin C, Verger P, Louis-Sylvestre J (1992). Dietary self-selection vs. complete diet: Body weight gain and meal pattern in rats. *Physiol. Behav.* 51(5): 995-999.

Lefkowith JB, Rogers M, Lennartz MR, Brown EJ (1991). Essential fatty acid deficiency impairs macrophage spreading and adherence. Role of arachidonate in cell adhesion. *J. Biol. Chem.* 266(2): 1071-1076.

Lemon PW (1996). Is increased dietary protein necessary or beneficial for individuals with a physically active lifestyle? *Nutr. Rev.* 54(4 Part 2): S169-175.

Linder MC (1991). Nutrition and metabolism of fats. In *Nutritional biochemistry and metabolism,* ed. MC Linder, pp. 90-91. Norwalk, CT: Appleton & Lange.

Ibid. pp. 104-105.

Ibid. pp. 87-108.

Litchtenstein AH (1996). Atherosclerosis. In *Present knowledge in nutrition,* eds. EE Ziegler, LJ Filer Jr, p. 435. Washington, DC: International Life Sciences Institute.

Liu GC, Coulston AM, Reaven GM (1983). Effect of high-carbohydrate-low-fat diets on plasma glucose, insulin and lipid responses in hypertriglyceridemic humans. *Metabolism* 32(8): 750-753.

MacLaren DPM, Reilly T, Campbell IT (1994). Hormonal and metabolic responses to glucose and malto-dextrin ingestion with or without the addition of guar gum. *Int. J. Sports Med.* 15: 466-471.

Maffetone P (1997). *In fitness and in health.* 3d ed., p. 46. Stamford, NY: David Barmore Productions.

Mantzioris E, James MJ, Gibson RA, Cleland LG (1995). Differences exist in the relationships between dietary linoleic and alpha-linolenic acids and their respective long-chain metabolites. *Am. J. Clin. Nutr.* 61: 320-324.

Maranesi M, Barzanti V, Coccheri S, Marchetti M, Tolomelli B (1993). Interaction between vitamin B6 deficiency and low EFA dietary intake on kidney phospholipids and PGE2 in the rat. *Prostaglandins Leukot. Essent. Fatty Acids* 49(1): 531-536.

Massey LK, Bergman EA, Wise KJ, Sherrard DJ (1994). Interactions between dietary caffeine and calcium on calcium and bone metabolism in older women. *J. Am. Coll. Nutr.* 13(6): 592-596.

Mattes RD (1997). Physiologic responses to sensory stimulation by food: Nutritional implications. *J. Am. Diet Assoc.* 97(4): 406-413.

McArdle WD, Katch FI, Katch VL (1991). *Exercise physiology.* 3d ed., p. 31. Philadelphia: Lea & Febiger.

McNamara DJ, Kolb R, Parker TS, Batwin H (1987). Heterogeneity of cholesterol homeostatis in man. Response to changes in dietary fat quality and cholesterol quantity. *J. Clin. Invest.* 79(6): 1729-1739.

Meyer K, Schwartz J, Crater D, Keyes B (1995). Zingiber officinale (ginger) used to prevent 8-Mop associated nausea. *Dermatol. Nurs.* 7(4): 242-244.

Miller CC, Tang W, Ziboh VA, Fletcher MP (1991). Dietary supplementation with ethyl ester concentrates of fish oil (n-3) and borage oil (n-6) polyunsaturated fatty acids induces epidermal generation of local putative anti-inflammatory metabolites. *J. Invest. Dermatol.* 96(1): 98-103.

Miller GD, Hrupka BJ, Gietzen DW, Rogers QR, Stern JS (1994). Rats on a macronutrient self-selection diet eat most meals from a single food group. *Appetite* 23: 67-78.

Miller WC, Bryce GR, Conles RK (1984). Adaptations to a high-fat diet that increase exercise endurance in male rats. *J. Appl. Physiol.* 56(1): 78-83.

Moller P, Wallin H, Knudsen LE (1996). Oxidative stress associated with exercise, psychological stress and life-style factors. *Chem. Biol. Interact.* 102(1): 17-36.

Moore CE, Hartung GH, Mitchell RE, Kappus CM, Hinderlitter J (1983). The relationship of exercise and diet on HDL cholesterol levels in women. *Metabolism* 32(2): 189-196.

Mosca L, Rubenfire M, Mandel C, Rock C, Tarshis T, Tsai A, Pearson T (1997). Antioxidant nutrient supplementation reduces the susceptibility of low density lipoprotein to oxidation in patients with coronary artery disease. *J. Am. Coll. Cardiol.* 30(2): 392-399.

Muoio DM, Leddy JJ, Horvath PJ, Awad AB, Pendergast DR (1994). Effect of dietary fat on metabolic adjustments to maximal $\dot{V}O_2$ and endurance in runners. *Med. Sci. Sports Exerc.* 26(1): 81-88.

National Cholesterol Education Program (1991). Report of the expert panel on population strategies for blood cholesterol reduction. *Circulation* 83: 2154-2232.

Nattiv A, Puffer JC, Green GA (1997). Lifestyles and health risks of collegiate athletes: A multi-center study. *Clin. J. Sport Med.* 7(4): 262-272.

Nestel PJ (1993). Contribution of fats and fatty acids to performance of the elite athlete. In *Nutrition and fitness for athletes,* eds. AP Simopoulos, KN Pavlou. *World Rev. Nutr. Diet.* Vol. 71, pp. 61-68. Basel: Karger.

Nordgaard I, Mortensen PB (1995). Digestive processes in the human colon. *Nutrition* 11(1): 37-45.

Nutter J (1991). Seasonal changes in female athlete's diets. *Int. J. Sport Nutr.* 1(4): 395-407.

Pariza MW (1996). Protein and amino acids. In *Present knowledge in nutrition,* eds. EE Ziegler, LJ Filer Jr, p. 567. Washington, DC: International Life Sciences Institute.

Pendergast DR, Horvath PJ, Leddy JJ, Venkatraman JT (1996). The role of dietary fat on performance, metabolism and health. *Am. J. Sports. Med.* 24(6): S53-S58.

Phillips SM, Atkinson SA, Tarnopolsky MA, MacDougall JD (1993). Gender differences in leucine kinetics and nitrogen balance in endurance athletes. *J. Appl. Physiol.* 75(5): 2134-2141.

Portanova JP, Zhang Y, Anderson GD, Hauser SD, Masferrer JL, Seibert K, Gregory SA, Isakson PC (1996). Selective neutralization of prostaglandin E2 blocks inflammation, hyperalgesia, and interleukin 6 production in vivo. *J. Exp. Med.* 184(3): 883-891.

Potter JD, Steinmetz K (1996). Vegetables, fruit and phytoestrogens as preventive agents. *IARC Sci. Publ.* 139: 61-90.

Rainey CJ, McKeown RE, Sargent RG, Valois RF (1996). Patterns of tobacco and alcohol use among sedentary, exercising, nonathletic, and athletic youth. *J. Sch. Health* 66(1): 27-32.

Reaven GM (1997). Do high carbohydrate diets prevent the development or attenuate the manifestations (or both) of syndrome X? A viewpoint strongly against. *Curr. Opin. Lipidol.* 8(1): 23-27.

Reed MJ, Cheng RW, Simmonds M, Richmond W, James VH (1987). Dietary lipids: An additional regulator of plasma levels of sex hormone binding globulin. *J. Clin. Endocrinol. Metab.* 64(5): 1083-1085.

Reeds PJ, Beckett PR (1996). Protein and amino acids. In *Present knowledge in nutrition,* eds. EE Ziegler, LJ Filer Jr, p. 67. Washington, DC: International Life Sciences Institute.

Rieth N, Larue-Achagiotis C (1997). Exercise training decreases body fat more in self-selecting than in chow-fed rats. *Physiol. Behav.* 62(6): 1291-1297.

Rossowska MJ, Nakamoto T (1994). Effects of chronic caffeine feeding on the activities of oxygen free radical defense enzymes in the growing rat heart and liver. *Experientia* 50(5): 465-468.

Sharma SS, Kochupillai V, Gupta SK, Seth SD, Gupta YK (1997). Antiemetic efficacy of ginger (Zingiber officinale) against cisplatin-induced emesis in dogs. *J. Ethnopharmacol.* 57(2): 93-96.

Shimizu S, Jareonkitmongkol S, Kawashima H, Akimoto K, Yamada H (1992). Inhibitory effect of curcumin on fatty acid desaturation in Mortierella alpina 1S-4 and rat liver microsomes. *Lipids* 27(7):509-512.

Sigleo S, Jackson M, Vahouny G (1984). Effects of dietary fiber constituents on intestinal morphology and nutrient transport. *Am. J. Physiol.* 246(1 Pt 1): G34-39.

Siguel EN, Lerman RH (1996). Prevalence of essential fatty acid deficiency in patients with chronic gastrointestinal disorders. *Metabolism* 45(1): 12-23.

Simi B, Sempore B, Mayet M, Favier RJ (1991). Additive effects of training and high-fat diet on energy metabolism during exercise. *J. Appl. Physiol.* 71(1): 197-203.

Simopoulos AP (1991). Omega-3 fatty acids in health and disease and in growth and development. *Am. J. Clin. Nutr.* 54(3): 438-463.

Srivastava KC, Mustafa T (1992). Ginger (Zingiber officinale) in rheumatism and musculoskeletal disorders. *Med. Hypotheses* 39(4): 342-348.

Standard Process, Inc. 1200 West Royal Lee Drive, Palmyra, WI 53516. 800-848-5061.

Sugawa M, Ikeda S, Kushima Y, Takashima Y, Cynshi O (1997). Oxidized low density lipoprotein caused CNS neuron cell death. *Brain Res.* 761(1): 165-172.

Sullivan GW, Luong LS, Carper HT, Barnes RC, Mandell GL (1995). Methylxanthines with adenosine alter TNF alpha-primed PMN activation. *Immunopharmacology* 31(1): 19-29.

Szepesi B (1996). Carbohydrates. In *Present knowledge in nutrition,* eds. EE Ziegler, LJ Filer Jr, p. 33. Washington, DC: International Life Sciences Institute.

Tarnopolsky MA, Atkinson SA, MacDougall JD (1992). Evaluation of protein requirements for trained strength athletes. *J. Appl. Physiol.* 73: 1986-1995.

Tarnopolsky MA, Atkinson SA, Phillips SM, MacDougall JD (1995). Carbohydrate loading and metabolism during exercise in men and women. *J. Appl. Physiol.* 78(4): 1360-1368.

Tarnopolsky MA, Bosman M, Macdonald JR, Vandeputte D, Martin J, Roy BD (1997). Postexercise protein-carbohydrate and carbohydrate supplements increase muscle glycogen in men and women. *J. Appl. Physiol.* 83(6): 1877-1883.

Tarnopolsky MA, MacDougall JD, Atkinson SA (1988). Influence of protein intake and training status on nitrogen balance and lean body mass. *J. Appl. Physiol.* 64(1): 187-193.

Thibault L. (1994). Dietary carbohydrates: Effects of self-selection, plasma glucose and insulin, and brain indoleaminergic systems in rat. *Appetite* 23: 275-286.

Thomas DE, Brotherhood JR, Brand JC (1991). Carbohydrate feeding before exercise: Effect of glycemic index. *Int. J. Sports Med.* 12: 10-186.

Thomas DE, Brotherhood JR, Miller JB (1994). Plasma glucose levels after prolonged strenuous exercise correlate inversely with glycemic response to food consumed before exercise. *Int. J. Sport Nutr.* 4: 361-373.

Thorsen K, Kristoffersson AO, Lerner UH, Lorentzon RP (1996). In situ microdialysis in bone tissue. Stimulation of prostaglandin E2 release by weight-bearing mechanical loading. *J. Clin. Invest.* 98(11): 2446-2449.

Tordoff MG, Friedman MI (1986). Hepatic portal glucose infusions decrease food intake and increase food preference. *Am. J. Physiol.* 251: 192-196.

Torre M, Rodriguez AR, Saura-Calixto F (1991). Effects of dietary fiber and phytic acid on mineral availability. *Crit. Rev. Food Sci. Nutr.* 1(1): 1-22.

Ulmann L, Blond JP, Poisson JP, Bezard J (1994). Incorporation of delta 6- and delta 5-desaturation fatty acids in liver microsomal lipid classes of obese Zucker rats fed n-6 or n-3 fatty acids. *Biochem. Biophys. Acta* 1214(1): 73-78.

Umeda-Sawada R, Takahashi N, Igarashi O (1995). Interaction of sesamin and eicosapentaenoic acid against delta 5 desaturation and n-6/n-3 ratio of essential fatty acids in rat. *Biosci. Biotechnol. Biochem.* 59(12): 2268-2273.

Venkatraman JT, Rowland JA, Denardin E, Horvath PJ, Pendergast D (1997). Influence of the level of dietary lipid intake and maximal exercise on the immune status in runners. *Med. Sci. Sports Exerc.* 29(3): 333-344.

Vukovich MD, Costill DL, Hickey MS, Trappe SW, Cole KJ, Fink WJ (1993). Effect of fat emulsion infusion and fat feeding on muscle glycogen utilization during cycle exercise. *J. Appl. Physiol.* 75(4): 1513-1518.

Welsh S (1996). Nutrient standards, dietary guidelines, and food guides. In *Present knowledge in nutrition,* ed. EE Ziegler, LJ Filer Jr, p. 641. Washington, DC: International Life Sciences Institute.

Welsh SO, Marston RM (1982). Review of trends in food use in the United States, 1909 to 1980. *J. Am. Diet. Assoc.* 81(2): 120-128.

Wiles JD, Bird SR, Hopkins J, Riley M (1992). Effect of caffeinated coffee on running speed, respiratory factors, blood lactate and perceived exertion during 1500-m treadmill running. *Br. J. Sports Med.* 26(2): 116-120.

Williams C (1995). Macronutrients and performance. *J. Sports Sci.* 13(Spec. no.): S1-10.

Wilmore JH, Costill DL (1994). *Physiology of sport and exercise,* p. 329. Champaign, IL: Human Kinetics.

Wilt TJ, Rubins HB, Robins SJ, Riley WA, Collins D, Elam M, Rutan G, Anderson JW (1997). Carotid atherosclerosis in men with low levels of HDL cholesterol. *Stroke* 28(10): 1919-1925.

Wolever TMS, Katzman-Relle L, Jenkins AL, Vuksan V, Josse RG, Jenkins DJA (1994). Glycaemic index of 102 complex carbohydrate foods in patients with diabetes. *Nutr. Res.* 14: 651-669.

World Health Organization/Food and Agriculture Organization of the United Nations (1985). Energy and protein requirements. WHO Technical Report Series, no. 724. Geneva: World Health Organization.

Yang MU, Van Itallie TB (1976). Composition of weight lost during short-term weight reduction. Metabolic responses of obese subjects to starvation and low-calorie ketogenic and nonketogenic diets. *J. Clin. Invest.* 58(3): 722-730.

Young VR (1994). Adult amino acid requirements: The case for a major revision in current recommendations. *J. Nutr.* 126: 1517S-1523S.

Zmarzty SA, Wells AS, Read NW (1997). The influence of food on pain perception in healthy human volunteers. *Physiol. Behav.* 62(1): 185-191.

CHAPTER 19

Aitken JC, Thompson J (1989). The effects of dietary manipulation upon the respiratory exchange ratio as a predictor of maximum oxygen uptake during fixed term maximal incremental exercise in man. *Eur. J. Appl. Physiol.* 58: 722-727.

Alessio HM, Goldfarb AH, Cao G (1997). Exercise-induced oxidative stress before and after vitamin C supplementation. *Int. J. Sport Nutr.* 7(1): 1-9.

Alston TA, Abeles RH (1987). Enzymatic conversion of the antibiotic metronidazole to an analog of thiamine. *Arch. Biochem. Biophys.* 257(2): 357-362.

Anderson SD (1996). Exercise-induced asthma and the use of hypertonic saline aerosol as a bronchial challenge. *Respirology* 1(3): 175-181.

Argov Z, De Stefano N, Arnold DL (1997). Muscle high-energy phosphates in central nervous system disorders. The phosphorus MRS experience. *Ital. J. Neurol. Sci.* 18(6): 353-357.

Aruoma OI, Reilly T, MacLaren D, Halliwell B (1988). Iron, copper and zinc concentrations in human sweat and plasma; the effect of exercise. *Clinica Chimica Acta* 177: 81-88.

Balon R, Jordan M, Pohl R, Yeragani VK (1989). Family history of anxiety disorders in control subjects with lactate-induced panic attacks. *Am. J. Psychiatry* 146: 1304-1306.

Berenshtein E, Mayer B, Goldberg C, Kitrossky N, Chevion M (1997). Patterns of mobilization of copper and iron following myocardial ischemia: Possible predictive criteria for tissue injury. *J. Mol. Cell. Cardiol.* 29(11): 3025-3034.

Bragg LE, Thompson JS, Rikkers LF (1991). Influence of nutrient delivery on gut structure and function. *Nutrition* 7(4): 237-243.

Brandi G, Pisi A, Biasco G, Miglioli M, Biavati B, Barbara L (1996). Bacteria in biopsies of human hypochlorhydric stomach: A scanning electron microscopy study. *Ultrastruct. Pathol.* 20(3): 203-209.

Brunner G, Luna P, Hartmann M, Wurst W (1996). Optimizing the intragastric pH as a supportive therapy in upper GI bleeding. *Yale J. Biol. Med.* 69(3): 225-231.

Buchman AL, Moukarzel AA, Bhuta S, Belle M, Ament ME, Eckhert CD, Hollander D, Gornbein J, Kopple JD, Vijayaroghavan SR (1995). Parenteral nutrition is associated with intestinal morphologic and functional changes in humans. *J. Parenter. Enteral. Nutr.* 19(6): 453-460.

Buller R, von Bardeleben U, Maier W, Benkert O (1989). Specificity of lactate response in panic disorder, panic with concurrent depression and major depression. *J. Affective Dis.* 16: 109-113.

Cao G, Sofic E, Prior RL (1997). Antioxidant and prooxidant behavior of flavonoids: Structure-activity relationships. *Free Radic. Biol. Med.* 22(5): 749-760.

Castell LM, Poortmans JR, Newsholme EA (1996). Does glutamine have a role in reducing infections in athletes? *Eur. J. Appl. Physiol.* 73(5): 488-490.

Cazzola P, Mazzanti P, Kouttab NM (1987). Update and future perspectives of a thymic biological response modifier (Thymomodulin). *Immunopharmacol. Immunotoxicol.* 9(2-3): 195-216.

Champagne ET (1989). Low gastric hydrochloric acid secretion and mineral bioavailability. *Adv. Exp. Med. Biol.* 249: 173-184.

Chan MM, Fong D, Ho CT, Huang HI (1997). Inhibition of inducible nitric oxide synthase gene expression and enzyme activity by epigallocatechin gallate, a natural product from green tea. *Biochem. Pharmacol.* 54(12): 1281-1286.

Chan MM, Ho CT, Huang HI (1995). Effects of three dietary phytochemicals from tea, rosemary and turmeric on inflammation-induced nitrite production. *Cancer Lett.* 96(1): 23-29.

Christen S, Woodall AA, Shigenaga MK, Southwell-Keely PT, Duncan MW, Ames BN (1997). Gamma-tocopherol traps mutagenic electrophiles such as NO(X) and complements alpha-tocopherol: Physiological implications. *Proc. Natl. Acad. Sci.* 94(7): 3217-3222.

Clarkson PM (1995). Micronutrients and exercise: Anti-oxidants and minerals. *J. Sports Sci.* 13: S11-S24.

Cohen HA, Neuman I, Nahum H (1997). Blocking effect of vitamin C in exercise-induced asthma. *Arch. Pediatr. Adolesc. Med.* 151(4): 367-370.

Corazza GR, Valentini RA, Andreani ML, D'Anchino M, Leva MT, Ginaldi L, De Feudis L, Quaglino D, Gasbarrini G (1995). Subclinical coeliac disease is a frequent cause of iron-deficiency anaemia. *Scand. J. Gastroenterol.* 30(2): 153-156.

Craig WJ (1997). Phytochemicals: Guardians of our health. *J. Am. Diet. Assoc.* 10(2): S199-S204.

Dager SR, Cowley DS, Dorsa DM, Dunner DL (1989). Plasma beta-endorphin response to lactate infusion. *Biol. Psychiatry* 25: 243-245.

Dekkers JC, van Doornen LJ, Kemper HC (1996). The role of antioxidant vitamins and enzymes in the prevention of exercise-induced muscle damage. *Sports Med.* 21(3): 213-238.

de Klerk A, Schulze KF, Kashyap S, Sahni R, Fifer W, Myers M (1997). Diet and infant behavior. *Acta Paediatr.* (Suppl.) 422: 65-68.

Demopoulos H (1983). The development of secondary pathology with free radical reactions as a threshold mechanism. *J. Am. Coll. Toxicol.* 2: 173-184.

Dickey W, Kenny BD, McMillan SA, Porter KG, McConnell JB (1997). Gastric as well as duodenal biopsies may be useful in the investigation of iron deficiency anaemia. *Scand. J. Gastroenterol.* 32(5): 469-472.

Doucet E, Tremblay A (1997). Food intake, energy balance and body weight control. *Eur. J. Clin. Nutr.* 51(12): 846-855.

Enright T (1996). Exercise-induced asthma and the asthmatic athlete. *Wis. Med. J.* 95(6): 375-378.

Ferraris RP (1997). Effect of aging and caloric restriction on intestinal sugar and amino acid transport. *Front. Biosci.* 2: E108-E115.

Fiocchi A, Borella E, Riva E, Arensi D, Travaglini P, Cazzola P, Giovannini M (1986). A double-blind clinical trial for the evaluation of the therapeutical effectiveness of a calf thymus derivative (Thymomodulin) in children with recurrent respiratory infections. *Thymus* 8(6): 331-339.

Food and Nutrition Board, National Academy of Sciences (1989) Recommended Daily Allowances, 10th ed. Washington, DC: National Academy Press.

Freston JW (1997). Long-term acid control and proton pump inhibitors: Interactions and safety issues in perspective. *Am. J. Gastroenterol.* 92(4 Suppl.): 51S-55S.

Gasbarrini G, Corazza GR (1993). Intestinal malabsorption and related clinical syndromes. *Ann. Ital. Med. Int.* 8(3): 185-188.

Gaur SN, Agarwal G, Gupta SK (1997). Use of LPC antagonist, choline, in the management of bronchial asthma. *Indian J. Chest Dis. Allied Sci.* 39(2): 107-113.

Genova R, Guerra A (1986). Thymomodulin in management of food allergy in children. *Int. J. Tissue React.* 8(3): 239-242.

Ghoshal UC, Kochhar R, Goenka MK, Chakravorty A, Talwar P, Mehta SK (1994). Fungal colonization of untreated peptic ulcer. *Indian J. Gastroenterol.* 13(4): 115-117.

Goldfarb AH (1992). Antioxidants: Role of supplementation to prevent exercise-induced oxidative stress. *Med. Sci. Sports Exerc.* 25(2): 232-236.

Graziani G, Como G, Badalamenti S, Finazzi S, Malesci A, Gallieni M, Brancaccio D, Ponticelli C (1995). Effect of gastric acid secretion on intestinal phosphate and calcium absorption in normal subjects. *Nephrol. Dial. Transplant.* 10(8): 1376-1380.

Gupta SK, Gaur SN (1997). A placebo controlled trial of two dosages of LPC antagonist—choline in the management of bronchial asthma. *Indian J. Chest Dis. Allied Sci.* 39(3): 149-156.

Guyton AC (1986). *Textbook of medical physiology,* p. 780. Philadelphia: Saunders.

Ibid. p. 778.

Halliwell B (1996). Antioxidants. In *Present knowledge in nutrition,* eds. EE Ziegler, LJ Filer Jr, pp. 596-603. Washington, DC: International Life Sciences Institute.

Hawkins CL, Davies MJ (1997). Oxidative damage to collagen and related substrates by metal ion/hydrogen peroxide systems: Random attack or site-specific damage? *Biochem. Biophys. Acta* 1360(1): 84-96.

Henriksson AE, Blomquist L, Nord CE, Midtvedt T, Uribe A (1993). Small intestinal bacterial overgrowth in patients with rheumatoid arthritis. *Ann. Rheum. Dis.* 52(7): 503-510.

Higashide S, Chu KU, Gomez G, Greeley GH Jr, Thompson JC, Townsend CM Jr (1997). Caloric restriction causes secretagogue specific changes of gastric acid secretion in rats. *Regul. Pept.* 68(3): 205-210.

Hirn J, Pekkanen TJ (1975). Quantitative analysis of thiaminase activity in certain fish species. *Nord. Vet. Med.* 27(12): 646-648.

Hirokawa K (1997). Reversing and restoring immune function. *Mech. Aging Dev.* 93(1-3): 119-124.

Hirokawa K, Utsuyama M, Kasai M, Kurashima C (1992). Aging and immunity. *Acta Pathol. Jpn.* 42(8): 537-548.

Houglum K, Ramm GA, Crawford DH, Witztum JL, Powell LW, Chojkier M (1997). Excess iron induces hepatic oxidative stress and transforming growth factor beta1 in genetic hemochromatosis. *Hepatology* 26(3): 605-610.

Humbert P, Lopez de Soria P, Fernandez-Banares F, Junca J, Boix J, Planas R, Quer JC, Domenech E, Gassull MA (1994). Magnesium hydrogen breath test using end expiratory sampling to assess achlorhydria in pernicious anaemia patients. *Gut* 35(9): 1205-1208.

Islam S, Mahalanabis D, Chowdhury AK, Wahed MA, Rahman AS (1997). Glutamine is superior to glucose in stimulating water and electrolyte absorption across rabbit ileum. *Dig. Dis. Sci.* 42(2): 420-423.

Jain P, Khanna NK (1981). Evaluation of anti-inflammatory and analgesic properties of L-glutamine. *Agents Actions* 11(3): 243-249.

Kamal-Eldin A, Appelqvist L (1996). The chemistry and antioxidant properties of tocopherols and tocotrienols. *Lipids* 31: 671-707.

Kelso TB, Shear CR, Max SR (1989). Enzymes of glutamine metabolism in inflammation associated with skeletal muscle hypertrophy. *Am. J. Physiol.* 257(6 Part 1): E885-E894.

Kidd JM 3d, Cohen SH, Sosman AJ, Fink JN (1983). Food-dependent exercise-induced anaphylaxis. *J. Allergy Clin. Immunol.* 71(4): 407-411.

Kouttab NM, Prada M, Cazzola P (1989). Thymomodulin: Biological properties and clinical applications. *Med. Oncol. Tumor Pharmacother.* 6(1): 5-9.

Kreider RB, Miriel V, Bertum E (1993). Amino acid supplementation and exercise performance—analysis of the proposed ergogenic value. *Sports Med.* 16: 190-209.

Krishnaswamy K (1996). Indian functional foods: Role in prevention of cancer. *Nutr. Rev.* 54(11): S127-S131.

Lacey JM, Wilmore DW (1990). Is glutamine a conditionally essential amino acid? *Nutr. Rev.* 48(8): 233-245.

Lehmann M, Huonker M, Dimeo F, Heinz N, Gastmann U, Treis N, Steinacker JM, Keul J, Kajewski R, Haussinger D (1993). Serum amino acid concentrations in nine athletes before and after the 1993 Colmar ultra triathlon. *Int. J. Sports Med.* 16(3): 155-159.

Linder MC (1991). Nutrition and metabolism of fats. In *Nutritional biochemistry and metabolism,* ed. MC Linder, pp. 339-348. Norwalk, CT: Appleton & Lange.

Ibid. p. 35.

Ibid. p. 167.

Ibid. p. 180.

Ibid. p. 123.

Ibid. p. 135.

Lukaski HC, Klevay LM, Milne DB (1988). Effects of dietary copper on human autonomic cardiovascular function. *Eur. J. Appl. Physiol.* 58(1-2): 74-80.

Lukaski HC, Penland J (1996). Functional changes appropriate for determining mineral element requirements. *J. Nutr.* 126(9 Suppl): 2354S-2364S.

Lukaski HC, Siders WA, Hoverson BS, Gallagher SK (1996). Iron, copper magnesium and zinc status as predictors of swimming performance. *Int. J. Sports Med.* 17(7): 535-540.

Maffetone P (1990). *The use of glutamine in small intestine dysfunction: A clinical observation.* Presentation at the International College of Applied Kinesiology, Winter Meeting, January, Vail, CO.

Mantzioris E, James MJ, Gibson RA, Cleland LG (1995). Dietary substitution with an alpha-linolenic acid-rich vegetable oil increases eicosapentaenoic acid concentrations in tissues. *Am. J. Clin. Nutr.* 59(6): 1304-1309.

Martinsen EW, Strand J, Paulsson G, Kaggestad J (1989). Physical fitness level in patients with anxiety and depressive disorders. *Int. J. Sports Med.* 10(1): 58-61.

May JM (1998). Ascorbate function and metabolism in the human erythrocyte. *Front. Biosci.* 3: 1-10. Abstract.

Mayes PA (1993a). Glycolysis & the oxidation of pyruvate. In *Harper's biochemistry,* eds. RK Murray, DK Granner, PA Mayes, VW Rodwell, p. 176. Norwalk, CT: Appleton & Lange.

Mayes PA (1993b). Oxidation of fatty acids: Ketogenesis. In *Harper's biochemistry,* eds. RK Murray, DK Granner, PA Mayes, VW Rodwell, p. 221. Norwalk, CT: Appleton & Lange.

Mayes PA (1993c). Structure & function of the lipid-soluble vitamins. In *Harper's biochemistry,* eds. RK Murray, DK Granner, PA Mayes, VW Rodwell, p. 594. Norwalk, CT: Appleton & Lange.

Mayes PA (1993d). Structure & function of the water-soluble vitamins. In *Harper's biochemistry,* eds. RK Murray, DK Granner, PA Mayes, VW Rodwell, pp. 577-579, 594. Norwalk, CT: Appleton & Lange.

McColl KE (1997). Helicobacter pylori and acid secretion: Where are we now? *Eur. J. Gastroenterol. Hepatol.* 9(4): 333-335.

McKinney CH, Antoni MH, Kumar M, Tims FC, McCabe PM (1997). Effects of guided imagery and music (GIM) therapy on mood and cortisol in healthy adults. *Health Psychol.* 16(4): 390-400.

McNeil D, Strauss RH (1988). Exercise-induced anaphylaxis related to food intake. *Ann. Allergy* 61(6): 440-442.

Meininger CJ, Wu G (1997). L-glutamine inhibits nitric oxide synthesis in bovine venular endothelial cells. *J. Pharmacol Exp. Ther.* 281(1): 448-453.

Meredith CN, Frontera WR, O'Reilly KP, Evans WJ (1992). Body composition in elderly men: Effect of dietary modification during strength training. *J. Am. Ger. Soc.* 40: 155-162.

Mero A, Pitkanen H, Oja SS, Komi PV, Pontinen P, Takala T (1997). Leucine supplementation and serum amino acids, testosterone, cortisol and growth hormone in male power athletes during training. *J. Sports Med. Phys. Fitness* 37(2): 137-45.

Messina M, Messina V (1996). Nutritional implications of dietary phytochemicals. *Adv. Exp. Med. Biol.* 401: 207-212.

Milam SB, Zardeneta G, Schmitz JP (1998). Oxidative stress and degenerative temporomandibular joint disease: A proposed hypothesis. *J. Oral Maxillofac. Surg.* 56(2): 214-223.

Miyajima H, Sakamoto M, Takahashi Y, Mizoguchi K, Nishimura Y (1989). Muscle carnitine deficiency associated with myalgia and rhabdomyolysis following exercise. *Rinsho Shinkeigaku* 29(1): 93-97.

Molina PE, Myers N, Smith RM, Lang CH, Yousef KA, Tepper PG, Abumrad NN (1994). Nutritional and metabolic characterization of a thiamine-deficient rat model. *J. Parenter. Enteral. Nutr.* 18(2): 104-111.

Moller P, Wallin H, Knudsen LE (1996). Oxidative stress associated with exercise, psychological stress and life-style factors. *Chem. Biol. Interact.* 102(1): 17-36.

Murray RK (1993). Metabolism of xenobiotics. In *Harper's biochemistry,* eds. RK Murray, DK Granner, PA Mayes, VW Rodwell, p. 706. Norwalk, CT: Appleton & Lange.

Nakasaki H, Ohta M, Soeda J, Makuuchi H, Tsuda M, Tajima T, Mitomi T, Fujii K (1997). Clinical and biochemical aspects of thiamine treatment for metabolic acidosis during total parenteral nutrition. *Nutrition* 13(2): 110-117.

Newsholme EA (1994). Biochemical mechanisms to explain immunosuppression in well-trained and overtrained athletes. *Int. J. Sports Med.* 15: S142-S147.

Nutri-West, Douglas, WY 82633. 800-443-3333.

Packer L (1997). Oxidants, antioxidant nutrients and the athlete. *J. Sports Sci.* 15(3): 353-363.

Parry-Billings M, Budgett R, Koutedakis Y, Blomstrand E, Brooks S, Williams C, Calder PC, Pilling S, Baigrie R, Newsholme EA (1992). Plasma amino acid concentrations in the overtraining syndrome: Possible effects on the immune system. *Med. Sci. Sports Exerc.* 24(12): 1353-1358.

Penland JG (1994). Dietary boron, brain function, and cognitive performance. *Environ. Health Perspect.* 102(Suppl. 7): 65-72.

Peuler JD, Morgan DA, Mark AL (1987). High calcium diet reduces blood pressure in Dahl salt-sensitive rats by neural mechanisms. *Hypertension* 9(6 Part 2): III159-III165.

Pfeifer MA, Weinberg CR, Cook D, Best JD, Reenan A, Halter JB (1983). Differential changes of autonomic nervous system function with age in man. *Am. J. Med.* 75(2): 249-258.

Pyne DB (1994). Exercise-induced muscle damage and inflammation: A review. *Aust. J. Sci. Med. Sport* 26(3-4): 49-58.

Ramani R, Ramani A, Kumari GR, Rao SA, Chkravarthy S, Shivananda PG (1994). Fungal colonization in gastric ulcers. *Indian J. Pathol. Microbiol.* 37(4): 389-393.

Rankin JW, Ocel JV, Craft LL (1996). Effect of weight loss and refeeding diet composition on anaerobic performance in wrestlers. *Med. Sci. Sports Exerc.* 28(10): 1292-1299.

Reeds PJ, Beckett PR. (1996). Protein and amino acids. In *Present knowledge in nutrition*, eds. EE Ziegler, LJ Filer Jr., p. 67. Washington DC: International Life Sciences Institute.

Rindi G (1996). Thiamin. In *Present knowledge in nutrition,* eds. EE Ziegler, LJ Filer Jr, pp. 161-164. Washington, DC: International Life Sciences Institute.

Rodwell VW (1993). Biosynthesis of the nutritionally nonessential amino acids. *In Harper's biochemistry,* eds. RK Murray, DK Granner, PA Mayes, VW Rodwell, p. 287. Norwalk, CT: Appleton & Lange.

Ibid. p. 288.

Rowbottom DG, Keast D, Morton AR (1996). The emerging role of glutamine as an indicator of exercise stress and overtraining. *Sports Med.* 21(2): 80-97.

Russell RM (1992). Changes in gastrointestinal function attributed to aging. *Am. J. Clin. Nutr.* 55(6 Suppl.): 1203S-1207S.

Russell TL, Berardi RR, Barnett JL, O'Sullivan TL, Wagner JG, Dressman JB (1994). pH-related changes in the absorption of dipyridamole in the elderly. *Pharm. Res.* 11(1): 136-143.

Salonen JT, Nyyssonen K, Korpela H, Tuomilehto J, Seppanen R, Salonen R (1992). High stored iron levels are associated with excess risk of myocardial infarction in eastern Finnish men. *Circulation* 86: 803-811.

Saltzman JR, Kemp JA, Golner BB, Pedrosa MC, Dallal GE, Russell RM (1994). Effect of hypochlorhydria due to omeprazole treatment or atrophic gastritis on protein-bound vitamin B12 absorption. *J. Am. Coll. Nutr.* 13(6): 584-591.

Savendahl L, Mar MH, Underwood LE, Zeisel SH (1997). Prolonged fasting in humans results in diminished plasma choline concentrations but does not cause liver dysfunction. *Am. J. Clin. Nutr.* 66(3): 622-625.

Scheppach W, Loges C, Bartram P, Christl SU, Richter F, Dusel G, Stehle P, Fuerst P, Kasper H (1994). Effect of free glutamine and alanyl-glutamine dipeptide on mucosal proliferation of the human ileum and colon. *Gastroenterology* 107(2): 429-434.

Schmitt WH Jr (1987a). The clorox test: A screening test for free radical pathology: Part I. *Digest of Chiropractic Economics* 30: 2.

Schmitt WH Jr (1987b). The clorox test: A screening test for free radical pathology: Part II. *Digest of Chiropractic Economics* 30: 3.

Schmitt, WH Jr (1990). *Compiled notes on clinical nutritional products,* pp. 155-156. Stamford, NY: David Barmore Productions.

Ibid. pp. 64-68.

Ibid. pp. 46-53.

Seacat AM, Kuppusamy P, Zweier JL, Yager JD (1997). ESR identification of free radicals formed from the oxidation of catechol estrogens by Cu2+. *Arch. Biochem. Biophys.* 347(1): 45-52.

Shabert JK (1997). *Glutamine: The ultimate nutrient.* Fourth International Symposium on Functional Medicine, May 15-17, Aspen, CO.

Skouby SO, Andersen O, Petersen KR, Molsted-Pedersen L, Kuhl C (1990). Mechanism of action of oral contraceptives on carbohydrate metabolism at the cellular level. *Am. J. Obstet. Gynecol.* 163: 343-348.

Snodgrass SR (1992). Vitamin neurotoxicity. *Mol. Neurobiol.* 6(1): 41-73.

Sobal J, Marquart LF (1994). Vitamin/mineral supplement use among athletes: A review of the literature. *Int. J. Sport Nutr.* 4(4): 320-334.

Song MK, Rosenthal MJ, Naliboff BD, Phanumas L, Kang KW (1998). Effects of bovine prostate powder on zinc, glucose, and insulin metabolism in old patients with non-insulin-dependent diabetes mellitus. *Metabolism* 47(1): 39-43.

Standard Process, Inc. 1200 West Royal Lee Drive, Palmyra, WI 53156. 800-848-5061.

Steen SN, Mayer K, Brownell KD, Wadden TA (1995). Dietary intake of female collegiate heavyweight rowers. *Int. J. Sport Nutr.* 5(3): 225-231.

Svintsyts'kyi AS, Horhol' VA, Kravchenko OI, Kolesova NA (1994). The functional-morphological status of the stomach in rheumatism patients (Ukrainian). *Lik. Sprava.* 1: 41-44. Abstract.

Taha AS, Angerson W, Nakshabendi I, Beekman H, Morran C, Sturrock RD, Russell RI (1993). Gastric and duodenal mucosal blood flow in patients receiving non-steroidal anti-inflammatory drugs—influence of age, smoking, ulceration and Helicobacter pylori. *Aliment. Pharmacol. Ther.* 7(1): 41-45.

Takahashi O (1995). Hemorrhagic toxicity of a large dose of alpha-, beta-, gamma- and delta-tocopherols, ubiquinone, beta-carotene, retinol acetate and L-ascorbic acid in the rat. *Food Chem. Toxicol.* 33(2): 121-128.

Tilles S, Schocket A, Milgrom H (1995). Exercise-induced anaphylaxis related to specific foods. *J. Pediatr.* 127(4): 587-589.

Toth MJ, Poehlman ET (1994). Sympathetic nervous system activity and resting metabolic rate in vegetarians. *Metabolism* 43(5): 621-625.

van der Beek EJ (1991). Vitamin supplementation and physical exercise performance. *J. Sports Sci.* 9 Spec No: 77-90.

van der Beek EJ, van Dokkum W, Schrijver J, Wedel M, Gaillard AWK, Wesstra A, van de Weerd H, Hermus RJJ (1988). Thiamin, riboflavin and vitamins B6 and C: Impact of combined restricted intake on functional performance in man. *Am. J. Clin. Nutr.* 48: 1451-1462.

van der Beek EJ, van Dokkum W, Wedel M, Schrijver J, van den Berg H (1994). Thiamin, riboflavin and vitamin B6: Impact of restricted intake on physical performance in man. *J. Am. Coll. Nutr.* 13(6): 629-640.

van der Hulst RR, van Kreel BK, von Meyenfeldt MF, Brummer RJ, Arends JW, Deutz NE, Soeters PB (1993). Glutamine and the preservation of gut integrity. *Lancet* 341(8857): 1363-1365.

van de Vijver LP, Kardinaal AF, Grobbee DE, Princen HM, van Poppel G (1997). Lipoprotein oxidation, antioxidants and cardiovascular risk: Epidemiologic evidence. *Prostaglandins Leukot. Essent. Fatty Acids* 57(4-5): 479-487.

Veera RK, Charles KT, Prasad M, Reddanna P (1992). Exercise-induced oxidant stress in the lung tissue: Role of dietary supplementation of vitamin E and selenium. *Biochem. Int.* 26(5): 863-871.

Verhagen H, de Vries A, Nijhoff WA, Schouten A, van Poppel G, Peters WH, van den Berg H (1997). Effect of Brussels sprouts on oxidative DNA-damage in man. *Cancer Lett.* 114(1-2): 127-130.

Veselov AI, Ruchkin VI (1987). Ulcer microflora and its antibiotic sensitivity in gastric and duodenal peptic ulcer. *Antibiot. Med. Biotekhnol.* 32(10): 785-789. Abstract.

Weiler JM (1996). Exercise-induced asthma: A practical guide to definitions, diagnosis, prevalence, and treatment. *Allergy Asthma Proc.* 17(6): 315-325.

Wilmore JH, Costill DL (1994). *Physiology of sport and exercise,* pp. 98-99. Champaign, IL: Human Kinetics.

Wolf G (1997). Gamma-tocopherol: An efficient protector of lipids against nitric oxide-initiated peroxidative damage. *Nutr. Rev.* 55(10): 376-378.

Young JB, Landsberg L (1997). Suppression of sympathetic nervous system during fasting. *Obes. Res.* 5(6): 646-649.

Yu BP (1996). Aging and oxidative stress: Modulation by dietary restriction. *Free Radic. Biol. Med.* 21(5): 651-668.

Zhu YI, Haas JD (1997). Iron depletion without anemia and physical performance in young women. *Am. J. Clin. Nutr.* 66(2): 334-341.

Ziegler TR, Szeszycki EE, Estivariz CF, Puckett AB, Leader LM (1996). Glutamine: From basic science to clinical applications. *Nutrition* 12(11-12 Suppl.): S68-S70.

CHAPTER 20

Armstrong LE, Maresh CM, Castellani JW, Bergeron MF, Kenefick RW, LaGasse KE, Riebe D (1994). Urinary indices of hydration status. *Int. J. Sport Nutr.* 4(3): 265-279.

Brouns F, Senden J, Beckers EJ, Saris WH (1995). Osmolarity does not affect the gastric emptying rate of oral rehydration solutions. *J. Parenter. Enteral. Nutr.* 19(5): 403-406.

Burke LM (1997). Fluid balance during team sports. *J. Sports Sci.* 15(3): 287-295.

Burke LM, Hawley JA (1997). Fluid balance in team sports. Guidelines for optimal practices. *Sports Med.* 24(1): 38-54.

Convertino VA, Armstrong LE, Coyle EF, Mack GW, Sawka MN, Senay LC Jr, Sherman WM (1996). American College of Sports Medicine position stand. Exercise and fluid replacement. *Med. Sci. Sports Exerc.* 28(1): I-VII.

DiBona GF (1994). Neural control of renal function in health and disease. *Clin. Auton. Res.* 4(1-2): 69-74.

Duchman SM, Ryan AJ, Schedl HP, Summers RW, Bleiler TL, Gisolfi CV (1997). Upper limit for intestinal absorption of a dilute glucose solution in men at rest. *Med. Sci. Sports Exerc.* 29(4): 482-488.

El-Sayed H, Hainsworth R (1996). Salt supplement increases plasma volume and orthostatic tolerance in patients with unexplained syncope. *Heart* 75(2): 134-140.

Frizzell RT, Lang GH, Lowance DC, Lathan SR (1986). Hyponatremia and ultramarathon running. *JAMA* 255: 772-774.

Guyton AC (1986). *Textbook of medical physiology,* pp. 909-914. Philadelphia: Saunders.

Ivaturi R, Kies C (1992). Mineral balances in humans as affected by fructose, high fructose corn syrup and sucrose. *Plant Foods Hum. Nutr.* 42(2): 143-151.

Lamb DR, Brodowicz GR (1986). Optimal use of fluids of varying formulations to minimise exercise-induced disturbances in homeostasis. *Sports Med.* 3(4): 247-274.

Luft FC (1996). Salt, water and extracellular volume regulation. In *Present knowledge in nutrition,* eds. EE Ziegler, LJ Filer Jr, p. 265. Washington, DC: International Life Sciences Institute.

Massicotte D, Peronnet F, Brisson G, Bakkouch K, Hillaire-Marcel C (1989). Oxidation of a glucose polymer during exercise: Comparison with glucose and fructose. *J. Appl. Physiol.* 66(1): 179-183.

Maughan RJ, Leiper JB, Shirreffs SM (1997). Factors influencing the restoration of fluid and electrolyte balance after exercise in the heat. *Br. J. Sports Med.* 31(3): 175-182.

McArdle WD, Katch FI, Katch VL (1991). *Exercise physiology,* 3d ed. p. 561. Philadelphia: Lea & Febiger.

Murray R, Eddy DE, Bartoli WP, Paul GL (1994). Gastric emptying of water and isocaloric carbohydrate solutions consumed at rest. *Med. Sci. Sports Exerc.* 26(6): 725-732.

Noakes TD (1992). The hyponatremia of exercise. *Int. J. Sport Nutr.* 2(3): 205-228.

Parker LN, Levin ER, Lifrak ET (1985). Evidence for adrenocortical adaptation to severe illness. *J. Clin. Endocrinol. Metab.* 60: 947-952.

Ravich WJ, Bayless TM, Thomas M (1983). Fructose: Incomplete intestinal absorption in humans. *Gastroenterology* 84(1): 26-29.

Savdie E, Prevedoros H, Irish A, Vickers C, Concannon A, Darveniza P, Sutton JR (1991). Heat stroke following Rugby League football. *Med. J. Aust.* 155(9): 636-639.

Sawka MN, Greenleaf JE (1992). Current concepts concerning thirst, dehydration, and fluid replacement: Overview. *Med. Sci. Sports Exerc.* 24(6): 643-644.

Selye H (1976). *The stress of life.* New York: McGraw-Hill.

Speedy DB, Faris JG, Hamlin M, Gallagher PG, Campbell RG (1997). Hyponatremia and weight changes in an ultradistance triathlon. *Clin. J. Sport Med.* 7(3): 180-184.

Surgenor S, Uphold RE (1994). Acute hyponatremia in ultra-endurance athletes. *Am. J. Emerg. Med.* 12(4): 441-444.

Wilmore JH, Costill DL (1994). *Physiology of sport and exercise,* p. 365. Champaign, IL: Human Kinetics.

Ibid. p. 365.

Ibid. p. 374.

Ibid. p. 366.

Yoshida T, Nakai S, Yorimoto A, Kawabata T, Morimoto T (1995). Effect of aerobic capacity on sweat rate and fluid intake during outdoor exercise in the heat. *Eur. J. Appl. Physiol.* 71(2-3): 235-239.

CHAPTER 21

Ahmaidi S, Granier P, Taoutaou Z, Mercier J, Dubouchaud H, Prefaut C (1996). Effects of active recovery on plasma lactate and anaerobic power following repeated intensive exercise. *Med. Sci. Sports Exerc.* 28(4): 450-456.

Bell GJ, Petersen SR, Wessel J, Bagnall K, Quinney HA (1991). Physiological adaptations to concurrent endurance training and low velocity resistance training. *Int. J. Sports Med.* 12(4): 384-390.

Bogdanis GC, Nevill ME, Lakomy HK, Graham CM, Louis G (1996). Effects of active recovery on power output during repeated maximal sprint cycling. *Eur. J. Appl. Physiol.* 74(5): 461-469.

Colliander EB, Dudley GA, Tesch PA (1988). Skeletal muscle fiber type composition and performance during repeated bouts of maximal, concentric contractions. *Eur. J. Appl. Physiol.* 58: 81-86.

Dudley G, Djamil R (1985). Incompatibility of endurance and strength training modes of exercise. *J. Appl. Physiol.* 59: 1446-1456.

Fry RW, Morton AR, Keast D (1991). Overtraining in athletes, an update. *Sports Med.* 12(1): 32-65.

Graves JE, Martin AD, Miltenberger LA, Pollock ML (1988). Physiological responses to walking with hand weights, wrist weights, and ankle weights. *Med. Sci. Sports Exerc.* 20(3): 265-271.

Hickson RC (1980). Interference of strength development by simultaneously training for strength and endurance. *Eur. J. Appl. Physiol.* 45(2-3): 255-263.

Hodgetts V, Coppack SW, Frayn KN, Hockadag DR (1991). Factors controlling fat mobilization from human subcutaneous adipose tissue during exercise. *J. Appl. Physiol.* 71: 445-451.

Horne L, Bell G, Fisher B, Warren S, Janowska-Wieczorek A (1997). Interaction between cortisol and tumour necrosis factor with concurrent resistance and endurance training. *Clin. J. Sport Med.* 7(4): 247-251.

Jacobs SJ, Berson BL (1986). A study of entrants to a 10,000 meter race. *Am. J. Sports Med.* 14: 151-155.

Jay G, Tetz D, Hartigan C, Lane L, Aghababian R (1995). Portable hyperbaric oxygen therapy in the emergency department with the Gamow bag. *Ann. Emerg. Med.* 26: 707-711.

Jones BH, Cowan DN, Knapik JJ (1994). Exercise, training and injuries. *Sports Med.* 18(3): 202-214.

Jones BH, Cowan DN, Tomlinson JP, Robinson JR, Polly DW, Frykman PN (1993). Epidemiology of injuries associated with physical training among young men in the army. *Med. Sci. Sports Exerc.* 25(2): 197-203.

Kasic J (1991). Treatment of acute mountain sickness: Hyperbaric versus oxygen therapy. *Ann. Emerg. Med.* 20: 1109-1112.

King S, Greenlee R (1990). Successful use of the Gamow hyperbaric bag in the treatment of altitude illness at Mt. Everest. *J. Wilderness Med.* 1: 193-202.

Leaf DA, Kleinman MT, Hamilton M, Barstow TJ (1997). The effect of exercise intensity on lipid peroxidation. *Med. Sci. Sports Exerc.* 29(8): 1036-1039.

Lehmann MJ, Lormes W, Opitz-Gress A, Steinacher JM, Netzer N, Foster C, Gastmann U (1997). Training and overtraining: An overview and experimental results in endurance sports. *J. Sports Med. Phys. Fitness* 37: 7-17.

Maffetone P (1996). *Training for endurance*, pp. 7-8. Stamford, NY: David Barmore Productions.

McArdle WD, Katch FI, Katch VL (1991). *Exercise physiology.* 3d ed., pp. 429-430. Philadelphia: Lea & Febiger.

Ibid. p. 513.

Ibid. pp. 132-133.

McCarthy JP, Agre JC, Graf BK, Pozniak MA, Vailas AC (1995). Compatibility of adaptive responses with combining strength and endurance training. *Med. Sci. Sports Exerc.* 27(3): 429-436.

Moon R (1988). Emergency treatment of diving casualties in remote areas. *Marine Tech. Soc. J.* 23: 50-55.

Newsholme EA (1994). Biochemical mechanisms to explain immunosuppression in well-trained and overtrained athletes. *Int. J. Sports Med.* 15: 142-147.

Safran MR, Garrett WE, Seaber AV, Glisson RR, Ribbeck BM (1988). The role of warmup in muscular injury prevention. *Am. J. Sports Med.* 16(2): 123-129.

Safran MR, Seaber AV, Garrett WE Jr (1989). Warm-up and muscular injury prevention. An update. *Sports Med.* 8(4): 239-249.

Sagiv M, Goldhammer E, Pollock ML, Graves JE, Schneewiss A, Ben-Sira D (1990). Comparative analysis of cardiopulmonary responses during dynamic exercise with wrist weights in the elderly versus young hypertensive responders. *Gerontology* 36(5-6): 333-339.

Shellock FG, Prentice WE (1985). Warming-up and stretching for improved physical performance and prevention of sports-related injuries. *Sports Med.* 2(4): 267-278.

Simoneau JA, Lortie G, Boulay MR, Marcotte M, Thibault MC, Bouchard C (1985). Human skeletal muscle fiber type alteration with high-intensity intermittent training. *Eur. J. Appl. Physiol.* 54: 250-253.

Skinner HB, Wyatt MP, Stone ML, Hodgdon JA, Barrack RL (1986). Exercise-related knee joint laxity. *Am. J. Sports Med.* 14(1): 30-34.

Taber R (1990). Protocols for the use of a portable hyperbaric chamber for the treatment of high altitude disorders. *J. Wilderness Med.* 1: 181-192.

Taoutaou Z, Granier P, Mercier B, Mercier J, Ahmaidi S, Prefaut C (1996). Lactate kinetics during passive and partially active recovery in endurance and sprint athletes. *Eur. J. Appl. Physiol.* 73(5): 465-470.

Van Mechelen W (1992). Running injuries. A review of the epidemiological literature. *Sports Med.* 14(5): 320-335.

Van Mechelen W, Hlobil H, Kemper HC, Voorn WJ (1993). Prevention of running injuries by warm-up, cool-down, and stretching exercises. *Am. J. Sports Med.* 21(5): 711-719.

Wiesler ER, Hunter DM, Martin DF, Curl WW, Hoen H (1996). Ankle flexibility and injury patterns in dancers. *Am. J. Sports Med.* 24(6): 754-757.

Wilmore JH, Costill DL (1994). *Physiology of sport and exercise,* p. 524. Champaign, IL: Human Kinetics.

Ibid. p. 525.

Wyndham C, Kok R, Strydom N, Rogers G, Zwi S (1971). Physiological effects of acute changes in altitude in a deep mine. *J. Appl. Physiol.* 30(2): 232-237.

Yee L, Brandon G (1983). Successful reversal of presumed carbon monoxide induced semi-coma. *Aviat. Space Environ. Med.* 54: 641-643.

Yoshida T, Watari H, Tagawa K (1996). Effects of active and passive recoveries on splitting of the inorganic phosphate peak determined by 31P-nuclear magnetic resonance spectroscopy. *NMR Biomed.* 9(1): 13-19.

CHAPTER 22

Costill DL, Flynn MG, Kirwan JP, Houmard JA, Mitchell JB, Thomas R (1988). Effects of repeated days of intensified training on muscle glycogen and swimming performance. *Med. Sci. Sports Exerc.* 20: 249-254.

Fry RW, Morton AR, Garcia-Webb P, Crawford GPM, Keast D (1992). Biological responses to overload training in endurance sports. *Eur. J. Appl. Physiol.* 64: 335-344.

Lehmann MJ, Lormes W, Opitz-Gress A, Steinacher JM, Netzer N, Foster C, Gastmann U (1997). Training and overtraining: An overview and experimental results in endurance sports. *J. Sports Med. Phys. Fitness* 37: 7-17.

McArdle WD, Katch FI, Katch VL (1991). *Exercise physiology.* 3d ed., p. 444. Philadelphia: Lea & Febiger.

Snyder AC, Kuipers H, Cheng B, Servais R, Fransen E (1995). Overtraining following intensified training with normal muscle glycogen. *Med. Sci. Sports Exerc.* 27: 1063-1070.

CHAPTER 23

Adlercreutz H, Harkonen M, Kuoppasalmi K, Naveri H, Huhtaniemi I, Tikkanen H, Remes K, Dessypris A, Karvonen J (1986). Effect of training on plasma anabolic and catabolic steroid hormones and their response during physical exercise. *Int. J. Sports Med.* 7: 27-28.

Arena B, Maffulli N, Maffulli F, Morleo MA (1995). Reproductive hormones and menstrual changes with exercise in female athletes. *Sports Med.* 19(4): 278-287.

Bale P, Doust J, Dawson D (1996). Gymnasts, distance runners, anorexics: Body composition and menstrual status. *J. Sports Med. Phys. Fitness* 36(1): 49-53.

Belanger A, Candas B, Dupont A, Cusan L, Diamond P, Gomez JL, Labrie F (1994). Changes in serum concentrations of conjugated and unconjugated steroids in 40- to 80-year-old men. *J. Clin. Endocrinol. Metab.* 79(4): 1086-1090.

Benson JE, Engelbert-Fenton KA, Eisenman PA (1996). Nutritional aspects of amenorrhea in the female athlete triad. *Int. J. Sport Nutr.* 6(2): 134-145.

Brandao-Neto J, de Mendonca BB, Shuhama T, Marchini JS (1990). Zinc acutely and temporarily inhibits adrenal cortisol secretion in humans. *Biol. Trace Elem. Res.* 24(1): 83-90.

Claassen N, Coetzer H, Steinmann CM, Kruger MC (1995). The effect of different n-6/n-3 essential fatty acid ratios on calcium balance and bone in rats. *Prostaglandins Leukot. Essent. Fatty Acids* 53(1): 13-19.

De Cree C, Lewin R, Barros A (1995). Hypoestrogenemia and rhabdomyelysis (myoglobinuria) in the female judoist: A new worrying phenomenon? *J. Clin. Endocrinol. Metab.* 80(12): 3639-3646.

Ding JH, Sheckter CB, Drinkwater BL, Soules MR, Bremner WJ (1988). High serum cortisol levels in exercise-associated amenorrhea. *Ann. Intern. Med.* 108(4): 530-534.

Dueck CA, Matt KS, Manore MM, Skinner JS (1996). Treatment of athletic amenorrhea with a diet and training intervention program. *Int. J. Sport Nutr.* 6(1): 24-40.

Fry AC, Kraemer WJ (1997). Resistance exercise overtraining and overreaching. *Sports Med.* 23(2): 106-129.

Hakkinen K, Pakarinen A, Alen M, Komi PV (1985). Serum hormones during prolonged training of neuromuscular performance. *Eur. J. Appl. Physiol.* 53(4): 287-293.

Johnson WG, Carr-Nangle RE, Bergeron KC (1995). Macronutrient intake, eating habits, and exercise as moderators of menstrual distress in healthy women. *Psychosom. Med.* 57(4): 324-330.

Kuipers H, Keizer HA (1988). Overtraining in elite athletes: Review and directions for the future. *Sports Med.* 6: 79-92.

Laughlin GA, Dominguez CE, Yen SS (1998). Nutritional and endocrine-metabolic aberrations in women with functional hypothalamic amenorrhea. *J. Clin. Endocrinol. Metab.* 83(1): 25-32.

Laughlin GA, Yen SS (1996). Nutritional and endocrine-metabolic aberrations in amenorrheic athletes. *J. Clin. Endocrinol. Metab.* 81(12): 4301-4309.

Lehmann MJ, Lormes W, Opitz-Gress A, Steinacher JM, Netzer N, Foster C, Gastmann U (1997). Training and overtraining: An overview and experimental results in endurance sports. *J. Sports Med. Phys. Fitness* 37: 7-17.

Lukaski HC, Penland JG (1996). Functional changes appropriate for determining mineral element requirements. *J. Nutr.* 126: 2354S-2364S.

McKay J, Selig S, Carlson J, Morris T (1997). Psychological stress in elite golfers during practice and competition. *Aust. J. Sci. Med. Sport* 29(2): 55-61.

O'Connor PJ, Morgan WP, Raglin JS, Barksdale CM, Kalin NH (1989). Mood state and salivary cortisol levels following overtraining in female swimmers. *Psychoneuroendocrinology* 14(4): 303-310.

Parmenter DC (1923). Some medical aspects of the training of college athletes. *Boston Med. Surg. J.* 4189: 45-50.

Ruderman NB, Schneider SH, Berchtold P (1981). The "metabolically-obese," normal-weight individual. *Am. J. Clin. Nutr.* 34: 1617-1621.

Selye H (1976). *The stress of life.* New York: McGraw-Hill.

Stone MH, Keith RE, Kearney JT (1991). Overtraining: A review of the signs, symptoms and possible causes. *J. Appl. Sports Sci. Res.* 5(1): 35-50.

Tegelman R, Aberg T, Pousette A, Carlstrom K (1992). Effects of a diet regimen on pituitary and steroid hormones in male ice hockey players. *Int. J. Sports Med.* 13(5): 424-430.

Urhausen A, Gabriel H, Kindermann W (1997). Blood hormones as markers of training stress and overtraining. *Sports Med.* 20(4): 251-276.

Weidner TG, Gehlsen G, Schurr T, Dwyer GB (1997). Effects of viral upper respiratory illness on running gait. *J. Athl. Training* 32(4): 309-314.

Wishart JM, Need AG, Horowitz M, Morris HA, Nordin BE (1995). Effect of age on bone density and bone turnover in men. *Clin. Endocrinol.* (Oxford) 42(2): 141-146. Abstract.

CHAPTER 24

Barrett J, Bilisko T (1995). The role of shoes in the prevention of ankle sprains. *Sports Med.* 20(4): 277-280.

Basmajian JV, Bentzon JW (1954). An electromyographic study of certain muscles of the leg and foot in the standing position. *Surg. Gynecol. Obstet.* 98: 662-666. Abstract.

Brizuela G, Llana S, Ferrandis R, Garcia-Belenguer AC (1997). The influence of basketball shoes with increased ankle support on shock attenuation and performance in running and jumping. *J. Sports Sci.* 15(5): 505-515.

Clark JE, Scott SG, Mingle M (1989). Viscoelastic shoe insoles: Their use in aerobic dancing. *Arch. Phys. Med. Rehabil.* 70(1): 37-40.

Gardner LI Jr, Dziados JE, Jones BH, Brundage JF, Harris JM, Sullivan R, Gill P (1988). Prevention of lower extremity stress fractures: A controlled trial of a shock absorbent insole. *Am. J. Public Health* 78(12): 1563-1567.

Grace TG, Skipper BJ, Newberry JC, Nelson MA, Sweetser ER, Rothman ML (1988). Prophylactic knee braces and injury to the lower extremity. *J. Bone Joint Surg.* 70(3): 422-427.

Guyton AC (1986). *Textbook of medical physiology,* pp. 580-581. Philadelphia: Saunders.

Hesse S, Luecke D, Jahnke MT, Mauritz KH (1996). Gait function in spastic hemiparetic patients walking barefoot, with firm shoes, and with ankle-foot orthosis. *Int. J. Rehabil. Res.* 19(2): 133-141.

Jorgensen U (1990). Body load in heel-strike running: The effect of a firm heel counter. *Am. J. Sports Med.* 18(2): 177-181.

Krivickas LS (1997). Anatomical factors associated with overuse sports injuries. *Sports Med.* 24(2): 132-146.

Leanderson J, Nemeth G, Eriksson E (1993). Ankle injuries in basketball players. *Knee Surg. Sports Traumatol. Arthrosc.* 1(3-4): 200-202.

Maffetone P (1996). *Training for endurance.* Stamford, NY: David Barmore Productions.

Perlman M, Leveille D, DeLeonibus J (1987). Inversion lateral ankle trauma: Differential diagnosis, review of literature, and prospective studies. *J. Foot Surg.* 26: 95-135.

Robbins S, Hanna AM (1987). Running-related injury prevention through barefoot adaptations. *Med. Sci. Sports Exerc.* 19(2): 148-156.

Robbins S, Waked E (1997a). Balance and vertical impact in sports: Role of shoe sole materials. *Arch. Phys. Med. Rehabil.* 78(5): 463-467.

Robbins S, Waked E (1997b). Hazard of deceptive advertising of athletic footwear. *Br. J. Sports Med.* 31(4): 299-303.

Robbins S, Waked E (1998). Factors associated with ankle injuries. *Sports Med.* 25(1): 63-72.

Robbins S, Waked E, Gouw GJ, McClaran J (1994). Athletic footwear affects balance in men. *Br. J. Sports Med.* 28(2): 117-122.

Robbins, S, Waked E, Rappel, R (1995). Ankle taping improves proprioception before and after exercise in young men. *Br. J. Sports Med.* 29(4): 242-247.

Rovere GD, Clarke TJ, Yates CS, Burley K (1988). Retrospective comparison of taping and ankle stabilizers in preventing ankle injuries. *Am. J. Sports Med.* 16(3): 228-233.

Rovere GD, Haupt HA, Yates CS (1987). Prophylactic knee bracing in college football. *Am. J. Sports Med.* 15(2): 111-116.

Teitz CC, Hermanson BK, Kronmal RA, Diehr PH (1987). Evaluation of the use of braces to prevent injury to the knee in collegiate football players. *J. Bone Joint Surg.* 69(1): 2-9.

Thonnard JL, Bragard D, Willems PA (1996). Stability of the braced ankle: A biomechanical investigation. *Am. J. Sports Med.* 24: 356-361.

Tomaro J, Burdett RG (1993). The effects of foot orthotics on the EMG activity of selected leg muscles during gait. *J. Orthop. Sports Phys. Ther.* 18(4): 532-536.

CHAPTER 25

Bassett DR, Block WD, Dean EN, White AA (1990). Recognition of borderline carbohydrate-lipid metabolism disturbance: An incipient form of Type IV hyperlipoproteinemia? *J. Cardio. Pharm.* 15(Suppl. 5): S8-S17.

Bergstrom E, Hernell O, Persson LA, Vessby B (1996). Insulin resistance syndrome in adolescents. *Metabolism* 45(7): 908-914.

Berkow MD (1992). *The Merck manual of diagnosis and therapy,* p. 1047. Rahway, NJ: Merck & Co, Inc.

Ibid. p. 1106-1107.

Bertelsen J, Christiansen C, Thomsen C, Poulsen PL, Vestergaard S, Steinov A, Rosmussen LH, Rosmussen O, Hermansen K (1993). Effect of meal frequency on blood glucose, insulin and free fatty acids in NIDDM subjects. *Diabetes Care* 16: 3-7.

Block CA, Clemons P, Sperling MA (1987). Puberty decreases insulin sensitivity. *J. Pediatr.* 110: 481-487.

Borkman ML, Storlien LH, Pan DA, Jenkins AB, Chisholm DJ, Campbell LV (1993). The relation between insulin sensitivity and the fatty-acid composition of skeletal-muscle phospholipids. *N. Engl. J. Med.* 328: 238-244.

Broughton DL, Taylor R (1991). Review: Deterioration of glucose tolerance with age: The role of insulin resistance. *Age and Ageing* 20: 221-225.

Campaigne BN, Lampman RM (1994). *Exercise in the clinical management of diabetes.* Champaign, IL: Human Kinetics.

Chan JC, Cockram CS, Critchley JA (1996). Drug-induced disorders of glucose metabolism. Mechanisms and management. *Drug Saf.* 15(2): 35-157.

Cononie CC, Goldberg AP, Rogus E, Hagberg JM (1994). Seven consecutive days of exercise lowers plasma insulin responses to an oral glucose challenge in sedentary elderly. *J. Am. Geriatr. Soc.* 42: 394-398.

Corbould AM, Judd SJ, Rodgers RJ (1998). Expression of types 1, 2, and 3 17 beta-hydroxysteroid dehydrogenase in subcutaneous abdominal and intra-abdominal adipose tissue of women. *J. Clin. Endocrinol. Metab.* 83(1): 187-194.

Coulston AM, Liu GC, Reaven GM (1993). Plasma glucose, insulin and lipid responses to high-carbohydrate low-fat diets in normal humans. *Metabolism* 32: 52-56.

Daly ME, Vale C, Walker M, Alberti KG, Mathers JC (1997). Dietary carbohydrates and insulin sensitivity: A review of the evidence and clinical implications. *Am. J. Clin. Nutr.* 66: 1072-1085.

Davy KP, Evans SL, Stevenson ET, Seals DR (1996). Adiposity and regional body fat distribution in physically active young and middle-aged women. *Int. J. Obes. Relat. Metab. Disord.* 20(8): 777-783.

de Jonge L, Bray GA (1997). The thermic effect of food and obesity: A critical review. *Obes. Res.* 5(6): 622-631.

Drummond S, Crombie N, Kirk T (1996). A critique of the effects of snacking on body weight status. *Eur. J. Clin. Nutr.* 50(12): 779-783.

Duncan BB, Chambless LE, Schmidt MI, Folsom AR, Szklo M, Crouse JR III, Carpenter MA (1995). Association of the waist-to-hip ratio is different with wine than with beer or hard liquor consumption. *Am. J. Epidemiol.* 142: 1034-1038.

Facchini F, Chen YD, Hollenbeck CM, Reaven GM (1991). Relationship between resistance to insulin-mediated glucose uptake, urinary uric acid clearance and plasma uric acid concentration. *JAMA* 266: 3008-3011.

Facchini FS, Stoohs RA, Reaven GM (1996). Enhanced sympathetic nervous system activity. The linchpin between insulin resistance, hyperinsulinemia, and heart rate. *Am. J. Hypertens.* 9(10 Part 1): 1013-1017.

Fagius J, Ellerfelt K, Lithell H, Berne C (1996). Increase in muscle nerve sympathetic activity after glucose intake is blunted in the elderly. *Clin. Auton. Res.* 6(4): 195-203.

Fahey PJ, Stallkamp ET, Kwatra S (1996). The athlete with type I diabetes: Managing insulin, diet and exercise. *Am. Fam. Physician* 53(5): 1611-1624.

Franks S, Robinson S, Willis DS (1996). Nutrition, insulin and polycystic ovary syndrome. *Rev. Reprod.* 1(1): 47-53.

Fry AC, Kraemer WJ (1997). Resistance exercise overtraining and overreaching. *Sports Med.* 23(2): 106-129.

Granner DK (1993). Hormones of the pancreas & gastrointestinal tract. In *Harper's biochemistry,* eds. RK Murray, DK Granner, PA Mayes, VW Rodwell, p. 568. Norwalk, CT: Appleton & Lange.

Grey N, Kipnis DM (1971). Effect of diet composition on the hyperinsulinemia of obesity. *N. Engl. J. Med.* 285(15): 827-831.

Griffiths AJ, Humphreys SM, Clark ML, Frayn KN (1994). Forarm substrate utilization during exercise after a meal containing both fat and carbohydrate. *Clin. Sci.* 86: 169-175.

Holden RJ (1995). Schizophrenia, suicide and the serotonin story. *Med. Hypotheses* 44(5): 379-391.

Hollmann M, Runnebaum B, Gerhard I (1997). Impact of waist-hip-ratio and body-mass-index on hormonal and metabolic parameters in young, obese women. *Int. J. Obes. Relat. Metab. Disord.* 21(6): 476-483.

Huang YJ, Fang VS, Juan CC, Chou YC, Kwok CF, Ho LT (1997). Amelioration of insulin resistance and hypertension in a fructose-fed rat model with fish oil supplementation. *Metabolism* 46(11): 1252-1258.

Hughes VA, Fiatarone MA, Ferrara CM, McNamara JR, Charnley JM, Evans WJ (1994). Lipoprotein response to exercise training and a low-fat diet in older subjects with glucose intolerance. *Am. J. Clin. Nutr.* 59: 820-826.

Ikemoto S, Takahashi M, Tsunoda N, Maruyama K, Itakura H, Ezaki O (1996). High-fat diet-induced hyperglycemia and obesity in mice: Differential effects of dietary oils. *Metabolism* 45(12): 1539-1546.

Iossa S, Lionetti L, Mollica MP, Barletta A, Liverini G (1996). Thermic effect of food in hypothyroid rats. *J. Endocrinol.* 148(1): 167-174.

Jenkins DJA (1997). Carbohydrate tolerance and food frequency. *Br. J. Nutr.* 77(Suppl. 1): S71-S81.

Jimenez CC (1997). Diabetes and exercise: The role of the athletic trainer. *J. Athl. Training* 32(4): 339-343.

Julius S, Nesbitt S (1996). Sympathetic overactivity in hypertension. A moving target. *Am. J. Hypertens.* 9(11): 113S-120S.

Kalmijn S, Feskens EJ, Launer LJ, Stijnen T, Kromhout D (1995). Glucose intolerance, hyperinsulinaemia and cognitive function in a general population of elderly men. *Diabetologia* 38(9): 1096-1102.

Katzel LI, Krauss RM, Goldberg AP (1994). Relationships of plasma TG and HDL-C concentrations to body composition and plasma insulin levels are altered in men with small LDL particles. *Arterioscler. Thromb.* 14: 1121-1128.

Keltikangas-Jarvinen L, Ravaja N, Raikkonen K, Lyytinen H (1996). Insulin resistance syndrome and autonomically mediated physiological responses to experimentally induced mental stress in adolescent boys. *Metabolism* 45(5): 614-621.

Kriketos AD, Pan DA, Lillioja S, Cooney GJ, Baur LA, Milner MR, Sutton JR, Jenkins AB, Bogardus C, Storlien LH (1996). Interrelationships between muscle morphology, insulin action, and adiposity. *Am. J. Physiol.* 270(6 Part 2): R1332-R1339.

Laakso M (1993). How good a marker is insulin level for insulin resistance? *Am. J. Epidemiol.* 137(9): 959-965.

Lambert EV, Speechly DP, Dennis SC, Noakes TD (1994). Enhanced endurance in trained cyclists during moderate intensity exercise following 2 weeks adaptation to a high fat diet. *Eur. J. Appl. Physiol.* 69: 287-293.

Lazarus R, Sparrow D, Weiss ST (1997). Handgrip strength and insulin levels: Cross-sectional and prospective associations in the Normative Aging Study. *Metabolism* 46(11): 1266-1269.

Lembo G, Vecchione C, Iaccarino G, Trimarco B (1996). The crosstalk between insulin and the sympathetic nervous system: Possible implications in the pathogenesis of essential hypertension. *Blood Press. Suppl.* 1: 38-42.

Lindgren F, Dahlquist G, Efendic S, Persson B, Skottner A (1990). Insulin sensitivity and glucose-induced insulin response changes during adolescence. *Acta Paediatr. Scand.* 79: 431-436.

McGrath SA, Gibney MJ (1994). The effects of altered frequency of eating on plasma lipids in free-living healthy males on normal self-selected diets. *Eur. J. Clin. Nutr.* 48: 402-407.

Mei G, Pugliese L, Rosato N, Toma L, Bolognesi M, Finazzi-Agro A (1994). Biotin and biotin analogues specifically modify the fluorescence decay of avidin. *J. Mol. Biol.* 242(4): 559-565.

Moan A, Eide IK, Kjeldsen SE (1996). Metabolic and adrenergic characteristics of young men with insulin resistance. *Blood Press. Suppl.* 1: 30-37.

Moy CS, Songer TJ, LaPorte RE, Dorman JS, Kriska AM, Orchard TJ, Becker DJ, Drash AL (1993). Insulin-dependent diabetes mellitus, physical activity, and death. *Am. J. Epidemiol.* 137: 74-81.

Muller MJ, Seitz HJ (1984). Thyroid hormone action on intermediary metabolism. Part I: Respiration, thermogenesis and carbohydrate metabolism. *Klin. Wochenschr.* 62(1): 11-18. Abstract.

Muoio DM, Leddy JJ, Horvath PJ, Awad AB, Pendergast DR (1994). Effect of dietary fat on metabolic adjustments to maximal $\dot{V}O_2$ and endurance in runners. *Med. Sci. Sports Exerc.* 26(1): 81-88.

Nestler JE (1994). Assessment of insulin resistance. *Scientific American,* Science & Medicine, September/October, 58-67.

Palatini P, Julius S (1997). Association of tachycardia with morbidity and mortality: Pathophysiological considerations. *J. Hum. Hypertens.* 11(Suppl. 1): S19-S27.

Pan DA, Lillioja S, Milner MR, Kriketos AD, Baur LA, Bogardus C, Storlien LH (1995). Skeletal muscle membrane lipid composition is related to adiposity and insulin action. *J. Clin. Invest.* 96(6): 2802-2808.

Parker DR, Weiss ST, Troisi R, Cassano PA, Vokonas PS, Landsberg L (1993). Relationship of dietary saturated fatty acids and body habitus to serum insulin concentrations: The Normative Aging Study. *Am. J. Clin. Nutr.* 58(2): 129-136.

Pendergast DR, Horvath PJ, Leddy JJ, Venkatraman JT (1996). The role of dietary fat on performance, metabolism and health. *Am. J. Sports. Med.* 24(6): S53-S58.

Perseghin G, Ghosh S, Gerow K, Shulman GI (1997). Metabolic defects in lean nondiabetic offspring of NIDDM parents: A cross-sectional study. *Diabetes* 46(6): 1001-1009.

Phillips DI, Barker DJ (1997). Association between low birthweight and high resting pulse in adult life: Is the sympathetic nervous system involved in programming the insulin resistance syndrome? *Diabet. Med.* 14(8): 673-677.

Pratley RE, Hagberg JM, Rogus EM, Goldberg AP (1995). Enhanced insulin sensitivity and lower waist-to-hip ratio in master athletes. *Am. J. Physiol.* 268(3 Part 1): E484-E490.

Preuss HG (1997). Effects of glucose/insulin perturbations on aging and chronic disorders of aging: The evidence. *J. Am. Coll. Nutr.* 16(5): 397-403.

Raitakari OT, Porkka KV, Ronnemaa T, Knip M, Uhari M, Akerblom HK, Viikari JS (1995). The role of insulin in clustering of serum lipids and blood pressure in children and adolescents. The Cardiovascular Risk in Young Finns Study. *Diabetologia* 38(9): 1042-1050.

Ravaja N, Keltikangas-Jarvinen L (1995). Temperament and metabolic syndrome precursors in children: A three-year follow-up. *Prev. Med.* 24(5): 518-527.

Ravaja N, Keltikangas-Jarvinen L, Viikari J (1996). Life changes, locus of control and metabolic syndrome precursors in adolescents and young adults: A three-year follow-up. *Soc. Sci. Med.* 43(1): 51-61.

Reaven GM (1988). Role of insulin resistance in human disease. *Diabetes* 37: 1595-1607.

Reaven GM (1997). Do high carbohydrate diets prevent the development or attenuate the manifestations (or both) of syndrome X? A viewpoint strongly against. *Curr. Opin. Lipidol.* 8(1): 23-27.

Report of the Expert Committee on the Diagnosis and Classification of Diabetes Mellitus (1997). *Diabetes Care* 20(7): 1183-1197.

Rogers MA, King DS, Hagberg JM, Ehsani AA, Holloszy JO (1990). Effect of 10 days of physical inactivity on glucose tolerance in master athletes. *J. Appl. Physiol.* 68(5): 1833-1837.

Rohner-Jeanrenaud F (1995). A neuroendocrine reappraisal of the dual-centre hypothesis: Its implications for obesity and insulin resistance. *Int. J. Obesity* 19: 517-534.

Rosolova H, Mayer O Jr, Reaven G (1997). Effect of variations in plasma magnesium concentration on resistance to insulin-mediated glucose disposal in nondiabetic subjects. *J. Clin. Endocrinol. Metab.* 82(11): 3783-3785.

Rubin MA, Miller JP, Ryan AS, Treuth MS, Patterson KY, Pratley RE, Hurley BF, Veillon C, Moser-Veillon PB, Anderson RA (1998). Acute and chronic resistive exercise increase urinary chromium excretion in men as measured with an enriched chromium stable isotope. *J. Nutr.* 128(1): 73-78.

Ruderman NB, Schneider SH, Berchtold P (1981). The "metabolically-obese," normal-weight individual. *Am. J. Clin. Nutr.* 34: 1617-1621.

Schiavon R, Altamirano-Bustamante N, Jimenez C, Calzada-Leon R, Robles-Valdes C, Larrea F (1996). Fasting and postprandial serum insulin in Mexican adolescents with menstrual disorders. *Rev. Invest. Clin.* 48(5): 335-342.

Schwille PO, Herrmann U, Schmiedl A, Kissler H, Wipplinger J, Manoharan M (1997). Urinary phosphate excretion in the pathophysiology of idiopathic recurrent calcium urolithiasis: Hormonal interactions and lipid metabolism. *Urol. Res.* 25(6): 417-426.

Seidell JC, Muller DC, Sorkin JD, Andres R (1992). Fasting respiratory exchange ratio and resting metabolic rate as predictors of weight gain: The Baltimore Longitudinal Study on Aging. *Int. J. Obesity* 16: 667-674.

Simmons RW, Richardson C, Deutsch K (1997). Limited joint mobility of the ankle in diabetic patients with cutaneous sensory deficit. *Diabetes Res. Clin. Pract.* 37(2): 137-143.

Simopoulos AP (1994). Is insulin resistance influenced by dietary linoleic acid and trans fatty acids? *Free Radic. Biol. Med.* 17(4): 367-372.

Skouby SO, Andersen O, Petersen KR, Molsted-Pedersen L, Kuhl C (1990). Mechanism of action of oral contraceptives on carbohydrate metabolism at the cellular level. *Am. J. Obstet. Gynecol.* 163: 343-348.

Song MK, Rosenthal MJ, Naliboff BD, Phanumas L, Kang KW (1998). Effects of bovine prostate powder on zinc, glucose, and insulin metabolism in old patients with non-insulin-dependent diabetes mellitus. *Metabolism* 47(1): 39-43.

Sparrow D, Borkan GA, Gerzof SG, Wisniewski C, Silbert CK (1986). Relationship of fat distribution to glucose tolerance. Results of computed tomography in male participants of the Normative Aging Study. *Diabetes* 35(4): 411-415.

Stoll BA (1997). Macronutrient supplements may reduce breast cancer risk: How, when and which? *Eur. J. Clin. Nutr.* 51(9): 573-577.

Stoohs RA, Facchini F, Guilleminault C (1996). Insulin resistance and sleep-disordered breathing in healthy humans. *Am. J. Respir. Crit. Care Med.* 154(1): 170-174.

Storlien LH, Kriketos AD, Calvert GD, Baur LA, Jenkins AB (1997). Fatty acids, triglycerides and syndromes of insulin resistance. *Prostaglandins Leukot. Essent. Fatty Acids* 57(4-5): 379-385.

Storlien LH, Pan DA, Kriketos AD, O'Connor J, Caterson ID, Cooney GJ, Jenkins AB, Baur LA (1996). Skeletal muscle membrane lipids and insulin resistance. *Lipids* 31(Suppl.): S261-S265.

Svec F, Nastasi K, Hilton C, Bao W, Srinivasan SR, Berenson GS (1992). Black-white contrasts in insulin levels during pubertal development. *Diabetes* 41: 313-317.

Swinburn BA, Gianchandani R, Saad MF, Lillioja S (1995). In vivo beta-cell function at the transition to early non-insulin-dependent diabetes mellitus. *Metabolism* 44(6): 757-764.

Taittonen L, Uhari M, Nuutinen M, Turtinen J, Pokka T, Akerblom HK (1996). Insulin and blood pressure among healthy children. Cardiovascular risk in young Finns. *Am. J. Hypertens.* 9(3): 194-199.

Tepperman J, Tepperman H (1987). *Metabolic and endocrine physiology,* pp. 249-296. Chicago: Year Book Medical.

Urhausen A, Gabriel H, Kindermann W (1997). Blood hormones as markers of training stress and overtraining. *Sports Med.* 20(4): 251-276.

VanHelder T, Radomski MW (1989). Sleep deprivation and the effect on exercise performance. *Sports Med.* 7(4): 235-247.

Van Reempts PJ, Wouters A, De Cock W, Van Acker KJ (1997). Stress response to tilting and odor stimulus in preterm neonates after intrauterine conditions associated with chronic stress. *Physiol. Behav.* 61(3): 419-424.

Velazquez EM, Mendoza S, Hamer T, Sosa F, Glueck CJ (1994). Metformin therapy in polycystic ovary syndrome reduces hyperinsulinemia, insulin resistance, hyperandrogenemia, and systolic blood pressure, while facilitating normal menses and pregnancy. *Metabolism* 43(5): 647-654.

Verwaerde P, Galinier M, Fourcade J, Massabuau P, Galitzky J, Senard JM, Tran MA, Berlan M, Montastruc JL (1997). Autonomic nervous system abnormalities in the initial phase of insulin resistance syndrome. Value of the study of variability of cardiac rate and blood pressure on a model of nutritional obesity. *Arch. Mal. Coeur. Vaiss.* 90(8): 1151-1154. Abstract.

Virkkunen M (1986). Reactive hypoglycemic tendency among habitually violent offenders. *Nutr. Rev.* 44(Suppl.): 94-103.

Walker KZ, O'Dea K, Johnson L, Sinclair AJ, Piers LS, Nicholson GC, Muir JG (1996). Body fat distribution and non-insulin-dependent diabetes: Comparison of a fiber-rich, high-carbohydrate, low-fat (23%) diet and a 35% fat diet high in monounsaturated fat. *Am. J. Clin. Nutr.* 63(2): 254-260.

Wolf SK (1998). Diabetes mellitus and predisposition to athletic pedal fracture. *J. Foot Ankle Surg.* 37(1): 16-22.

Xie H, Lautt WW (1996). Insulin resistance caused by hepatic cholinergic interruption and reversed by acetylcholine administration. *Am. J. Physiol.* 271(3 Part 1): E587-E592.

Zhang H, Osada K, Maebashi M, Ito M, Komai M, Furukawa Y (1996). A high biotin diet improves the impaired glucose tolerance of long-term spontaneously hyperglycemic rats with non-insulin-dependent diabetes mellitus. *J. Nutr. Sci. Vitaminol.* (Tokyo) 42(6): 517-526.

Ziegler D, Gries FA (1997). Alpha-lipoic acid in the treatment of diabetic peripheral and cardiac autonomic neuropathy. *Diabetes* 46(Suppl. 2): S62-S66.

Zimmet PZ, Collins VR, Dowse GK, Knight LT (1992). Hyperinsulinaemia in youth is a predictor of Type 2 (non-insulin-dependent) diabetes mellitus. *Diabetologia* 35: 534-541.

CHAPTER 26

Abraham S (1996). Eating and weight controlling behaviours of young ballet dancers. *Psychopathology* 29(4): 218-222.

Aitken JC, Thompson J (1989). The effects of dietary manipulation upon the respiratory exchange ratio as a predictor of maximum oxygen uptake during fixed term maximal incremental exercise in man. *Eur. J. Appl. Physiol.* 58: 722-727.

Bar-Or O, Foreyt J, Bouchard C, Brownell KD, Dietz WH, Ravussin E, Salbe AD, Schwenger S, St Jeor S, Torun B (1998). Physical activity, genetic, and nutritional considerations in childhood weight management. *Med. Sci. Sports Exerc.* 30(1): 2-10.

Carmichael HE, Swinburn BA, Wilson MR (1998). Lower fat intake as a predictor of initial and sustained weight loss in obese subjects consuming an otherwise ad libitum diet. *J. Am. Diet. Assoc.* 98(1): 35-39.

Clarys JP, Martin AD, Drinkwater DT, Marfell-Jones MJ (1987). The skinfold: Myth and reality. *J. Sports Sci.* 5(1): 3-33.

Doucet E, Tremblay A (1997). Food intake, energy balance and body weight control. *Eur. J. Clin. Nutr.* 51(12): 846-855.

Drummond S, Crombie N, Kirk T (1996). A critique of the effects of snacking on body weight status. *Eur. J. Clin. Nutr.* 50(12): 779-783.

Elbers JM, Haumann G, Asscheman H, Seidell JC, Gooren LJ (1997). Reproducibility of fat area measurements in young, non-obese subjects by computerized analysis of magnetic resonance images. *Int. J. Obes. Relat. Metab. Disord.* 21(12): 1121-1129.

Elliot DL, Goldberg L, Kuehl KS, Bennett WM (1989). Sustained depression of the resting metabolic rate after massive weight loss. *Am. J. Clin. Nutr.* 49(1): 93-96.

Ferraro R, Lillioja S, Fontvieille AM, Rising R (1992). Lower sedentary metabolic rate in women compared with men. *J. Clin. Invest.* 90(3): 780-784.

Fogelholm GM, Sievanen HT, van Marken Lichtenbelt WD, Westerterp KR (1997). Assessment of fat-mass loss during weight reduction in obese women. *Metabolism* 46(8): 968-975.

Golay A, Eigenheer C, Morel Y, Kujawski P, Lehmann T, de Tonnac N (1996). Weight-loss with low or high carbohydrate diet? *Int. J. Obes. Relat. Metab. Disord.* 20(12): 1067-1072.

Kohrt WM (1998). Preliminary evidence that DEXA provides an accurate assessment of body composition. *J. Appl. Physiol.* 84(1): 372-377.

Kriketos AD, Pan DA, Lillioja S, Cooney GJ, Baur LA, Milner MR, Sutton JR, Jenkins AB, Bogardus C, Storlien LH (1996). Interrelationships between muscle morphology, insulin action, and adiposity. *Am. J. Physiol.* 270(6 Part 2): R1332-R1339.

Lamarche B, Despres JP, Pouliot MC, Moorjani S, Lupien PJ, Theriault G, Tremblay A, Nadeau A, Bouchard C (1992). Is body fat loss a determinant factor in the improvement of carbohydrate and lipid metabolism following aerobic exercise training in obese women? *Metabolism* 41(11): 1249-1256.

Martin M, Schlabach G, Shibinski K (1998). The use of non-prescription weight loss products among female basketball, softball, and volleyball athletes from NCAA Division I Institutions: Issues and concerns. *J. Athl. Training* 33: 41-44.

McArdle WD, Katch FI, Katch VL (1991). *Exercise physiology.* 3d ed., p. 659. Philadelphia: Lea & Febiger.

Ibid. p. 627.

McNeill G, Bruce AC, Ralph A, James WPT (1988). Inter-individual differences in fasting nutrient oxidation and influence of diet composition. *Int. J. Obesity* 12: 455-464.

Molnar D, Schutz Y (1997). The effect of obesity, age, puberty and gender on resting metabolic rate in children and adolescents. *Eur. J. Pediatr.* 156(5): 376-381.

Oppliger RA, Landry GL, Foster SW, Lambrecht AC (1998). Wisconsin minimum weight program reduces weight-cutting practices of high school wrestlers. *Clin. J. Sport Med.* 8(1): 26-31.

Pichard C, Kyle UG, Gremion G, Gerbase M, Slosman DO (1997). Body composition by x-ray absorptiometry and bioelectrical impedance in female runners. *Med. Sci. Sports Exerc.* 29(11): 1527-1534.

Rankin JW, Ocel JV, Craft LL (1996). Effect of weight loss and refeeding diet composition on anaerobic performance in wrestlers. *Med. Sci. Sports Exerc.* 28(10): 1292-1299.

Ranneries C, Bulow J, Buemann B, Christensen NJ, Madsen J, Astrup A (1998). Fat metabolism in formerly obese women. *Am. J. Physiol.* 274(1 Part 1): E155-E161.

Ravussin E, Swinburn BA (1993). Metabolic predictors of obesity: Cross-sectional versus longitudinal data. *Int. J. Obes. Relat. Metab. Disord.* 17(Suppl. 3): S28-S31.

Reaven GM (1997). Do high carbohydrate diets prevent the development or attenuate the manifestations (or both) of syndrome X? A viewpoint strongly against. *Curr. Opin. Lipidol.* 8(1): 23-27.

Rolls BJ, Miller DL (1997). Is the low-fat message giving people a license to eat more? *J. Am. Coll. Nutr.* 16(6): 35-543.

Seidell JC, Muller DC, Sorkin JD, Andres R (1992). Fasting respiratory exchange ratio and resting metabolic rate as predictors of weight gain: The Baltimore Longitudinal Study on Aging. *Int. J. Obesity* 16: 667-674.

Standard Process, Inc. 1200 West Royal Lee Drive, Palmyra, WI 53516. 800-848-5061.

Stout JR, Housh TJ, Johnson GO, Housh DJ, Evans SA, Eckerson JM (1995). Validity of skinfold equations for estimating body density in youth wrestlers. *Med. Sci. Sports Exerc.* 27(9): 1321-1325.

Talbott SM, Rothkopf MM, Shapses SA (1998). Dietary restriction of energy and calcium alters bone turnover and density in younger and older female rats. *J. Nutr.* 128(3): 640-645.

Valtuena S, Sola R, Salas-Salvado J (1997). A study of the prognostic respiratory markers of sustained weight loss in obese subjects after 28 days on VLCD. *Int. J. Obes. Relat. Metab. Disord.* 21(4): 267-273.

Wannamethee G, Shaper AG (1990). Weight change in middle-aged British men: Implications for health. *Eur. J. Clin. Nutr.* 44(2): 133-142.

CHAPTER 28

Nutri-West, Douglas, WY 82633. 800-443-3333.

Standard Process, Inc. 1200 West Royal Lee Drive, Palmyra, WI 53516. 800-848-5061.

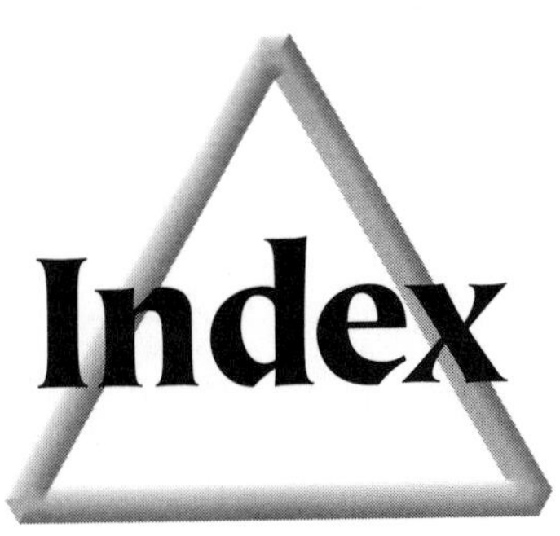

Index

A
abdominal muscles
  external oblique 132-133
  relationships 192, 193*t*
Abeles, R.H. 305
Abernathy, P. 30
Abraham, S. 366
academic (term) 9
Achilles tendinitis 254, 257
active recovery 322-323
active warm-up 320-322
  case histories 322, 323
  in competition 323
acupuncture
  beginning and end points 269, 269*f*, 269-270
  meridians 21, 106
  for pain control 265-266
  points 105-106
    CV 8 232-233
    on foot 234, 234*f*
    KI 27 232-233
    locations of 106
    muscle relationships 192, 193*t*, 233
    relationships with nutrients, organs and glands, nerves, and 192, 193*t*
  tonification points 266-268, 267*f*, 268*t*
Adams, P. 288
addictions 387
adductor brevis 154
adductor longus 154
adductor magnus 154
adductor relationships 192, 193*t*
adrenal hormones 41-43
  effects on sodium 313-314
  training effects on 43-44
aerobic (term) 12-13
aerobic challenge 207-208
aerobic deficiency syndrome 210-211
  causes 208
  signs and symptoms 208
aerobic function
  assessment of 207-211
  building 324-326
  walking and 326
aerobic imbalances 209
aerobic intervals 326
aerobic speed 13-14
aerobic system 28-29
aerobic system nutrition 304
AeroSport, Inc. 73*f*
  gas analyzer 80, 80*f*
  TEEM 100 metabolic analyzer 80, 81*t*
Ahmaidi, S. 323
Aitken, J.C. 305, 366
Alessio, H.M. 308
Ali, M. 283
Allen 82, 222
Allen, Mark 11, 11*f*, 325
allergic substances 200
all-or-none phenomenon 33
Almekinders, L.C. 49, 282
Alpher, V.S. 76
Alston, T.A. 305
alternative medicine 1
Alvarez-Mon, M. 51
Amadio, P. 50, 263
Amadio, P., Jr. 50, 263
amenorrhea 340-341
American College of Sports Medicine 314
American Medical Association 6
amino acids
  conditionally essential 307
  essential 306-307
  nonessential 306-307
  semiessential 307
  supplementation 306-307
Anacin 3 264
anaerobic (term) 12-13
anaerobic challenge 209
anaerobic function
  assessment of 207-211
  building 327-328
  case history 210
anaerobic imbalances 209
anaerobic system 29-30
Anderson, L.C. 71
Anderson, S.D. 308
androgens 42
anemia
  dilutional 77
  sports 76, 304
ankle dysfunction 347-349
ankle problems 251-256
antioxidants 308-309
Antronex 265
Appelqvist, L. 302
applied kinesiology 17, 17*t*, 21-22
  assessment 191-205
  differentiating primary and secondary problems 203-204
  muscle testing 191-192
Aragao, W. 229
arch function 346
Arena, B. 278, 340, 341
Argov, Z. 304
Armentia, Z. 195
Armstrong, L.E. 312
Aruoma, O.I. 304
assessment(s)
  of aerobic and anaerobic function 207-211
  applied kinesiology 191-205
  of autonomic function 203
  of body fat 365
  heart rate monitor 213-223
  methods of 16-17
  muscle evaluation 96-97
  nutritional 294
  of overtraining 337, 341-342
  of oxidative stress 309
  of posture, gait, and neuromuscular system 85-104
  routine office 69-77, 83*t*
  specialized tests 77-83, 83*t*
  of temporomandibular joint dysfunction 229
  vertebral, non-force 250-251
asthma, exercise-induced 74-75, 307-308
Asztely, A. 71
athlete-designed competition schedules 334-335
athletes 5-6
  amenorrhea in 340-341
  carbohydrate intolerance in 351-362
  competitive 365-366
  with predetermined competition schedules 332-333
  with type 1 diabetes 362
athlete's diet 358
athletic dysfunction, triad of 369-374, 379
  noteworthy factors 373, 374*t*

athletic dysfunction, triad of (*continued*)
stage 1 372, 374*t*
stage 2 372-373, 374*t*
stage 3 373, 374*t*
stages of 372-373
athletic shoes 345-350
Austin, M.A. 280
autonomic balance 39-40
and nutrition 305-306
testing procedures for 203
autonomic function
assessment of 203
challenge procedure 203
awareness, sport 22-23

B

balance. *See also* imbalance
autonomic 39-40, 305-306
body fat 364
macronutrient 288-292
between pro- and anti-inflammatory effects 283-286
sodium and potassium 315
balanced care 8
Bale, P. 340
Balon, R. 305
Bannister, Roger 22
Barbeau, W.E. 281
Barker, D.J. 353
Barletta, A. 76
Barnes, B. 72
Barnes, C. 72
Baron, S. 54
Bar-Or, O. 363
Barrett, J. 348
Barron, J.L. 43, 78
Basmajian, J.V. 346
Bassett, D.R. 45, 352
Bassey, E.J. 214
Baumgarten, C.R. 194
Beckett, P.R. 281, 294
Belanger, A. 43, 340
Bell, G.J. 324, 328
Bell, J.M. 214
Bellinger, L.L. 275
Benfante, R. 74
Benson, J.E. 274, 340
Bentley, S. 271
Bentzon, J.W. 346
Berenshtein, E. 308
Bergman, E.A. 287
Bergstrom, E. 354
Bergstrom, J. 281
Berkow, M.D. 45, 70, 352, 359, 361
Bernardis, L.L. 275
Bernstein, J.H. 15
Bernton, E. 42
Berson, B.L. 324
Bertelsen, J. 359
Betaine Hydrochloride 300, 383, 385
beverages
caffeine levels in 287, 287*t*
sports drinks 311, 315-317
Bezard, J. 46, 47, 49, 282
Biasioli, S. 194
biceps brachii muscle 118-119
facilitation and inhibition 35-36, 36*f*
relationships 192, 193*t*
testing 119, 119*f*
Bilisko, T. 348
Bingham, S.A. 56
Bird, S.R. 219, 278
Bjorntorp, P. 278
Bland, J.S. 43, 282
Block, C.A. 352
Block, G. 286
Blond, J.P. 46, 49, 282
blood pressure
exercise 71, 83*t*
postural 69-71, 83*t*
blood tests 77
body fat
assessment of 365
balance 364
excess 363-365
body language 33
body temperature. *See* temperature
Bogdanis, G.C. 323
Bonde-Petersen, F. 29
Boone, T. 214
Bordia, A. 280, 283
Bordia, T. 283
Bordoni, A. 49
Borensztajn, J. 26, 278
Borg scale 222
Borg-Stein, J. 231
Borkman, M.L. 352
Bosch, A.N. 278
Boulay, M.R. 213
Bouziane, M. 49, 284
Bove, A.A. 43
Bragg, L.E. 295
Brandao-Neto, J. 343
Brandi, G. 296
Brandon 78, 328
Brandt, K.D. 264
Bray, G.A. 357
breath-holding endurance 75
breath-holding time 75-76, 83*t*
Brener, J. 213
Brizuela, G. 348
Broadhurst, C.L. 279
Brodowicz, G.R. 314
Broughton, D.L. 44, 360
Brouns, F. 316
Brunner, G. 296
buccinator muscle 230, 230*f*
Buchman, A.L. 296
Buller, R. 305
Bunch, T.W. 76
Burchfiel, C.M. 75
Burdett, R.G. 347
Burke, L.M. 312
Burkitt, D.P. 7
Burrows, B. 74
Butterfield, G.E. 280

C

caffeine 287, 287*t*
calcaneal dysfunction 254
case history 255
correction of 254, 254*f*
Calcium Lactate 384
Calderon, L. 96, 192
Callahan, R.J. 201
Campaigne, B.N. 361
Campbell, S.S. 72
Canfield, R.C. 231
Cao, G. 309
carbohydrate intolerance 44-45, 351
in athletes 351-362
case histories 356, 357, 358
dietary fats and 359
factors associated with 360, 361*t*
nutritional factors 359-360
Stage 1 353-356, 361*t*
Stage 2 356-357, 361*t*
Stage 3 357-358, 361*t*
stages of 353
terms for 351
treatment of 358-360
carbohydrates 27, 276-278
dietary excess 289
kilocalories derived from 79, 79*t*
nutrients important for metabolism of 301
care
balanced 8
patient 319-320
Carlston, M. 23
Carmichael, H.E. 366
carpal tunnel syndrome 258
Carranza-Madrigal, J. 280
Cashman, S.J. 15
Castaneda, C. 281
Castell, L.M. 297
Cataplex B 306
Cataplex E 303
Cataplex G 306
catecholamines 42-43
Cavanagh, P.R. 219
Cazzola, P. 299
challenge 192
aerobic 207-208
autonomic function 203
chemical 195, 198-200

mental/emotional 195-196, 200-202
neurological sensory receptor 194-196
oral, potassium/sodium 315
structural (physical) 195, 196-198
Chamberlite bag 328*f*
Champagne, E.T. 296
Chan, J.C. 356
Chan, M.M. 298
Chang, M.S. 70
Chapman, Frank 19
Chapman's reflexes 19, 106, 235
Chardigny, J.M. 282
Chavali, S.R. 49, 282, 283
chemical balance 4
chemical challenges 195, 198-200
oral
with allergic substances 200
with noxious substances 200
with nutrient remedies 199
chemical injuries 375-387
treatment of 375, 376*t*
chemicals, naturally occurring in pain control 265
Chen, Y. 75
chewing food 274-275
Chinese medicine 17, 17*t*, 21
chiropractic 17, 17*t*, 18
cholesterol 279-280
choline 307-308
Chorot, P. 71
Christen, S. 302
Christensen, L. 288
Christie, V.M. 15
Chyou, P.H. 75
Claassen, N. 48, 282, 341
Clark, J.E. 347
Clarkson, P.M. 270, 271, 294
Clarys, J.P. 365
Cleak, M.J. 270, 271
Clemons, P. 352
clinical (term) 9
Clyman, B. 264
Cohen, H.A. 308
cold pressor test 77-78, 83*t*
Colliander, E.B. 29, 208, 322, 323, 328
competition
active warm-up and recovery in 323
Maximum Aerobic Function test and 219-220
practitioner's role in 319-329
predetermined season 333
competition schedules 331, 332-335
athlete-designed 334-335
case history 335
predetermined 332-333
competitive athletes 365-366
competitive footwear 345-350
complaints, subjective 82, 82*t*
complementary sports medicine
as art and science 6-7
case history 5
definitions vii, 9-14
disciplines 17, 17*t*
philosophy 1-8
specialties 15-23
today 1-2
concussion 243
Connor, W.E. 280
Cononie, C.C. 360
Convertino, V.A. 70, 314, 317
Cook, N.E. 275
cooling-down 322
Corazza, G.R. 295
Corbould, A.M. 356
Cordero, D.L. 220
Cordova, A. 51
Cori cycle 27
correction
of calcaneal dysfunction 254, 254*f*
of cranial respiratory faults 246
of cranial sagittal suture faults 242, 242*f*
of cuboid bone dysfunction 256, 256*f*
of expiration-assisted faults 239-240
of inspiration-assisted faults 239
of lateral talus distortion 253, 253*f*
of navicular bone dysfunction 255-256, 256*f*
of pelvic faults 245, 245*f*, 246*f*, 246-247
respiratory method 256-257
of sphenobasilar expiration-assisted faults 241-242
vertebral, non-force 250-251
of wrist joint dysfunction 258-259, 259*f*
Costill, D.L. 12, 13, 43, 79, 214, 221, 287*t*, 304, 312, 313, 320, 323, 328, 335
Coulston, A.M. 44, 49, 276, 358
Craig, B.W. 45
Craig, W.J. 273, 297, 298, 309
cranial dysfunction 237-238, 378
treatment of 237-248
cranial faults
respiratory 246
sagittal suture 242, 242*f*, 243
cranial-sacral respiratory faults 238-239
Crapo, L. 11, 11*f*
Croft, A.C. 72
Crossman, J. 22
cuboid bone dysfunction 256, 256*f*
Cummings, J.H. 286
Cunningham, R.B. 77
CV 8 232-233, 233*f*

D
Dager, S.R. 305
daily menus
with 15 grams of fiber 286
with 25 grams of fiber 286-288
Dajani, E.Z. 48, 264
Daly, M.E. 351
Davi, G. 280
David, M.J. 264
Davies, M.J. 308
Davis, C.M. 275
Davy, K.P. 360
de Alaniz, M.J. 49
DeAndrade, J.R. 35
De Castro, J.M. 56
De Cree, C. 43, 78, 340
definitions 9-14
DeJarnette, M.B. 18, 237
de Jonge, L. 357
Dekkers, J.C. 51, 308
de Klerk, A. 305
delayed-onset muscle soreness (DOMS) 270, 271
De Lorenzo, F. 70
delta-5-desaturase 302, 302*f*
deltoid muscles 164-165
relationships 192, 193*t*
testing 165, 165*f*
Demaison, L. 278
Demopoulos, H. 308
Denyer, C.V. 283
Deschaumes-Molinaro, C. 200
Desimone, D.P. 48, 282
Despret, S. 49
Deuster, P.A. 279
de Wijer, A. 229
diabetes, type 1 360-361, 362
dialogue, patient 53-67
diaphragm muscle 190
Diaz, M.N. 280
DiBattista, D. 275
DiBona, G.F. 313
Dickey, W. 295
Dickson, D.N. 77
Dieppe, P. 264
diet(s) 364, 379
athlete's diet 358
fatty acid profile 284, 284*t*
imbalance 288-289
mental and emotional aspects of 288
and nutrition 17, 17*t*, 19-20, 366-367
pancreatic hormones and 44
diet (term) 364
Dietary Analysis 56, 57*f*, 67*f*
dietary decision making 289
dietary factors 286-288
affecting inflammation 282-286
balancing pro- and anti-inflammatory effects of 283-286
in overtraining syndrome 343
dietary fats 278-279
and carbohydrate intolerance 359
conversion to eicosanoids 46, 47*f*
imbalance in 48-50
dietary fiber 286-288
dietary macronutrients 276, 276*f*
diet therapy 273-292
differentiating primary and secondary problems 203-204
Dillard, C.J. 51

dilutional anemia 77
Ding, J.H. 43, 78, 340
Di Pietro, S. 44
disciplines 17, 17*t*
Djamil, R. 327
Doll, R. 288
DOMS. *See* delayed-onset muscle soreness
Dorland's Illustrated Medical Dictionary 18, 191, 194, 213
Doucet, E. 305, 367
Douglas, P.D. 76
Dreon, D.M. 279
Drew, L.M. 286
drugs 264
  nonsteroidal anti-inflammatory 263-264
  over-the-counter 287, 287*t*
Drummond, S. 359, 366
Duchman, S.M. 316
Dudkin, M.S. 286
Dudley, G. 327
Dueck, C.A. 340, 341
Duncan, B.B. 76, 355, 360
Duncan, J.R. 49
dysfunction 7-8, 75
  calcaneal 254, 254*f*, 255
  cranial 237-248, 378
  cuboid bone 256
  extravertebral 249-259
  fibula 257-258
  foot 256-257
  joint complex 377-378
  muscle 225-235
  navicular bone 255-256, 256*f*
  neurological 225, 232-235
  pelvic 237, 243-248
  rib joint 258
  spinal 250-251
  talus 252-253
  temporomandibular joint 228-231
  triad of 369-374, 379
  vertebral 249-259
  wrist joint 258-259, 259*f*

E
Eder, K. 49
eicosanoids 45-48
  conversion of dietary fats to 46, 47*f*
  conversion of Group B fats to 283, 283*f*
  Series 1 and 3 302, 302*f*
Series 2 47-48, 48*f*
Eisenberg, D.M. 15
Elbers, J.M. 365
electrolytes 313-315
Elliot, D.L. 364
Elmquist, J.K. 194
El-Sayed, H. 314
emotional challenges 195-196, 200-202
emotional injuries 375-387, 379-380
emotional problems, secondary 380
emotional wellness. *See* mental/emotional wellness
endurance
  breath-holding 75
  definition of 13
energy
  bodily functions used 274
  from food 273-274
  from macronutrients 25-26
energy bars 311, 317-318, 359
energy production 26-28
energy systems 25, 28-30
  training effects on 30-31
Enright, T. 308
Erasuas, U. 285*t*
ergogenic nourishment 311-318
Escherichia coli 46
Eston, R.G. 270, 271
evaluation. *See also* assessment(s)
  muscle 96-97
exercise
  effects on water regulation 312
Blood Cholesterol in Adults 279
expiration-assisted faults 238
  correction of 239-240
  sphenobasilar 240, 241-242
external oblique abdominal muscles 132-133, 133*f*
external pterygoid muscle 230, 231*f*
extravertebral dysfunction 251
  treatment of 249-259

F
Facchini, F. 354
Facchini, F.S. 355
facilitation 33
  normal 35-36, 36*f*
    during gait 37, 37*t*
    during head positions 235
  overfacilitated muscles
    Golgi tendon organ therapy for 227, 227*f*
    muscle spindle cell therapy for 228, 228*f*
Fagius, J. 355
Fahey, P.J. 361
Fasano, M.L. 78
fat control 363-368
fatigue 379
fats 26-27. *See also* body fat
  dietary 278-279
    and carbohydrate intolerance 359
    conversion to eicosanoids 46, 47*f*
    imbalance in 48-50
  Group A 46-47
    in common foods 285, 285*t*
    foods containing 284, 284*t*
  Group B 47-48
    conversion to eicosanoids 283, 283*f*
    foods containing 284, 284*t*
  Group C 48
    in common foods 285, 285*t*
    foods containing 284, 284*t*
  kilocalories derived from 79, 79*t*
  unsaturated and saturated 285, 285*t*
fatty acids 45-48
  foods high in 280
  profile 284, 284*t*
faults 237
  cranial, sagittal suture 242, 242*f*, 243
  expiration-assisted 238
    correction of 239-240
    sphenobasilar 240, 241-242
  inspiration-assisted 238
    case history 243
    correction of 239
    sphenobasilar 240, 241
  pelvic
    Category I 243-244, 244*f*, 245, 245*f*, 246
    Category II 246*f*, 246-247, 247-248
  respiratory
    cranial 246
    cranial-sacral 238-239
    sphenobasilar 240-242
fears 202
Feiner, J.R. 75
Fern, E.B. 281
Ferraris, R.P. 295
Ferraro, R. 364
Ferrofood 384
fiber
  daily menu with 15 grams of fiber 286
  daily menu with 25 grams of fiber 286-288
  dietary 286-288
fibula dysfunction 257-258
Field, T. 19
fight-or-flight mechanism 42
Fiocchi, A. 299
Fisher, N.M. 35
fitness 9-10
Fluori-Methane 231
Fogelholm, G.M. 365
Foldes, J. 72
food(s)
  chewing 274-275
  concencrated carbohydrate 289
  concentrates 297-298
  energy from 273-274
  glycemic index 276-277, 277*t*
  Group A and C fats in 285, 285*t*
Group A, B, and C fat-containing 284, 284*t*
  high in fatty acids 280
  sources of nutrients related to carbohydrate metabolism 301
  therapeutic effects of 273
  unsaturated and saturated fat percentages 285, 285*t*
Food and Nutrition Board 294
foot
  function 345-346

gait reflexes (acupuncture points) on 234, 234*f*
foot problems 251-256
non-force respiratory correction of 256-257
footwear 345-350
forms
basal temperature 73*f*
Dietary Analysis 67*f*
General Inventory 59*f*-60*f*
General Survey 59*f*-60*f*
history 54-55
Nutrition Questionnaire 65*f*-66*f*
Symptom Survey 61*f*-64*f*
Foster, C. 29, 278
Foster-Powell, K. 277
Fowler, P.B. 53
Fox, E.L. 30
Franks, S. 357
Franzblau, A. 54
Freeman, R. 203
Freston, J.W. 296
Friedman, J.E. 280
Friedman, M.I. 275
Fries, J. 11, 11*f*
Frizzell, R.T. 314
Fromentin, G. 275
Fry, A.C. 220, 337, 353
Fry, R.W. 327, 335
Fuchs, C.S. 288
function 7-8, 39
functional capacity 74
functional carpal tunnel syndrome 258
functional injury 7*f*, 7-8
functional overtraining 337-338
functional testing 69-84
Funk, C.D. 48

G
Gaesser, G.A. 222
gait
abnormal 38
assessing 85-104
manual muscle testing in 37, 38*f*
muscle–acupuncture point relationships during 233
muscles normally facilitated and inhibited during 37, 37*t*
muscle testing and 102-104
neurological influences on 85-86
neuromuscular relationships with 36-39
normal 37, 37*f*
normal actions that affect 86
gait reflexes 233-234
assessment of 234-235
on foot 234, 234*f*
gait testing
with latissimus dorsi muscles 102-103, 103*f*
with pectoralis major clavicular muscles 102*f*, 102-103
Gallaher, D.D. 286
Gamow, R. Igor 328
Gamow hyper bags 328, 329*f*
Gardiner, N.S. 49
Garner, William 237
gas analyzers 80, 80*f*
Gasbarrini, G. 295
gastrocnemius relationship 192, 193*t*
Gaur, S.N. 303, 307
Gay, S.B. 75
Gaziano, J.M. 280
Geddes, N. 16
General Inventory 55, 59*f*-60*f*
General Survey 59*f*-60*f*
Genova, R. 299
Gerwin, R.D. 231
Ghiselli, A. 51
Ghoshal, U.C. 296
Gibney, M.J. 359
glandular preparations 299-300
glucocorticoids 41-42
L-Glutamine 296-297
L-Glutamine Plus 300, 385
gluteus muscles
maximus 174-175, 175*f*
medius 156-157, 157*f*
minimus 158-159, 159*f*
relationships 192, 193*t*
glycemic index 276-277, 277*t*
Golay, A. 279, 366
Goldberg, L. 222
Goldfarb, A.H. 309
Golgi tendon organs 35, 35*f*
Golgi tendon organ therapy 225-228
general procedure 226
for inhibition 226, 226*f*
for overfacilitated muscles or muscle spasms 227, 227*f*
Gollnick, P.K. 28
Goodheart, George 19, 22, 192
Goodheart, G.J., Jr. 230, 266
Gottlieb, D.J. 75
Grace, T.G. 347
gracilis muscle 178-179
relationships 192, 193*t*
testing 179, 179*f*
Graham, Sylvester 6
Graham, T.E. 287
Gram, Hans 20
Grandjean, A.C. 276
Granner, D.K. 44, 50, 276, 360
Graves, J.E. 326
Gray, J.B. 46
Gray's Anatomy 190
Graziani, G. 296
Greenleaf, J.E. 314
Greenlee, R. 328
Grey, N. 358
Gries, F.A. 359
Griffiths, A.J. 278, 358
groin pull 255, 257
Gronbaek, M. 288
Groop, L. 45
Grundy, S.M. 278, 280
Grynberg, A. 278
Guerra, A. 299
Gupta, S.K. 307
Guskiewicz, K.M. 85
Guyton, A.C. 34, 40, 72, 86, 194, 220, 274, 280, 295, 296, 313, 346

H
Haas, J.D. 304
Hagberg, J.M. 74
Haggmark, T. 30
Hahnemann, Samuel 20
Hainsworth, R. 314
Hajek, P. 75
Hakkinen, K. 43, 337
Hall, H. 200
Halliwell, B. 308, 309
Halstead, C.H. 288
Hampf, G. 22
hamstrings 176-177
relationships 192, 193*t*
testing 177, 177*f*
Hanai, H. 286
Hanna, A.M. 346
Harman, Willis W. 2
Harper, A.E. 275
Hawkins, C.L. 308
Hawkins, H. 71
Hawley, J.A. 276, 312
Hay, S. 219, 278
head positions, normal 235
health
definition of 9-10
structural 3-4
heart rate 214-215
changes during warm-up and recovery 321, 321*f*, 322, 322*f*
maximum aerobic
180-formula for 221
220-formula for 222
neurological aspects of 214
180-formula for 220
and respiratory quotient 82, 82*t*
220-formula for 221
heart rate monitoring 213-223
case history 223
during exercise 214, 214*f*
manual vs electronic 213-214
use of 213
Heinert, L.D. 219
Heinrichs, S.C. 275
Hendrix, T.R. 71
Henriksson, A.E. 296
Henry, J.K. 16
Herkenhoff, F. 78
Hermansen, L. 72
Hertel, J. 263, 264
Hesse, S. 347

Hickson, R.C. 327
Higashide, S. 295
Hill, E.G. 284
Himmel, W. 15
hip adductor muscles 154-155, 155*f*
Hippocrates 20
Hirn, J. 305
Hirokawa, K. 299, 308
history 53-67
  forms 54-55
  training diary and 57-58
Hitsuda, Y. 74
Hodgetts, V. 208, 320
Holden, R.J. 354, 357
Holder, M.D. 275
holistic view 2-3, 3*f*, 3-4
Hollmann, M. 357
Holman, R.T. 284
Holt, S. 277
homeopathy 17, 17*t*, 20
Hong, C.Z. 231
Hoogeveen, A.R. 42, 43, 50
Horak, F.B. 86
hormones 41-52
  adrenal 41-43
    effects on sodium 313-314
    training effects on 43-44
  pancreatic 44-45
  salivary 83*t*
  salivary tests 78-79
Horne, L. 327
Houglum, K. 298
Hourihane, J.O.B. 194
Hsieh, C.Y. 101
Huang, Y.J. 359
Hubinger, L. 77
Hugenberg, S.T. 264
Hughes, V.A. 29, 45, 352, 355
Humbert, P. 295
Hurley, B.F. 28
hydration 312-313
hydrochloric acid 295-296
hyperbaric chambers 328-329
Hyperbaric Technologies Incorporated 328*f*, 329*f*
hyperinsulinemia 44
hyponatremia 314

I
Ikemoto, S. 359
iliacus muscle 136-137
  relationships 192, 193*t*
  testing 137, 137*f*
iliotibial band syndrome 256, 257
imbalance
  aerobic and anaerobic 209
  dietary 288-289
  dietary fat 48-50
  postural 87-88, 89*f*-95*f*
immunity 50-51
impingement syndrome 169
inflammation 45-48, 378-379
  dietary factors affecting 282-286
  diminishing effects 282-283
  increasing responses 282
  nutrients important for anti-inflammatory activity 301-303
infraspinatus muscle 172-173
  relationships 192, 193*t*
  testing 173, 173*f*
inhibition 33
  assessment of cranial-sacral respiratory faults with 238
  assessment of sphenobasilar respiratory faults with 240
  Golgi tendon organ therapy for 226, 226*f*
  normal 35-36, 36*f*
    during gait 37, 37*t*
    during head positions 235
  piriformis 246
  secondary 377
  spindle cell therapy for 227, 227*f*
injury 375-387
  black and white model of 7*f*, 7-8
  case histories 381, 382-383, 383, 384, 385-386, 386*t*
  chemical 375, 376*t*
  clinical notes 381-386
  definition of 7*f*, 7-8
  functional 7*f*, 7-8
  mental/emotional 375, 376*t*, 379-380
  pain as 380-381
  physical 375-387
  structural 375, 376*t*, 376-377
Innis, S.M. 46
inspiration-assisted faults 238
  case history 243
  correction of 239
  sphenobasilar 240, 241
International College of Applied Kinesiology 22
Iossa, S. 357
Ironson, G. 19
Irving, R.A. 77
Ishii, H. 229
Islam, S. 296
Ivaturi, R. 317

J
Jacob, G. 70
Jacobs, I. 278
Jacobs, S.J. 324
Jacobson, B.H. 287
Jain, P. 297
Jakubowicz, D.J. 44
jamming 257
Janda, V. 17, 35
Jay, G. 328
Jenkins, D.J.A. 289, 358
Jenkins, R.R. 51
Jeong, B.Y. 86
Jeppesen, J. 279
Jimenez, C.C. 361, 362
Joannic, J.L. 276
Johnson, L.R. 231
Johnson, M.M. 49
Johnson, W.G. 341
joint complex dysfunction 96, 377-378
joint support 347
Jones, B.H. 324
Jones, D.A. 78
Jorda, A. 281
Jorgensen, U. 80, 346
Julius, S. 356, 357
Jull, G. 35

K
Kalmijn, S. 357
Kamal-Eldin, A. 283, 302
Kaminogawa, S. 281
Karlsson, J. 28
Karvonen, J. 222
Karvonen, M.J. 222
Karvonen method 222
Kasic, J. 328
Kasper, S. 44
Katch, F. 79*t*
Katch, V. 79*t*
Katzel, L.I. 354
Kaufman, J.J. 7
Keast, D. 213
Keizer, H. 43, 78
Keizer, H.A. 214
Kellogg, John 6
Kelso, T.B. 297
Keltikangas-Jarvinen, L. 354, 355
Kendall, F.P. 37, 96, 101, 126, 128, 190
Kesavachandran, C. 74
Khan, M.I. 264
Khanna, N.K. 297
KI 27 232-233, 233*f*
Kidd, J.M. 308
Kies, C. 317
kilocalories 79, 79*t*
kinesiology, applied 17, 17*t*, 21-22
  assessment 191-205
King, J.C. 194
King, S. 328
Kipnis, D.M. 358
Kirchgessner, M. 49
Kirwan, J.P. 43
Klatsky, A.L. 288
Koester, M.C. 48, 264, 283
Kohrt, W.M. 365
Kolopp-Sarda, M.N. 77, 282
Komaroff, A.L. 203
Konig, D. 45, 46, 50
Koob, G.F. 275
Kouttab, N.M. 299
Kraemer, W.J. 220, 337, 353
Kram, R. 219

Krebs cycle 26, 26*f*
Kreider, R.B. 306
Krieger, N.S. 48, 282
Kriketos, A.D. 360, 367
Krishnaswamy, K. 309
Krivickas, L.S. 347
Kronenberg, F. 15
Kuipers, H. 214, 271
Kummerow, F.A. 49
Kynast-Gales, S.A. 287

L
Laakso, M. 354
Laaksonen, D.E. 51
laboratory tests 76-77
labyrinthine reflexes 235
Lacey, J.M. 296, 307
lactic acid 304-305
Laemmel, K. 22, 53
Lairon, D. 286
Lamarche, B. 368
Lamb, D.R. 314
Lambert, E.V. 28, 278, 358
Lampman, R.M. 361
Landsberg, L. 305
Lange, P. 75
Larue-Achagiotis, C. 275
lateral talus distortion 253-254
lateral talus joint dysfunction 253, 253*f*
latissimus dorsi 100, 184-185
  gait testing with 102-103, 103*f*
  relationships 192, 193*t*
  testing 100, 100*f*, 185, 185*f*
Lattanzio, P.J. 86
Laubli, T. 54
Laughlin, G.A. 341
Lautt, W.W. 355, 360
Lawler, J.M. 51
law of similars 20
Lawson, A. 96, 192
Lazarus, R. 355
Leadbetter, J.D. 1, 6, 8
Leadbetter, W.B. 1, 6, 8
Leaf, D.A. 82, 222, 320
Leanderson, J. 347
Lee, J.Y. 213
Lefkowith, J.B. 282
Lehmann, M. 306
Lehmann, M.J. 39, 213, 220, 327, 335, 338, 339, 341
Leisman, G. 21, 96, 97, 101, 192
Lembo, G. 355
Lemon, P.W. 280, 281
Lemon, P.W.R. 280
Lepers, R. 86
Lerman, R.H. 284
levator scapulae muscle 162-163, 163*f*
Levine, B.D. 70
Lewit, K. 19
Li, X. 86
Liebenson, C. 35, 96
light touch reflexes, stimulating 200-201, 201*f*
Linder, M.C. 280, 281, 285*t*, 287*t*, 294, 299, 301, 302, 304, 307
Lindgren, F. 352, 353
Linum B6 367, 384
Litchtenstein, A.H. 279
Liu, G.C. 279
Lombardi, E. 194
Lopez Jimenez, J.A. 49
Luft, D. 78
Luft, F.C. 312, 314
Lukaski, H.C. 77, 194, 210, 293, 305, 341

M
Macfarlane, G.T. 286
MacLaren, D.P.M. 278
macronutrients 274-276
  balance 288-292
    Two-Week test 289-292
  dietary 276, 276*f*
  energy from 25-26
  quality of 276, 289
  quantity of 289
  self-selection 275-276
Madanmohan, D. 76
Maenpaa, J. 43
Maffetone, P. 44, 45, 51, 74, 82, 207, 210, 213, 257, 278, 283, 287*t*, 289, 296, 325, 349
MAF test. *See* Maximum Aerobic Function test
Magnesium Lactate 367
Mahajan, K.K. 77
Mahfouz, M.M. 49
Malmberg, L.P. 75
Maniongui, C. 49
Mantzioris, E. 47, 283, 303
manual muscle testing 96-101
  in gait position 37, 38*f*
  types of 101-102
manufactured nutritional supplements 298-299
Maranesi, M. 49, 284
Marino, M. 101
Marquart, L.F. 293
Marra, C.A. 49
Marston, R.M. 284
Martin, M. 366
Martinovic, A.M. 46
Martinsen, E.W. 305
massage therapy 17, 17*t*, 19
masseter muscle 230, 230*f*
Massey, L.K. 287
Massicotte, D. 316
Mathias, C.J. 70
Mattes, R.D. 194, 274
Maughan, R.J. 312, 313
Maximum Aerobic Function test 213, 215-217
  adjusting time and distance 217
  case history 216
  and competition 219-220
  example 215, 215*f*
  first-mile vs 5-km average mile times 219, 219*t*
  5-mile 216, 216*t*
frequency of 217
  performing 215-216
  plateau 217
  results 216, 218-219
  weather effects on 218
May, J.M. 308
Mayes, P.A. 26, 27, 45, 46, 49, 71, 294, 301, 304, 306, 308
McArdle, W.D. 13, 28, 43, 71, 72, 75, 79, 79*t*, 215, 221, 270, 281, 316, 320, 327, 334, 363
McCarthy, J.P. 70, 328
McColl, K.E. 40, 295
McGee, H. 6
McGrath, S.A. 359
McKay, J. 339
McKinney, C.H. 297
McNamara, D.J. 279
McNeil, D. 308
McNeill, G. 366
McNeill, M.E. 200
mechanical challenge
  extravertebral 198
  for spinal vertebrae 198
Medeiros, L.C. 47, 49
Mei, G. 360
Meigal, A.Y. 86
Meininger, C.J. 297
mental/emotional challenge 195-196, 200-202
  case history 205
  general procedure 201-202
  for phobias, fears, stress 202
mental/emotional problems
  diet aspects 288
  injuries 375, 376*t*, 379-380
  secondary 380
mental/emotional therapy
  case history 202
  light touch reflex stimulation for 200-201, 201*f*
mental/emotional wellness 4
mental imagery 200
Meredith, C.N. 306
meridians 21, 106
Mero, A. 306
Messina, M. 298
Messina, V. 298
metabolic analyzers 80, 81*t*
metabolic obesity 339
metabolism 25-31
metatarsal problems 257
Meyer, K. 283
Michelangelo 6
Milam, S.B. 308
mild hyperbaric chambers 328*f*, 328-329, 329*f*
Miles, M.P. 270, 271
Miller, C.C. 279

Miller, D.L. 366
Miller, G.D. 275
Miller, J.B. 277
Miller, W.C. 221, 278
Mills, D.E. 50
Mills, P.C. 51
mineralocorticoids 42
Mishra, N. 77
Miyajima, H. 77, 294, 304
Moan, A. 355
Molina, P.E. 305
Moller, P. 52, 288, 308
Molnar, D. 364
monitors, heart rate 213-223
Moon, R. 328
Moore, A.D., Jr. 213
Moore, C.E. 280
Mortensen, P.B. 286
Mosca, L. 280
Motyka, T. 192
Mountcastle, V.B. 29
Moy, C.S. 361
Muller, M.J. 74, 353
multiple supplements 299
Mundal, R. 69, 71
Muoio, D.M. 28, 278, 358
Murphy, P.J. 72, 264
Murray, R. 316
Murray, R.K. 309
muscle(s). *See also specific muscles by name*
  neurological mechanisms in 34-35
  neurological reaction of 195
  normally facilitated and inhibited during gait 37, 37*t*
  overfacilitated
    Golgi tendon organ therapy for 227, 227*f*
    muscle spindle cell therapy for 228, 228*f*
  relationships 192-194
    acupuncture point 192, 193*t*, 233
    with nutrients, organs and glands, nerves 192, 193*t*
  temporomandibular joint 190
  tested indirectly 190
muscle dysfunction 225-235
muscle evaluation 96-97
muscle fibers 29, 29*t*
muscle inhibition. *See* inhibition
muscle pain 270-271
muscle spasms
  Golgi tendon organ therapy for 227, 227*f*
  muscle spindle cell therapy for 228, 228*f*
muscle spindle cells 34, 34*f*
muscle spindle cell therapy
  for inhibition 227, 227*f*
  for overfacilitated muscles or muscle spasms 228, 228*f*
muscle testing
  applied kinesiology 191-192
  example tests 97-101
  and gait 102-104
  interpreting 101
  manual 96-101
    in gait position 37, 38*f*
    performing 96-97
    types of 101-102
  procedures 105-190
  treatment of reflex points with 107
muscle testing devices 101
muscular imbalances 35-36
Mustafa, T. 283
myofascial trigger points 231-232

N
Nakamoto, T. 287
Nakamura, T. 86
Nakasaki, H. 305
National Academy of Sciences 294
National Cholesterol Education Program (NCEP) 278, 279
Nattiv, A. 287
naturally occurring chemicals 265
natural pain control 263
naturopathy 17, 17*t*, 20
navicular bone dysfunction 255-256, 256*f*
Nazar, K. 71
NCEP. *See* National Cholesterol Education Program
neck extensors 188-189
  relationships 192, 193*t*
  testing 189, 189*f*
neck flexors
  medial 110-111, 111*f*
  relationships 192, 193*t*
nerve relationships 192, 193*t*
Nesbitt, S. 357
Nestel, P.J. 278
Nestler, J.E. 43, 44, 76, 352, 354, 355, 362
neurological disorganization 232
neurological dysfunction 225, 232-235
neurological sensory receptor challenge 194-196
neuromuscular junction 33-34
neuromuscular systems 33-40
  assessing 85-104
  relationships with gait and posture 36-39
Newsholme, E. 28, 51
Newsholme, E.A. 22, 192, 213, 296, 320
Ng, A.V. 78
Niacinamide B6 384
Nicholas, J.A. 101
Nicolaidis, S. 275
Nieman, D.C. 51
Noakes, T.D. 314
nonsteroidal anti-inflammatory drugs (NSAIDs) 263-264
  effectiveness of 264
  side effects 264
Nordgaard, I. 286
Northover, B. 72
nourishment 311-318
noxious substances 200
NSAIDs. *See* nonsteroidal anti-inflammatory drugs
NutrAnalysis, Inc. 276*f*, 277*t*, 284*t*
nutrients
  absorption 295-297
  important for anti-inflammatory activity 301-303
  important for carbohydrate metabolism 301
  important for production of Series 1 and 3 eicosanoids 302, 302*f*
  macronutrients 25-26, 274-276
  oral chemical challenge with 199
  relationships 192, 193*t*
nutrition 17, 17*t*
  aerobic system 304
  autonomic balance and 305-306
  carbohydrate intolerance and 359-360
  diet and 19-20, 366-367
  functional 293-294
  lactic acid and 304-305
  overtraining syndrome and 343
nutritional assessment 294
nutritional supplements 293-310
  case histories 300, 303
  manufactured 298-299
  types of 297-300
Nutrition Questionnaire 56, 65*f*-66*f*
Nutri-West 300, 385
Nutter, J. 279

O
obesity, metabolic 339
O'Connor, P.J. 78, 341
office assessments 69-77, 83*t*
oils 285, 285*t*
Oldridge, N.B. 214
O'Malley, B.P. 74
180-formula 220
  to calculate heart rate 220
  training relationships and 222-223
onion (*Allium cepa*) 283
Oppliger, R.A. 366
opponens digiti minimi muscle 124-125, 125*f*
opponens pollicis muscle 122-123, 123*f*
oral challenges
  with allergic substances 200
  with noxious substances 200
  with nutrient remedies 199
  potassium/sodium 315
oral pH 71, 83*t*
Orentreich, N. 43
Orlando, P. 77
orthotics 347
Osler, Sir William 53
osteopathy 17, 17*t*, 18-19
overfacilitated muscles
  Golgi tendon organ therapy for 227, 227*f*
  muscle spindle cell therapy for 228, 228*f*
over-the-counter drugs 287, 287*t*
overtraining
  assessment of 337, 341-342
  case history 342
  definition of 12

dietary factors 343
functional 337-338, 344*t*
functional signs and symptoms 338-339
nutritional factors 343
parasympathetic 340, 344*t*
preventing 336
recovery from 343-344
stages of 344, 344*t*
sympathetic 339-340, 344*t*
syndrome of 337-344
treatment of 342
oxidative stress 51-52
assessment of 309

P
Packer, L. 51, 308, 309
pain 261-271
as assessment tool 262
benefits of 261
drugs and 264
as injury 380-381
muscle 270-271
nonsteroidal anti-inflammatory drugs and 263-264
origins of 261-262
quality 262
sources of 261-262
visceral referred 263
words used to describe 262
pain control 261-271
acupuncture therapy for 265-266
beginning and end point 270
case history 266
natural 263
naturally occurring chemicals in 265
tonification point 269
Palatini, P. 356
pancreatic hormones 44-45
Pariza, M.W. 282
Parker, D.R. 359
Parker, L.N. 42, 313
Parmenter, D.C. 338
Parry-Billings, M. 192, 297
patient care 319-320
patient history 53-67
forms 54-55
taking 53-54
training diary and 57-58
Pavlov, I.P. 194
Pawelczyk, J.A. 70
pectineus 154
pectoralis major clavicular muscle (PMC) 98-99, 112-113
gait testing with 102*f*, 102-103
relationships 192, 193*t*
testing 99, 99*f*, 113, 113*f*
pectoralis major sternal muscle (PMS) 114-115, 115*f*
Pedersen, B.K. 50
Pekkanen, T.J. 305
Peluffo, R.O. 49
pelvic dysfunction 243-248
treatment of 237
pelvic faults
Category I 243
assessment of 243-244, 244*f*
correction of 245, 245*f*, 246
Category II 246-247
assessment of 247-248
case history 248
correction of 246*f*, 246-247
treatment of 247-248
Pendergast, D.R. 276, 278, 358
Penland, J. 293
Penland, J.G. 77, 294, 341
Perez-Padilla, R. 75
Perlman, M. 347
peroneus muscles
longus and brevis 150-151, 151*f*
relationships 192, 193*t*
tertius 152-153, 153*f*
Perot, C. 96, 101, 192
Perseghin, G. 353
Peters, J.C. 275
Peters, J.R. 78
Petrella, R.J. 86
Peuler, J.D. 305
Pfeifer, M.A. 305
pH, oral 71, 83*t*
Phillips, D.I. 353
Phillips, R.B. 101
Phillips, S.M. 281
philosophy 1-8
phobias 202
physical challenge 195, 196-198
physical injuries 375-387
phytochemicals 297-298
Pichard, C. 365
Pichichero, D.M. 194
Pichichero, M.E. 194
Pigg, Mike 325
piriformis muscle 186-187
inhibition 246
relationships 192, 193*t*
testing 187, 187*f*
piriformis syndrome 186
PMC. *See* pectoralis major clavicular muscle
PMS 192, 193*t*
Poehlman, E.T. 305
Poisson, J.P. 49
Polinsky, R.J. 70
Portanova, J.P. 263, 282
postural blood pressure 69-71, 83*t*
postural imbalance 87-88, 89*f*-95*f*
posture
abnormal 39
assessing 85-104
lateral view 87, 87*f*, 88, 88*f*
neurological influences on 85-86
neuromuscular relationships with 36-39
normal 38-39, 88, 88*f*
normal actions that affect 86
posterior view 86, 87*f*, 88, 88*f*
static 86-96
potassium
requirements 314-315
sodium balance 315
potassium/sodium oral challenge 315
power 39
practitioner role 319-329
Pratley, R.E. 360
Prentice, W.E. 321, 324
Preuss, H.G. 359, 360
prevention 10-11
primary vs secondary problems 203-204
protein(s) 27-28, 280-282
psoas major muscle 134-135
relationships 192, 193*t*
testing 135, 135*f*
psychology, sport 17, 17*t*, 22-23
Pulkkinen, M.O. 43
Puvi-Rajasingham, S. 70
Pyne, D.B. 271, 308

Q
quadriceps femoris muscles
rectus femoris 142-143, 143*f*
relationships 192, 193*t*
vastus lateralis, intermedialis, and medialis 144-145, 145*f*

R
Radomski, M.W. 354
Rainey, C.J. 287
Raitakari, O.T. 354
Ramani, R. 296
Rankin, J.W. 294, 365
Ranneries, C. 365
Rashed, H.M. 78
Ravaja, N. 354
Raven, P.B. 70
Ravich, W.J. 317
Ravussin, E. 365
Reaven, G.M. 44, 276, 351, 358, 366
Rebuck, D.A. 75
recovery
active 322-323
heart rate changes during 321, 321*f*, 322, 322*f*
from overtraining 343-344
rectus abdominis 130-131, 131*f*
rectus femoris 142-143, 143*f*
Reed, M.J. 279
Reeds, P.J. 281, 294
referred pain 263
reflexes
gait
assessment of 234-235
on foot 234, 234*f*

reflexes (*continued*)
labyrinthine 235
light touch, stimulating 200-201, 201*f*
reflex points 107
Report of the Expert Committee on the Diagnosis and Classification of Diabetes Mellitus 360
respiratory correction
method 256-257
non-force, of foot dysfunction 256-257
respiratory faults
cranial 246
cranial-sacral 238-239
sphenobasilar 240-242
respiratory quotient 79, 83*t*
heart rate and 82, 82*t*
nonprotein equivalents 79, 79*t*
subjective complaints and 82, 82*t*
using 79-83
rib joint dysfunction 258
Rieth, N. 275
Rijcken, B. 75
Rindi, G. 305
Ring, C. 213
Rinzler, S.H. 19
Robbins, S. 86, 345, 346, 347, 348, 349, 350
Roberts, A.C. 43
Robertson, C.H., Jr. 29
Rodwell, V.W. 307
Rogers, M.A. 45, 360
Rohner-Jeanrenaud, F. 354
Rolls, B.J. 366
Rosen, L.W. 44
Rosenthal, N.E. 43, 44
Rosolova, H. 360
Rossowska, M.J. 287
rotator cuff 169
rotator cuff syndrome 169
Rovere, G.D. 347, 348
Rowbottom, D.G. 297
Rubin, M.A. 360
Ruchkin, V.I. 296
Ruderman, N.B. 339, 354
Rudin, D.O. 49
Ruegg, R.G. 194
Russell, R.M. 296
Russell, T.L. 296

S
Saco Occipital Technique 18
Safran, M.R. 225, 271, 320, 321, 327
sagittal suture cranial faults 242, 242*f*, 243
Sagiv, M. 326
Sahrmann, S. 35
Saito, I. 72
Sakai, K. 78
Sakellari, V. 86
salivary hormones 83*t*
salivary hormone tests 78-79
Salonen, J.T. 298, 304
Salonen, M.A. 231
Saltin, B. 72
Saltzman, J.R. 296
Sanderson, J.E. 78
Sandvik, L. 214
sartorius muscle 140-141
relationships 192, 193*t*
testing 141, 141*f*
Savdie, E. 312
Savendahl, L. 307
Sawka, M.N. 314
Saxton, J.M. 86
scalenus anticus, medius, and posticus 110-111
schedules
competition 331, 332-335
training 331-332
case history 336
one-year 333
Scheppach, W. 297
Schiavon, R. 354, 357
Schiff, T. 53
Schmitt, W.H., Jr. 101, 203, 264, 265, 269, 299, 302, 306, 309
Schneeman, B.O. 286
Schoene, R.B. 75
Schutz, Y. 364
Schwaiblmair, M. 194
Schwille, P.O. 354
sciatica 186
Seacat, A.M. 308
Seals, D.R. 45, 78
Seaman, D.R. 18, 96
seasonal affective disorder 44
Seaward, B.L. 213
secondary muscle inhibition 377
secondary problems
differentiating 203-204
emotional 380
structural 369-371
Sehnert, K.W. 72
Seidell, J.C. 357, 365
Seitz, H.J. 74, 353
self-selection, macronutrient 275-276
Selye, Hans 8, 40, 314, 338
Sen, C.K. 51
serratus anterior muscle 116-117, 117*f*
Shabert, J.K. 296
Shadick, N.A. 75
Shaper, A.G. 363
Sharma, S.S. 283
Shashidhar, S. 74
Shek, P.N. 50
Shellock, F.G. 321, 324
Shepard, R.J. 50
Shimizu, M. 77
Shimizu, S. 282
shinsplints, posterior 146
Shlik, J. 194
shoes 345-350
Shupert, C.L. 86
Shuval, J.T. 15
Siffert, R.S. 7
Sigleo, S. 286
Siguel, E.N. 284
Simi, B. 278
Simmons, R. 86
Simmons, R.W. 362
Simoneau, J.A. 30, 328
Simons, D.G. 231
Simopoulos, A.P. 46, 49, 352
Sisto, S.A. 208
Skinner, H.B. 324
Skouby, S.O. 301, 356
small-intestine efficacy 296-297
Smit, A.J. 77
Smith, L.L. 19, 271
Smith, R.L. 264
Snodgrass, S.R. 298, 302, 308
Snook, G. 1
Snyder, A.C. 335
Sobal, J. 293
sodium
adrenal hormone effects on 313-314
potassium balance 315
soleus muscle 192, 193*t*
Somers, S. 288
Song, M.K. 48, 299, 360
Sparrow, D. 74, 75, 355
spasms
Golgi tendon organ therapy for 227, 227*f*
muscle spindle cell therapy for 228, 228*f*
specialized tests 77-83, 83*t*
specialties 15-23
contemporary 15-16
examples of 17*t*, 17-23
major categories 16
Speedy, D.B. 314
Spencer, J.D. 35
Sperling, M.A. 352
sphenobasilar expiration-assisted faults 240, 241-242
sphenobasilar inspiration-assisted faults 240, 241
sphenobasilar respiratory faults 240-242
assessment of
with muscle inhibition 240
with normal muscle function 240-241
spinal dysfunction 250-251
spinal vertebrae. *See* vertebrae
spindle cell therapy 225-228
for inhibition 227, 227*f*
for overfacilitated muscles or muscle spasms 228, 228*f*
spirometric reading 83*t*
sport psychology 17, 17*t*, 22-23
sports anemia 76, 304
sports drinks 311, 315-317
case history 317
customizing 316

suggestions to consider 316-317
sports medicine. *See* complementary sports medicine
Spriet, L.L. 287
Spruijt, R.J. 229
squaring the survival curve 11, 11*f*
Srivastava, K.C. 283
Stallknecht, B. 43
Standard Process, Inc. 265, 300, 303, 306, 367, 382, 383, 384, 385
Stanley, N.N. 75, 76
Staubli, M. 76
Steen, S.N. 294
Stein, J. 231
Steinmetz, K. 273
sternocleidomastoid muscle 108-109, 109*f*
Still, Andrew Taylor 18
Stoll, B.A. 359
stomatognathic system 229
Stone 220, 338, 340
Stoohs, R.A. 356
Storlien, L.H. 49, 359, 360
Stout, J.R. 365
Strauss, J.F. 44
Strauss, R.H. 308
strength 39
stress
effects on nutrient absorption 295
mental/emotional challenge procedure for 202
oxidative 51-52, 309
stress (term) 371
stress fracture 257
stretching 323-324
structural (physical) challenges 195, 196-198
structural health 3-4
structural injuries 375, 376*t*, 376-377
structural problems
primary 249-250
secondary 249-250, 369-371
subluxation 18
subscapularis muscle 168-169
relationships 192, 193*t*
testing 168-169, 169*f*
Sugawa, M. 280
Sullivan, G.W. 287
supplements
amino acid 306-307
glandular preparations 299-300
multiple 299
nutritional 293-310
supraspinatus 166-167, 167*f*
Suraci, C. 44
Surgenor, S. 314
Sutherland, L.R. 15
Sutherland, William 18
Svec, F. 351
Svintsyts'kyi, A.S. 296
Swaak, A.J. 264
swimmer's shoulder 169
Swinburn, B.A. 45, 352, 365
Symptom Survey 55-56, 61*f*-64*f*
Group Ten 284
Szabo, A. 200
Szepesi, B. 276

T
Taber, R. 328
Taha, A.S. 264, 295
Taittonen, L. 354
Takahashi, O. 302
Talbott, S.M. 365
talus joint
dysfunction 252-253
lateral distortion 253*f*, 253-254
Taoutaou, Z. 323
tapering 333
taping 347
Tarnopolsky, M.A. 278, 279, 280, 281
Taskar, V. 75
Taylor, R. 44, 360
team training 332
Tegelman, R. 343
Teitz, C.C. 347
Telford, R.D. 77
temperature 72, 83*t*
basal 73*f*
higher or raised 72, 321
lowered 72
temporomandibular joint dysfunction 228-231
assessment of 229, 230
closed problems 230, 230*f*
open problems 230-231, 231*f*
temporomandibular joint muscles 190
tennis elbow 258
tensor fascia lata muscle 138-139
relationships 192, 193*t*
testing 139, 139*f*
Tepperman, H. 40, 353
Tepperman, J. 40, 353
teres minor muscle 170-171
relationships 192, 193*t*
testing 171, 171*f*
Terezhalmy, G.T. 53
terminology vii, 9-14
carbohydrate intolerance 351
diet 364
stress 371
tests and testing
autonomic balance 203
functional testing 69-84
gait
with latissimus dorsi muscles 102-103, 103*f*
with pectoralis major clavicular muscles 102*f*, 102-103
hormone tests 78-79
laboratory tests 76-77
Maximum Aerobic Function test 213, 215-217, 218-219, 219-220
muscle
applied kinesiology 191-192
and gait 102-104
manual 37, 38*f*, 96-101, 101-102
procedures for 105-190
treatment of reflex points with 107
routine office assessments 69-77, 83*t*
specialized tests 77-83, 83*t*
Two-Week test 289-292
therapeutic massage. *See* massage therapy
therapy localization 192, 195
case history 205
procedure 196-197
Thibault, L. 275
Thomas, D.E. 278
Thompson, J. 305, 366
Thomson, M. 283
Thonnard, J.L. 347
Thorsen, K. 282
tibialis anterior muscle 148-149
relationships 192, 193*t*
testing 149, 149*f*
tibialis posterior muscle 146-147
relationships 192, 193*t*
testing 147, 147*f*
Tiidus, P.M. 51
Tilles, S. 308
Tomaro, J. 347
tonification points 106, 266-268
location 266, 267*f*, 268, 268*t*
pain control with 269
Tordoff, M.G. 275
Torre, M. 286
Toth, M.J. 305
training 360, 367-368
definition of 11-12
effects 74
effects on adrenal hormones 43-44
effects on energy systems 30-31
effects on immunity 50-51
equation for 11
footwear for 345-350
formula for 332
and 180-formula 222-223
overtraining 12, 337-344
practitioner's role in 319-329
team 332
training diaries 57-58, 332
training schedules 331-332
case history 336
one-year 333
year-long plan 334-335
trapezius muscles
lower 182-183, 183*f*, 192, 193*t*
middle 180-181, 181*f*, 192, 193*t*
upper 160-161, 161*f*, 192, 193*t*
Travell, J. 19, 231
Tremblay, A. 305, 367

triad of athletic dysfunction 369-374, 379
triceps brachii muscle 120-121
  normal facilitation and inhibition with 35-36, 36*f*
  relationships 192, 193*t*
  testing 121, 121*f*
220-formula 221-222
Two-Week test 289-292
  case history 291
  steps 289-292
Tylenol 264

U
Ulmann, L. 49, 284
Umeda-Sawada, R. 48, 49, 282, 283
Uphold, R.E. 314
Upledger, J. 237
Urhausen, A. 50, 78, 338, 339, 343, 352
U.S. Food Guide Pyramid 276
Utriainen, T. 27

V
Vacek, L. 75, 194
Valium 264
Valtuena, S. 365
Vana, S. 72
Van Antwerpen, V.L. 75
van den Berg, A. 77
van der Beek, E.J. 293, 304, 305
van Der Hulst, R.R. 297
van de Vijver, L.P. 303
VanHelder, T. 354
Van Itallie, T.B. 290
Van Mechelen, W. 324
Van Reempts, P.J. 353
vastus lateralis, intermedialis, and medialis 144-145, 145*f*
Veera, R.K. 308
Velazquez, E.M. 357
Venkatraman, J.T. 278
Verhagen, H. 298
Verhoef, M.J. 15
vertebrae
  mechanical challenge procedure 198
  non-force assessment and correction 250-251
vertebral dysfunction
  case history 251
  treatment of 249-259
Verwaerde, P. 355
Veselov, A.I. 296
Ves-Losada, A. 49
Virkkunen, M. 354
visceral referred pain 263
vital capacity 74, 75, 83*t*
Vredevoogd, J. 237
Vukovich, M.D. 29, 278
Vuorimaa, T. 222

W
Wabeke, K.B. 229
Wada, L. 194
Wadsworth, C.T. 101
waist-to-hip ratio 76
Waked, E. 345, 347, 348, 349, 350
Walker, K.Z. 358
walking 326
Walther, D. 229, 231, 232, 237
Walther, D.S. 3, 3*f*, 17, 37, 70, 96, 101, 190
Wannamethee, G. 363
warming-down 322
warm-up
  active 320-322, 323
  heart rate changes during 321, 321*f*, 322, 322*f*
Warner, J.O. 200
Wasserman, D.H. 44
water 311-313
water regulation 312
weather effects 218
Weidner, T.G. 50, 86, 192, 219, 338
weight and fat control 363-368
weight loss 365-366
weight-loss programs 363
Weiler, J.M. 74, 308
Weiss, S.T. 75
wellness 4
Welsh, S. 276
Welsh, S.O. 284
Westling, L. 229
Westrum, L.E. 231
Whaley, M.H. 221
Wiesler, E.R. 324
Wiles, J.D. 287
Williams, C. 276
Wilmore, D.W. 296, 307
Wilmore, J.H. 13, 43, 79, 214, 221, 287*t*, 304, 312, 313, 320, 323, 328
Wilson, L.A. 222
Wilt, T.J. 280
Winkler, P. 53
Wishart, J.M. 340
Wolever, T.M.S. 276
Wolf, G. 302
Wolf, S.K. 362
workouts 326
World Health Organization 280
Wright, V. 263, 264
wrist extensor muscles 126-127, 127*f*
wrist flexor muscles 128-129, 129*f*
wrist joint dysfunction 258-259, 259*f*
Wu, G. 297
Wyndham, C. 328

X
Xanax 264
Xie, H. 355, 360

Y
Yang, M.U. 290
Yang, T.M. 70
Yanuck, S. 192
Yee, L. 328
Yen, S.S. 341
Yoshida, T. 312, 323
Young, J.B. 305
Young, V.R. 280
Yu, B.P. 51, 309

Z
Zhang, H. 360
Zhu, Y.I. 304
Ziegler, D. 359
Ziegler, T.R. 296, 297
Zimmet, P.Z. 45, 352, 357
Zinc Liver Chelate 303, 382
Zmarzty, S.A. 279
Zonderland, M.L. 42, 43, 50

About the Author

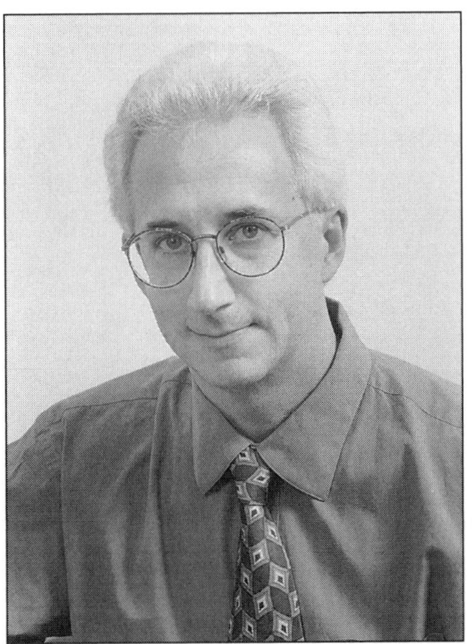

Philip Maffetone, DC, has more than 20 years of experience in private practice treating and training athletes in all sports including many world class and professional athletes. He lectures extensively on the topics of health and fitness, diet and nutrition, and lifestyle and stress management, and he serves as a consultant to athletes, sport teams, and corporations.

Author of several books on sport for general audiences, Dr. Maffetone is a member and former chairman of the International College of Applied Kinesiology—a complementary medicine organization devoted to education and research.

In 1994, he was named Coach of the Year by *Triathlete Magazine*. He is a member of the National Athletic Trainers Association and the Foundation for Allied Conservative Therapies Research. He attained his DC from the National College of Chiropractic in Lombard, Illinois.

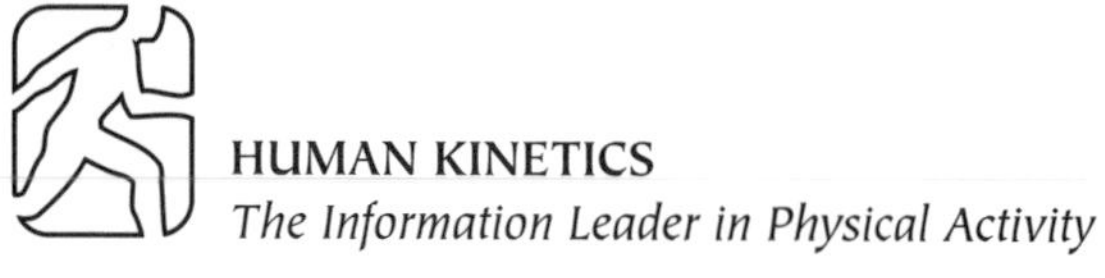